CLINICAL
GYNECOLOGIC IMAGING

CLINICAL GYNECOLOGIC IMAGING

Arthur C. Fleischer, M.D.
Professor, Department of Radiology and Radiological Sciences
Professor, Department of Obstetrics and Gynecology
Chief, Diagnostic Sonography
Vanderbilt University Medical Center
Nashville, Tennessee

Marcia C. Javitt, M.D.
Associate Professor, Department of Radiology
The George Washington University Medical Center
Washington, D.C.

R. Brooke Jeffrey, Jr., M.D.
Professor, Department of Radiology
Stanford University Medical Center
Stanford, California

Howard W. Jones III, M.D.
Professor, Department of Obstetrics and Gynecology
Director, Gynecologic Oncology
Department of Obstetrics and Gynecology
Vanderbilt University Medical Center
Nashville, Tennessee

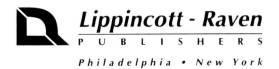

Lippincott - Raven
PUBLISHERS

Philadelphia • New York

Acquisitions Editor: James Ryan
Developmental Editor: Emilie Linkins
Project Editor: Patricia Connelly
Production Manager: Caren Erlichman
Production Coordinator: MaryClare Malady
Design Coordinator: Melissa Olson
Indexer: Gloria R. Hamilton
Compositor: Maryland Composition Company, Inc.
Printer: Worzalla Publishing

Library of Congress Cataloging-in-Publication Data

Clinical gynecologic imaging / [edited by] Arthur C. Fleischer . . . [et
  al.]. — 1st ed.
      p.   cm.
  Includes bibliographical references and index.
  ISBN 0-397-51706-8 (alk. paper)
  1. Generative organs, Female—Imaging. 2. Gynecology—Diagnosis.
I. Fleischer, Arthur C.
  [DNLM: 1. Genital Diseases, Female—diagnosis. 2. Diagnostic
  Imaging—methods.   WP 141 C641 1997]
RG107.C55 1997
618.1'0754—dc20
DNLM/DLC
for Library of Congress   96-8780
                                                CIP

9 8 7 6 5 4 3 2 1

Dedicated to those who work toward improving women's health.

Contributors

Ted L. Anderson MD, PhD
Department of Obstetrics and Gynecology
Vanderbilt University School of Medicine
21st Ave. South at Garland Ave.
Nashville, TN 37232

Mostafa Atri, MD
Department of Radiology
Montreal General Hospital
1650 Cedar Avenue
Montreal, QC H3G 1A4

Marcela Böhm-Vélez, MD
Chief, Ultrasound Section
Clinical Associate Professor of Diagnostic
  Radiology
University of Pittsburgh School of Medicine
Department of Radiology
The Western Pennsylvania Hospital
4800 Friendship Avenue
Pittsburgh, PA 15224

Mike Bourne, FRCR
c/o Martin Quinn
Obstetrics and Gynecology
University of Wales, College of Medicine
Heath Park, Cardiff CF4 4XN
United Kingdom

Jeanne A. Cullinan, MD
Assistant Professor, Departments of Radiology
  and
Radiological Sciences and Obstetrics and
  Gynecology
Vanderbilt University Medical Center
21st Ave. South at Garland Ave.
Nashville, TN 37232

Michael P. Diamond, MD
Professor, Department of Obstetrics and
  Gynecology
Director, Division of Reproductive
  Endocrinology and Infertility
Hutzel Hospital, Detroit Medical Center
4727 St. Antoine
Detroit, MI 48201-1498

Stephen Entman, MD
Professor and Chairman
Department of Obstetrics and Gynecology
School of Medicine
Vanderbilt University
21st Ave. South at Garland Ave.
Nashville, TN 37232

Arthur C. Fleischer, MD
Department of Radiology
Vanderbilt University School of Medicine
21st Ave. South at Garland Ave.
Nashville, TN 37232

Murray A. Freedman, MD
818 St. Sebastian Way, Suite 400
Augusta, GA 30901

Marta Hernanz-Schulman, MD
Associate Professor, Department of Radiology
  and Radiological Sciences
School of Medicine
Vanderbilt University
21st Ave. South at Garland Ave.
Nashville, TN 37232

Marcia C. Javitt, MD
Department of Radiology
School of Medicine and Health Sciences
George Washington University
2300 Eye Street, NW
Washington, D.C. 20037

R. Brooke Jeffrey, Jr., MD
Department of Radiology
Stanford University Medical Center
300 Pasteur Drive, H-1307
Stanford, CA 94305

Howard W. Jones III, MD
Department of Obstetrics and Gynecology
School of Medicine
Vanderbilt University
21st Ave. South at Garland Avenue
Nashville, TN 37232

Donna Kepple, RDMS
Chief Sonographer
Department of Radiology and Radiological
* Sciences*
Vanderbilt University Medical Center
Nashville, TN 37232-2675

Eric K. Outwater, MD
Associate Professor, Department of Radiology
* and Radiological Sciences*
Thomas Jefferson University Hospital
132 South Tenth Street, 1096 Main
Philadelphia, PA 19107-5244

Anna K. Parsons, MD
Department of Radiology
University of South Florida
12901 Bruce B. Downs Boulevard
Tampa, FL 33612-4799

Martin Quinn, MB, ChB
Senior Registrar in Obstetrics and Gynecology
University of Wales, College of Medicine
Heath Park, Cardiff CF4 4XN
United Kingdom

Miles Reid, MD
Department of Radiology, C5-163
Montreal General Hospital
1650 Cedar
Montreal, Quebec, H3G1A4
Canada

Deidre Russell, MD
Assistant Professor, Department of Obstetrics
* and Gynecology*
Vanderbilt University Medical Center
Nashville, TN 37232-2675

David Tait, MD
Department of Obstetrics and Gynecology
School of Medicine
Vanderbilt University
21st Ave. South at Garland Ave.
Nashville, TN 37232

Amy S. Thurmond, MD
Clinical Professor, Department of Obstetrics and
* Gynecology*
Oregon Health Sciences University Hospital
12031 SW Breyman Avenue
Portland, OR 97219

Kaori Togashi, MD
Department of Radiology and Nuclear Medicine
Faculty of Medicine, Kyoto University
54 Kawaramachi, Shogoin, Sakyoi-ku, Kyoto 606
Japan

Jaime Vasquez, MD
Center for Reproductive Health
Nashville, TN 37203

James W. Walsh, MD
Department of Radiology
UMHC, Box 293
University of Minnesota
420 Delaware Street SE
Minneapolis, MN 55455

Preface

This book describes and illustrates the use of medical imaging in gynecologic disorders. Each chapter begins with a discussion by a clinician of the clinically pertinent parameters of a particular gynecologic disorder. This is followed with presentation and correlation of the applications of the primary and secondary diagnostic modalities, including pelvic sonography, magnetic resonance imaging, and computed tomography. It is hoped that the presentation of the material in this fashion is useful, both to the clinician and imager, in that the imaging aspects of each gynecologic disorder are presented from a clinically pertinent standpoint.

Each diagnostic modality that is used for gynecologic disorders has its strengths and limitations. Even when the diagnostic accuracy of a particular modality is considered, repetitive and redundant imaging with the various modalities should be minimized, since it is desirable to optimize cost-effectiveness. Intelligent selection of a single series of diagnostic modalities is in everyone's interest. It can tailor management and preclude unnecessary procedures. It is hoped that this book will also serve as a guide to cost-effective and coordinated imaging of gynecologic disorders.

As an overview, the authors recommend the following as a guideline to gynecologic imaging. In general, sonography is the first diagnostic modality of choice in most benign gynecologic disorders, whereas MRI and CT are best used for gynecologic malignancies. Imaging efficacy takes into account the cost of the procedure, as well as the likelihood that the sensitivity and specificity of the test will result in clinically pertinent information.

DIAGNOSTIC MODALITIES FOR VARIOUS GYNECOLOGIC DISORDERS

	1° dx Modality	2° dx Modality	Comments
Adnexal Masses	TAS/TVS	MRI	CT for tumor extent
Ovarian Cancer	TVS	MRI/TV-CDS	CT for tumor extent
Endometrial Disorders	TVS	MRI	MRI diagnostic for adenomyosis
Myometrial Disorders	TAS/TVS	MRI	
		MRI	
Cervical Cancer	MRI		CT for parapelvic extent
Pelvic Inflammatory Disease	TAS/TVS		TAS/CT useful for guided procedures
Pelvic Pain	TVS/TV-CDS	MRI	TV-CDS diagnosis of torsion
Fertility Disorders	TVS	HSG	SHG can detect adhesions, polyps, submucosal fibroids. Sono HSG can be used in place of SHG.
Lower Urinary Tract Disorders	TVS/TPS/TRS	MRI	MRI depicts detailed anatomy but is not real-time such as TVS/TPS/TRS
Pediatric Gynecologic Disorders	TAS		TVS usually not needed

The information contained within this book will discuss and illustrate the advantages and limitations of each diagnostic modality relative to those clinically pertinent parameters that affect management. It is intended to assist the practicing gynecologist and imaging specialist, as well as trainees in these disciplines in making intelligent choices concerning the diagnostic evaluation of the most common gynecologic disorders.

Arthur C. Fleischer, M.D.
Marcia C. Javitt, M.D.
R. Brooke Jeffrey, Jr., M.D.
Howard W. Jones, III, M.D.
October 24, 1995

Acknowledgments

The authors would like to acknowledge several people whose contributions were significant and appreciated. Paul Gross, M.S.'s artistic talent is appreciated for his illustrations, Alice Hammond and Claire S. Brown for their editorial efforts, and John Bobbitt for his photographic skills.

Contents

Clinical Gynecologic Imaging, edited
by Arthur C. Fleischer, Marcia C. Javitt,
R. Brooke Jeffrey, Jr., and Howard W. Jones III,
Lippincott-Raven Publishers, Philadelphia © 1997.

CHAPTER 1

Gynecologic Imaging: Instrumentation, Techniques, and Normal Anatomy

Gynecologic Sonography: Instrumentation and Techniques

Arthur C. Fleischer, MD

In this chapter, the clinically pertinent aspects of instrumentation and techniques for sonography, MRI, and CT are presented, as well as the normal pelvic anatomy portrayed by each modality.

There are a variety of approaches that can be used for sonographic examination of a region of interest within the pelvis. These include transabdominal sonography through a fully distended bladder or transvaginal, transperineal, or transrectal sonography. Selection of the optimal sonographic approach involves the proximity of the region of interest to the variety of sonographic probes. Sonographic evaluation can include transabdominal sonography using large field-of-view curvilinear- or linear-array probes, transvaginal sonography using convex linear or flat footprint probes, and transvaginal color Doppler sonography using curvilinear or straight linear probe technology. In some instances, transrectal sonography or transperineal sonography can be used for specialized examination, such as evaluation of the cervix and uterus during guided intraoperative procedures. Each approach has its advantages and limitations.

TRANSABDOMINAL SONOGRAPHY

Transabdominal sonography is performed by linear- or phased-array probes that afford large fields of view (Fig. 1-1). A distended urinary bladder is required for adequate penetration of the incident beam into the deeper pelvic struc-

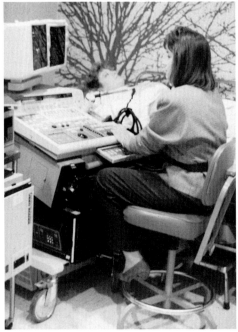

A

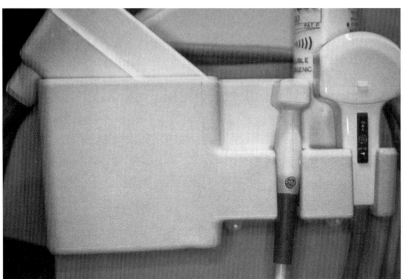

B

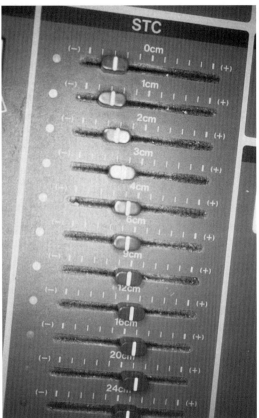

C

FIG. 1-1. Scanners. **(A)** Typical sonographic scanner with alphanumeric keyboard, two monitors, and several selectable function keys. **(B)** Transabdominal sonographic probes. The large probe in the probe holder affords the largest field of view compared with the phased array sector probe, which can access smaller places such as between the ribs. **(C)** Close-up of time gain compensation control panel. These controls optimize the image from a particular depth.

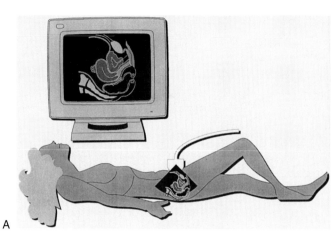
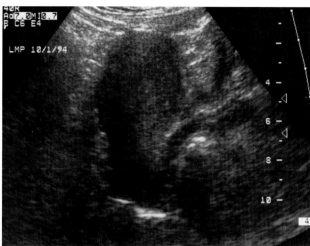

FIG. 1-2. Transabdominal pelvic sonography. **(A)** Diagram showing sagittal imaging plane and orientation of image on the monitor. **(B)** Typical midline sagittal image shows anteflexed uterus superior to a nondistended bladder. (**A,** courtesy of P. Jeanty, MD.)

tures. A distended bladder also accomplishes displacement of small bowel from the pelvis and places the uterus in a more horizontal orientation than when examined in the nondistended state. Transabdominal sonography affords global depiction of the pelvic organs in their long and short axis and demonstrates the relationship of a structure to the major pelvic organs such as the uterus and ovaries (Fig. 1-2).[1] Most linear-array probes allow adjustment of time gain compensation and focusing to optimize an area of interest. Transabdominal sonography is usually used before transvaginal sonography to globally delineate pelvic structures. The images obtained by transabdominal sonography should document the uterus and adnexal regions.

In some patients, the images obtained by transabdominal sonography may be sufficient and transvaginal sonography is not necessary. Transabdominal sonography may occasionally be more useful than transvaginal sonography in these patients, such as those who have undergone hysterectomy in whom the ovaries cannot be delineated with transvaginal sonography. In these situations, transabdominal sonography with a distended bladder may better delineate the ovaries.

TRANSVAGINAL SONOGRAPHY

Transvaginal sonographic probes use mechanical sector curvilinear-array or linear-phased array (Fig. 1-3). Because of the anatomic confines, the transvaginal probes have a small footprint; but because of the proximity of the structures to the probe, high-frequency transducers (over 5 MHz) can be used. The curved linear-array has optimal line density because it has the most send and receive elements and thus affords greatest detail in the small transvaginal sonographic field of view.

Transvaginal sonography allows detailed delineation of a relatively limited (10 cm) field of view.[2] Images are oriented with the apex of the image at the top of the scan, which corresponds to the long axis in the sagittal plane imaged as if the patient were placed on her head (Fig. 1-4). When the transducer is turned 90 degrees, semicoronal or oblique images are obtained of the adnexa. Abdominal palpation can be used during transvaginal sonography to displace bowel loops. It also provides an assessment of the mobility of organs that may relate to the presence or absence of pelvic adhesions.

Needle guides can be attached to the shaft of the probe for guiding follicular aspiration, cyst aspiration, and other pelvic interventional techniques (see Fig. 1-4). A guide that attaches flush to the probe is usually preferred over one that is outrigged. The needle path should be clearly shown on the monitor, and the use of either a scored needle tip or a Teflon-coated needle may improve its visualization.

Transvaginal sonographic examinations usually begin in the sagittal plane with depiction of the uterus. Then the probe is directed toward the adnexal regions with depiction of the internal iliac vein and artery as well as the ovaries. The probe then can be retracted out of the vaginal fornices to the midvaginal area and directed anteriorly for an anteflexed uterus to depict the uterus in ''short axis'' or in a semicoronal plane. Before removing the probe from the vagina, one can image the cervix and cul-de-sac. To optimize imaging, abdominal palpation can be applied by the examiner or the patient can be asked to put pressure on her lower abdomen while scanning is performed.

Before the examination, a condom is placed over the shaft of the probe and secured with rubber bands. After each usage, the probe must be wiped with a SaniTowel or placed in an approved sterilizing and disinfecting solution.

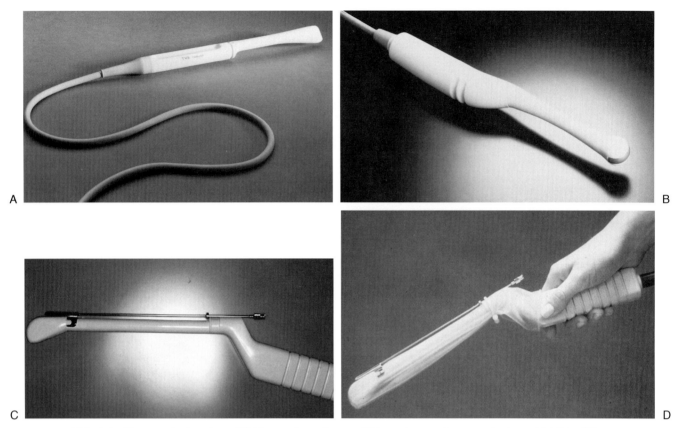

FIG. 1-3. Transvaginal probes. **(A)** Linear phased array. This probe can image at 5, 6, and 7 MHz. **(B)** Curvilinear array can easily be manipulated from sagittal to coronal imaging phases. **(C)** A needle guide can be attached to shaft of transvaginal probe for guided procedures. **(D)** The needle guide is placed over the condom and secured to the shaft of the probe. (**A,** courtesy of Acuson, Inc., Mountain View, CA; **B,** courtesy of Toshiba America Medical Systems, Inc., Tastin, CA.)

TRANSVAGINAL COLOR DOPPLER SONOGRAPHY

Transvaginal color Doppler sonography involves depiction of anatomy as well as the detection of flow by colorization of pixels that have Doppler shifts (Fig. 1-5).[3] Red is arbitrarily chosen to denote flow toward the transducer, blue shows flow away from the transducer, and higher velocity is shown in whiter shades. Low pulse repetition frequencies are used for detection of slow flow, and a wall filter is typically low, which limits depiction of vessel motion but allows display of true flow.

Transvaginal color Doppler sonography can usually be performed by the same probe that is used for transvaginal sonography. The difference is in the image processing, which decreases the frame rate of gray scale images to utilize color Doppler interrogation. The image display should be large enough to identify the location of colorized pixels, and a simultaneous waveform is preferred that includes the region of interest. The gain with color priority setting is of the utmost importance in evaluation of areas of interest with transvaginal color Doppler sonography. Overcompensation for gray scale may negate depiction of colorized areas, whereas colorized areas may be artifactually generated if the color gain setting is set high. The smallest sample volume is usually used; and if the vessel course is visualized, the Doppler angle is set between 20 and 60 degrees for optimal display of the waveforms. Calculation of impedance using resistive index (systolic peak minus diastolic over systolic velocities) or by pulsatility index (systolic peak minus diastole over the mean) can be used.

Newer developments involving power Doppler imaging have greatly enhanced the detection sensitivity of flow but do not allow quantification of direction of flow or velocities. This may be used to evaluate whether a particular area has any vascularity or has reduced flow, such as in areas of infarction. In the near future, this type of scanning may allow quantification of flow to make transvaginal color Doppler sonography more objective than it is in its current state.

TRANSRECTAL AND TRANSPERINEAL SONOGRAPHY

Transrectal sonography is used for guidance of certain intraoperative procedures that are performed vaginally, such

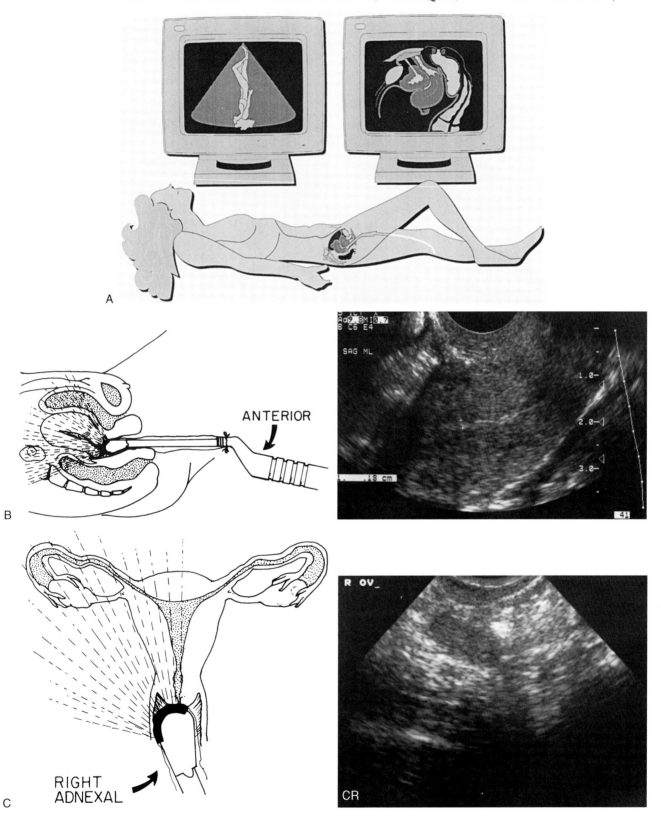

FIG. 1-4 Transvaginal imaging planes and typical transvaginal images. **(A)** Orientation of image with apex at top of monitor. The patient is scanned in the sagittal plane as if she is on her head. **(B)** In midline sagittal imaging, the probe is anteriorly directed for depicting the uterus and endometrium in long axis *(left)*. Transvaginal sonogram *(right)* showing uterus in long axis and thin endometrium measured in anteroposterior dimension *(area between cursors - bilayer thickness)*. Right transvaginal view **(C)** shows right ovary, and left adnexal view.

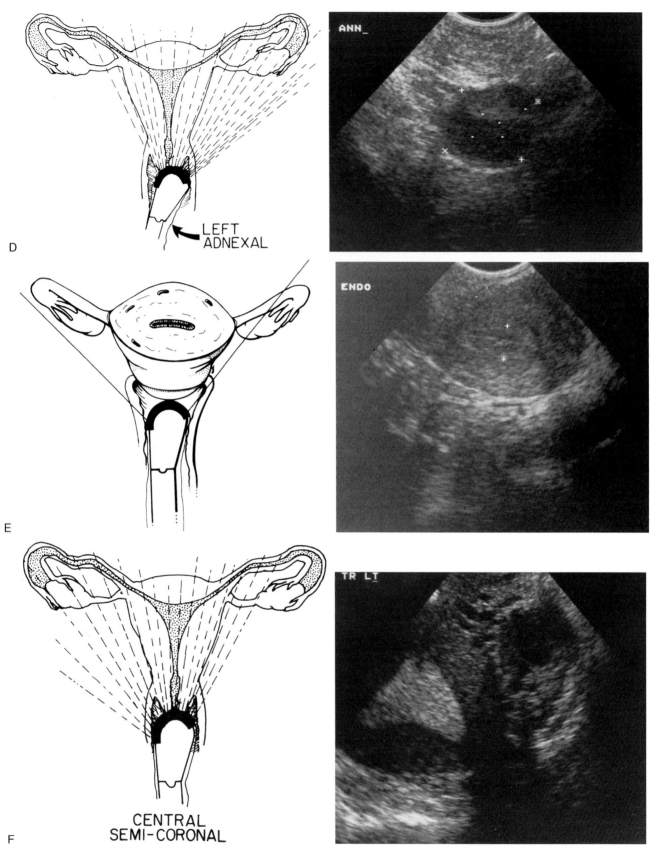

FIG. 1-4 *Continued.* **(D)** shows left ovary, which contains an involuting corpus luteum depicted as a hypoechoic area. **(E)** Short axis view of the uterus. Transvaginal sonography shows a multilayered endometrium *(between cursors).* **(F)** Semicoronal view. Transvaginal sonography demonstrates the entire endometrium, especially the endometrium in the cornual regions.

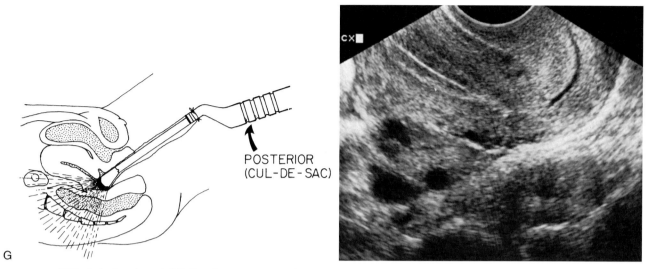

FIG. 1-4 *Continued.* **(G)** Cervix, cul-de-sac. This sonogram shows hypoechoic mucus within the endocervical canal and a multilayered endometrium. (**A,** courtesy of P. Jeanty, MD.)

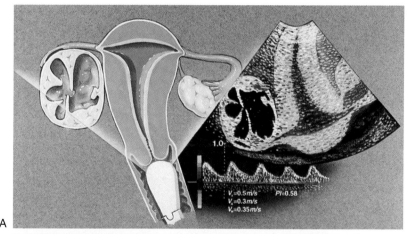

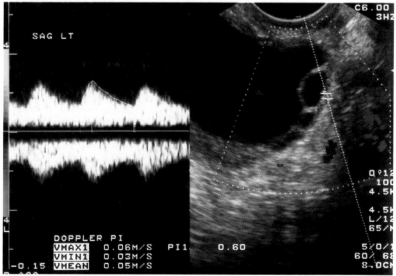

FIG. 1-5. Transvaginal color Doppler sonography. **(A)** Diagram shows the transvaginal image, a phased Doppler range gate, and the Doppler waveform. **(B)** Sonogram of a cystic mass with low impedance, low velocity flow.

as dilatation and curettage, intrauterine tandem placement, or cerclage.[4] It is particularly helpful in patients with cervical stenosis or obscured cervices for which dilatation and curettage or placement of an intracavitary tandem for radiation therapy is required. A biplane transrectal probe is recommended because one may image in both long and short axes to confirm the placement of a dilator (Fig. 1-6).

Transperineal sonography can be used in evaluation of the cervix, lower uterine segment, and low-lying placenta (Fig. 1-7).[5,6] A nondistended bladder is recommended, and standard probes can be used covered by a glove for this procedure. Imaging only in the sagittal plane is possible, but this is usually sufficient for delineation of the cervix and lower uterine segment throughout pregnancy.

SUMMARY

There are a variety of approaches that can be used for sonographic evaluation of the pelvis. Each should be used according to the proximity of the region of interest relative to the incident ultrasound beam.

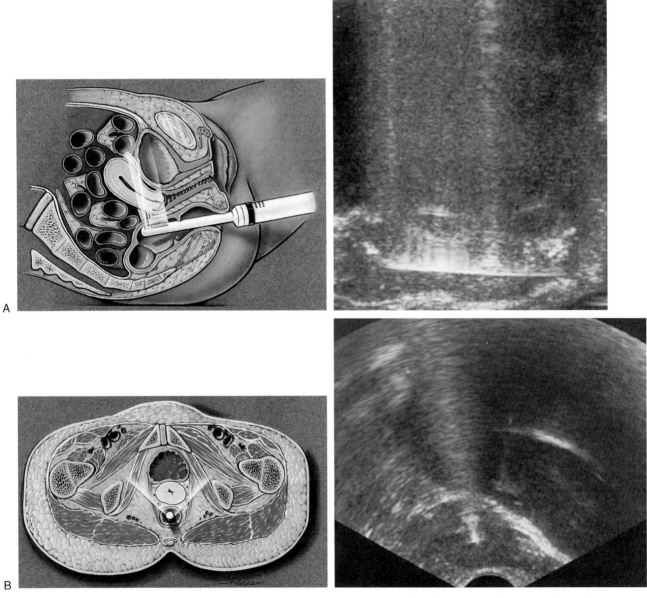

FIG. 1-6. Transrectal sonography. **(A)** Long axis of the longitudinally oriented transducer array is activated to depict the cervix *(left)*. An intracavitary tandem was guided to be within the uterine lumen *(right)*. **(B)** Short axis of the curvilinear transducer is mounted on the tip of the probe to depict anatomy in the axial orientation *(left)*. The axially oriented image confirms the central location of the tandem *(right)*.

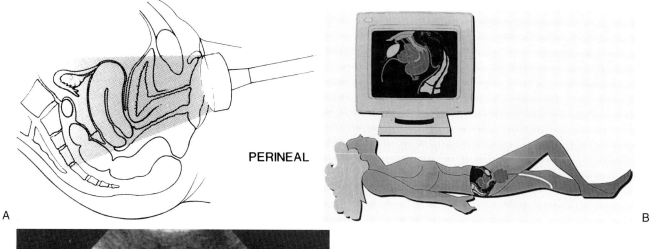

PERINEAL

A

B

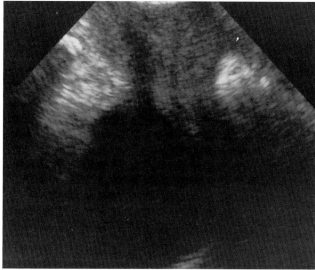

C

FIG. 1-7. Transperineal sonography. **(A)** Diagram shows field of view depicted with transperineal sonography. **(B)** Orientation of image. **(C)** Sonogram showing the urethra, inferior to symphysis pubis. (**B,** courtesy of P. Jeanty, MD.)

REFERENCES

1. Fleischer A, Entman S. Transabdominal vs transvaginal sonography of pelvic masses. Ultrasound Med Biol 1989;8:51.
2. Fleischer A, Kepple D. Transvaginal sonography: a clinical atlas, ed 2. Philadelphia, JB Lippincott, 1995.
3. Fleischer A, Emerson D. Color Doppler sonography in obstetrics and gynecology. New York, Churchill-Livingstone, 1993.
4. Fleischer A, Cullinan J, Burnett L, Jones H. Transrectal and transperineal sonographic guidance of intraoperative procedures. J Ultrasound Med 1995;14:135.
5. Hertzberg BS, Bowie JD, Weber TM, et al. Sonography of the cervix during the third trimester of pregnancy: value of the transperineal approach. AJR 1991;157:73.
6. Hertzberg BS, Bowie JD, Carroll BA, et al: Diagnosis of placenta previa during the third trimester: role of transperineal sonography. AJR 1992;159:83.

Normal Pelvic Anatomy as Depicted by Various Sonographic Techniques

Arthur C. Fleischer, MD and Donna M. Kepple, RDMS

There are a variety of sonographic techniques available for depiction of pelvic anatomy. Transabdominal approaches require a fully distended bladder and afford a global depiction of the pelvic anatomy (Fig. 1-8). Transvaginal sonography, on the other hand, provides only a limited field of view but depicts the major pelvic structures, such as the uterus and ovaries, in great detail. Transvaginal color Doppler sonography affords depiction of major vessels around and within the pelvic structures. It is important for the sonographer and sonologist to realize differences in these sonographic techniques as they relate to what is depicted sonographically.

This subchapter is divided into the depiction of major pelvic structures and their anatomic variants. The discussion of the sonographic appearance of these structures by the various sonographic approaches is emphasized. This material is presented from the aspect of the normal pelvic cavity that is routinely and readily depicted by ultrasound.

UTERUS

The uterus forms the central landmark for sonographic evaluation of the pelvis (Figs. 1-8 through 1-11). The size and shape of the uterus varies according to the age and hormonal status of the patient. In the child, the cervix is larger than the fundus, whereas after puberty the uterine fundus enlarges. During the childbearing years, the uterine corpus and fundus are larger than the uterine cervix. After menopause, however, the uterus atrophies, with the fundus and corpus becoming approximately equal in size to the cervix. The relative size and shape of the uterus is variable as well. Although it would be best to describe the uterus in a three-dimensional volume, the uterus is typically described in its length or long-axis and short-axis or transverse fundal dimensions. Table 1-1 lists the relative sizes of the uterus in different stages and parity. In general, the prepubertal and postmenopausal uterus measures 4 to 6 cm in length and 3 to 5 cm in anterior position and transverse dimension. The uterus in menstruating women varies according to parity status, but in general is 6 to 8 cm in length by 5 to 6 cm in transverse and anteroposterior dimensions (Table 1-2).

The uterus is made up of three layers of myometrial fibers.

The most predominant is the middle layer, which runs in a more circular or spiral fashion. The inner layer immediately beneath the basal layer of the endometrium runs in a longitudinal fashion and has a role in stripping the endometrium during menses and promoting sperm transport to the fundus in the mid cycle. The outer myometrium extends into the tubal musculature and forms the "pacemaker." Between the outer and middle layers are the arcuate vessels.

The vascular supply to the uterus is derived from the anterior branch of the internal iliac artery. Once it courses toward the internal cervical os, the uterine artery courses along the lateral aspects of the corpus and is a very tortuous structure, allowing for enlargement of the uterus in the gravid state. The arteries then penetrate the capsule of the uterus and form the arcuate network of vessels. The radial branches traverse the myometrium, giving off spiral branches within the endometrium. Many of these larger vessels can be depicted on color Doppler sonography.

Impedance values within the uterine artery vary somewhat during the cycle, with lower impedance during the secretory phase. Blood flow in the postmenopausal uterus demonstrates higher impedance than in premenopausal women. Unopposed estrogen treatment may be associated with lower impedance than in patients on combined estrogen and progesterone treatment (Sladkevicius, 1995; Zalud, 1992). The layers of the endometrium can be depicted particularly in the mid cycle in the patient of childbearing years. In the preovulatory period, a multilayered appearance can be seen. The outer echogenic interface represents the basal layer, with the inner hypoechoic area representing the functionalis layer. The central interface represents a median echo from refluxed cervical mucus. During luteal phase, the endometrium thickens and becomes more echogenic. In the menstrual phase, irregular interfaces and thinning of the endometrium are present. The endometrium in the postmenopausal woman is typically thin (~5 mm bilayer thickness). A small amount of intraluminal fluid may be present. The combined thickness of the endometrial layers should be no greater than 8 mm (4 mm single layer) (Goldstein, 1994). For further discussion of normal endometrial patterns and thicknesses, please refer to the first subchapter in Chapter 4.

The uterus may be anteflexed or retroflexed. Retroflexion

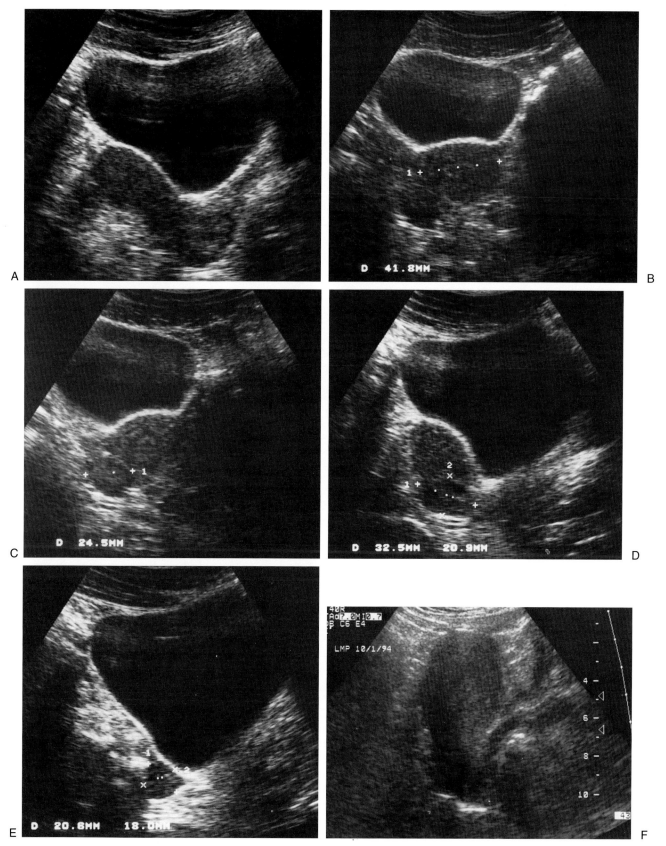

FIG. 1-8. Transabdominal sonography of normal uterus and ovaries. **(A)** Sagittal sonogram shows anteflexed uterus in a patient with a distended urinary bladder. **(B)** Transverse sonogram shows uterine width *(between cursors)*. **(C)** Transverse sonogram shows right ovary *(between cursors)*. **(D)** Parasagittal sonogram of right ovary *(between cursors)*. **(E)** Parasagittal sonogram of left ovary *(between cursors)*. **(F)** Sagittal sonogram of anteflexed uterus in a patient with a nondistended urinary bladder. Note how anteflexed the normal uterus is when the bladder is empty.

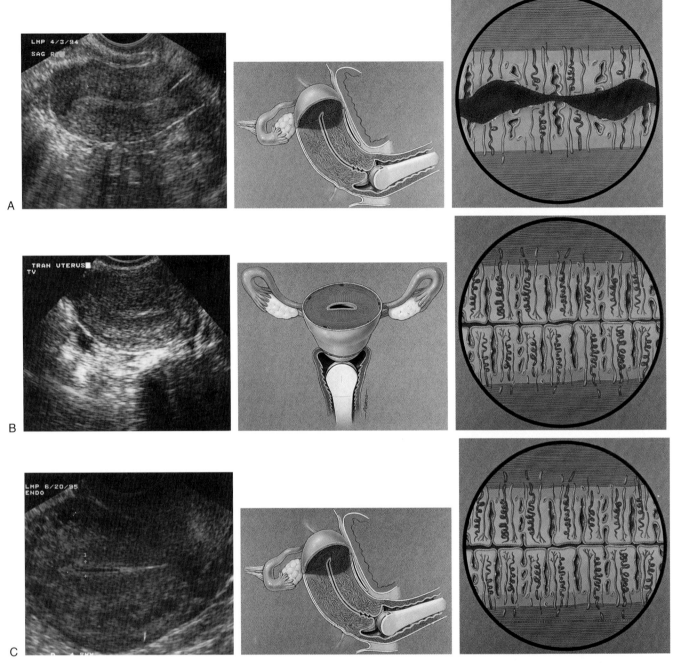

FIG. 1-9. Transvaginal sonography *(left)* of normal uterus and endometrium with accompanying diagram of scan plane *(middle)* and microscopic anatomy *(right)*. **(A)** Long-axis transvaginal sonogram of menstrual and early proliferative-phase endometrium. **(B)** Short-axis transvaginal sonogram showing proliferative-phase endometrium. **(C)** Long-axis transvaginal sonogram of periovulatory endometrium. There is a small intraluminal fluid collection.

is common in women who have had children, whereas anteflexion is common in nulliparous patients. Version refers to the angle of the cervix relative to the vagina.

Anatomic variants of the uterus are described in Chapter 9. Most involve abnormal fusion. Small cystic areas in the outer myometrium may represent remnants of Gartner's duct or possibly distended veins in the arcuate system (see Fig. 1-9C).

It is common to find cervical inclusion cysts appearing as 2- to 5-mm cystic structures within the endocervical canal. These represent obstructed glands that contain mucus material.

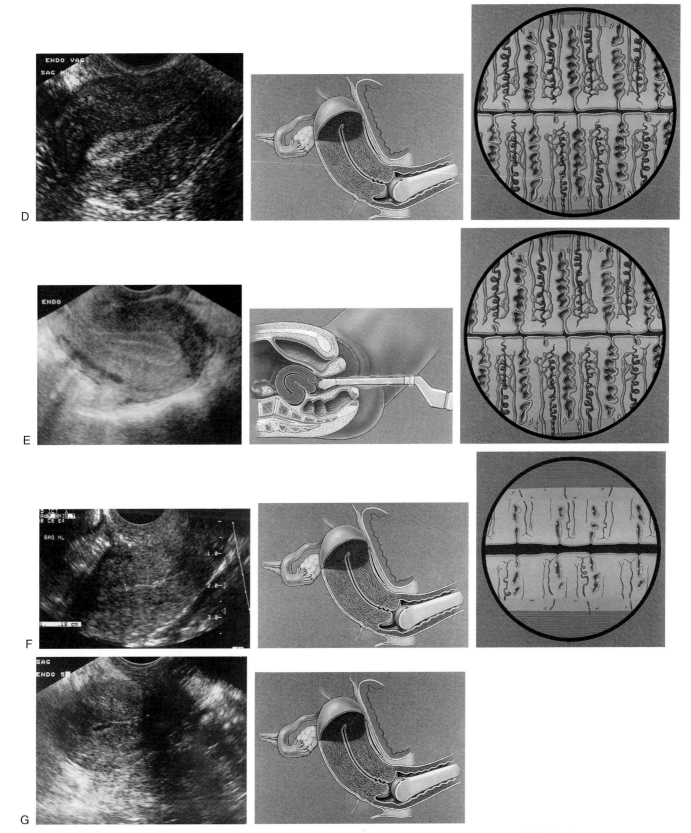

FIG. 1-9. (D) Sagittal transvaginal sonogram showing secretory-phase endometrium. **(E)** Sagittal transvaginal sonogram showing retroflexed uterus with secretory-phase endometrium. Distended arcuate veins are seen at the junction of the middle and outer myometrial layers. **(F)** Transvaginal sonogram of normal postmenopausal endometrium that measured only 2-mm bilayer thickness. **(G)** Transvaginal sonogram of normal postmenopausal endometrium with a small amount of intraluminal fluid. The endometrial layers are thin and regular surrounding the fluid.

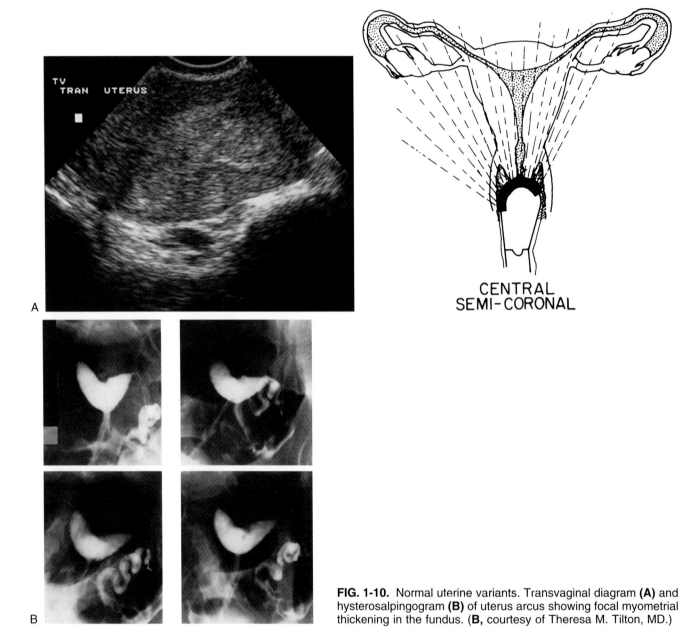

FIG. 1-10. Normal uterine variants. Transvaginal diagram **(A)** and hysterosalpingogram **(B)** of uterus arcus showing focal myometrial thickening in the fundus. **(B,** courtesy of Theresa M. Tilton, MD.)

TABLE 1-1. *Average uterine size (cm)*

	Length	Width	AP	Volume	Cx: Fundus
Prepubertal	3.0	1.5	1.0	2.25	2:1
Postpubertal	7.0	2.5	2.0	17.50	1:1
Nulliparous	8.0	5.0	2.5	50.00	1:2
Multiparous	11.0	6.0	3.0	99.00	1:3
Menopausal	5.0	2.0	2.0	10.00	1:1

Data from Sample W. Radiology 1977;125:477; Ferenczy A. Blaustein's Pathology of the female genital tract. New York, Springer Verlag, 1982:258; and Platt J, Bree R. Davidson D. Ultrasound of the normal non-gravid uterus: Correlations with gross and histopathology. J Clin Ultrasound 1990;18:15.

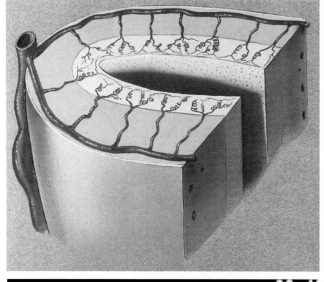

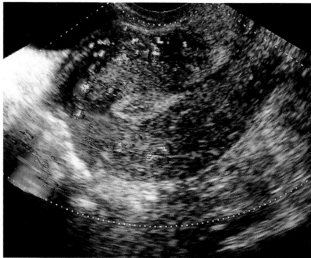

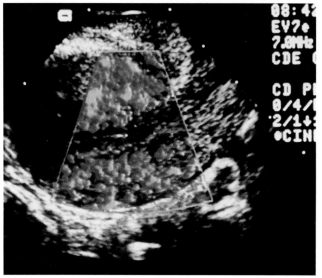

FIG. 1-11. Transvaginal color Doppler sonography of uterine blood flow. **(A)** Diagram of uterine blood flow shows relative size and location of main arteries and arcuate, radial, and spiral arteries. **(B)** Frequency color Doppler sonogram shows myometrial vessels. **(C)** Amplitude color Doppler sonogram shows myometrial vascularity. **(A,** drawn by Paul Gross, MS; **C,** courtesy of Acuson, Inc., Mountain View, CA.)

OVARIES

The ovaries vary in size and texture, depending on the presence or absence of follicular development (Cohen, 1993) (Figs. 1-12 through 1-14 and Table 1-3). During childbearing years, a hypoechoic structure representing a follicle can be identified in most ovaries. Mature follicles range from 18

TABLE 1-2. *Uterine size proportional to parity*

Parity	Weight (g)	2 SD above mean
0	60 ± 20	100
1	109 ± 26	161
2	108 ± 28	164
4	121 ± 35	191
>4	130 ± 37	200

From Platt J. Bree R, Davidson D. Ultrasound of the normal nongravid uterus: correlations with gross and histopathology. J Clin Ultrasound 1990; 18:15.

to 25 mm and have thin, smooth walls. On the other hand, corpora lutea have irregular "crenated" or serrated walls.

The ability to delineate normal ovaries is dependent on the presence or absence of follicles. Their position relates to bowel and size. Although most premenopausal ovaries can be delineated with transabdominal or transvaginal sonography, only approximately 60% of normal postmenopausal ovaries are readily detectable (Fleischer, 1990). The size of the ovary varies according to age (Diagram 1-1). In general, normal ovaries of childbearing age measure 3 × 2 × 2 cm and are oblong. Postmenopausal women have smaller ovaries.

The ovary has a dual blood supply, one derived from the uterine circulation and the other directly from the aorta. The main ovarian artery is derived from the aorta and courses through the infundibulopelvic ligament to join with the adnexal branch of the uterine artery. Multiple small twigs penetrate the capsule of the ovary. In areas of follicular development, flow can be depicted on color Doppler sonography.

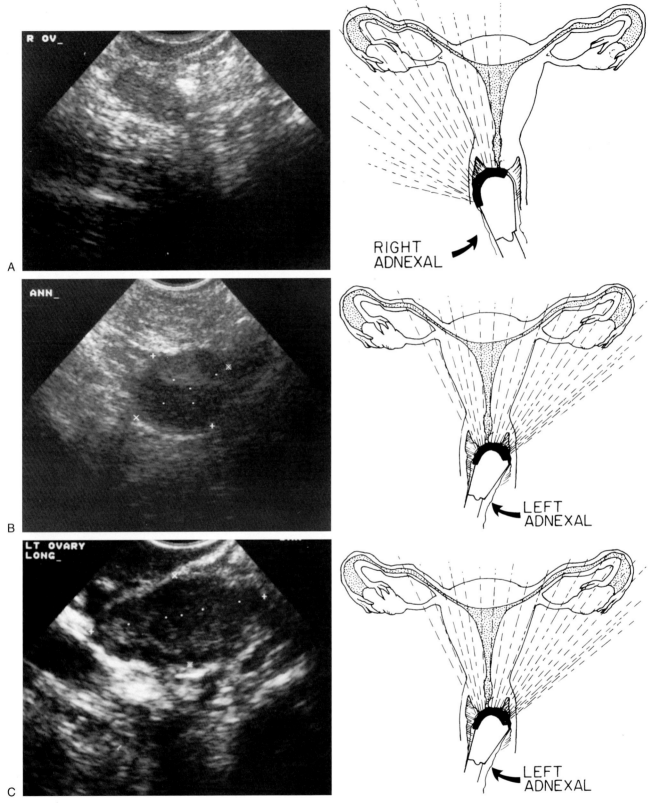

FIG. 1-12. Transvaginal sonography of normal ovaries. **(A)** Transvaginal sonogram of normal right ovary devoid of maturing follicle. **(B)** Transvaginal sonogram of normal left ovary containing a corpus luteum. **(C)** Transvaginal sonogram of normal ovary containing corpus luteum. Note focal enlargement of the ovary due to the corpus luteum.

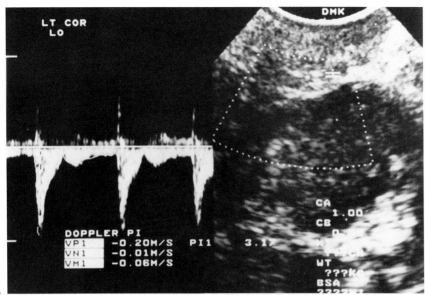

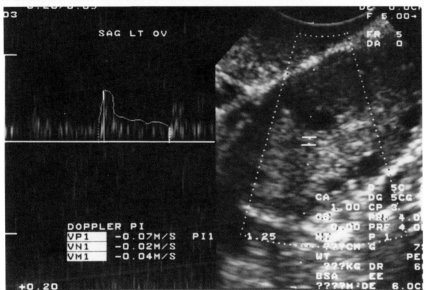

FIG. 1-13. Transvaginal color Doppler sonography of normal variant ovaries. **(A)** Transvaginal sonogram of polycystic ovary with left feeder vessels showing high impedance. **(B)** Sonogram of polycystic ovary with intraovarian waveforms showing lower impedance.

However, in quiescent ovaries that do not have follicular development, typically no intraovarian flow is depicted. As the corpus luteum forms, circumferential flow is present that has a typical low impedance waveform. Veins surrounding the ovaries can distend, particularly if there is incompetence of the ovarian vein valves near their origin on the left near the left renal vein and on the right near the inferior vena cava. The ovarian vein can occasionally be depicted, particularly when it is distended (over 5 mm). Variants of this vascular arrangement include distended periuterine and parovarian veins that have been associated with "pelvic congestion syndrome" (Fig. 1-15). For a further discussion of this, the reader is referred to Chapter 8.

TABLE 1-3. *Average ovarian size (greatest dimension)*

	Range (cm)	Mean (cm)
Transverse	2.5–5.0	3.00
Longitudinal	0.1–1.5	1.00
Anteroposterior	1.5–3.0	1.70
Volume (cm³)		
Prepubertal (>12 y)		0.46
Postpubertal (13–20 y)		4.00
Childbearing (20–50 y)		10.00
Postmenopausal (<50 y)		8.00

FALLOPIAN TUBES

The fallopian tubes are typically not depicted with transvaginal sonography in normal patients. However, when contrast medium enhancement is used, they can be depicted as

(*text continued on p. 20*)

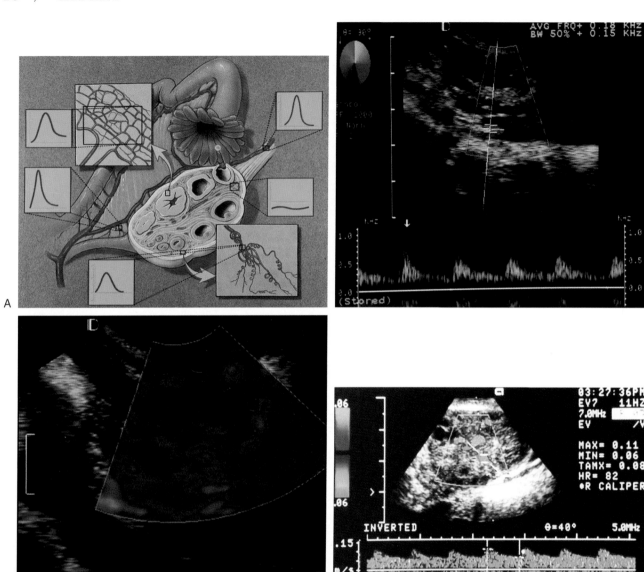

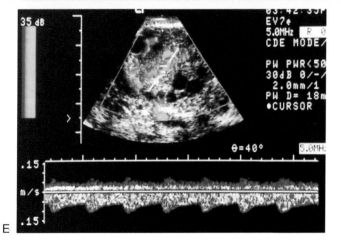

FIG. 1-14. Transvaginal color Doppler sonography of normal ovarian flow. **(A)** Diagram showing dual blood supply to ovary, one from the aorta, the other from the uterine artery. Within the ovary, the vessel arrangement varies according to the presence of a corpus luteum. The impedance also varies according to which vessels are sampled, with vessels within the corpus luteum having lowest impedance compared with intraovarian vessels remote from a developing follicle or corpus luteum. **(B)** Frequency Color-Doppler sonogram shows intermediate impedance flow within an intraovarian arteriole. **(C)** Amplitude Color Doppler sonogram of same ovary showing flow *(whiter areas).* **(D)** Frequency Color Doppler sonogram of a corpus luteum showing low impedance flow. **(E)** Amplitude Color Doppler sonogram showing low impedance intraovarian arterial flow. **(D** and **E,** courtesy of Acuson, Inc., Mountain View, CA.)

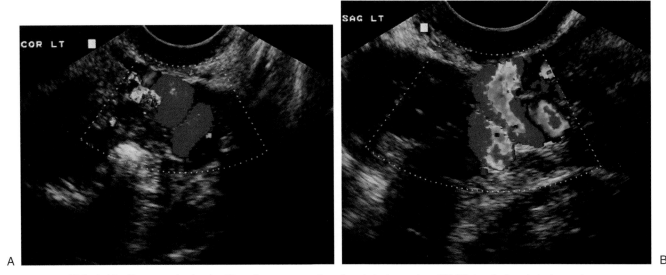

FIG. 1-15. Transvaginal color Doppler sonography of periuterine veins. **(A)** Distended periuterine veins (long axis). **(B)** Distended periuterine veins (short axis). This patient did not have any symptoms suggesting pelvic congestion syndrome.

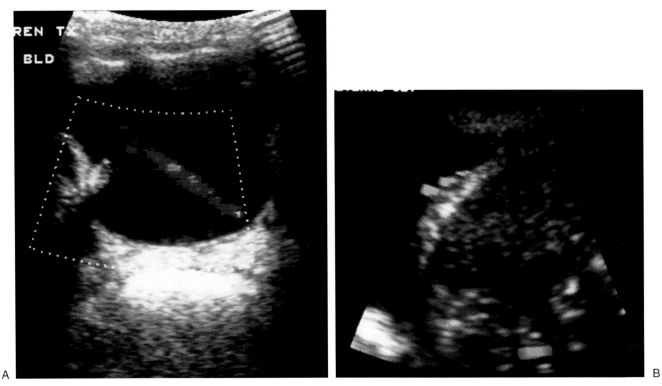

FIG. 1-16. Transabdominal and transvaginal color Doppler sonography of ureteral orifices. **(A)** Sonogram shows ureteral jet from left uterovesical orifice. **(B)** Sonogram of ureteral jet.

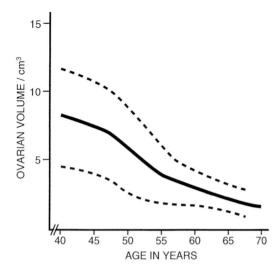

Diagram 1-1. Mean and standard deviation of normal ovarian volume versus age. (From Andolf E. Normal ovarian size versus age. Acta Obstet Gynecol Scand 1987;66:387.)

they course from the tubal ostia to the fimbriated end of the tube. Tubal anatomy as depicted on contrast medium—enhanced transvaginal sonography is discussed in detail in the first subchapter in Chapter 10.

OTHER STRUCTURES

Other pelvic structures that are well depicted on sonography include the urinary bladder, the distal ureters, the supporting ligaments, and the bowel. The ureteral orifice can be seen particularly on color Doppler sonography when a ureteral jet is recognized (Fig. 1-16). The distal ureter lies relatively posterior and inferior and can be depicted well on transvaginal sonography (Laing, 1995).

Bowel occasionally is seen in the pelvis and can mimic the sonographic appearance of a pelvic mass. Bowel typically has peristaltic motion, but occasionally the fat surrounding bowel loops can be echogenic and appear as a mass (Fig. 1-17).

Other structures that can be depicted in the pelvis include pelvic musculature and fascial planes. These include the obturator internis muscle, which forms the lateral aspect of the pelvic sidewall, and the piriformis muscle, which runs posteriorly and can simulate the appearance of an ovary.

Transperineal sonography can also be used to depict the urethra (Fig. 1-18).

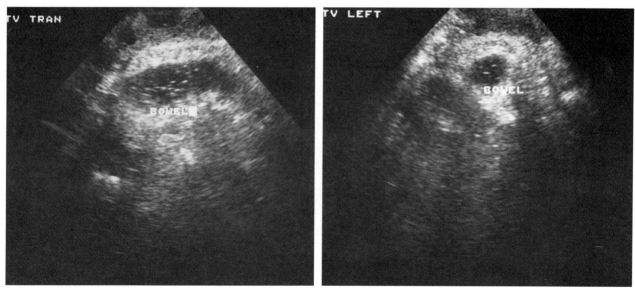

A   B

FIG. 1-17. Transvaginal sonography of peristaltic bowel loop in long **(A)** and short **(B)** axis.

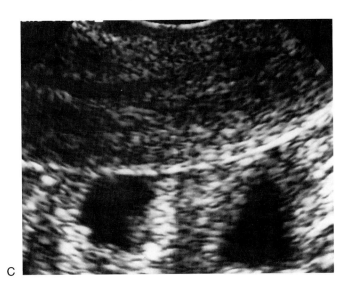

C

FIG. 1-17. *Continued.* **(C)** Transvaginal sonogram shows fluid-filled bowel loops posterior to uterus.

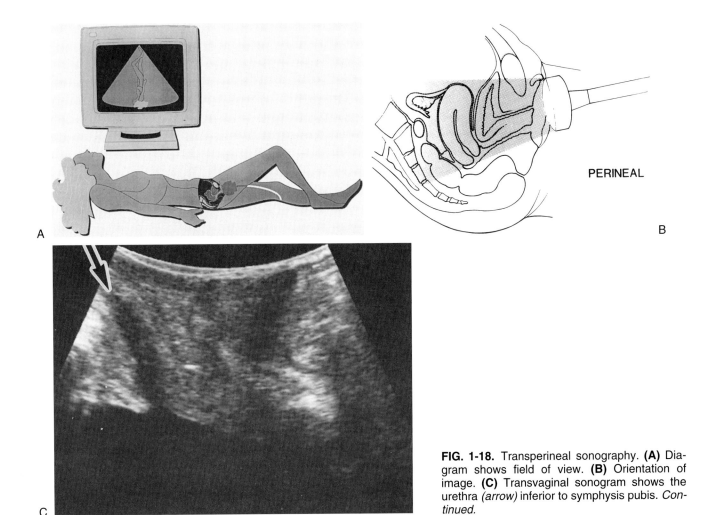

PERINEAL

A

B

C

FIG. 1-18. Transperineal sonography. **(A)** Diagram shows field of view. **(B)** Orientation of image. **(C)** Transvaginal sonogram shows the urethra *(arrow)* inferior to symphysis pubis. *Continued.*

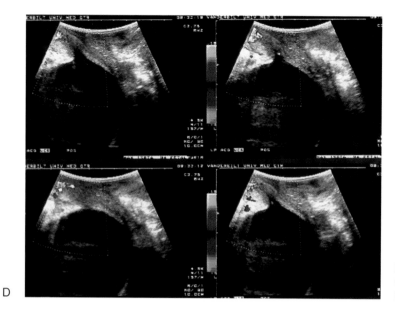

FIG. 1-18. *Continued.* **(D)** Composite transvaginal color Doppler sonogram of bladder and urethra. (**B,** courtesy of P. Jeanty, MD.)

SUMMARY

This subchapter outlines the sonographic appearance of normal anatomy and some of the variants that can be depicted by transabdominal, transvaginal, and transvaginal color Doppler sonography. With improved resolution, finer anatomic detail will become apparent.

BIBLIOGRAPHY

Cohen HL, Tice HM, Mandel FS. Ovarian volumes measured by US: bigger than we think. Radiology 1990;177:189.

Fleischer A, McKee M, Gordon A, et al. Transvaginal sonography of post-menopausal ovaries with pathologic correlation. J Ultrasound Med 1990; 9:637.

Goldstein SR. Postmenopausal endometrial fluid collections revisited: look at the doughnut rather than the hole. Obstet Gynecol 1994;83:738.

Goswamy RK, Campbell S, Royston JP, et al. Ovarian size in postmenopausal women. Br J Obstet Gynecol 1988;95:795.

Holt S. Normal anatomy of female pelvis. In: Callen P, ed. Ultrasound in Obstetrics and Gynecology. Philadelphia, WB Saunders, 1995:548.

Laing F, Benson C, DiSalvo D. Distal ureteral calculi: detected with vaginal ultrasound. Radiology 1994;192:545.

Sladkevicius P, Valentin L, Marsal K. Blood flow velocity in uterine and ovarian arteries during the normal menstrual cycle. Ultrasound Obstet Gynecol 1993;3:199.

Sladkevicius P, Valentin L, Marsal K. Transvaginal gray-scale and Doppler ultrasound examinations of the uterus and ovaries in healthy postmenopausal women. Ultrasound Obstet Gynecol 1995;6:81.

Zalud I, Conway C, Schulman H, Trinca D. Endometrial and myometrial thickness and uterine blood flow in postmenopausal women: the influence of hormonal replacement therapy and age. J Ultrasound Med 1993; 12:737.

Gynecologic Imaging With Magnetic Resonance Imaging: Instrumentation and Technique

Marcia C. Javitt, MD

The advantages of MRI in the pelvis are lack of ionizing radiation, exquisite soft tissue contrast, direct multiplanar imaging, tissue characterization, and extent of disease evaluation for tumors. These advantages are offset by the higher cost of MRI compared with sonography and CT. Sonography is an inexpensive screening procedure and should remain the study of choice for initial investigation of a pelvic mass, but it cannot reliably define the fat planes surrounding a mass or deep adenopathy. CT requires use of ionizing radiation and often intravenous contrast material and lacks comparable soft tissue contrast to MRI in depicting the zonal anatomy of the pelvic organs.

Faster scanning sequences including fast spin-echo imaging have allowed faster acquisition times, thereby increasing utilization. Newer techniques such as chemical shift imaging, especially when combined with dynamic bolus enhancement with gadolinium, have yielded better definition of abnormal from surrounding normal tissue not only in the pelvis but also in the entire body. Advances in hardware, most notably pelvic coil technology with the advent of the pelvic phased-array coil, show improved spatial resolution and better signal-to-noise ratio than the conventional single-loop surface coils (Fig. 1-19). The basic techniques for performing MRI of the female pelvis are reviewed here.

BASIC SCANNING TECHNIQUES

No special patient preparation is used. Patients are usually scanned supine using a pelvic phased-array multicoil.[1–3] A localizer sequence is run as rapidly as possible usually in the coronal plane (Fig. 1-20). Axial relatively short repetition time (TR), short echo time (TE) spin-echo scans (TR, 800–1000 ms; TE min) are obtained usually with 10-mm slice thickness, 20 cm field of view, and 192 × 256 matrix with 4 NEX to achieve a T1-weighted scan with adequate coverage in a reasonable acquisition time. A presaturation

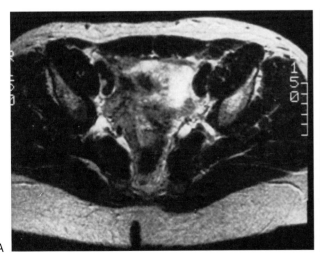
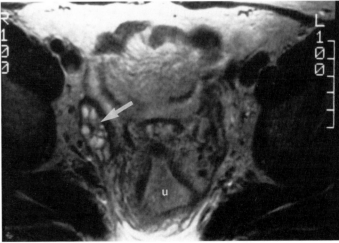

A   B

FIG. 1-19. Pelvic phased-array coil. **(A)** Body coil T2-weighted fast spin-echo axial image. **(B)** Pelvic phased-array coil T2-weighted fast spin-echo image. Note the retroverted uterus (u) and normal right ovary *(arrow)* containing bright signal follicles. The phased-array coil provides improved signal-to-noise ratio and better spatial resolution.

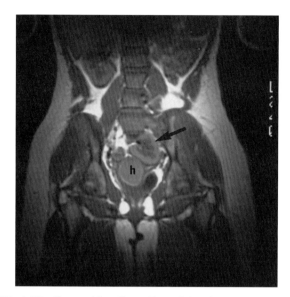

FIG. 1-20. Coronal localizer. T1-weighted coronal localizer is routinely obtained and should include the kidneys, especially in cases with suspected müllerian duct anomalies. This patient has hematocolpos (h) with an ectopic left kidney *(arrow)* located in the pelvis. The right kidney is normotopic.

band is placed above and below the imaged volume to saturate the signal in arteries and veins. These images are useful for definition of adenopathy from surrounding bright signal fat and for fat planes surrounding solid pelvic organs.

Axial fast spin-echo scan is performed with long repetition time and long echo time (TR, 4000 ms; TE, 108 ms) 256 × 256 matrix, 2 NEX, echo train length 8, 5-mm skip, 2.5-mm section thickness, no phase wrap (gradient moment nulling), with superior and inferior saturation bands, and 20-cm field of view. Fast spin-echo scans use multiple refocusing pulses (the echo train) to form multiple phase-encoded signals in a single repetition time, thereby significantly shorten-

ing the acquisition time of the scan. The zonal anatomy of the pelvic organs that is shown on these T2-weighted images includes the endometrium, junctional zone, and myometrium in the uterus; the endocervix with surrounding fibrous stroma in the cervix; and the follicles and ovarian stroma in the ovaries. A second plane with fast spin-echo imaging in the sagittal or sometimes coronal plane is usually acquired and is most useful for uterine and cervical evaluation (Fig. 1-21).[1] Respiratory compensation techniques use a bellows to acquire images at predictable times in the respiratory cycle to reduce phase-related artifacts from respiratory motion of the abdominopelvic wall.

Use of endocervical coils for the cervix and vaginal canal have been developed and provide exquisite signal-to-noise ratios at the expense of a limited field of view and must be accompanied by pelvic phased-array coil or body coil images to cover the remainder of the pelvis, especially nodal chains.[4,5]

The pelvic phased-array coil uses a multicoil technology composed of multiple receiver coils used to generate a composite image with a larger area of coverage but preserving improved signal-to-noise ratio.[2,6–8] The images are susceptible to motion artifact from phase shifts with respiration because these coils operate within a band fastened around the pelvis that contains the coils. Endoluminal coils can be combined with the phased-array coils for better signal-to-noise ratios with a larger field of view.[3]

Chemical shift imaging may be added to the imaging described earlier to identify fat and separate it from other similar-appearing substances such as blood. This can be accomplished by using frequency selective fat suppression, or by use of modified Dixon methods with in-phase and out-of-phase images for fat and water, or by using STIR imaging. STIR imaging is not specific for fat and has lesser signal-to-noise ratios.[1,9–13]

The frequency-selective fat-suppression technique has

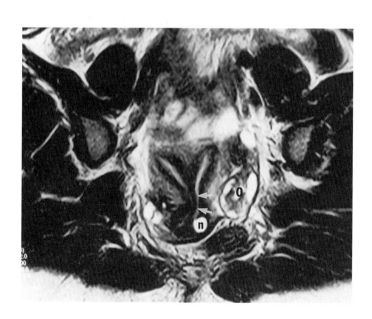

FIG. 1-21. Off-axis coronal scan. T2-weighted off-axis coronal scans can be obtained using graphic prescription along the long axis of the uterus from sagittal scans. The zonal anatomy of the uterus and cervix are shown to advantage as in this case of a septate uterus. Note the uterine contour is relatively normal, but there is a low signal defect *(arrows)* from the septum in the lower uterine segment. nabothian cyst (n); left ovary (o).

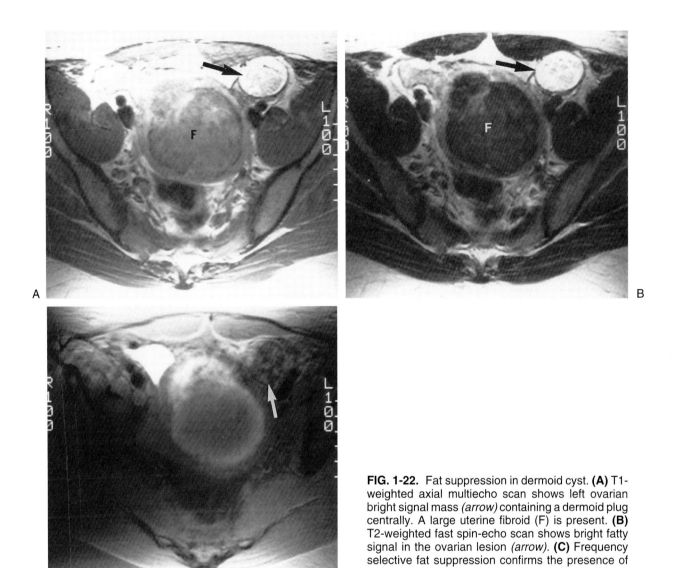

FIG. 1-22. Fat suppression in dermoid cyst. **(A)** T1-weighted axial multiecho scan shows left ovarian bright signal mass *(arrow)* containing a dermoid plug centrally. A large uterine fibroid (F) is present. **(B)** T2-weighted fast spin-echo scan shows bright fatty signal in the ovarian lesion *(arrow)*. **(C)** Frequency selective fat suppression confirms the presence of fatty contents within the dermoid cyst *(arrow)*.

been widely used to identify fat-containing masses such as dermoid cysts (Fig. 1-22) and to differentiate them from blood elements, as well as to identify bright signal endometriosis (Fig. 1-23), which can be obscured on T1-weighted and fast spin-echo images by surrounding fat.[9,14,15] When intravenous gadolinium is added to fat suppression there is improved conspicuousness of abnormal processes infiltrating the fat. Opposed-phase images can be made either by using spin-echo sequences or gradient-echo sequences by appropriate choice of echo time such that the echo generated occurs out of phase or by using hybrid techniques.[16]

When intravenous gadolinium is added to fat suppression, there is improved conspicuousness of abnormal processes infiltrating the fat. The information obtained from enhanced fat-suppressed images for tumor staging may not be available on sonography or CT scans. These scans provide accu-

rate information about tumor margins, necrosis as differentiated from viable tumor, peritoneal implants, and mature fibrosis versus residual or recurrent tumor in an operated or irradiated field (Fig. 1-24).[17–23] Use of a very rapid scan sequence after 0.1 mmol/kg of intravenous gadolinium diethylenetriaminepentaacetic acid (Gd-DTPA) such as a fast multiplanar spoiled gradient-echo scan may be substituted for the T1-weighted fat-suppressed images to obtain early postcontrast scans within 20 or 30 seconds of the injection.

Use of gastrointestinal positive and negative luminal contrast agents has been attempted, but many of these agents have some side effects. In addition, the gut can usually be identified on MRI by virtue of the signal characteristics of luminal contents, which usually differ from surrounding pelvic viscera and fat, rendering the benefit from use of these agents less important on MRI than on CT.[1] Some success

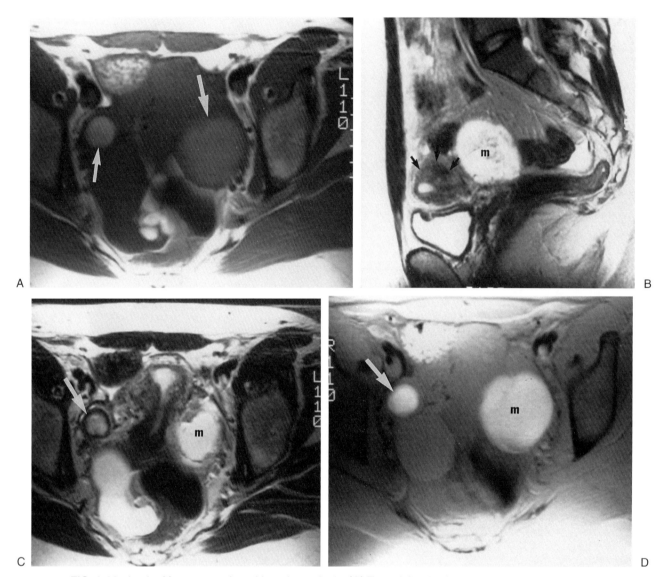

FIG. 1-23. Lack of fat suppression with endometriosis. **(A)** T1-weighted axial scan shows a bright lesion within the right ovary *(arrow)* as well as a large bright signal left adnexal mass *(large arrow)*. **(B)** T2-weighted fast spin-echo sagittal scan. There is diffuse thickening of the junctional zone of the uterus due to adenomyosis *(arrows)*. The left adnexal mass with septations is hyperintense. **(C)** T2-weighted axial fast spin-echo scan shows bilateral adnexal masses with bright signal. There is shading within the right ovarian lesion *(arrow)* that is strongly suggestive of T2-shortening seen in endometriosis from recurrent bleeding. **(D)** Fat-suppressed image. Both ovarian lesions are endometriomas that do not demonstrate fat saturation.

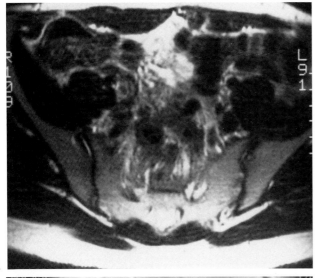

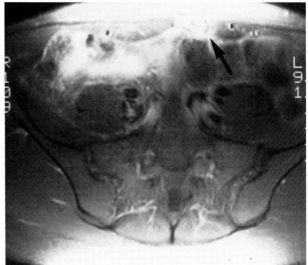

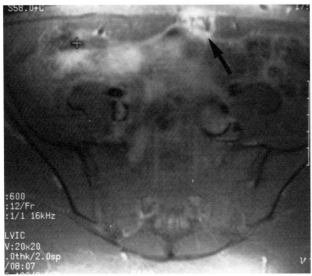

FIG. 1-24. Abdominal wall mass and bright signal fat subjacent to the anterior and posterior pelvic phased-array coils. **(A)** T2-weighted axial scan. Note the bright signal fat in the anterior abdominal wall due to the location of the pelvic phased-array coils against the anterior abdominal wall. The left rectus abdominis mass is inapparent. **(B)** With typical windowing for the pelvic contents, the abdominal wall mass *(arrow)* could be missed on this fat-suppressed gadolinium-enhanced axial T1-weighted image. **(C)** With proper windowing, the mass *(arrow)* is easily identified on the same image as in **B.**

has been achieved with perfluorocarbons, which render the lumen black from signal void. Although they are commercially available and approved for human use, there is no uniform policy regarding reimbursement for these agents.[1,24,25]

REFERENCES

1. Outwater EK, Mitchell DG. Magnetic resonance imaging techniques in the pelvis. In: Mezrich R, guest ed. MRI Clin North Am 1994:2: 161.
2. Hayes CE, Dietz MJ, King BF, et al. Pelvic imaging with phased-array coils: quantitative assessment of signal-to-noise improvement. J Magn Reson Imaging 1992;2:321.
3. Schnall MD, Connick T, Hayes CE, et al. MR imaging of the female pelvis with an endorectal-external multicoil array. J Magn Reson Imaging 1992;2:229.
4. Baudoin CJ, Soutter WP, Gilderdale DJ, et al. Magnetic resonance imaging of the uterine cervix using an intravaginal coil. Magn Reson Med 1992;24:196.
5. Mielstone BN, Schnall MD, Lenkinski RE, et al. Cervical carcinoma: MR imaging with an endorectal surface coil. Radiology 1991;180:91.
6. Smith RC, Reinhold C, Lange RC, et al. Fast spin echo MR imaging of the female pelvis: I. Use of a whole volume coil. Radiology 1992; 184:665.
7. Smith RC, Reinhold C, McCauley TR, et al. Multicoil high-resolution fast spin-echo MR imaging of the female pelvis. Radiology 1992;184: 671.
8. McCauley TR, McCarthy S, Lange R. Pelvic phased-array coil: image quality assessment for spin-echo MR imaging. Magn Reson Imaging 1992;10:513.
9. Kier R, Smith RC, McCarthy SM. Value of lipid- and water-suppression MR images in distinguishing between blood and lipid within ovarian masses. AJR 1992;158:321.
10. Keller PJ, Hunter WW, Schmalbrock P. Multisection fat-water imaging with chemical shift selective presaturation. Radiology 1987;164:539.
11. Wehrli FW. Chemical shift effect. In: Wehrli FW, ed. Fast scan magnetic resonance: principles and applications. New York, Raven Press, 1990.
12. Wehrli FW, Perkins TG, Shimakawa A, et al. Chemical shift–induced

amplitude modulations in images obtained with gradient refocusing. Magn Reson Imaging 1987;5:157.

13. Mitchell DG. Chemical shift magnetic resonance imaging: applications in the abdomen and pelvis. Top Magn Res 1992;4:46.

14. Stevens SK, Hricak H, Campos Z. Teratomas versus cystic hemorrhagic adnexal lesions: differentiation with proton-selective fat-saturation MR imaging. Radiology 1993;186:481.

15. Sugimura K, Okizuka H, Imaoka I, et al. Pelvic endometriosis: detection and diagnosis with chemical shift MR imaging. Radiology 1993; 188:435.

16. Szumowski J, Eisen JK, Vinitski S, et al. Hybrid methods of chemical shift imaging. Magn Reson Med 1989;9:379.

17. Hricak H, Kim B. Contrast enhanced MR imaging of the female pelvis. J Magn Reson Imaging 1993;3:297.

18. Hamm B, Laniado M, Saini S. Contrast enhanced magnetic resonance imaging of the abdomen and pelvis. Magn Reson Q 1990;6:108.

19. Thurner SA. MR imaging of pelvic masses in women: contrast enhanced versus unenhanced images. AJR 1992;159:1243.

20. Semelka RC, Lawrence PH, Shoenut JP, et al. Primary ovarian cancer: prospective comparison of contrast-enhanced CT and pre- and post-contrast fat suppressed MR imaging, with histologic correlation. J Magn Reson Imaging 1993;3:99.

21. Sironi S, Colombo E, Villa G, et al. Myometrial invasion by endometrial carcinoma: assessment with plain and gadolinium-enhanced MR imaging. Radiology 1992;185:207.

22. Stevens SK, Hricak H, Stern JL. Ovarian lesions: detection and characterization with gadolinium enhanced MR imaging at 1.5 T. Radiology 1991;181:481.

23. Yamashita Y, Harada M, Sawada T, et al. Normal uterus and FIGO stage I endometrial carcinoma: dynamic gadolinium enhanced MR imaging. Radiology 1993;186:495.

24. Mattry RF, Trambert MA, Brown JJ, et al. Oral contrast agents of magnetic resonance imaging, result of phase III trials with Imagent;® GI as an oral magnetic resonance contrast agent. Invest Radiol 1991; 26:S65.

25. Brown JJ, Duncan JR, Heiken JP, et al. Perfluoroctylbromide as a gastrointestinal contrast agent for MR imaging: use with and without glucagon. Radiology 1991;181:455.

Magnetic Resonance Imaging of Anatomy of the Female Pelvis

Eric K. Outwater, MD

For the past decade, the advent of high-frequency transvaginal transducers has permitted high-resolution sonographic imaging of the female pelvis. These devices have vastly expanded the diagnostic power and applications of sonography, particularly for characterization of adnexal masses, Doppler analysis and imaging, and in vitro fertilization procedures. The anatomic detail that becomes apparent with increased resolution is, of course, far greater than that with transabdominal scanning and in some cases may be at variance with that of transabdominal images, particularly in regard to the details of endometrial structure, internal morphology of the ovary and its cysts, and the fine detail of fallopian tubes.

Advances in MRI of the female pelvis have similarly led to increased resolution for imaging the female pelvis. These improvements include fast spin-echo imaging and the development of phased array surface coils for imaging the pelvis.[1-4] This brief introduction to imaging features of the uterus and adnexae focuses on the high-resolution details attainable with these techniques and correlates the appearance on MRI with the sonographic appearance and the underlying normal anatomy.

CERVIX

The cervix has an echogenicity similar to that of the myometrium. The endocervical canal in general appears as a thin hyperechoic line.[5] Small anechoic cystic structures are frequently identified along the endocervical canal within the cervix and represent dilated endocervical glands (Nabothian cysts) or tunnel clusters; these are without clinical significance.[5] Rarely, carcinoma can arise within these cysts (adenoma malignum), but this is difficult to distinguish from normal cysts.[5-7] The most prominent periuterine vessels visible with transvaginal sonography or MRI are the pericervical venous plexus line to the right and the left sides of the cervix. These can be distinguished from dilated fallopian tubes by their location lateral to the cervix and not at the cornua, by the presence of flow demonstrable within them by color Doppler imaging, and by their high signal intensity on T2-weighted images.

Unlike the uterine myometrium, the cervical stroma is composed predominantly of connective tissue, with a lesser degree of smooth muscle.[8,9] The uterine myometrium is composed almost exclusively of smooth muscle and intervening vessels, whereas cervical stroma is composed of about 80% fibrous connective tissue and 15% smooth muscle.[8] The cervical mucosa is composed of columnar epithelium with deep glands and clefts dividing the mucosa and forming the plicae palmatae.[8,9] The deep glands frequently become cystic in appearance. The appearance on MRI of the cervix differs from that of the uterine corpus, in contrast to their appearance on sonography. Cervical anatomy is best displayed with a combination of the sagittal and axial views on T2-weighted images. On T1-weighted images, the cervix has intermediate signal intensity similar to the corpus. The signal intensity on T2-weighted images is very low except for a thinner outer layer of cervix, which is somewhat intermediate in signal intensity (Fig. 1-25).[8] Unlike on transvaginal sonography, which generally only visualizes the coapted mucosa and endocervical canal, MRI visualizes the entire extent of the endocervical mucosa. Numerous dilated endocervical glands are frequently seen by MRI (see Fig. 1-25). Thus, on MRI four layers can frequently be seen: (1) mucus of very high signal intensity in the endocervical canal; (2) high signal intensity endocervical mucosa; (3) very low signal intensity of the inner cervical stroma; and (4) slightly higher signal intensity of the outer cervical stroma. During pregnancy the outer one half of the cervical stroma shows significantly higher signal intensity and the low signal intensity submucosal zone becomes thinner.[10]

ENDOMETRIUM

The endometrium consists of the superficial functional layer (which includes the zona functionalis, which is composed of the zona compacta and the zona spongiosa), which undergoes cyclic growth and shedding with the menstrual cycle, and the deep basal endometrium (the zona basalis), which does not undergo cyclic changes. Transvaginal sonography generally displays three sonographic features related to the endometrium. In the center of the endometrium is a thin echogenic line representing the coapted surfaces of the anterior and posterior endometrial surfaces. Deep to this is a slightly more hypoechoic region representing the bulk of

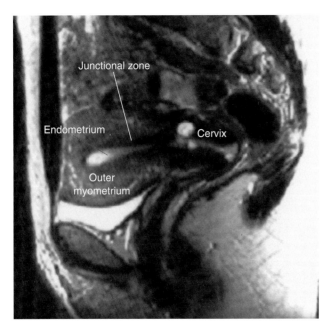

FIG. 1-25. Sagittal anatomy of the uterus on T2-weighted fast spin-echo image. The junctional zone of the myometrium is of lower signal intensity than the outer myometrium and contrasts to the high signal intensity of the endometrium. Most of the cervix demonstrates signal intensity similar to that of the junctional zone. Several dilated endocervical glands of high signal intensity are present. Note the high signal intensity of the arcuate vessels in the outer myometrium.

the endometrium. The echogenicity of this region changes during the cycle, and during the secretory phase it becomes hyperechoic and obscures the other echogenic interfaces.[5] In the postmenopausal woman the endometrial thickness (double layer thickness) measures 5 mm ± 5 mm (standard deviation) in women not taking estrogens and is slightly thicker in those who are on estrogen therapy.[11]

During the proliferative phase the endometrium gradually thickens, progressing from a width of 4 to 8 mm or less to a thickness of 6 to 10 mm at the start of the secretory phase. During the secretory phase, the endometrial thickness generally measures between 7 and 14 mm.[5] Deep to the endometrium is a slightly hypoechoic zone around the endometrium that represents the innermost myometrium.[5] This zone should be excluded for the purposes of endometrial thickness measurements.

On MRI the endometrium appears as a uniformly hyperintense layer (see Fig. 1-25).[12] Generally, fluid within the endometrial cavity displays even higher signal intensity, unless hemorrhagic. On MRI there is no correlate to the echogenic interfaces seen at the coapted endometrial surfaces and at the endometrial-myometrial interface as in sonography. Rather, the high signal intensity of the homogeneous endometrium contrasts sharply to the low signal intensity of the inner myometrium (Fig. 1-26; see also Fig. 1-25). The endometrial layer on MRI is thicker compared with the endometrium when imaged by sonography, possibly because

of inclusion of the endometrial-myometrial interface on sonographic measurements.[13]

The endometrium enhances with injected gadolinium compounds more slowly and in a delayed fashion relative to the myometrium. On delayed images (1 minute or more), the endometrium usually enhances equal to or greater than the myometrium.

MYOMETRIUM

Functionally, the uterine myometrium has three muscle layers. The outer layer is very thin and consists of longitudinal fibers extending from the cervix to the cornua. The very thick intermediate layer is composed of spiral bands of muscle that rise from each uterine cornua and insert into the cervix. In the intermediate layer, generally in the periphery, are numerous arcuate veins that can be appreciated by transvaginal sonography and MRI. The innermost layer of the myometrium consists of longitudinal and circular fibers and lies just beneath the endometrium.

Transvaginal sonography displays a portion of the inner layer as a hypoechoic halo surrounding the endometrium. The remainder of the uterus appears uniformly echogenic. On MRI the inner myometrium is shown as a discrete hypointense layer termed the *junctional zone* (see Fig. 1-26). The junctional zone has lower water content and a higher degree of smooth muscle cellularity, which accounts for the lower signal intensity on MRI.[14,15] It normally measures less than 12 mm on MRI[16] and is thicker on MRI than the subendome-

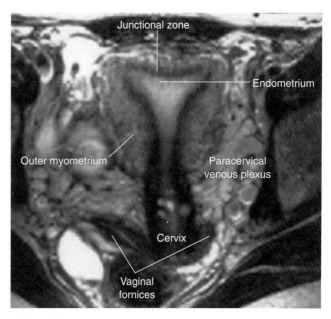

FIG. 1-26. Axial anatomy of the uterus and parametrium on T2-weighted fast spin-echo image. Note the large veins of the paracervical plexus and broad ligament. Hemorrhagic cul-de-sac fluid is present on the right.

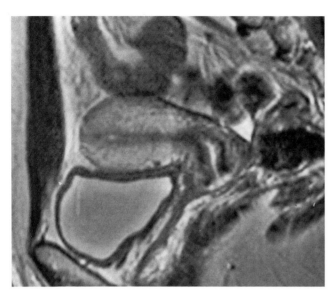

FIG. 1-27. Alteration of signal intensity of the uterus in a woman taking oral contraceptives. The myometrial signal intensity is higher than usual, and the junctional zone and endometrium are thin.

trial halo on sonography.[13] In addition, there is a subserosal thin zone demonstrable on MRI that also shows compact smooth muscle and is lower in signal intensity than the bulk of the myometrium. MRI shows the arcuate uterine vessels as having high signal intensity (see Fig. 1-25). Flow in these is not normally sufficient to produce signal voids on MRI.

The signal intensity of the myometrium changes with the menstrual cycle and with the use of oral contraceptives. During the secretory phase the signal intensity of the myometrium increases, becoming maximally hyperintense in the midsecretory phase (Fig. 1-27).[17–19] The junctional zone remains of low signal intensity (see Fig. 1-27).[17,19] Similar changes to this are seen in users of oral contraceptives, with increased myometrial signal intensity.[19] In contrast to a normal secretory phase, however, in oral contraceptive users the endometrium is not thickened but appears as a thin line of high signal intensity. The junctional zone appears to be somewhat thinner in users of oral contraceptives.

Myometrial contractions can be seen on MRI as localized areas of low signal intensity within the normally higher signal intensity myometrium outside the junctional zone.[20] Such contraction waves cannot normally be seen on transvaginal sonography but can be appreciated on real-time sonography with prolonged viewing.[5]

OVARIES

Ovaries can be identified by identifying the region of the cornua of the uterus and searching laterally and superiorly toward the pelvic sidewall (Fig. 1-28). In most women the ovaries are tethered to the region of the bifurcation of the

common iliac artery lying in the fossa between the internal and external iliac artery. Occasionally the ovaries may lie somewhat posterior toward the cul-de-sac. In addition, with uterine enlargement due to pregnancy or fibroids the ovaries will be drawn up outside the inner pelvis and lie anterior to the iliac arteries.

High-resolution MRI of the ovary shows slightly more ovarian structure than evident on transvaginal sonography. The ovarian stroma appears as intermediate signal intensity or slightly high signal intensity in premenopausal women. The periphery of the ovary (ie, ovarian cortex) is of very low signal intensity on T2-weighted images.[21] In gadolinium-enhanced images, the ovaries generally enhance less than the myometrium.[21] This is particularly true for premenopausal women, in whom a majority of ovaries enhance to an equal degree as the myometrium.

The ovaries are easily identified in the vast majority of premenopausal women by the presence of small follicles within the ovary. The average ovarian volume in premenopausal women is approximately 10 cm, but the range is wide. In the postmenopausal woman the ovary is seen as an oval structure of uniformly intermediate low signal intensity (Fig. 1-29). The ovaries can be identified in most postmenopausal women because of their small size and nonspecific characteristics.

Numerous follicles can be identified in normal premenopausal women by MRI (see Fig. 1-28). The appearance of the normal ovary with follicles may be difficult to distinguish from polycystic ovary syndrome on imaging characteristics alone.[21] In polycystic ovary syndrome the follicles are typically very small and displaced to the periphery of the ovary owing to the hypertrophied central ovarian stroma (Fig. 1-30).[22] Small follicular cysts of the ovary show a thin enhancing rim on gadolinium enhancement (Fig. 1-31). Corpus luteum cysts demonstrate a thicker wall than other functional ovarian cysts or follicles, reflecting the increased vascularity of the thick luteinized lining of the corpus luteum cysts. This is reflected on the Doppler analysis of these structures as increased diastolic flow, which may be a pitfall in the evaluation of ovarian cysts by Doppler waveform analysis. These cysts are frequently hemorrhagic; the hallmark of hemorrhage on MRI is the presence of high signal intensity on T1-weighted images.

Dominant preovulatory follicles can be seen as 1.5- to 2.5-cm discrete thin-walled cysts. With formation of the corpus luteum the wall may involute and become irregular, and diffuse echoes within the cyst representing hemorrhage can be identified. Corpus lutea may be cystic or involuted and noncystic. With high enough resolution thin rims representing the follicle wall and surrounding ovarian stroma can be identified around these as well as around functional cysts. Generally, these are of very high signal intensity on T2-weighted images, although the presence of hemorrhage within a functional cyst may modify this appearance.

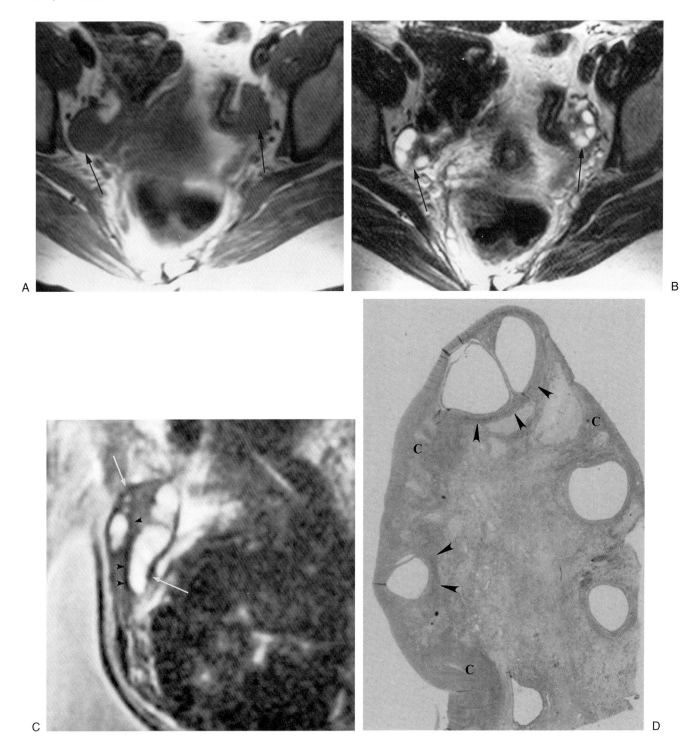

FIG. 1-28. Normal premenopausal ovaries on axial T1-weighted spin-echo **(A)** and T2-weighted fast spin-echo **(B)** images. The ovaries *(arrows)* appear homogeneous on the T1-weighted image. Note high signal intensity of multiple cystic follicles evident on the T2-weighted image. Sagittal T2-weighted fast spin-echo image in another patient **(C)**, with corresponding histologic section **(D)**, demonstrates the low signal intensity of the cortex *(long arrows)* and stroma surrounding the cystic follicles *(arrowheads)*, corresponding to the ovarian cortex (C) and stromal rims in the histologic section *(arrowheads,* **D**). (Fig. 1-28C, D reprinted with permission from: Outwater EK, Mitchell DG. Normal ovaries and functional cysts: MR appearance. Radiology, in press.)

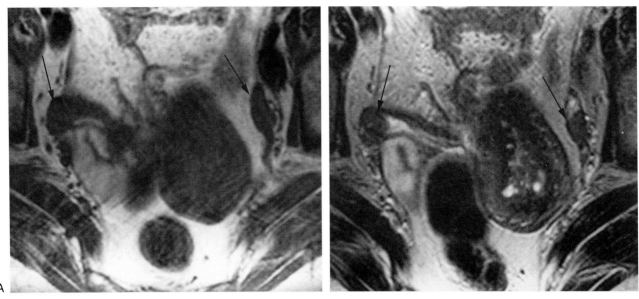

FIG. 1-29. Normal postmenopausal ovaries on axial T1-weighted spin-echo **(A)** and T2-weighted fast spin-echo **(B)** images. The ovaries (arrows) are homogeneous and of somewhat low signal intensity on both images.

FALLOPIAN TUBES

Normal fallopian tubes are not well identified by either transvaginal sonography or MRI. The normal fallopian tubes contain a small amount of intraluminal fluid that is dispersed within innumerable infoldings of the fallopian tube mucosa.

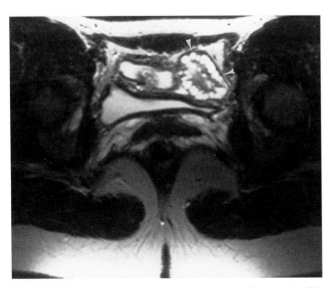

FIG. 1-30. Polycystic ovary syndrome as shown by T2-weighted fast spin-echo image of the left ovary (arrowheads). Note the relatively uniform size and peripheral distribution of the cystic follicles compared with the normal ovaries in Figure 1-28. (Reprinted with permission from: Outwater EK. MR imaging of the pelvis. In: Haaga J, Lanzieri C, Sartoris D, Zerhouni E, eds. Computed tomography and magnetic resonance imaging of the whole body. vol 2. St. Louis, CV Mosby Co., 1994:1393.

These infoldings prevent visualization of the tube as a discrete fluid-filled structure. With dilatation, the tube can be identified as a discrete structure. With increasing degrees of distention, the tube will fold over on itself, which will facilitate identification both by MRI and transvaginal sonography. On a sonogram the tube may resemble periuterine veins, but it can generally be distinguished by the absence of color flow. In addition, as the tube dilates, the mucosal infoldings become attenuated against the wall of the tube and appear as small linear projections across the tubal inner surface. These can be identified both by transvaginal sonography and by high-resolution MRI. A discrete wall to the tube can generally be seen.

PELVIC FLUID

Pelvic fluid is a frequent finding on transvaginal sonography and MRI. On transvaginal sonography pelvic fluid is most commonly identified in the cul-de-sac, although by MRI scattered pockets throughout the pelvis are often identified. Pelvic fluid is a common finding in women throughout the menstrual cycle and tends to peak in the secretory phase.[23] Longitudinal sonographic studies of women throughout the cycle show that, although some of the fluid may be related to ovarian cyst rupture, clearly most of the fluid is not directly related to cyst rupture. Pelvic fluid is a frequent finding in women with benign and malignant gynecologic disease.[24] Only larger amounts are suggestive of a malignant tumor or peritoneal spread of tumor.[24] On MRI, peritoneal enhancement may be an important finding to indicate the presence of peritoneal spread of tumor in malignancies. Normal peritoneum does not enhance with gadolinium.

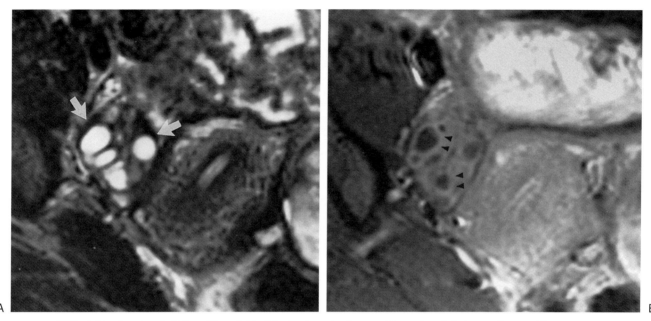

FIG. 1-31. Ovarian follicles. T2-weighted fast spin-echo image **(A)** and gadolinium-enhanced fat-saturated T1-weighted image **(B)** show numerous cystic follicles of the right ovary. Note the low signal intensity of the cortex *(arrows)*. The rims of the cysts on the T2-weighted image show enhancement *(arrowheads)* on the gadolinium-enhanced image.

Peritoneal enhancement may not be specific; however, it may be seen in benign disease.[24]

VAGINA

MRI displays vaginal anatomy to the best advantage when acquired in the sagittal or axial planes with T2-weighted sequences. The muscular wall of the vagina appears as a low signal intense structure between the rectovaginal septum and the bladder neck and urethra anteriorly (Figs. 1-32 and 1-33). On T2-weighted images and gadolinium-enhanced images, a thin higher signal intensity rim on the interior of this low signal intensity muscularis represents the mucosa and submucosa. This layer may appear to increase in thickness during the secretory phase during estrogen stimulation.[25] The muscular wall of the vagina is surrounded by the veins of the perivaginal venous plexus. These have high signal inten-

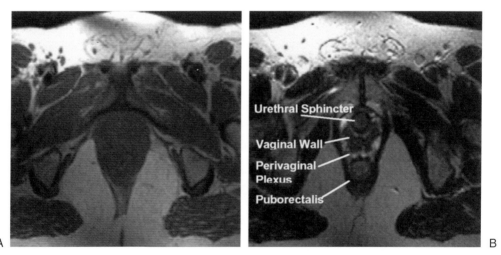

FIG. 1-32. Axial vaginal anatomy on axial T1-weighted spin echo **(A)** and T2-weighted fast spin-echo **(B)** images. The urethra, vagina, rectum, and perivaginal venous plexuses cannot be differentiated on the T1-weighted image, analogous to a CT image of the same structures. In contrast, the T2-weighted image shows the low signal intensity of the urethral sphincter, vaginal muscularis, and muscularis propria of the rectum distinct from the high signal intensity of the perivaginal plexus.

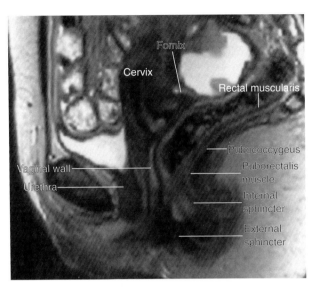

FIG. 1-33. T2-weighted fast spin-echo image of midline sagittal perineal anatomy. The muscular walls of the urethral sphincter, vagina, rectum, and anal sphincter are identified as structures of low signal intensity.

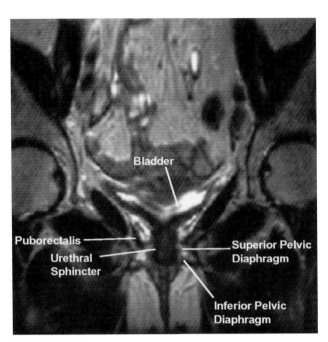

FIG. 1-34. Coronal perineal anatomy on a T2-weighted fast spin-echo image at the level of the urethral sphincter.

sity on T2-weighted images and fill the space between the vagina and the levator muscle.

SUPPORTING LIGAMENTS AND STRUCTURES

The main supporting structures of the uterus and vagina can be identified by MRI. The round ligaments project anteriorly from the uterine cornua at the superior edge of the broad ligament and course anteriorly toward the internal inguinal ring and through the inguinal canal, where the round ligament terminates diffusely on the mons pubis. The round ligament appears as low signal intensity and is well defined on T2-weighted images.[26] The broad ligament itself is not identified because of the paucity of connective tissue fibers.[27] The broad ligament is a peritoneal reflection around the round ligament, fallopian tube, and periuterine arterial and venous plexus. On MRI these appear as high signal intensity serpiginous structures on T2-weighted images (see Fig. 1-26). Flow in the intrauterine and periuterine veins and vessels is not sufficient to produce a signal void in these sequences from time-of-flight effects. Therefore, high signal intensity results from the stagnant blood in these veins (see Fig. 1-26).

The uterosacral ligaments can be identified as thin strands projecting from the junction of the low uterine segment of the cervix posteriorly around the perirectal space and appear to merge with the perirectal fascia.[26,27] These are much more prominent when abnormal, such as from invasion by cervical carcinoma. The so-called cardinal ligaments, which are supporting structures for the cervix, are ill defined pathologically and not identified on MRI.[26] Anatomic studies have

shown that there is not organized connective tissue in the area of these ligaments.[26] Inferiorly on either side of the lower vagina and introitus are the two layers of low signal intensity that indicate the pelvic diaphragm (Fig. 1-34).[28] This structure is most evident on coronal images. Just inferior to this, coursing out to the side just medial to the inferior pubic rami, are the crura of the clitoris. These are shown as areas of high signal intensity. They lie medial to the inferior pubic rami and project anteriorly toward the anterior vulva.[28] The vulva and labia appear as structures of intermediate signal intensity on T2-weighted images that are best displayed in the coronal plane (see Fig. 1-34).

REFERENCES

1. Hayes CE, Hattes N, Roemer PB. Volume imaging with MR phased arrays. Magn Reson Med 1991;18:309.
2. Hayes CE, Dietz MJ, King BF, Ehman RL. Pelvic imaging with phased-array coils: quantitative assessment of signal-to-noise ratio improvement. J Magn Reson Imaging 1992;2:321.
3. Nghiem HV, Herfkens RJ, Francis IR, et al. The pelvis: T2-weighted fast spin-echo MR imaging. Radiology 1992;185:213.
4. Smith RC, Reinhold C, McCauley TR, et al. Multicoil high-resolution fast spin-echo MR imaging of the female pelvis. Radiology 1992;184:671.
5. Lyons EA, Gratton D, Harrington C. Transvaginal sonography of normal pelvic anatomy. Radiol Clin North Am 1992;30:663.
6. Yamashita Y, Takahashi M, Katabuchi H, et al. Adenoma malignum: MR appearances mimicking nabothian cysts. AJR 1994;162:649.
7. Daya D, Young RH. Florid deep glands of the uterine cervix: Another mimic of adenoma malignum. Am J Clin Pathol 1995;103:614.
8. Scoutt LM, McCauley TR, Flynn SD, et al. Zonal anatomy of the cervix: correlation of MR imaging and histologic examination of hysterectomy specimens. Radiology 1993;186:159.
9. Ferenczy A, Wright TC. Anatomy and histology of the cervix. In: Kurman RJ, ed. Blaustein's pathology of the female genital tract. New York, Springer-Verlag, 1994:185.

10. Holland GA, Ludmir J, Holland LD, et al. Evaluation of the uterine cervix with MR imaging in the nonpregnant, pregnant, and postpartum states. Radiology 1993;189(P):370.
11. Lin MC, Gosink BB, Wolf SI, et al. Endometrial thickness after menopause: effect of hormone replacement. Radiology 1991;180:427.
12. Lee JKT, Gersell DJ, Balfe DM, et al. The uterus: in-vitro MR-anatomic correlation of normal and abnormal specimens. Radiology 1985;157:175.
13. Mitchell DG, Schonholz L, Hilpert PL, et al. Zones of the uterus: discrepancy between US and MR images. Radiology 1990;174:827.
14. Scoutt LM, Flynn SD, Luthringer DJ, et al. Junctional zone of the uterus: correlation of MR imaging and histologic examination of hysterectomy specimens. Radiology 1991;179:403.
15. Brown HK, Stoll BS, Nicosia SV, et al. Uterine junctional zone: correlation between histologic findings and MR imaging. Radiology 1991;179:409.
16. Reinhold C, McCarthy S, Bret M, et al. Uterine adenomyosis: a prospective comparative analysis with endovaginal US and MR imaging. Radiology 1993;189(P):300.
17. Occhipinti KA. Magnetic resonance imaging of the uterus under hormonal stimulation. In: Jaffe R, Pierson R, Abramowicz J, eds. Imaging in infertility and reproductive endocrinology. Philadelphia, JB Lippincott, 1994:269.
18. Demas BE, Hricak H, Jaffe RB. Uterine MR imaging: effects of hormonal stimulation. Radiology 1986;159:123.
19. McCarthy S, Tauber C, Gore J. Female pelvic anatomy: MR assessment of variations during the menstrual cycle and with use of oral contraceptives. Radiology 1986;160:119.
20. Togashi K, Kawakami S, Kimura I, et al. Sustained uterine contractions: a cause of hypointense myometrial bulging. Radiology 1993;187:707.
21. Outwater EK, Mitchell DG. Normal ovaries and functional cysts: MR appearance. Radiology 1996;198:397.
22. Mitchell DG, Gefter WB, Spritzer CE, et al. Polycystic ovaries: MR imaging. Radiology 1986;160:420.
23. Davis JA, Gosink BB. Fluid in the female pelvis: cyclic patterns. J Ultrasound Med 1986;5:75.
24. Outwater EK, Wilson KM, Siegelman ES, Mitchell DG. MR imaging of benign and malignant gynecologic disease: significance of fluid and peritoneal enhancement in the pelvis. Radiology 1996, in press.
25. Hricak H, Chang Y, Thurnher S. Vagina: evaluation with MR imaging: I. Normal anatomy and congenital anomalies. Radiology 1988;169:169.
26. Fritsch H, Hotzinger H. Tomographical anatomy of the pelvis, visceral pelvic connective tissue, and its compartments. Clin Anat 1995;8:17.
27. Pawlina W, Larkin LH, Masterson BJ, Ross MH. Subperitoneal layer of elastic fibers in the female pelvis. Clin Anat 1991;4:447.
28. Vanneuville G, Lenck LC, Garcier JM, et al. Contribution of imaging to the understanding of the female pelvic fasciae. Surg Radiol Anat 1992;14:147.

Pelvic Computed Tomography: Instrumentation, Technique, and Normal Anatomy

R. Brooke Jeffrey, Jr., MD

The primary advantages of CT of the pelvis are speed of examination, ease of interpretation, and technical consistency. With the development of rapid scanning techniques using spiral (helical) CT, an entire pelvic examination requires only 15 to 20 minutes for patient preparation, scan acquisition, and image reconstruction. The overall examination times for pelvic CT are considerably shorter than for pelvic MRI, which often requires 45 minutes to an hour to complete. Another advantage of CT of the pelvis is its relative ease of interpretation. Pelvic MRI may be complex and time consuming to interpret because it requires analyzing a large number of images obtained in multiple planes. With CT, only axial images are required for most routine scanning and the number of images acquired is significantly less than with pelvic MRI. Compared with sonography and MRI, CT more clearly depicts the rectosigmoid colon and pelvic small bowel because of its ability to opacify the luminal gastrointestinal tract with oral or rectal contrast medium. Because of the relatively short examination time and the exquisite spatial resolution of state-of-the-art spiral scanners there is remarkable technical consistency to the CT studies of the pelvis.

However, CT has a number of significant limitations in gynecologic imaging. To a large degree, transvaginal sonography and MRI have supplanted CT as the initial imaging method of choice. One clear disadvantage is that CT uses ionizing radiation. For this reason alone CT is often not the primary imaging modality in adolescents and young women of childbearing age. Intravenous contrast medium is routinely required for optimal CT visualization of pelvic vessels. A very small percentage of patients may develop a significant allergic reaction to iodinated contrast media. CT excels at identifying fascial planes and pelvic muscles separated by fat and, thus, the image quality of pelvic CT is often dependent on the degree of intraperitoneal and extraperitoneal fat. In patients with little or no fat, it may be exceedingly difficult to clearly distinguish normal adnexal structures on CT. Furthermore, because the tissue attenuation of the cervix, uterus, and fallopian tubes is similar, pelvic CT provides considerably less anatomic detail than MRI. CT is not able to discriminate the zonal anatomy of the uterus, and it is often difficult in thin patients to visualize the normal ovary. Finally, the true multiplanar imaging capability of MRI may be a distinct advantage in selected patients.

COMPUTED TOMOGRAPHIC SCANNING TECHNIQUE

The development of spiral (helical) CT has greatly facilitated evaluation of the pelvis. Spiral CT takes advantage of slip-ring technology, which combines a continuous gantry rotation with a continuous table feed (Fig. 1-35).[1] Compared with conventional CT, spiral CT greatly increases the speed of scan acquisition by entirely eliminating any interscan delay.[1] Therefore, routine pelvic scans can be obtained with a single breathhold, thus eliminating respiratory and motion artifacts. If desired, three-dimensional editing of the CT data set can be performed to produce three-dimensional angiographic studies or multiplanar re-formations with superior resolution compared with conventional CT.[2]

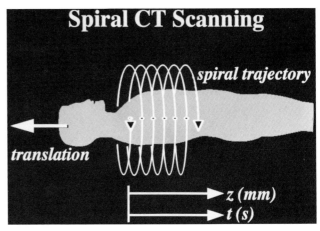

FIG. 1-35. Schematic of spiral CT. Unlike conventional CT, spiral CT uses slip-ring technology to combine a continuous table translation with a continuous gantry rotation. This results in a spiral trajectory for CT data acquisition that completely eliminates interscan delay.

For most routine pelvic CT examinations, a slice collimation of 5 to 8 mm is used. For specialized studies, such as three-dimensional CT arteriography, scans are obtained using 3-mm collimation. Increased anatomic coverage can be obtained with spiral CT by increasing the pitch greater than 1 during scan acquisition. Pitch represents the ratio of table speed to slice collimation multiplied by the time required for gantry rotation. Whenever a pitch greater than 1 is used the images must be reconstructed at least at the same interval as the scan collimation to minimize partial volume effects.

Both oral and intravenous contrast media are used routinely for pelvic CT.[3,4] At least 1½ hours before CT 500 to 800 mL of dilute barium or water-soluble contrast medium is administered.[3,4] For many outpatient scans, oral contrast medium can be given the night before to opacify the colon. In selected patients, 200 mL of rectal contrast medium may be used to more clearly delineated the distal colon and to avoid misinterpreting the rectosigmoid colon as a pelvic mass (Fig. 1-36).

For intravenous contrast medium injection, 150 mL of 60% iodinated contrast medium is injected at a rate of 2 to 3 mL/s. Because spiral CT is considerably faster than conventional dynamic CT, initial scans must be delayed until 80 to 90 seconds after the initiation of the contrast medium bolus to ensure opacification of the pelvic veins. Because the spiral CT images are obtained during the nephrogram phase before significant renal excretion, selected delayed images at 5 to 8 minutes after the initial scan acquisition must be obtained to identify the pelvic ureters opacified with contrast medium. Evaluation of bladder pathology is often best performed with moderate distention of the bladder with urine. Lesions that infiltrate the bladder wall can often be identified to better advantage with the urine as a negative contrast agent. Therefore, moderate distention of the urinary bladder may be helpful in evaluating bladder wall invasion.

NORMAL CT ANATOMY OF THE FEMALE PELVIS

Cervix

Unlike MRI, CT cannot reliably distinguish the endocervical canal and endocervical mucosa from the surrounding cervical stroma. With bolus contrast medium administration, the cervical epithelium enhances to a greater degree than the surrounding cervical stroma and has a ringlike appearance (Fig. 1-37).[5] Enhancing vessels representing the cervical vascular plexus can be identified in the paracervical fat just lateral to the cervix. Because the cervix enhances significantly with contrast medium administration, most carcinomas appear as low attenuating lesions because of their decreased vascularity compared with the normal cervix. Nabothian cysts and dilated endocervical glands may be clearly identified on CT as water-density masses. However, these are of no clinical significance. The normal cardinal ligaments extend laterally from the cervix and have a triangular appearance (see Fig. 1-37).

Uterus

After intravenous contrast medium is injected, the myometrium demonstrates intense enhancement owing to its abundant blood supply. In many patients the endometrial cavity may be identified as a low-attenuating central area (Fig. 1-38).[5] However, this is an inconsistent finding and CT cannot reliably delineate the zonal anatomy of the uterus. Specifically, the junctional zone cannot be identified as a discrete layer, owing to its similar attenuation to the myometrium. Masses within the myometrium, such as fibroids, generally are of lower attenuation than the

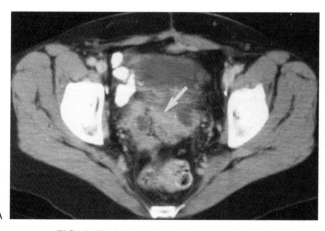
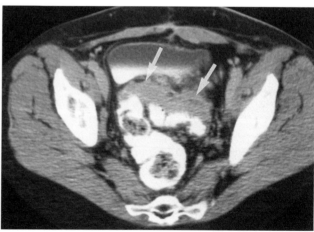

FIG. 1-36. Value of rectal contrast in identifying pelvic mass. The patient was status post laparotomy for ovarian carcinoma. CT was performed before second-look laparotomy. Questionable pelvic mass is seen in **(A)** *(arrow)*. After instillation of rectal contrast medium **(B)** there is a clearly defined pelvic mass adjacent to the sigmoid colon representing recurrent ovarian carcinoma *(arrows)*. This obviated the need for second-look laparotomy.

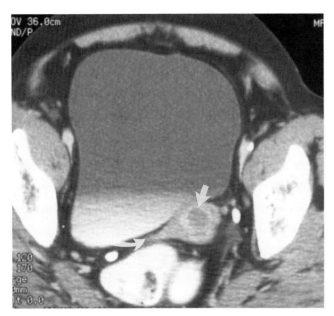

FIG. 1-37. CT of the normal cervix and cardinal ligaments. Note the enhancing ring of the cervical epithelium *(straight arrow)*. The normal cardinal ligaments extend laterally from the cervix and have a triangular configuration *(curved arrow)*.

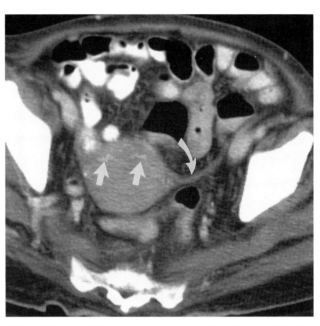

FIG. 1-39. Calcified spiral arteries of the uterus. Note the serpiginous calcifications representing calcified spiral arteries *(straight arrows)*. The normal round ligament is identified on the left *(curved arrow)*.

contrast medium–enhanced myometrium. However, the CT appearance of fibroids is variable because they may be calcified or demonstrate fatty degeneration or hemorrhage.[6] In elderly patients and especially in diabetics, calcification of spiral arteries of the uterus is often readily apparent with CT (Fig. 1-39).

Fallopian Tubes and Ovaries

The normal fallopian tube cannot be reliably identified with CT. Although the ovary most often lies in the ovarian

fossa near the common iliac artery bifurcation, its position is variable.[7,8] The boundaries of the ovarian fossa include the ureter and internal iliac vessels posteriorly, the ovarian ligament medially, and the broad ligament mesovarium and the hilus of the ovary anteriorly.[9] In some individuals, identification of prominent low-attenuating follicles can be helpful in delineating the location of the ovary.[5] In other patients the normal ovary is an oval soft tissue structure 1.5×2.5 cm adjacent to the broad ligament or in the cul-de-sac (Fig. 1-40). In the absence of discrete follicles or normal func-

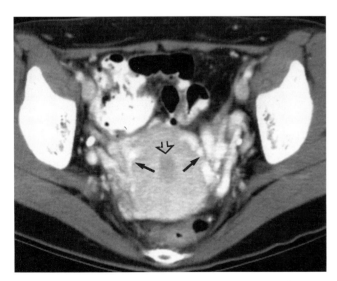

FIG. 1-38. Normal endometrial cavity and parametrial vascular plexus. Note the low attenuation centrally within the uterus representing the endometrial cavity *(open arrow)*. Because of the excellent vascular opacification, the parametrial vascular plexus *(arrows)* is well delineated.

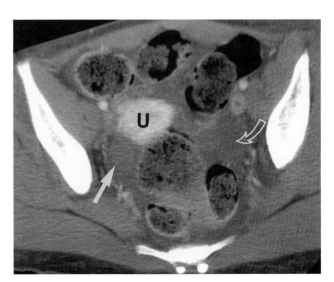

FIG. 1-40. CT of the normal ovary surrounded by ascites. The normal ovary *(straight arrow)* is seen adjacent to the uterus (U). Note the pelvic ascites *(curved arrow)*.

tional cysts it is often difficult to confidently visualize the normal ovary on CT. This is particularly true in thin patients with little pelvic fat.

Pelvic Ligaments

In patients with ample pelvic fat or ascites, it may be possible to identify on CT the supporting ligaments of the uterus, including the broad ligament, round ligament, and uterosacral ligaments. The broad ligament is composed of two layers of peritoneum. It reflects over the uterus and courses laterally to the pelvic sidewall (Fig. 1-41).[10,11] The broad ligament terminates caudad as the cardinal ligament and superiorly as the suspensory ligament of the ovary. The loose connective tissue of the broad ligament is referred to as the parametrium. It contains the fallopian tube, the round ligament, the uterine and ovarian blood vessels, lymphatics, and a portion of the ureter.[12,13] The parametrium is often ill defined on CT. It may be identified primarily by its position lateral to the uterus and lower uterine segment.[13] In patients without ascites the broad ligament is not commonly visualized on CT (see Fig. 1-41). The location of the broad ligament can be inferred, however, by visualizing the normal structures it contains. The fibromuscular round ligament may be identified as it extends from the anterolateral aspect of the fundus of the uterus to the pelvic sidewall (see Fig. 1-39).[14] It courses anterior to the external iliac vessels and extends to the anterior abdominal wall through the inguinal canal. At its origin from the uterine fundus, the round ligament has a characteristic triangular configuration. On axial CT images it may be difficult to distinguish the cardinal ligament (see Fig. 1-37) from the endopelvic fascia or the

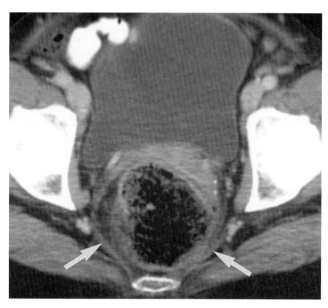

FIG. 1-42. Normal uterosacral ligaments. Note the normal uterosacral ligaments extending laterally and posterior from the lower corpus of the uterus to the presacral area *(arrows)*.

uterosacral ligaments, which both extend posteriorly from the lateral margin of the vagina and cervix extending toward the anterior aspect of the sacrum at the level of S2 or S3.[14,15] Often the normal uterosacral ligaments are only a few millimeters thick (Fig. 1-42). However, they may become thickened by tumor infiltration or after radiation therapy for pelvic malignancy.

Pelvic Vessels

With contrast medium enhancement the pelvic vasculature can be clearly displayed with CT even in patients with minimal fat. The paired uterine arteries can be visualized along the lateral aspect of the uterus coursing medially above the cardinal ligament in the base of the broad ligament.[8,11] The vessels course anterior to the ureter and bifurcate into a smaller cervical vaginal branch along the inferior margin of the cervix. The uterine artery then branches in the corpus of the uterus into branches to the fallopian tube, uterine fundus, and ovary. The parametrial plexus can readily be identified with contrast medium–enhanced spiral CT (see Fig. 1-38).

REFERENCES

1. Napel SA. Basic principles of spiral CT. In: Fishman EK, Jeffrey RB Jr., eds. Spiral principles, techniques and clinical applications. New York, Raven Press, 1994:1.
2. Rubin GD, Dake MD, Napel S, et al. Three-dimensional spiral CT angiography of the abdomen: initial clinical experience. Radiology 1993;186:147.
3. Walsh JW. Computed tomography of gynecologic neoplasms. Radiol Clin North Am 1992;30:817.

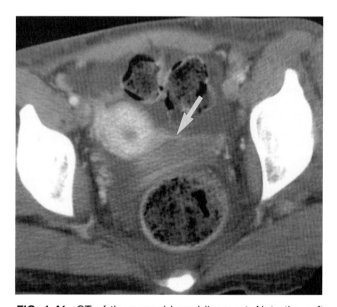

FIG. 1-41. CT of the normal broad ligament. Note the soft tissue density of the ligament extending laterally from the cervix surrounded by ascites *(arrow)*.

4. Ammann AM, Walsh JW. Normal anatomy and techniques of examination. In: Walsh JW, ed. Computed Tomography of the Pelvis. New York, Churchill Livingstone, 1985:1.
5. Foshager MC, Walsh JW. CT anatomy of the female pelvis: a second look. Radiographics 1994;14:51.
7. Pritchard JA, MacDonald PC, Gant NF. Williams obstetrics, ed 17. Norwalk, CT, Appleton-Century-Crofts, 1985:7.
8. Gardner E, Gray DJ, O'Rahilly R. Anatomy. Philadelphia, WB Saunders, 1960:568, 596.
9. Snell RS. Gross anatomy dissector: a companion for atlas of clinical anatomy. Boston, Little, Brown & Co, 1978:83.
10. Jones HW, Jones GS. Novak's textbook of gynecology, ed 10. Baltimore, Williams & Wilkins, 1981:8.
11. Netter FG. The CIBA collection of medical illustrations, vol 2, reproductive system. New York, Colorpress, 1965:89.
12. Sciarra JJ, McElin TW. Gynecology and obstetrics. Cambridge, MA, Harper & Row, 1980:1.
13. Vick CW, Walsh JW, Wheelock JB, Brewer WH. CT of the normal and abnormal parametria in cervical cancer. AJR 1984;143:597.
14. Walsh JW. Computed tomography of the pelvis. New York, Churchill-Livingstone, 1985:851.
15. Lee JK, Sagel SS, Stanley RJ. Computed body tomography. New York, Raven Press, 1989:851.

Clinical Gynecologic Imaging, edited
by Arthur C. Fleischer, Marcia C. Javitt,
R. Brooke Jeffrey, Jr., and Howard W. Jones III,
Lippincott-Raven Publishers, Philadelphia © 1997.

CHAPTER 2

Adnexal Mass—Detection and Evaluation

Clinical Overview

Deidre J. Russell, MD

The clinician is often called on to evaluate a pelvic mass in a female patient. The problem may come to light during the course of a routine physical examination, as an incidental finding after imaging studies for unrelated conditions, or secondary to specific patient complaints. Because pelvic masses are commonly encountered in female patients, it is essential for today's physician to be familiar with the tools available to facilitate diagnosis and treatment.

Because the source may be either gynecologic or nongynecologic and because of the complex anatomy of the area, the differential diagnosis of a pelvic mass in a female patient is extensive. In the female reproductive tract, the adnexal region is composed of the ovary, fallopian tube, broad ligament, and the associated blood and nervous supply. Masses can also arise from the uterus, round ligament, and uterosacral ligaments (Fig. 2-1). Nongynecologic sources of abdominopelvic masses must also be considered. Possible sources include the bladder, ureter, rectum, colon, small intestine, peritoneum, omentum, blood vessels, and nerves of the pelvis (Table 2-1). The process that creates the mass may be congenital, functional, hemorrhagic, neoplastic, obstructive, or inflammatory.

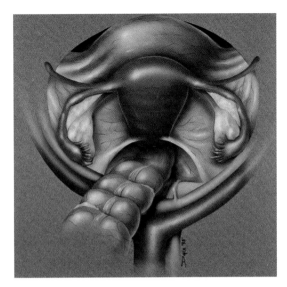

FIG. 2-1. The female pelvis as viewed from above.

Because of the prevalence and importance of masses in the adnexal region, attention is specifically directed toward this area. Masses are commonly encountered here owing to the number of structures present and to the ovary itself. By virtue of its anatomic structure and function, it is not surprising that the ovary is often the source of a mass in the pelvis. After menarche, normal cyclic ovarian function involves the formation of increasingly large follicles, follicular rupture followed by oocyte expulsion, and the development of the corpus luteum. Normally, only one follicle becomes dominant and progresses toward maturation, while the others regress. The mature follicle can contain a large quantity of

TABLE 2-1. *Classification of adnexal masses*

Gynecologic origin	Nongynecologic origin
Nonneoplastic	Nonneoplastic
Ovarian	Appendiceal abscess
Physiologic cysts	Diverticulosis
Follicular	Adhesions of bowel
Corpus luteum	and omentum
Theca lutein cyst	Peritoneal cyst
Luteoma of pregnancy	Feces in rectosigmoid
Polycystic ovaries	Urine in bladder
Endometriosis	Pelvic kidney
Inflammatory cysts	Urachal cyst
Nonovarian	Anterior sacral
Ectopic pregnancy	meningocele
Congenital anomalies	Neoplastic
Embryologic remnants	Carcinoma
Tubal	Sigmnoid
Pyosalpinx	Cecum
Hydrosalpinx	Appendix
Neoplastic	Bladder
Ovarian	Retroperitoneal spasm
Nonovarian	Presacral teratoma
Leiomyoma	
Paraovarian cyst	
Endometrial carcinoma	
Tubal carcinoma	

antral fluid, causing it to become palpable on physical examination. Additionally, if the dominant or "graffian" follicle fails to rupture and extrude the oocyte or other follicles fail to regress, a follicle cyst of the ovary may develop. Similarly, the corpus luteum, under normal nonpregnant conditions, should undergo regression; however, if this does not occur, or if hemorrhage occurs into the corpus luteum, a cyst or hematoma may develop and persist.

Once an adnexal mass has been identified, the main question that needs to be answered is whether the tumor requires treatment, and, if so, what approach is most appropriate. For example, a simple physiologic cyst usually resolves with time, whereas an ovarian tumor requires prompt surgical intervention. An ectopic pregnancy may be managed by laparoscopy, laparotomy, or medical therapy depending on various circumstances. Because treatment options vary considerably depending on etiology, accurate diagnosis is of paramount importance. There are several criteria that assist in guiding the physician toward an accurate diagnosis. These include patient age, patient history, physical examination, laboratory tests, and diagnostic imaging studies.

PATIENT AGE

Patient age is perhaps the first parameter that should be considered when an adnexal mass has been identified. Based on reproductive function, patients should be thought of in the following categories: childhood, adolescence, the reproductive years, and the perimenopausal and postmenopausal period.

Childhood

Ovarian cysts are found in 2% to 5% of otherwise healthy prepubertal females and occasionally are present in the newborn. In general, these are caused by the stimulatory effect of maternal hormones on otherwise normal ovaries, resulting in true functional cysts. Thus, when the infant is removed from the maternal hormonal milieu, the cysts regress. Resolution usually occurs within the first few months of life. After this period, because ovulation does not normally occur in this age group, functional cysts are extremely rare and the finding of an adnexal mass should raise concerns of a neoplastic process—malignant or benign. Most gynecologic neoplasms in this age group arise from germ cell origin and should be surgically explored. Most are small (<1 cm); however, they can be 10 cm or larger. In one study, Milar and colleagues[1] looked at 99 premenarchal females diagnosed with ovarian cysts. The great majority of large cysts (>2 cm) occurred during the first year of life, and all were benign.

Adolescence

With the onset of menses, the differential diagnosis of an adnexal mass becomes more extensive. At this time the ovary becomes functional, entering into the cyclic phases of follicle development, oocyte release, and corpus luteum development. The majority of adnexal masses in this age group are physiologic cysts (those related to ovarian function).

Neoplasm is always a possibility and must be considered. The most common neoplasm found in this age group is the benign cystic teratoma or dermoid cyst. These tumors are slow growing and usually asymptomatic. They are generally between 5 and 10 cm in diameter and have a 15% chance of bilaterality. Because they arise from pluripotential germ cells, they can give rise to a number of structures and often contain hair, teeth, sebaceous material, and neural elements. Other germ cell tumors, including dysgerminomas and malignant teratomas, are much less common. Occasionally, cysts arising from mesonephric remnants are found associated with the ovary or the fallopian tube or both. These are benign, are thin walled, and contain no solid elements.

A discussion of adnexal masses in this age group would be incomplete without inclusion of ectopic pregnancy. This is a potentially life-threatening condition that should always be considered in a patient of reproductive age with a pelvic mass. Classically, these patients present with a positive pregnancy test, an adnexal mass, pain, and vaginal bleeding. Timely diagnosis and treatment may serve to preserve reproductive function and avoid major abdominal surgery; therefore, prompt evaluation is indicated whenever this diagnosis is considered.

The Reproductive Years

Adnexal masses in this age group are most often ovarian and primarily represent physiologic cysts. Cystadenomas are the most common neoplasms found here, followed by benign teratomas. Additionally, patients can develop endometriosis (implants of endometrial tissue outside of the endometrium). This condition is seen most commonly in white, nulliparous women between the ages of 35 and 45 years. Occasionally, these implants are present on one or both ovaries and can coalesce to form cysts filled with viscous fluid. These endometriomas or "chocolate cysts," so called because of the thick, brown fluid they contain, usually cause the patient to be symptomatic, complaining of cyclic pelvic pain, pressure, and dyspareunia.

Once again, ectopic pregnancy must be considered in this age group. Risk factors for the development of an ectopic pregnancy include a history of pelvic inflammatory disease, previous ectopic pregnancy, tubal surgery, and assisted reproductive technology. If a patient presents with a positive pregnancy test after a tubal ligation, she has a 50% chance of having an ectopic pregnancy.

Leiomyomas (fibroids) are solid masses most commonly seen in the uterus, although they can be present essentially anywhere in the pelvis. Approximately 30% of women in their reproductive years will have developed one or many

of these benign tumors. For unclear reasons, they are three times more common in blacks than whites. Although often asymptomatic, they can be responsible for pelvic pain, pressure, and vaginal bleeding. They vary in size from very small (several millimeters) to huge, filling the entire abdominal cavity with resultant ureteral and bowel compression. Leiomyosarcoma can occur in these tumors but is rare (<0.1%) and presents at a mean age of 50 to 55 years.

Ovarian torsion should be considered whenever a patient presents with a negative result of a pregnancy test, severe pelvic pain, and an adnexal mass. Classically, the patient has an ovarian cyst, which because of its size and position causes the ovary to rotate, or torse, around its blood supply. This process can evolve over several days, with the symptoms waxing and waning until complete torsion occurs. When torsion is complete, arterial flow continues while venous flow is occluded, resulting in ovarian engorgement and pain. If complete torsion occurs and is not treated promptly, ischemia and necrosis may result, necessitating oopherectomy.

Infectious processes are also possible. In the course of the development of pelvic inflammatory disease, pathogens from the cervix extend to the uterine corpus and onto the fallopian tube, which becomes distended with purulent material. The ovary may also become involved, creating a tuboovarian abscess. Tubal scarring, often the sequel of pelvic inflammatory disease, can lead to blockage and clubbing of the fimbriated end of the tube. As tubal secretions build up within the blocked tubal lumen, distention occurs, forming a hydrosalpinx, which can be detected as a tubular pelvic mass.

Nongynecologic sources for infection should also be considered. In Ehren's study, the most commonly missed diagnosis in adolescents presenting with pelvic pain was appendicitis.[2]

As patient age increases so does the concern for malignancy. Ovarian cancer is unusual before age 40; however, the diagnosis must be considered in a patient presenting with an adnexal mass. The lifetime risk for a woman in the United States of developing ovarian cancer is approximately 1 in 70,[3] which increases to 4% to 6% if there is a family history of the disease (one first-degree relative).[4] The disease incidence increases from 4 per 100,000 in women aged 25 to 29 to 15.7 per 100,000 women aged 40 to 44 to 54 per 100,000 women aged 75 to 79.[5,6] Unfortunately, more than two thirds of women continue to be diagnosed with advanced disease. The most common ovarian malignancy is the cystadenocarcinoma. The second most common ovarian malignancy is actually metastatic from a nongynecologic source such as the gastrointestinal tract or from a primary breast lesion.

Nonmalignant masses arising from nongynecologic sources must also be considered. One of the most common conditions mistaken for a neoplastic process is a pelvic kidney.

The Perimenopausal and Postmenopausal Period

In this age group, estrogen-sensitive neoplasms often undergo regression. Such is the case with leiomyomas and endometriosis. This regression is seen even in light of estrogen replacement therapy. Adnexal masses in this age group are most often benign, but the incidence of malignancy increases with age. Physiologic or "functional cysts" are rarely seen in the postmenopausal patient, because the ovary is essentially no longer functioning. Occasionally ovulation will occur in women in their 50s who have stopped menstruating so that rarely a simple small physiologic cyst may be seen. Nevertheless, any adnexal mass in the postmenopausal patient deserves prompt evaluation. Masses from a nonreproductive origin should be considered. Colon cancer is particularly common in the United States and is responsible for 30,000 deaths annually among women, more than double that of ovarian cancer.[7]

HISTORY

It is important to obtain a thorough patient history, including a complete menstrual history, when considering the etiology of a adnexal mass. In a patient with regular menses, it is important to establish in which half of the menstrual cycle she presents. The first day of menses is considered the first cycle day. Ovulation occurs at approximately cycle day 14. Thus, a patient who presents with a mass around mid cycle could have a follicular cyst. If she is in the latter portion of the cycle, a corpus luteum cyst could be present. A patient with a long history of irregular menses with bilaterally enlarged, tender ovaries could have polycystic ovary syndrome. Pelvic inflammatory disease usually presents 7 to 10 days after menstruation. A contraceptive history should also be obtained. Patients on oral contraceptive pills are unlikely to develop functional cysts, because ovulatory function is suppressed. Patients with multiple sexual partners or who do not use barrier contraception are at increased risk of developing pelvic inflammatory disease.

Associated symptoms are also important to obtain. The characterization of pelvic pain can give the astute clinician many clues regarding its etiology. The acute onset of severe abdominopelvic pain is consistent with ovarian torsion, hemorrhage into a cyst, rupture of a cyst or abscess, ectopic pregnancy, and appendicitis. Cyclic lower abdominal pain with dyspareunia and heavy menses should bring to mind endometriosis or adenomyosis. The patient with pelvic inflammatory disease and resultant tuboovarian abscess or hydrosalpinx often complains of pelvic discomfort. The gradual development of increasing discomfort suggests a neoplastic process.

The postmenopausal patient with a pelvic mass requires specific attention to other organ systems. Questions should be directed toward evaluating the breasts and gastrointestinal and genitourinary systems as possible primary sources for metastatic disease. The family history should be explored as it pertains to heritable malignancies such as breast, ovary, endometrium, and colon.

PHYSICAL EXAMINATION

Although patient size, mobility, and cooperation can all be limiting factors in performing an adequate examination, there are several characteristics of adnexal masses, determined by physical examination, that can contribute valuable information to the differential diagnosis and should not be overlooked. The external genitalia should be examined for signs of hormonal imbalance (eg, clitoral hypertrophy, degree of estrogenization). The vagina and cervix should be visually inspected for abnormalities, including signs of infection. The bimanual examination can provide information regarding the size, location, shape, consistency, tenderness, and mobility of the mass. An irregular, firm, immobile adnexal mass raises concerns for malignancy, whereas a smooth, mobile, cystic structure is more consistent with a benign process. Nodularity and tenderness in the cul-de-sac behind the uterus or thickened, tender uterosacral ligaments are typical of endometriosis. Fixed masses in the cul-de-sac with associated ascites are very worrisome for malignancy.

LABORATORY TESTS

Laboratory tests are generally not helpful in the diagnosis of pelvic masses. The urinary or blood pregnancy test is an exception and should be used liberally in patients of reproductive age with pelvic masses. To determine whether a pregnancy is present, the urine test is adequate because it detects the presence of urinary beta-human chorionic gonadotropin and gives a qualitative result. If an ectopic pregnancy is being considered, a serum beta-human chorionic gonadotropin sample should be obtained because this will give a quantitative result that then can be followed serially. A complete blood cell count with differential is often useful in patients suspected of having pelvic inflammatory disease because it can assess for leukocytosis and other indicators of acute infection.

Several tumor markers are available for laboratory analysis and are generally not very helpful for initial evaluation. The CA 125 (cancer antigen 125) is one that can be helpful when used in the appropriate setting. The CA 125 determinant is expressed by epithelial ovarian tumors and other normal and abnormal tissues of müllerian origin. It is often elevated in many benign conditions such as endometriosis, adenomyosis, leiomyoma, pregnancy, diverticulitis, cirrhosis, and pelvic infection. Because of its elevation with commonly encountered benign conditions seen in the premenopausal patient, its usefulness is greatly limited in this population. The CA 125 level is also elevated in pancreatic, breast, and colorectal cancer. Additionally, when an ovarian cancer is present, the CA 125 value is not reliably elevated in all serous tumors, less so in mucinous tumors, and only positive in 50% of patients with early disease; therefore, a normal level does not rule out the presence of an ovarian cancer and an elevated level does not diagnose ovarian cancer. With these facts in mind, the CA 125 is best reserved for those postmenopausal patients with adnexal pathology and not as a screening test. The cutoff value for CA 125 is accepted as 35 units/mL. Postmenopausal patients with CA 125 values greater than 35 units/mL in association with an ovarian cyst are considered to have ovarian cancer until proven otherwise.

DIAGNOSTIC IMAGING STUDIES

Unfortunately, even with the most careful history and physical examination, the precise cause of a pelvic mass often remains uncertain. Consider the case of a 250-kg 33-year-old woman who presented to her physician with complaints of increasing abdominal girth. Her physician was skeptical regarding the source of her complaints, which were initially attributed to her size alone. During the course of her evaluation, a sonogram was obtained that demonstrated a 60-cm cystic pelvic mass. At laparotomy, a 64-kg left ovarian cyst was removed. The final diagnosis was a low-grade adenocarcinoma.[8] There are several different imaging modalities available that can help direct diagnosis and aid in management of pelvic masses. These include CT, MRI, and sonography. Although abdominal x-ray is sometimes employed, its usefulness is limited in this area because it does not define the soft tissues of the pelvis adequately.

CT provides transaxial imaging based on radiographic attenuation of tissues. Because it employs ionizing radiation, it should be used with caution in the pregnant patient. It allows excellent spatial resolution and readily detects calcifications, but it provides relatively little soft tissue contrast, it requires intravenous iodinated contrast injection, and the image can be degraded in the pelvis by bowel loops that obscure the adnexa. It is therefore not the initial imaging technique recommended when an adnexal mass is suspected.

MRI provides anatomic imaging based on differences in the magnetic properties of various tissues. In contrast to CT, it does not use ionizing radiation. Although the anatomic depiction and soft tissue contrast of MRI are usually much better than those of CT, it is not ideal for imaging adnexal structures because adjacent muscle and bowel have similar signals to that of the ovary. Additionally, MRI is expensive and not widely available.

Sonography, which has been shown to depict the gross anatomic features of the pelvis with excellent detail, is the procedure of choice for the evaluation of pelvic masses.[9] It offers many additional advantages, including lack of ionizing radiation, relative low cost, transportability, and widespread availability. Sonographic imaging of an adnexal mass provides many useful characteristics that can aid the physician in determining the etiology of the mass and in directing treatment.

The principal task of a clinician when presented with a patient in whom an adnexal mass has been detected is to determine whether the tumor requires treatment and, if so, what approach is most appropriate. Because the source of the mass can be gynecologic or nongynecologic, and may be either congenital, functional, hemorrhagic, neoplastic, obstructive, or inflammatory, the clinician needs to be familiar with the tools available to best direct diagnosis and treatment. Careful attention should be paid to the age of the patient, her history, and the physical examination findings. Laboratory tests may aid in diagnosis but should be ordered with discretion. Selection of the imaging studies that will be most useful in this decision should be based on the clinical findings as well as on a thorough understanding of the limitations and advantages of the various studies available. The cost, availability, and clinician's previous experience with the techniques available should also be considered.

REFERENCES

1. Milar DE, Blake JM, Stringer DA, et al. Prepubertal ovarian cyst formation. Obstet Gynecol 1993;81:434.
2. Ehren IM. Benign and malignant ovarian tumors in children and adolescents. Am J Surg 1984;147:339.
3. Andolf E. Ultrasound screening in women at risk for ovarian cancer. Clin Obstet Gynecol 1993;36:423.
4. Goldstein SR. Conservative management of small, postmenopausal cystic masses. Clin Obstet Gynecol 1993;36:395.
5. Boente MP, Godwin AK, Hogan WM. Screening, imaging, and early diagnosis of ovarian cancer. Clin Obstet Gynecol 1994;37:377.
6. Schwarts PE. The role of tumor markers in the preoperative diagnosis of ovarian cysts. Clin Obstet Gynecol 1993;36:384.
7. American College of Obstetricians and Gynecologists Committee on Gynecologic Practice. Routine cancer screening (Committee Opinion No. 128). Washington, DC, American College of Obstetricians and Gynecologists, 1993.
8. Poole SY, Malone JM Jr, Jaques SM, et al. Giant mucinous ovarian tumor with low malignant potential with foci of well-differentiated mucinous adenocarcinoma masked by massive obesity: a case report. J Reprod Med 1994;39:982.
9. Fleischer AC, Walsh JW, Jones HW III, et al. Sonographic evaluation of pelvic masses: methods of examination and role of sonography relative to other imaging modalities. Radiol Clin North Am 20:397, 1982.

Sonographic Evaluation of Adnexal Masses with Transabdominal or Transvaginal Sonography

Arthur C. Fleischer, MD

Sonography is the diagnostic modality of choice for evaluation of patients with a pelvic mass. This is particularly true for pelvic masses thought, on a clinical basis, to be benign. MRI and CT can add additional diagnostic information if the findings of sonography are nondiagnostic or equivocal.

Although the sonographic features of a pelvic mass frequently do not permit a specific histopathologic diagnosis, sonography usually provides clinically important parameters for the pelvic mass.[1] These include

- Confirmation of the presence of a pelvic mass
- Delineation of the size, internal consistency, and contour of the mass
- Establishment of the origin and anatomic relationship of the mass to other pelvic structures
- A survey to establish the presence of abnormalities associated with malignant disease, such as ascites or metastatic lesions
- Guidance for aspiration or biopsy of selected pelvic masses

Each of these parameters is discussed here, as well as specific types of pelvic masses. This subchapter is structured to emphasize the way sonographic evaluation of pelvic masses proceeds from evaluation of clinically pertinent parameters to consideration of specific lesions. Color Doppler sonography provides additional information concerning the chance of malignancy or torsion in some cases.

Information gained by sonography is useful in guiding the gynecologic surgeon through decisions regarding surgical intervention. In general, masses that are larger than 5 cm in average dimension, contain irregular solid components, or are associated with significant amounts (over 20 mL) of intraperitoneal fluid require surgical treatment.[2] Similarly, pelvic masses that are associated with acute pelvic pain may require immediate surgical intervention because they may be associated with adnexal torsion.[3] On the other hand, masses that are completely cystic and smaller than 4 to 5 cm may be observed over a few months with repeat sonograms to document any change in size. Although small (less than 5 cm) adnexal masses can be detected in postmenopausal women, only a low percentage (approximately 3%) will represent a malignant neoplasm.[4,5] In patients with recurrent ovarian carcinoma, sonography has been found to be highly accurate in the detection of ascites but is a poor predictor of the presence of diffuse small peritoneal implants.[6]

The role of MRI and CT relative to sonography must be considered. In general, CT and MRI are more accurate than sonography in staging histologically proven neoplastic tumors such as cervical carcinoma.[7] Because of their high operational costs and limited availability, however, these modalities are not as frequently used in the initial evaluation of a pelvic mass as sonography. CT and MRI are usually used as secondary adjunctive examinations when the characteristics of the mass raise concern about malignancy.

The use of transvaginal sonography can add specificity in certain areas to the conventional transabdominal sonographic examination. The limited field of view of most transvaginal transducer probes confines their use in the pelvis where global delineation of structures is of diagnostic importance. However, the added information regarding tumor composition and location can add specificity to the sonographic examination.

Color Doppler sonography seems to be helpful in distinguishing benign from malignant ovarian masses as well as in the evaluation of adnexal torsion.[8] It is particularly useful as an adjunct to morphologic assessment of ovarian lesions.[9] This topic is covered in detail in the next subchapter.

Accordingly, here the intent is to familiarize the reader with certain differential points that are clinically important when evaluating a patient with a pelvic mass by means of transabdominal or transvaginal sonography.

SONOGRAPHIC PARAMETERS

Presence of a Pelvic Mass

Pelvic sonography has an important role in establishing the presence of a pelvic mass that may be palpated or suspected on pelvic examination. It is particularly useful in patients in whom an adequate pelvic examination cannot be performed or in whom an ill-defined pelvic mass is found on physical examination.

Because some masses may be outside the range of the examiner's finger, sonography may occasionally detect masses that cannot be palpated adequately. In this situation, a real-time sonographic examination during pelvic examination may be used to demonstrate the presence or absence of a mass.[10] Transvaginal sonography can be used to particular advantage in delineation of the uterus and ovaries in obese patients. In fact, sonography has been found to be more reliable than palpation in identification of normal-sized ovaries—even in the postmenopausal woman.[11]

The change in configuration in bowel loops associated with peristalsis is helpful in distinguishing true pelvic masses from those created by bowel. A fecal-filled cecum may occasionally simulate the appearance of a solid adnexal mass, as well as matted omentum or fat that is in the adnexal region. Transvaginal sonography may be helpful in these cases to distinguish true pelvic masses from those created by bowel.

Size and Location

The uterus serves as a central landmark for identifying the location of a mass within the pelvis. The echogenic endometrial interface within the uterus serves as an additional landmark for delineation of its borders.[12] Masses within the ovary can usually be identified by the rim of compressed parenchyma (''beak'') that is present between the mass and the remaining portion of the ovary. This feature is particularly well depicted with transvaginal scanning. Abnormally distended tubes can be identified by their origin from the lateral aspect of the uterine cornu and their fusiform enlargement as they extend from the uterus into the pelvis. In addition, the origin of the tube can be identified on semiaxial or coronal transvaginal examinations by delineating the portion of the endometrium that extends into the cornu.

The size of the pelvic mass occasionally can be helpful in distinguishing its differential diagnosis. Physiologic cysts, for example, are rarely larger than 3 to 5 cm in average dimension; ovarian tumors have generally enlarged to about 10 cm before they are symptomatic. Exceptions to this may be encountered in acute hemorrhage or torsion of the ovary, when it can quickly enlarge over a 24- to 48-hour time period.

In some large patients, it may be difficult to palpate some masses that are over 10 cm in size. Size alone, however, is not a specific criterion because it depends on when the patient presents for an examination relative to the growth pattern of the mass.

The origin of a mass may be further elucidated by applying gentle pressure with the operator's hand or with the probe between the mass and the uterus. For example, pedunculated subserosal fibroids can be identified by the presence of a pedicle attaching to the uterus, whereas an adnexal mass would be separable from the uterus.

Internal Consistency

Sonography allows detailed delineation of the internal consistency of a pelvic mass. A cystic mass can be inferred when mass has no internal echoes, has smooth borders, and is enhanced through transmission. Occasionally, low-level echoes may be present within a cyst arising from proteinaceous fluid, blood, or cellular debris. A truly solid mass typically contains internal echoes, whereas a complex mass contains both solid and cystic components.

In general, ovarian masses tend to be cystic, whereas nonovarian masses tend to be solid. Thin and echogenic internal septations suggest the diagnosis of an epithelial ovarian neoplasm—usually a mucinous cystadenoma. The internal interfaces can also be found in hemorrhagic cysts, the result of partial coagulation of an internal clot. Echogenic material within an area can be seen in some dermoid cysts that contain sebaceous material. Areas of hemorrhagic necrosis can be seen as irregular anechoic regions within a mass. The more solid and irregular components that are present within a mass suggest it is more likely to be malignant.[2,13]

With most scanners that use high-frequency transducers, it is now possible to detect proteinaceous and mucinous material suspended within fluid collections. This material appears as echogenic particles within predominantly fluid structures that, overall, demonstrate enhanced transmission. Echogenic internal contents, such as endometriomas that contain clotted blood, may also be encountered in a mass. Irregularities and disruption in the borders of the mass suggest that malignant spread or rupture through the capsule has occurred. Papillary excrescences usually suggest the possibility of malignancy.

Detection of Associated Findings

Sonography is very accurate in the detection of intraperitoneal fluid that can be associated with adnexal masses. Although a small amount (3 to 5 mL) of fluid may be present due to physiologic processes, it is uncommon to have more than 10 mL of fluid in the cul-de-sac or peritoneal cavity. Intraperitoneal fluid associated with pelvic masses increases the likelihood of a neoplastic lesion and the possibility of malignant spread or rupture. However, in some cases (eg, ovarian torsion) the fluid can represent a transudate related to obstructed venous and lymphatic return.[3,14] Rarely, intraperitoneal fluid can be associated with an ovarian fibroma or other benign adnexal mass.

Sonographic Guidance for Aspiration or Biopsy

Sonography has a major role in directing guided aspiration or biopsy of pelvic masses. Guided biopsy may be indicated in cases in which loculated fluid collections are present or when drainage of a mass, such as a tuboovarian abscess, is indicated.[15] Occasionally, this can be accomplished by the transvaginal route. In these cases, a transvaginal transducer probe with needle guide attachment provides guided aspiration or biopsy.

TRANSVAGINAL SONOGRAPHY OF PELVIC MASSES

Transvaginal sonography has an important role in the evaluation of the uterus and adnexa. However, because of its limited field of view and unusual image orientation, it is best used as an adjunct to a standard transabdominal scan. In particular, transvaginal sonography is indicated for

- Determination of the presence, and evaluation of, relatively small (less than 5- to 10-cm) adnexal masses
- Determination of the origin of a mass (uterine, ovarian, or tubal) and whether it has torsed
- Detailed evaluation of its internal consistency with particular emphasis on the presence of polypoid excrescences, septations, or internal consistencies (blood, pus, serous fluid)
- Guiding transvaginal aspiration of certain masses
- Evaluation of endometrial or myometrial disorders related to pelvic masses

For masses less than 10 cm in size, transvaginal sonography can afford detailed delineation of the mass and determine its origin.[16–19] Specifically, masses that arise or are contained within the ovary can be differentiated from those of uterine origin. In addition, anatomic distortion of the tube by dilatation or inflammatory thickening can be identified with this technique. This is particularly helpful in differentiating inflammatory disease that may involve the tube or ovary—such as a tuboovarian abscess—from simple hydrosalpinx. The relative mobility of the pelvic organs can also be assessed when the probe comes into contact with the uterus or ovary.

Transvaginal sonography is particularly helpful in patients with fibroids because the ovaries can be identified as separate from the uterine abnormality. Conversely, some masses that are associated with uterine disorders (such as tuboovarian abscess with associated endometritis) can be identified.

Transvaginal sonography has been used as a means to guide abscess drainage.[20] It is conceivable that simple cysts with serous fluid could be safely aspirated using this procedure. However, intraperitoneal spillage of the contents of "complicated" cysts, such as endometriomas, dermoid cysts, or neoplastic cysts, might produce peritonitis or peritoneal spread from rupture, and such cysts probably should not be aspirated.

Similarly, transvaginal sonography affords a means to consider transvaginal aspiration of those pelvic masses thought to be benign serous cysts. These masses should demonstrate a smooth and well-defined border with no internal echoes. The sonographer should be aware that low-level artifactual echoes can be observed most with higher-frequency transducer probes—even with completely serous cysts. But sonographic findings of calcification, gravity-dependent layering material, or papillary excrescences should dissuade consideration of transvaginal aspiration because these may indicate "complicated" cysts. Accepting these limitations, however, there may be a role for transvaginal aspiration with or without instillation of sclerosing agents for simple serous cysts. More extensive experience with follow-up after aspiration is needed before the clinical utility and indications for this procedure are known.

Although it is tempting to speculate about the use of sonography as a means to screen for ovarian carcinoma in postmenopausal women, the incidence of this disorder would require that hundreds of patients be scanned for a single positive examination. In addition, most masses that are less than 5 cm are benign, according to one study demonstrating a 3% incidence of malignancy in masses of less than 5 cm.[21] Clearly, however, transvaginal sonography has a role in delineation of the ovaries in obese, postmenopausal women in whom the incidence of carcinoma is high and pelvic examination is less than optimal.[22]

Additional investigation is necessary to determine whether the improved resolution afforded by transvaginal sonography of the internal content of a mass would aid in its diagnostic specificity. Our experience indicates that transvaginal sonography adds diagnostically specific information in more than three fourths of women studied.[23] It is particularly helpful in determining the origin of a pelvic mass (intraovarian or extraovarian) and in documenting tubal, endometrial, and myometrial disorders. It also adds sensitivity over transabdominal sonography, particularly in obese patients.

On transvaginal sonography, masses that appear hypoechoic on transabdominal sonography may demonstrate echogenic material suspended within the mass. The echogenic material most frequently represents blood in various degrees of coagulation. However, pus, mucus, or sebaceous material can be echogenic. Thus, it can be difficult to distinguish hemorrhagic from neoplastic cysts with transvaginal sonography, and transvaginal aspiration may be warranted.

In summary, the major roles of transvaginal sonography for evaluation of adnexal masses include demonstration of the origin and internal consistency and provision of a means for guided aspiration. Transvaginal aspiration may have a role in guided aspiration of those masses that by clinical and sonographic criteria appear to be benign. However, because of the remote possibility of peritoneal spillage after an aspiration procedure, one should limit the application of transvaginal aspiration to only those masses that appear to be completely cystic with well-defined borders within adnexal structures that are freely mobile.

SONOGRAPHIC DIFFERENTIAL DIAGNOSIS OF PELVIC MASSES

This discussion of the sonographic differential diagnosis of pelvic masses is organized according to the most frequently seen sonographic appearance of particular types of pelvic mass. If a particular pelvic mass has a spectrum of sonographic appearances, it is mentioned in more than one category. Masses that are difficult to localize relative to a particular organ or category are considered "indetermi-

TABLE 2-2. *Sonographic differential diagnoses of pelvic masses**

Cystic	Complex	Solid
COMPLETELY CYSTIC	PREDOMINATELY CYSTIC	UTERINE
Physiologic ovarian cysts	Cystadenomas	Leiomyoma (sarcoma)
Cystadenomas	Tuboovarian abscess	Endometrial carcinoma, sarcoma
Hydrosalpinx	Ectopic pregnancy	
Endometrioma	Cystic teratoma	EXTRAUTERINE
Parovarian cyst		Solid ovarian tumor
Hydatid cyst of Morgagni	PREDOMINATELY SOLID	
	Cystadenoma (carcinoma)	
MULTIPLE	Germ cell tumor	
Endometriomas		
Multiple follicular cysts		
SEPTATED		
Cystadenoma (carcinoma)		
Mucinous		
Serous		
Papillary		

* Based on most common appearance.

nant.'' These may represent lesions related to the bowel, for example.[24,25]

This scheme for differential diagnosis should be used only as a general approach to the sonographic characterization of a pelvic mass (Table 2-2). Sonographic findings must be correlated with the clinical ones. The sonographic depiction of morphology is helpful in determining the chance that a mass is malignant. The presence of wall or septal irregularity or papillary excrescences correlates with the chance of malignancy. Each of four parameters is assessed, including inner wall structure, wall thickness, septa, and echogenicity. Malignancies tend to have high scores (over 12)[39]

Cystic Masses

Several types of pelvic masses can appear as cystic adnexal masses on sonography (Figs. 2-2 and 2-3). They include physiologic (follicular or luteal) ovarian cysts, hydrosalpinges, cystadenomas, parovarian cysts, and endometriomas. In general, physiologic cysts are the most common mass to appear as a well-defined anechoic, adnexal mass. Luteal cysts usually have a thicker wall than follicular cysts and tend to contain hemorrhagic areas. Rarely, cysts that do not arise from the ovary (eg, parovarian cysts or cysts of Morgagni) can mimic the sonographic features of an ovarian cyst.[26,27] These cysts do not demonstrate a rim of ovarian tissue, however. It may be helpful to use transvaginal scanning to determine whether a mass is surrounded by a rim of ovarian tissue to confirm its intraovarian location.

Even with the similar sonographic appearance of several types of cystic adnexal masses, the diagnostic possibilities can usually be narrowed to one or two entities based on clinical presentation and evaluation. In general, most cystic masses that arise within the pelvis are of ovarian origin. Depending on the referral population, physiologic ovarian cysts or hydrosalpinges are the most common cystic pelvic masses encountered by the sonologist. Acute enlargement of a mass is usually the result of internal hemorrhage or venous engorgement secondary to adnexal (ovarian) torsion. The echoes that can be observed within some cystic masses arise from cellular debris, pus, organized blood, proteinaceous fluid, cholesterol crystals, or sebaceous material encountered in some dermoid cysts.[28,29] Irregular thickening of a cyst wall may be the result of inflammatory or neoplastic processes involving the wall or vasculogenic edema due to torsion of the cystic mass on its pedicle. Clot adhered to the wall of a hemorrhagic ovarian cyst may also produce an irregular wall.[30,31]

Certain conditions are usually associated within a single cyst as opposed to those disorders that are associated with multiple pelvic cysts. For example, single cystic lesions are frequently physiologic ovarian cysts, whereas conditions such as endometriosis are associated with multiple pelvic cysts.[32] An enlarged (over 10- to 15-mL) rounded ovary containing multiple immature follicles in the 5- to 7-mm range can be recognized in patients with polycystic ovary disease.[4]

Physiologic Ovarian Cysts

Several types of cystic masses can result from abnormalities that occur at different stages of folliculogenesis. In general, follicular cysts occur either due to failure of a mature follicle to rupture at the time of ovulation or to collection of blood within the follicle after ovulation occurs, resulting in a corpus luteum cyst. In most individuals, a mature follicle ranges from 15 to 20 mm in average dimension.[5,33] Follicular cysts of the ovary are usually larger than a mature follicle, ranging from 3 to 8 cm. They may regress spontaneously or after a clinical trial of hormonal suppression. Luteal cysts may form from continued hemorrhage with a corpus luteum and usually have a thicker wall than follicular cysts. Sono-

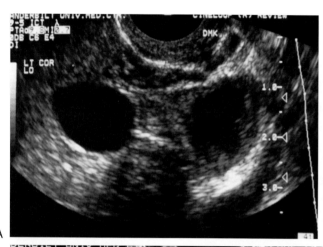

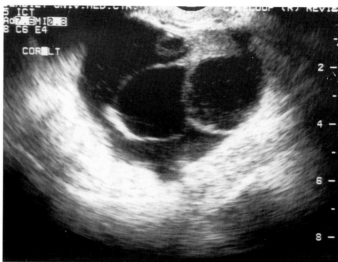

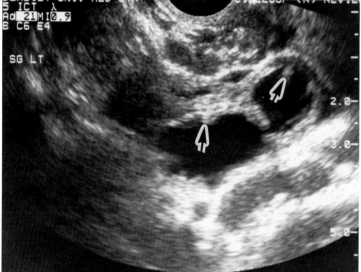

FIG. 2-2. Cystic masses. **(A)** Transvaginal sonogram shows the differences between a smooth-walled follicular cyst in the right ovary and a hypoechoic, irregular thick-walled hemorrhagic corpus luteum in the left ovary. **(B)** On this transvaginal sonogram, intraperitoneal fluid outlines the lateral aspects of a peritoneal cyst adjacent to a hemorrhagic cyst within the left ovary. **(C)** Transvaginal sonogram of bilobulated cystic masses in left adnexa shows a mucosal fold *(arrows)*. This finding is helpful in identifying this as a hydrosalpinx.

graphy has an important role in documenting any change in size of the cyst during and after clinical observation or treatment. This is particularly important when considering hemorrhagic ovarian cysts that have a spectrum of sonographic appearances—depending on the amount and organization of internal clot. Indeed, some hemorrhagic ovarian cysts can mimic the sonographic features of solid ovarian masses such as a teratoma. However, in most cases of hemorrhagic ovarian cysts, the degree of through-transmission is greater than in truly solid masses and the mass will regress in size over a 2- to 3-week period.[34]

Patients with hemorrhagic ovarian cysts may experience the abrupt onset of lower abdominal or pelvic pain.[30,31] Because this history can also be elicited in cases of ruptured ectopic pregnancy, it is important to obtain an accurate pregnancy test on these patients. Other conditions such as ovarian torsion and acute appendicitis can mimic the clinical presentation of patients with a hemorrhagic ovarian cyst.

On sonography, the most common appearance of a hemor-

rhagic ovarian cyst is a complex mass with internal echoes but with enhanced through-transmission. Although fibrinolyzed clot is typically hypoechoic, acute intraparenchymal hemorrhage frequently appears as an irregular echogenic area. The cyst wall may be irregular in contour due to clot that is adherent to it. Occasionally, mildly echogenic interfaces can be seen within a hemorrhagic cyst, most likely representing partially solid clot.[30,31]

Hydrosalpinx/Tuboovarian Abscesses

Hydrosalpinges occur when an inflammatory process produces adhesions of the fimbriated end of the tube, trapping intraluminal secretions. The fluid that is secreted distends the tube, resulting in a fusiform anechoic adnexal mass. The tapered fusiform shape and lack of peristalsis of a hydrosalpinx usually allows differentiating it from fluid-filled small bowel loops. In addition, the typical configuration of a hydrosalpinx—tapering as it enters the uterus and enlarging distally—is helpful in its sonographic recognition. Typically, a hydrosalpinx can be traced to its origin along the lateral aspects of cornual area of the uterus. The origin of the tube can also be identified on transvaginal scanning by the pointed configuration of the endometrium in the cornu. The isthmic portion of the tube lies immediately posterior to the round ligament.

If the inflammatory process involves the ovary as a part of the wall, a tuboovarian abscess may be produced. It may be difficult to differentiate a simple hydrosalpinx that does not involve the ovary from a tuboovarian abscess on the basis of sonography. However, in our experience, the tuboovarian abscess has a more complex internal appearance, with low-level echoes arising from inflammatory fluid. In addition, the ovary can be identified in some patients as a border to the inflammatory mass in patients with a tuboovarian mass. In most cases, tuboovarian abscesses can be distinguished from other pelvic masses by means of sonography by determining that the abscess cavity is indeed within the confines of the ovary. This can be recognized by the abscess forming a rim of compressed tissue or a "beak" within the ovary.

Endometriosis

Endometriosis is a condition resulting from ectopic location of endometrial tissue within the peritoneal cavity and on the surface of abdominal and pelvic organs and pelvic ligaments. Endometriotic implants typically locate on the uterosacral ligaments and serosal surfaces of the bowel and peritoneum. These implants are difficult to depict with sonography because they are typically very small (5 mm) and in a position that is difficult to image sonographically posterior to the uterine surface.[32] Occasionally, they can be recognized as echogenic areas within the cul-de-sac on transvagi-

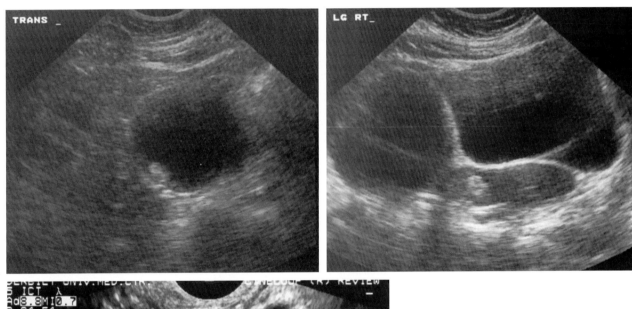

A   B

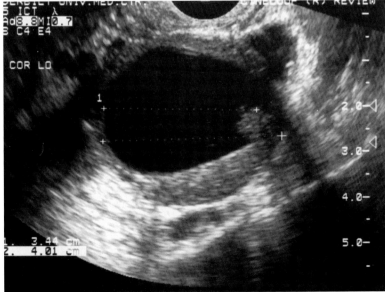

C

FIG. 2-3. Predominately cystic masses. **(A)** Transvaginal sonogram of a cystic mass with focal irregularity in the wall indicates a dermoid cyst. **(B)** Transabdominal sonogram of same patient as in **A** shows a cystic mass arising from the right ovary. The right ovary contains an echogenic focus that was found to represent a fat nodule within the wall of this dermoid cyst. **(C)** Transvaginal sonogram of a cystic mass with a papillary excrescence denotes an ovarian cystadenocarcinoma. Papillary excrescences are suggestive of malignancy but can be seen in benign lesions as well.

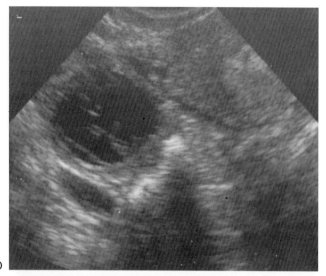

D

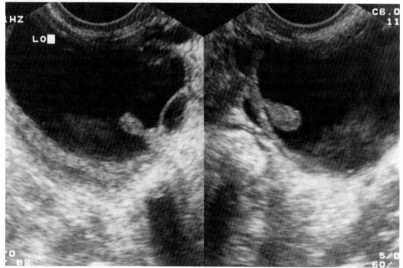

E   F

FIG. 2-3 *Continued.* **(D)** Transvaginal sonogram of a "fresh" corpus luteum with hemorrhagic area shows "lacy" interfaces within hypoechoic area. Long-axis **(E)** and short-axis **(F)** transvaginal sonograms show a cystic mass containing a polypoid-like solid area. This was retained placenta from a chronic ectopic pregnancy.

nal sonography. The ectopic endometrial tissue undergoes cyclical changes and bleeds during the menstrual cycle. Diffuse, low-level echoes can be observed within these masses arising from the clotted blood (Fig. 2-4).

Endometriosis can also cause obstructive uropathy by implanting near the ureters and, rarely, can cause bowel obstruction secondary to implantation on the serosal surfaces of the bowel. The periodic bleeding that occurs within the mass causes pain, and extravasated blood can result in fibrosis around the region of the endometriotic implant. Rupture

of an intraperitoneal endometrioma that contains clotted blood may result in acute peritonitis.

In up to 40% of patients with endometriosis, endometrial implants that are present within the peritoneum are associated with endometrial implants within the myometrium. This condition is termed *adenomyosis.* Although the involved uterus may not be noticeably enlarged, there is usually an irregularly thickened and echogenic or hypoechoic texture of the inner portion of the myometrium. There is a spectrum of sonographic findings in endometriosis, depending on the

FIG. 2-4. Predominately solid masses. **(A)** Transvaginal sonogram shows a mostly solid mass with an echogenic foci *(arrow).* The echogenic form was a "hair ball" within a dermoid cyst. **(B)** Transvaginal sonogram of a large solid mass *(between cursors)* denotes a dysgerminoma. **(C)** Transvaginal sonogram of a solid mass combining numerous echogenic foci indicates a dermoid cyst with multiple teeth. **(D)** Transvaginal sonogram of an irregularly shaped echogenic area within the left ovary represents hemorrhage within a corpus luteum. **(E)** Transvaginal sonogram shows a "ground glass" texture of an endometrioma. **(F)** Transvaginal sonogram shows an echogenic ill-defined area posterior to the ovary that was found to represent a "deflated" endometrioma by an area of fibrosis.

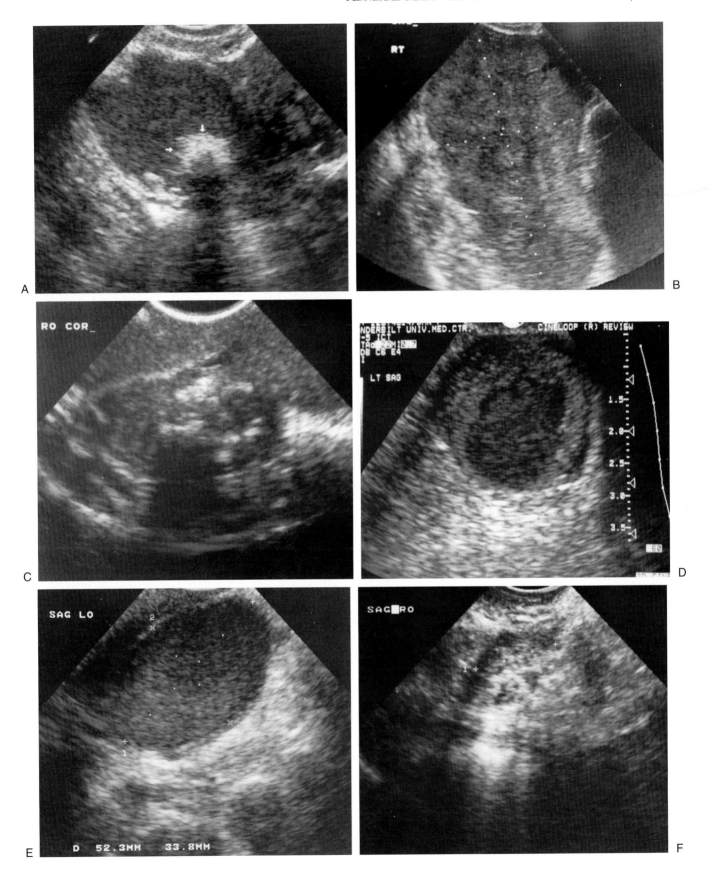

size and number of endometriomas present and their internal contents.[32] In some patients with endometriosis, no recognizable sonographic findings are observed because the endometriosis results in fibrosis and thickening of the adnexal ligaments without production of definite masses. When the endometriomas become greater than 1 to 2 cm, they can be identified as multiple cystic masses by sonography. Low-level echoes may be observed in some endometriomas arising from clotted blood contained within these masses. Intraovarian endometriomas have a similar sonographic appearance to hemorrhagic corpus luteum cysts and occasionally cannot be confidently distinguished from them. Rupture of endometriomas that contain clotted blood can result in diffuse peritoneal inflammatory response. Endometriosis can be encountered in patients who are febrile and thought to have a tuboovarian abscess because masses can become secondarily infected. Sonography is a useful means to monitor the effectiveness of medical therapy of the more extensive cases.

Cystadenomas

Cystadenomas are the most common type of cystic ovarian tumors. Although they are most frequently encountered in postmenopausal women, they can occasionally be encountered in women of childbearing age. These tumors arise from cells of the coelomic peritoneum that covers the ovary. The cells that line these tumors can secrete either a mucinous or a serous substance. Papillary tumors tend to have irregular solid areas and projections of solid tissue internally (see Fig. 2-3). In general, the more solid and irregular the internal morphology of an epithelial tumor, the more likely it is malignant.

In the early stages of development, cystadenomas may have a similar appearance to other cystic adnexal masses. When they enlarge, they frequently contain characteristic internal components, such as septations or papillary excrescences, that allow their sonographic recognition. These tumors metastasize by extending through the capsule of the tumor and spreading to peritoneal, serosal, omental, and diaphragmatic surfaces. Ascitic fluid may be cytologically negative, but its presence raises concern that spread beyond the tumor capsule has occurred. Because ascitic fluid is usually produced in response to peritoneal implantation and obstruction of transdiaphragmatic lymph drainage, the lack of ascites does not ensure that the mass is benign. Sonography is not accurate in depicting tumor invasion into the bladder or rectum or the presence or absence of associated lymphadenopathy.

Other Less Common Cystic Masses

A variety of masses that do not arise directly from the uterus or ovaries can appear as adnexal cystic masses. The most common one is the paraovarian cyst, which arises from wolffian duct remnants in the mesovarium. This type of mass usually measures from 3 to 5 cm but can be as large as a pelvoabdominal cystadenoma. Occasionally, these cysts contain hemorrhage; rarely they contain internal septations.[26,27] Like other adnexal cysts, these masses may potentiate torsion of the adnexa.

Another cystic mass that can be encountered in the patient with previous surgery is a peritoneal inclusion cyst. The cysts result from serous fluid collections that become entrapped by adhesions or overlaps of pelvic peritoneum related to previous pelvic surgery. Cysts arising from the fimbriated end of the tube (cysts of Morgagni) may appear as cystic adnexal masses. Retention cysts of the cervix (nabothian cysts) can usually be distinguished from other adnexal cysts in that they can be delineated to be within the confines of the uterine cervix and endocervical canal. Nabothian cysts are typically a few millimeters in size and can be distinguished from Gartner's duct cysts, which appear as tubular cystic structures in the upper vagina and less frequently within the uterine wall. Distended arcuate veins that course along the outer third of the myometrium can also appear as punctate cystic structures within the confines of the uterus. Calcifications within the arcuate arteries can be observed, particularly in postmenopausal women.

Complex Masses

Complex masses are defined as those that contain both fluid and solid areas (see Figs. 2-2 and 2-3). These masses can be further subdivided into those that are predominately cystic and those that are predominately solid. As stated previously, some cystic masses that have pus, cellular debris, sebum, suspended proteinaceous material, or organized clot may appear as echogenic material within a complex mass. In some cases, these internal echoes within masses can be identified as being dependent by varying orientation of the layer of echogenic material as imaged when the patient is scanned in the right- and left-anterior oblique positions. Ovarian tumors that contain solid components or irregular septations may also be classified into this complex-mass category. In addition, those masses that usually contain areas of internal hemorrhagic degeneration (eg, granulosa cell tumors) are categorized as complex pelvic masses.

Dermoid Cysts

Neoplasms that arise from the germinal tissue within and around the ovary are generally described as germ cell tumors of the ovary. The most common type of germ cell tumor is the benign cystic teratoma or dermoid cyst. Malignant varieties of germ cell tumors include the teratocarcinoma, malignant dysgerminoma, and endodermal sinus tumor.

Dermoid cysts are the most common type of germ cell tumor encountered in patients of childbearing age.[35] These masses contain a variety of internal components consisting of fat, skin, teeth, and hair. Because the internal components of a dermoid cyst vary, their sonographic appearance differs depending on their internal consistency. In general, the most common sonographic appearance of a dermoid cyst is a complex, predominately solid mass with echogenic internal components arising from fat and calcified portions of the mass. Less common appearances of dermoid cysts range from the totally cystic dermoid cyst, encountered in those dermoid cysts lined by neuroectoderm, to the almost completely solid dermoid cysts that have a large amount of soft tissue component within. Similarly, other germ cell tumors have a variety of appearances. The granulosa cell tumor—which may be associated with precocious puberty in the child and a variety of disorders related to hyperestrogenism in the adult—usually has a complex, predominately cystic appearance with multiple cystic areas within the mass corresponding to hemorrhagic areas.

One must be aware that dermoid cysts can mimic the findings of gas- or feces-containing bowel loops within the pelvis. Because the majority of dermoid cysts form pedunculated ovarian masses—and because they contain high fat content—they typically are located superior to the uterine fundus. This location may contribute to initial failure to recognize the presence of a dermoid cyst because of confusing a highly echogenic focus (arising from fat within the dermoid cyst) with gas-filled bowel loops. However, real-time scanning will demonstrate peristaltic activity in an echogenic area within bowel loops, as opposed to the relatively stationary configuration of fat within a dermoid cyst. Occasionally, the sebum with a dermoid cyst will be layered within the mass, producing an internal interface between more serous components of the cyst and the sebaceous fluid. Changes in orientation in this interface that are gravity dependent can also be documented with real-time scanning. The presence of distal acoustical shadowing, associated with some dermoid cysts that contain a large amount of fat, may also be a helpful indicator of the presence of a dermoid cyst. A pelvic radiograph may be helpful in confirming the sonographic impression of a dermoid cyst because calcification and radiolucency associated with the fat of a dermoid cyst may be apparent radiographically.

Ectopic Pregnancy

This subject is mentioned here to emphasize that an ectopic pregnancy can present as a complex and sometimes solid adnexal mass in women of childbearing age. The topic of ectopic pregnancy is extensively covered in Chapter 9.

Cystadenoma and Cystadenocarcinoma

The discussion of cystadenoma is repeated here because some of these ovarian tumors demonstrate a complex sonographic appearance. As mentioned previously, the greater the amount of internal solid area or irregular septation, the more likely is it that these types of tumors are malignant.[13]

The presence of ascites usually indicates the tumor has extended beyond its capsule and has implanted on the peritoneal, diaphragmatic, or omental surfaces. Rarely, ascites is associated with a benign tumor such as the ovarian fibroma (Meigs' syndrome). Very rarely, ascites may be associated with uterine fibroids (probably the result of a transserosal exudate).

Torsed Ovary

An enlarged ovary has the potential for attenuating its pedicle and torsing along its axis (see Fig. 2-4). Masses within the ovary, such as those resulting from hemorrhagic corpus luteum, can potentiate torsion. There are no specific sonographic findings in ovarian torsion.[3,14] Usually, the ovary is enlarged and contains a single hypoechoic area representing a hemorrhagic area. If the torsion is intermittent and incomplete, massive stromal edema of the ovary can result. In these cases, the ovary is diffusely enlarged and contains multiple hypoechoic and echogenic areas resulting from hemorrhagic infarcts. Intraperitoneal fluid may be present related to obstruction of venous and lymphatic return, resulting in a transudate from the capsule of the ovary. Duplex Doppler examination of the ovarian blood supply along the ovarian and infundibulopelvic ligaments may facilitate the specific diagnosis of ovarian torsion by demonstrating absent or high impedance arterial flow and absent venous flow. The full spectrum of findings on transvaginal color Doppler sonography is presented in detail in the next subchapter.

Solid Pelvic Masses

In general, most solid pelvic masses are of uterine, rather than ovarian, origin. Therefore, distinction of the internal consistency of a pelvic mass is indirectly helpful in establishing a uterine or ovarian origin. The sonographic findings in leiomyomas are covered in the chapter on uterine disorders.

Uterine Leiomyomas

Uterine leiomyomas are the most common masses to appear as solid masses on sonography. These tumors typically have a hypoechoic texture and can usually be traced to be within the borders of the uterus.[36] However, a subserosal fibroid may be pedunculated or even parasitize to the broad ligament bowel or omentum, creating the impression of an extrauterine mass. Uterine (myometrial) masses are discussed in detail in Chapter 5.

Ovarian Masses

Compared with the frequency of solid masses representing uterine leiomyomas, ovarian solid masses are less common. Solid ovarian tumors include adenocarcinoma, fibromas, and

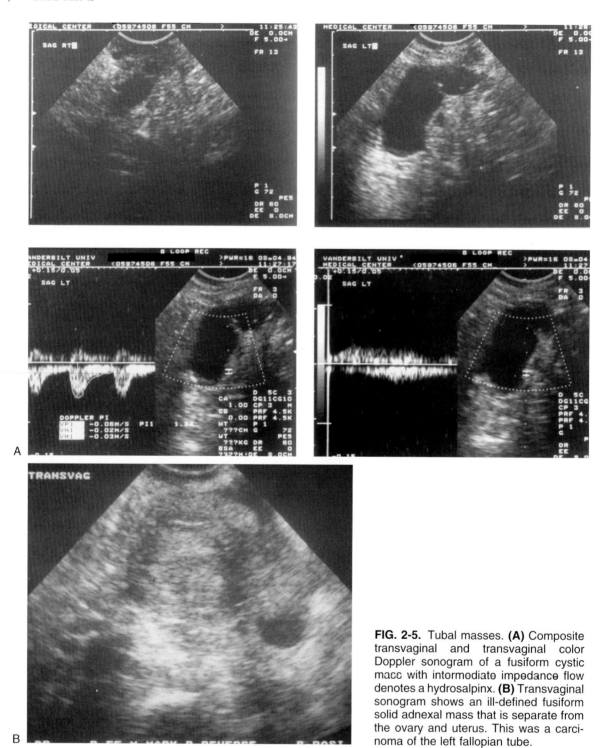

FIG. 2-5. Tubal masses. (A) Composite transvaginal and transvaginal color Doppler sonogram of a fusiform cystic mass with intermediate impedance flow denotes a hydrosalpinx. (B) Transvaginal sonogram shows an ill-defined fusiform solid adnexal mass that is separate from the ovary and uterus. This was a carcinoma of the left fallopian tube.

thecomas. Some rapidly growing epithelial tumors of the ovary, such as cystadenofibromas, may also appear as solid. Fibromas and thecomas may be associated with benign ascitic fluid.

Ovaries that undergo partial or intermittent torsion may appear as a solid mass. These ovaries are usually extremely edematous, related to the obstruction in venous return (Figs. 2-5 and 2-6) Fibromas typically appear as solid masses that demonstrate marked attenuation owing to the fibrous tissue elements.[37] Cystadenofibromas may appear as solid masses with areas of calcification, similar to the sonographic findings of a extrauterine fibroid. Other less common solid ovarian tumors can arise from metastasis from the gastrointestinal tract, lymphomas, and other primary neoplasms.

Other Solid Masses

Rarely, tubal disorders such as carcinomas produce solid adnexal masses. These are best depicted using transvaginal sonography. Some nongynecologic masses that can appear solid include lymphadenopathy or masses related to bowel. Lymphadenopathy can be recognized by its typical location in the iliac or paraaortic regions. Only massively enlarged groups of lymph nodes can be detected on sonography and usually appear as a lobulated, hypoechoic mass in the expected region of a major lymph node chain. Solid masses resulting from bowel tumors can be diagnosed by the typical echogenic center arising from the bowel lumen.[38] Ectopic pelvic kidneys may be located superior to the bladder dome and have a reniform shape with an echogenic central interface arising from the collecting system. Loculated fluid collection can mimic the sonographic features of some pelvic

masses. However, their irregular shape and unusual location can be depicted by transvaginal or transabdominal sonography.

BENIGN VERSUS MALIGNANT DETERMINATION BASED ON SONOGRAPHIC MORPHOLOGY

Scoring systems have been developed that quantitate the probability of benignancy or malignancy based on sonographic morphology.[39] In one system, inner wall, structure, wall thickness, septa, and echogenicity were the major categories, with grades from 1 to 5, depending on the sonographic feature. Malignancies had scores over 9, with dermoid cyst showing the greatest propensity for overlap.

This type of system is helpful for standardizing sonographic assessment of pelvic masses by their morphology.

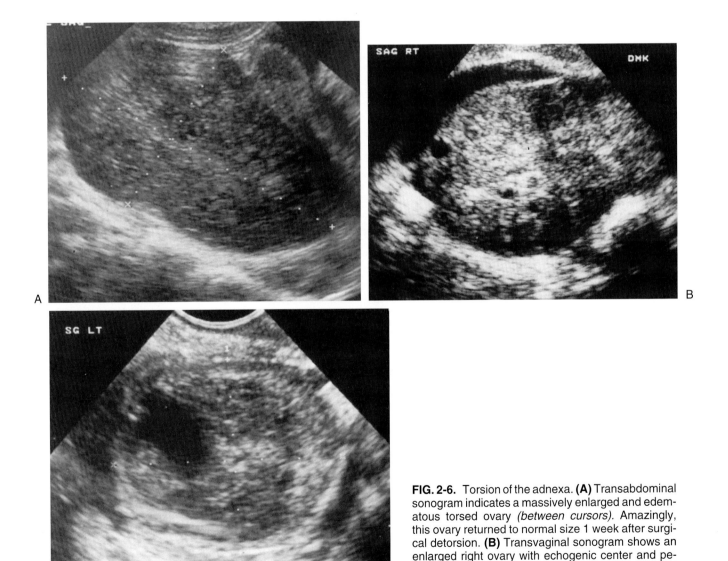

FIG. 2-6. Torsion of the adnexa. **(A)** Transabdominal sonogram indicates a massively enlarged and edematous torsed ovary *(between cursors).* Amazingly, this ovary returned to normal size 1 week after surgical detorsion. **(B)** Transvaginal sonogram shows an enlarged right ovary with echogenic center and peripheral follicles in a torsed ovary. **(C)** Transvaginal sonogram shows an enlarged left ovary containing a cystic area.

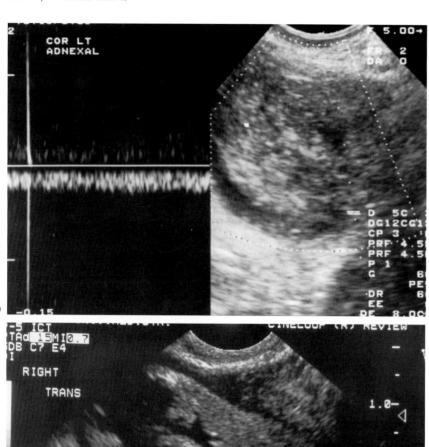

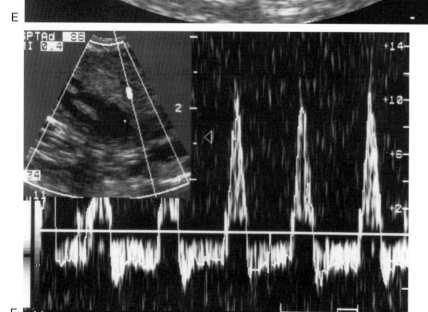

FIG. 2-6 *Continued.* **(D)** Transvaginal color Doppler sonogram of patient in **C** shows peripheral venous and arterial flow. At surgery, the cystic area was aspirated and the ovary was detorsed and was considered viable. **(E)** Transvaginal sonogram denotes a fusiform adnexal mass with thickened walls. **(F)** Transvaginal color Doppler sonogram of patient in **E** shows high-impedance, reversed diastolic flow in this torsed fallopian tube. This was a unilaterally torsed hydrosalpinx in a patient after bilateral tubal ligation.

It should also serve as a reminder to the sonologist and sonographer as to which parameters need to be assessed.

SUMMARY

Although the sonographic features of a pelvic mass may not allow a specific diagnosis, clinically useful information can usually be obtained. In general, transvaginal sonography is a useful adjunct to transabdominal sonography because it adds specificity in determining intraovarian versus extraovarian masses and endometrial and myometrial disorders. Transvaginal sonography affords an accurate means for evaluation of the ovaries and is particularly useful in obese, postmenopausal women in whom the incidence of ovarian carcinoma is especially high.[11,22]

REFERENCES

1. Fleischer A, James AE Jr, Millis J, et al. Differential diagnosis of pelvic masses by gray-scale sonography. AJR 1978;131:469.
2. Moyle J, Rochester D, Sider L, et al. Sonography of ovarian tumors: Predictability of tumor type. AJR 1983;141:985.
3. Warner M, Fleischer A, Edell S, et al. Uterine adnexal torsion: sonographic findings. Radiology 1985;154:773.
4. Swenson M, Sauerbrei E, Cooperberg P. Medical implications of ultrasonographically detected polycystic ovaries. J Clin Ultrasound 1981; 9:219.
5. Fleischer A, Daniell J, Rodier J, et al. Sonographic monitoring of ovarian follicular development. J Clin Ultrasound 1981;9:275.
6. Khan O, Cosgrove DO, Fried AM, Savage PE. Ovarian carcinoma follow-up: US versus laparotomy. Radiology 1986;159:111.
7. Mitchell DG, Mintz MC, Spritzer CE, et al. Adnexal masses: MR imaging observations at 1.5T, with US and CT correlation. Radiology 1987; 162:319.
8. Fleischer AC, Rodgers WH, Kepple DM, et al. Color Doppler sonography of benign and malignant ovarian masses. Radiographics 1992;12; 879.
9. Kurjak A, Shalan H, Kupesic S, et al. Transvaginal color Doppler sonography in the assessment of pelvic tumor vascularity. Ultrasound Obstet Gynecol 1993;3:137.
10. Bluth E, Ferrarri B, Sullivan M. Real-time ultrasonography of the pelvis as an adjunct to the digital examination. Radiology 1984;153:789.
11. Granberg S, Wikland M. A comparison between ultrasound and gynecologic examination for detection of enlarged ovaries in a group of women at risk for ovarian carcinoma. J Ultrasound Med 1988;7:59.
12. Callen P, DeMartins W, Filly R. The central uterine cavity echo: a useful anatomic sign in ultrasonographic evaluation of the female pelvis. Radiology 1979;131:187.
13. Meire J, Ferant P, Guha T. Distinction of benign from malignant ovarian cysts by ultrasound. Br J Obstet Gynecol 1978;85:893.
14. Graif M, Shalev J, Strauss S, et al. Torsion of the ovary: sonographic features. AJR 1984;143:1331.
15. Worthen NJ, Gunning JE. Percutaneous drainage of pelvic abscesses: management of the tubo-ovarian abscess. J Ultrasound Med 1986;5: 551.
16. Mendelson EB, Bohm-Velez M, Joseph N, Neiman HL. Gynecologic imaging: comparison of transabdominal and transvaginal sonography. Radiology 1988;166:321.
17. Lande IM, Hill MC, Cosco FE, Kator NN. Adnexal and cul-de-sac abnormalities: transvaginal sonography. Radiology 1988;166:325.
18. Vilaro MM, Rifkin MD, Pennell RG, et al. Endovaginal ultrasound: a technique for evaluation of nonfollicular pelvic masses. J Ultrasound Med 1987;6:697.
19. Timor-Tritsch I, Rottem S (eds). Transvaginal sonography. New York, Elsevier Science Publishing Company, 1988:125.
20. Nosher JL, Winchman HK, Needell GS. Transvaginal pelvic abscess drainage with US guidance. Radiology 1987;165:872.
21. Rulin M, Preston A. Adnexal masses in postmenopausal women. Obstet Gynecol 1987;70:578.
22. Campbell S, Goswamy R. Screening for ovarian carcinoma with ultrasound. Clin Obstet Gynecol 1984;10:621.
23. Fleischer A, Entman S, Gordon A. TV and TA US of pelvic masses. J Ultrasound Med Biol 1989;15:529.
24. Schnur P, Symmonds R, Williams T. Intestinal disorders masquerading as gynecologic problems. Surg Gynecol Obstet 1969;128:1016.
25. Rifkin MD, Needleman L, Kurtz AB, et al. Sonography of nongynecologic cystic masses of the pelvis. AJR 1984;142:1169.
26. Alpern M, Sandler M, Madrazo B. Sonographic features of paraovarian cysts and their complications. AJR 1984;143:157.
27. Athey P, Cooper N. Sonographic features of paraovarian cysts. AJR 1985;144:83.
28. Guttman P. In search of the elusive benign cyst in teratoma "tip of the iceberg sign." J Clin Ultrasound 1977;5:403.
29. White E, Filly R. Cholesterol crystals as the source of both diffuse and layered echoes in a cystic ovarian tumor: case report. J Clin Ultrasound 1980;8:241.
30. Baltarowich OH, Kurtz AB, Pasto ME, et al. The spectrum of sonographic findings in hemorrhagic ovarian cysts. AJR 1987;148:901.
31. Reynolds T, Hill MC, Glassman LM. Sonography of hemorrhagic ovarian cysts. J Clin Ultrasound 1986;14:449.
32. Friedman H, Vogelzang R, Mendelson E, et al. Endometriosis detection by ultrasound with laparoscopic correlation. Radiology 1985;157:217.
33. Hall D, Hann L, Ferrucci J, et al. Sonographic morphology of the normal menstrual cycle. Radiology 1979;133:185.
34. Bass I, Haller J, Freidman A, et al. The sonographic appearance of hemorrhagic ovarian cysts in adolescents. J Ultrasound Med 1984;3: 509.
35. Towne B, Maholar H, Wooley M, et al. Ovarian cysts and tumors in infancy and childhood. J Pediatr Surg 1975;10:311.
36. Gross B, Silver T, Jaffe M. Sonographic features of uterine leiomyomas: analysis of 41 proven cases. J Ultrasound Med 1983;2:401.
37. Stephenson WM, Laing FC. Sonography of ovarian fibromas. AJR 1985;144:1239.
38. Chang TS, Böhm-Vélez M, Mendelson EB. Nongynecologic applications of transvaginal sonography. AJR 1993;160:87.
39. Sassone AM, Timor-Tritsch IE, Artner A, et al. Transvaginal sonographic characterization of ovarian disease: evaluation of a new scoring system to predict ovarian malignancy. Obstet Gynecol 1991;78:70.

Color Doppler Sonography of Adnexal Masses

Arthur C. Fleischer, MD, Jeanne A. Cullinan, MD, and
Donna M. Kepple, RDMS

The ability to assess the flow to and within pelvic masses expands the capability of diagnostic sonography to include pathophysiologic parameters. Although differential diagnosis of pelvic masses by their morphology can achieve accuracies of 80% to 90%, a secondary test such as transvaginal color Doppler sonography is occasionally needed to further characterize masses that have nonspecific morphologic sonographic features.[1] By depiction of their vascular supplies, ovarian masses can be distinguished from uterine masses. In addition, areas of abnormal vascularity (tumor neovascularity) can be used as a means to distinguish benign from malignant masses.

As greater experience with color Doppler sonography is obtained, its role in the evaluation of pelvic masses is becoming more clear. Its practical role as an adjunct to morphologic assessment by traditional transvaginal imaging in the evaluation of pelvic masses has been verified in several published studies.[2-7] One study indicated that color Doppler imaging added important clinical information in approximately 40% of patients scanned because of a pelvic mass.[8]

The information obtained from color Doppler sonography can potentially add to the clinical management of patients by

- Adding confidence for the observation of masses that may represent hemorrhagic masses that may spontaneously regress
- Confirming the sonographic diagnosis of ovarian torsion, which requires immediate surgical intervention
- Differentiating those patients whose masses may be treated with a minimally invasive approach (such as pelvoscopic surgery) versus those who need standard laparotomy and extensive cancer surgery

This subchapter emphasizes those areas in which Doppler sonography can significantly assist in the differential diagnosis of pelvic masses beyond that information obtained with conventional transabdominal or transvaginal sonography.

INSTRUMENTATION AND TECHNIQUE

Doppler sonography can be obtained with either transabdominal or transvaginal transducer probes. Once a line of sight is established, the sample volume should be tailored to the size of the vessel examined (Diagrams 2-1 and 2-2). Large feeding vessels should have their entire volume sampled, whereas small intraparenchymal vessels need only the smallest sample volume that encompasses the entire vessel. The waveform shape gives a rough indication to the type of flow within the vessel. With major feeding vessels, the flow is of more uniform velocity, thus giving a thinner frequency envelope rather than the turbulent flow of smaller intraparenchymal vessels, which gives a larger range of velocities, as evidenced by the width of the waveform. Resistance is typically higher the farther into the parenchymal bed the blood flows.

Maximum systolic velocity can be estimated if the Doppler angle is kept between 20 and 60 degrees of the actual course of the vessel. When the vessel is visualized, angle correction is recommended. Wall filters should be set at a minimum so that even lowest velocities can be determined.

Analysis of waveforms can be accomplished using standard indices such as the resistive index (maximum systolic velocity minus diastolic peak velocity divided by maximum systolic velocity) or pulsatility index (maximum systolic velocity minus diastolic velocity divided by the mean velocity). Although there is some debate as to which of these indices is more accurate, both are sufficient if diastolic flow is present. If diastolic flow is absent or reversed, resistive indices cannot be used and pulsatility indices are needed. We prefer the pulsatility index because it takes into account more of the shape of the waveform. Another index that can be used is the perfusion index, which is the area under the waveform in systole divided by the area under the waveform in diastole. Future systems may allow assessment of the relative perfusion similar to that on a scintigraphic camera with quantification of the number of excited pixel elements per unit time. Infusion of contrast media may also prove to be useful in assessment of perfusion by color Doppler sonography.

The transvaginal approach is recommended if the lesion is within 5 to 10 cm of the cul-de-sac. Transabdominal scanning is needed if the lesion is over 10 cm or superior to the uterine fundus. Gentle pressure can be applied to the mass in an attempt to determine whether the mass is intrauterine or extrauterine or adherent or freely mobile.

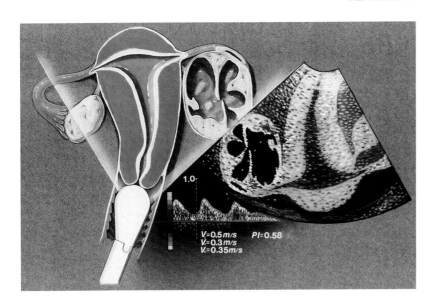

DIAGRAM 2-1. Diagram of triplex color Doppler sonography of an ovarian neoplasm. The image consists of a real-time image of the anatomy and pulsed and color Doppler with a waveform. (Drawing by Paul Gross, MS.)

BASIC DIAGNOSTIC PRINCIPLES

The waveform obtained from Doppler assessment of flow indicates the relative resistance to flow within an organ or area within a particular structure (Diagram 2-3). Waveforms can be analyzed by their resistive index or pulsatility index,

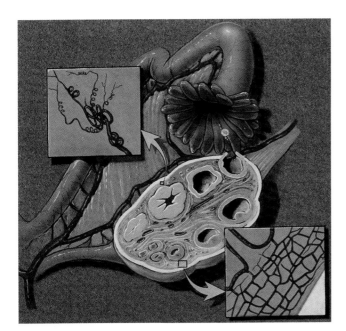

DIAGRAM 2-2. Diagram of arterial blood supply of the ovary. The ovary has a dual arterial blood supply arising from the adnexal branch of the uterine artery and the main ovarian artery, which is derived from the aorta. The intraovarian arterial supply is derived from the numerous branches of the feeding vessels and varies, depending on the presence of developing follicles. In areas remote from follicles, the intraovarian vessels are coiled and tortuous, having high impedance flow. However, in areas near a corpus luteum, the vascular arcade provides low impedance, high velocity flow within the wall of a functioning corpus luteum.

location and distribution of vessels, maximum systolic velocity, and presence or absence of a diastolic notch.

Diagram 2-1 shows a transvaginal color Doppler sonogram of abnormal vessels within an ovarian tumor. Normal arterioles have a layer of muscular lining that is not present in the vessels of tumors. This muscular lining has a role in regulating parenchymal perfusion and is thereby typically associated with a flow pattern that has relatively high pulsatility. With a paucity or lack of this muscular lining seen in tumor vessels, there is continuous diastolic flow and less of a difference in systolic and diastolic peaks and low pulsatility. There is usually a lack of a diastolic notch as well. The presence of a diastolic notch usually indicates initial resistance to forward flow during the initial diastolic phase. It is also seen as the branch points in major vessels. When a vessel is vasodilated, the pulsatility is reduced as a reflection of decreased resistance to forward flow. This pattern simulates that of a tumor vessel.

Tumor vessels typically have high diastolic flow related to the multiple areas of stenosis and vasodilatation within the network of tumor vessels. Their branching pattern is nonuniform as well.[9] The velocities may also be increased related to the requirements of tumor perfusion and arteriovenous communications within the network of tumor vessels.

A clear understanding of these principles is needed in analysis of pelvic masses with Doppler sonography. With this basis for understanding, it is clear that some nonneoplastic tumors may demonstrate blood flow characteristics of truly malignant masses (Tables 2-3 and 2-4). Future developments may include more precise determination of the blood flow characteristics of these vessels as depicted by their Doppler waveforms.

ACCURACY AND SPECIFICITY

Diagnostic accuracies of 90% and higher have been reported in several series in differentiating benign from malig-

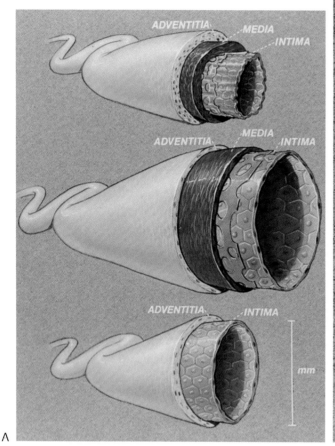
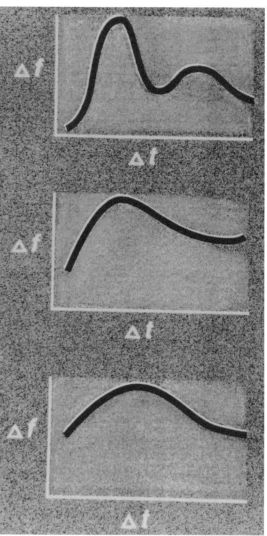

DIAGRAM 2-3. (A) Diagram of normal arteriole *(top)* with muscular media, vasodilated normal arteriole *(middle),* and tumor vessel without muscular media *(bottom).* **(B)** Corresponding waveforms from these vessels. The waveform from the normal arteriole shows a large difference in systolic and diastolic flow and frequently a notch during diastole owing to initial resistance to forward flow by the media. The tumor vessel lacks this media and has little difference in systolic and disastolic peaks and relatively high diastolic flow without a "notch." The vasodilated vessel may demonstrate features of both extremes. (Drawings by Paul Gross, MS.)

TABLE 2-3. *Typical transvaginal color doppler sonographic parameters*

BENIGN

PI greater than 1.0 (high impedance flow)
Flow seen in periphery, not in center
Diastolic "notch"

MALIGNANT

PI less than 1.0 (low impedance flow)
Flow in periphery and center
Absent diastolic "notch"

PI, pulsatility index.

TABLE 2-4. *Typical impedance of ovarian masses*

High (PI greater than 1.5)
  Cystadenomas
  Hemorrhagic cysts
Intermediate and/or variable (PI between 1.0 and 1.5)
  Dermoid cyst
  Endometrioma*
Low (PI less than 1.0)
  Ovarian malignancies
  Inflammatory masses
  Metabolically "active" masses
  Corpus luteum

PI, pulsatility index.
* May vary with menstrual cycle.

nant ovarian lesions using these diagnostic principles,[3,4] whereas other studies are less accurate (Table 2-5, Diagram 2-4). Variation in results can be related to studies that involved different patient population (some included premenopausal women whereas others attempted to include only postmenopausal women), different scanners, and measurement parameters. There seems to be the highest accuracy in postmenopausal women. This is probably due to physiologic changes in the adnexa (arterioles), giving higher impedance than in perimenopausal women.

In general, true-positive (percentage of malignant masses with low impedance) results are 90% to 95% whereas the false-positive results (percentage of benign lesions with low pulsatility index) range from 2% to 5%.[14] Even though transvaginal color Doppler sonography may not improve actual detection of mass, it seems to improve specificity in differentiating benign from malignant masses. The figures from these studies substantiate the use of transvaginal color Doppler sonography in selected cases as a means to differentiate benign versus malignant masses.

Using cutoff values of pulsatlity index less than 1.0 as indicative of malignancies, our series documented a very high negative predictive value of 98% and nearly had a high positive predictive value of 85%.[4] Thus, transvaginal color Doppler sonography seems to accurately exclude the possibility of malignancy, thereby allowing for less minimally invasive surgery, such as pelvoscopic surgery, to be considered. Analysis of multiple parameters such as vessel location, maximum systolic velocity, the presence of a notch, and vessel arrangement and density may also enhance specificity[4,15] (Table 2-6).

Retrospective analysis of 93 patients who underwent surgery and pathologic evaluation of the excised tissue after transvaginal sonography and color Doppler sonography indicates that in approximately 40% of cases studied, color Doppler sonography provided enhanced specificity concerning the organ of origin and histologic type of mass over those findings obtained with transvaginal sonography.[8] In particular, the enhanced specificity of color Doppler sonography was most evident in detection of the presence of ovarian malignancy, adnexal torsion, and ectopic pregnancy. In 40% of the cases the specificity of color Doppler sonography and transvaginal sonography were considered equal, whereas in 6% of cases transvaginal sonography was more

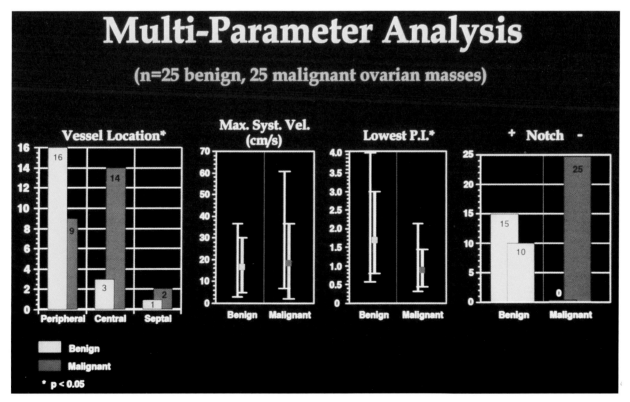

DIAGRAM 2-4. Multiparameter analysis of twenty-five benign and twenty-five malignant ovarian lesions. Most benign tumors had central flow, low velocity, and high impedance, whereas malignant tumors tended to have central flow, higher velocities, and lower impedance. The notch was absent in all malignancies but also absent in ten of twenty-five benign lesions. (From Fleischer A, Kepple D, Rodgers W. Color Doppler Sonography of Ovarian Masses: a multiparameter analysis. J Ultra Med 1993;12:41.)

TABLE 2-5. *Transvaginal color Doppler sonography*

Author (yr)	No. of patients	No. Benign/ malignant	Index	Value	Malignant ± SD (range)	No. of stage I CaO
Kurjak (1989)	20	5/15	RI	0.4	0.33 ± 0.08	5
Bourne (1989)	18	8/10	PI	—	(0.3–0.9)	3
Kurjak (1991)	680	56/624	RI	0.4	0.28–0.40	16
Fleischer (1991)	43	11/32	PI	1.0	0.8 ± 0.6 (0.7–1.0)	7
Fleischer (1991)	26	3/23	PI	1.0	0.7 ± 0.2	
Campbell (1992)	7	7/0	PI	—	0.61 (0.40–0.96)	
			RI	—	0.46 (0.33–0.78)	5
Weiner (1992)	53	17/36	PI	1.0	(0.75–0.81)	4
Kawai (1992)	24	9/15	1/PI	1.25	0.93 ± 0.65	
Hata (1991)	20	8/12	RI	—	0.50 ± 0.12	
Timor-Tritsch (1992)	80	13/67	PI	—	0.45	2
			RI	—	0.48	
Tekay (1992)	72	11/61	RI	0.6 0.5	(0.4–0.6)	1
			PI	—	(0.5–0.9)	
Kurjak (1992)	83	29/54	RI	0.4	0.37 ± 0.08	18
Hamper (1992)	31	6/24	PI		0.77 ± 0.33 (0.31–1.09)	
Schneider (1993)	55	16/39	RI	0.8		
Lin (1994)	370	90/280	RI	0.4		21
Bromley (1993)	33	12/21	RI	0.6		4
Valentin (1994)	149	28/121	Vel; PI; morph			4
Brown (1994)	44	24/36	PI	1.0		
			RI	0.4		
Levine (1994)	36	19/17	RI	0.4	0.47 ± 0.1 (0.32–0.66)	
Wu (1994)	410	103/307	RI	0.4		24
Wu (1994)	222	70/152	RI	0.4		
			Morph +			
Carter (1994)	167	88/79	RI	0.4	0.6 ± 0.2	
			PI	1.0	2.3 ± 1.5	
Prömpter (1994)	83	41/42	RI	0.4	0.4 (0.2–0.7)	
			PI; Vel	1.0	47 (15–105)	

RI, resistive index; PI, pulsatility index; SD, standard deviation; vel, velocity; morph, morphology.

specific than color Doppler sonography. In 14% of cases, however, neither color Doppler sonography nor transvaginal sonography was histologically specific. These cases included a patient in whom a 2-cm metastatic ovarian cancer was not diagnosed and a patient with necrotic leiomyosarcoma that was misdiagnosed as an ovarian neoplasm.

The true sensitivity of color Doppler sonography awaits studies that compare preoperative to postoperative findings in women undergoing surgery for conditions not related to the ovary. This requires studies similar to those done with conventional transvaginal sonography in women undergoing urologic surgery or hysterectomy and oophorectomy secondary to endometrial carcinoma.[14,16] In general, it is thought that the added specificity afforded by color Doppler sonogra-

phy substantiates its use in selected cases in which transvaginal sonography is equivocal or nondiagnostic.[10,15,17]

OVARIAN MASSES

The ovary is the source of a variety of pelvic masses, ranging from benign cysts to solid neoplasms (Figs. 2-7 through 2-9). It can also be the site of metastases, usually from gastrointestinal tract primary lesions. Some pelvic masses may also simulate the appearance of an ovarian mass. These include endometriomas and paraovarian cysts that are adjacent to but not within the substance of the ovary. The waveforms seen in the ovary vary in women of reproductive age according to the phase of the menstrual

of ovarian masses: reported series

RI ± SD (PI, range) [Vel]	Sensitivity (%)	Specificity (%)	Positive predictive value (%)	Negative predictive value (%)	Accuracy (%)
—	100	97	87	100	98
3.2–7.0	—	—	—	—	—
>0.40	96	99	98	99	99
(1.8 ± 0.8)	83	95	71	92	
(0.7–4.0)	73	100	100		
1.9 ± 0.7	95	71	92		
(0.6–2.8)	83	73	100	100	
—	—	—	—	—	—
	94	97	97	94	—
(1.45 ± 0.05)	—	—	—	—	—
0.88 ± 0.22	—	—	—	—	—
(1.15)	—	—	—	—	—
0.64	—	—	—	—	—
0.4–1.0	82	72	35	96	74
	46	89	42	90	82
0.5–3.5	—	—	—	—	—
0.62 ± 0.11	90	95	96	95	—
(1.93 ± 1.02)	97	100	100	99	99
(0.23–3.99)					
	94	56	47	76	—
	69	97	89	91	—
	91	52	—	—	—
	—	—	—	—	—
	100	46	—	—	—
	50	96	—	—	—
0.57 ± 0.17	—	—	—	—	—
(0.33–0.87)	—	—	—	—	—
0.23–0.82	68	97	—	—	—
0.8 ± 0.2					
1.1 ± 0.6	83	95	91	90	—
0.6 (0.6–1.0)	77	77	—	80	—
17.5 (5.2)[62]	85	83	—	84	—

TABLE 2-6. *Color Doppler sonographic parameters*

IMPEDANCE
High (PI > 1.5)
Intermediate (PI 1.0–1.4)
Low (PI < 0.9)

MAXIMUM SYSTOLIC VELOCITY
High (>25 cm/s)
Intermediate (15–25 cm/s)
Low (>15 cm/s)

VESSEL LOCATION
Central
Peripheral
Other

VESSEL DENSITY
High
Low

VESSEL DISTRIBUTION
Clustered
Sparse

PI, pulsatility index.

cycle. During the menstrual and follicular phase, there is high resistance flow. With formation of the corpus luteum, low resistance waveforms are seen as the result of newly formed vessels within the walls of the corpus luteum.

Although the morphology as depicted by conventional transvaginal sonography can be used in the majority of cases to determine their probable histologic composition, there clearly are overlaps so that an adjunctive test such as Doppler sonography can be helpful in further clarifying the etiology of some pelvic masses. For example, complex masses containing cystic and solid areas may represent either benign hemorrhagic corpus luteum or ovarian tumors (see Figs. 2-7 through 2-9). Some irregularities in the wall of a mass may be due to benign causes such as dermoid cysts or a reflection of malignant change. Thus, Doppler sonography is most useful in these cases that have nonspecific morphologic features as well as in cases where torsion is suspected.

The waveforms obtained from vessels using Doppler sonography give a general impression of the distribution and

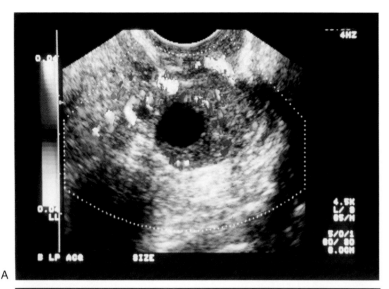

A

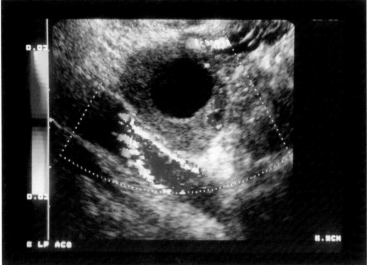

B

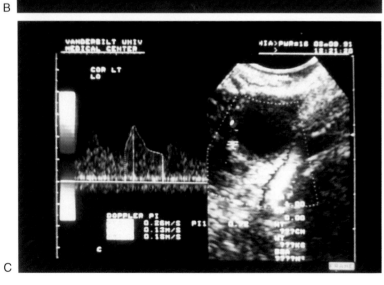

C

FIG. 2-7. Physiologic masses. **(A)** Transvaginal color Doppler sonogram of ovary containing a corpus luteum. Note flow within wall as well as in the major branches of the uterine and ovarian arteries. **(B)** Same as **A** in coronal section. **(C)** Corpus luteum with low impedance flow within wall.

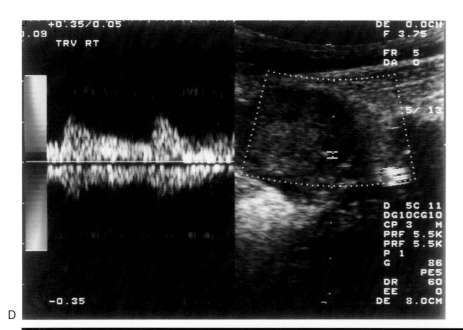

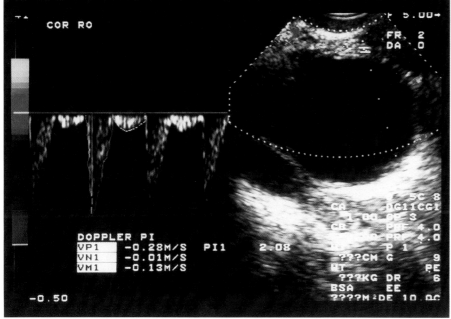

FIG. 2-7. *Continued.* **(D)** Focal area within normal-sized ovary showing low impedance related to an imperceptible corpus luteum. **(E)** Physiologic cyst showing high impedance flow.

The feeding arteries, mainly the adnexal branch of the uterine artery and the main ovarian artery, have a muscular coating that is present in both benign and malignant lesions. However, vessels located within the mass typically are low flow and high impedance, with the important exception of the corpus luteum. In the corpus luteum there are vessels along the wall that have a paucity of muscular lining and high diastolic flow that is clearly suggestive of tumor neovascularity.

In patients in whom a corpus luteum is suspected clinically, it is highly recommended that these patients be rescanned in the late menstrual phase of the next cycle to exclude the possibility of a corpus luteum. If low impedance flow persists after rescanning or cessation of hormone replacement medications, an abnormal mass is probably present and surgery is indicated.

There are a variety of lesions that may demonstrate low impedance, high diastolic flow (see Table 2-4, Diagram 2-4). These include inflammatory masses such as tuboovarian abscesses, actively hemorrhaging luteal cysts, and some dermoid cysts. These masses have in common enlarged and vasodilated normal vessels that can simulate the flow pattern seen in some ovarian tumors (see Fig. 2-9). It is important to determine whether the waveform has a diastolic notch, because this is an indication that there is initial resistance to

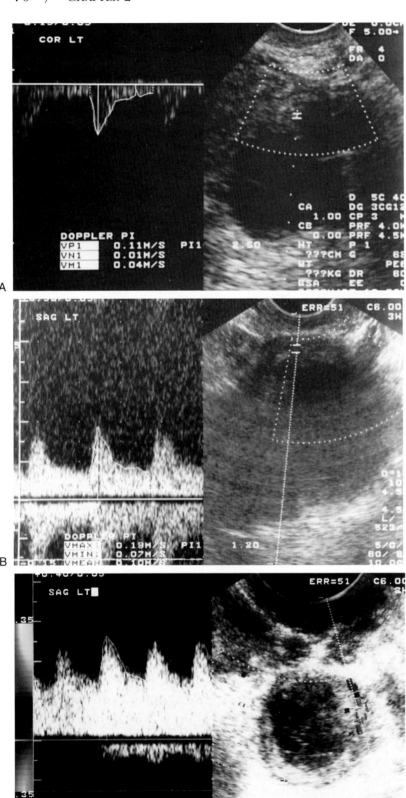

FIG. 2-8. Hemorrhagic masses. **(A)** Initial transvaginal color Doppler sonogram shows an irregularly thickened wall within a cystic adnexal mass. **(B)** Same patient as in **A** presented with pain 3 weeks later. The flow now demonstrates low impedance. At surgery an actively hemorrhaging corpus luteum was found. **(C)** Transabdominal color Doppler sonogram shows low impedance flow within a hemorrhagic corpus luteum.

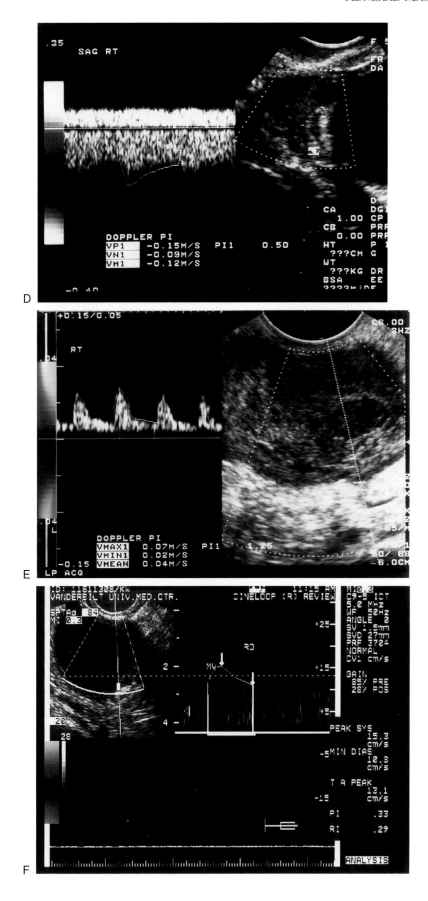

FIG. 2-8. *Continued.* **(D)** Endometrioma showing low impedance flow. **(E)** "Stable" endometrioma with organized low and high impedance peripheral flow. **(F)** Initial transvaginal color Doppler sonogram of a solid mass in a patient with lymphoma.

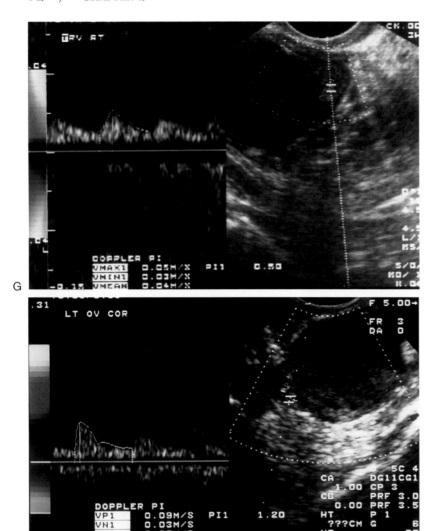

G

H

FIG. 2-8. *Continued.* **(G)** Same patient as in **F**; 6 weeks later there is no change. At surgery, an endometrioma was found. **(H)** Hypoechoic area within ovary was organized hemorrhage.

forward flow offered by the muscular lining of the arteriole. Intraovarian arterioles may not demonstrate a diastolic notch. Because resistance typically is greater as the vessel courses toward the center of an organ, the absence of a notch in a feeder vessel probably has higher predictive value than if it was obtained on an intraparenchymal branch. Malignancies tend to demonstrate clustered groups of low impedance, high velocity vessel flow in the solid areas in the center portion of the mass or in papillary excrescences or in irregular areas of the wall (see Fig. 2-9). This flow typically has a low pulsatility index (<1.0) and lacks a diastolic notch.[15] Some metabolically active tumors and germ cell tumors demonstrate this pattern as well. In general, tumors have more vessels than benign lesions (see Table 2-6).

There are a group of lesions that demonstrate a range of Doppler flow from high resistance to low resistance. These include dermoid cysts and endometriomas (Fig. 2-10; see also Fig. 2-9). Dermoid cysts may have low impedance flow

when they are actively dividing cells within the dermoid cysts, as opposed to relatively stagnant growth in established masses. Endometriomas may demonstrate low impedance flow when there is hemorrhage in the menstrual phase of the cycle.

Although there are only approximately 60 stage I cancers detected by color Doppler sonography at this time, it is clear that most of these are recognizable by their characteristic low pulsatility flow patterns.[3,18,19] In one study, 16 of 17 malignancies had a pulsatility index of less than 1 whereas benign lesions had an index greater than 1 in 35 of 36 examples.[5] The overall accuracy of color Doppler sonography appears to be better than that of CA 125 and probably is greatest in rapidly growing tumors that require significant blood flow, such as in some aggressive stage I and II lesions.

The transvaginal color Doppler sonographic findings in ovarian tumors seem to depend on several factors, most importantly the growth of the tumor and its ability to incite tumor neovascularity. Rapidly growing tumors tend to display more vessels and low impedance flow, whereas large tumors that have either outgrown their blood supply or become necrotic do not display tumor neovascularity.

Various studies have reported variable sensitivities and specificities of transvaginal color Doppler sonography in diagrams of ovarian malignancies.[11–13,19–23] Some studies show poor discriminating power of impedance values whereas others observe adequate accuracies. Much of the variation in results is related to different sensitivities of the scanning system used and measurement differences related to variable detection of intraovarian flow. There is common agreement that tumors tend to demonstrate low impedance flow; and when this is combined with morphologic assessment, sufficiently accurate diagnosis can be made.

EXTRAOVARIAN MASSES

A variety of lesions may mimic the morphologic and Doppler features of ovarian masses. These include pedunculated uterine fibroids, some tubal masses, paraovarian cysts, and, rarely, bowel lesions (Fig. 2-11). Gentle pressure may be exerted manually or with the probe between the uterus and the mass to differentiate pedunculated uterine lesions from those arising in the adnexa. Vascular fibroids tend to have low pulsatility characteristics similar to ovarian neoplasms. Tubal cancers, although extremely rare, may also demonstrate low pulsatility. Paraovarian lesions tend to be cystic and only when infected have low pulsatility. Some bowel lesions may simulate the appearance of adnexal pathology owing to their multiloculated appearance if matted.

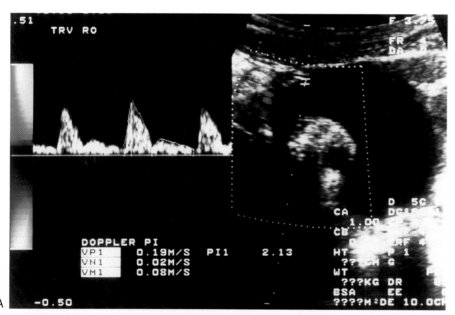

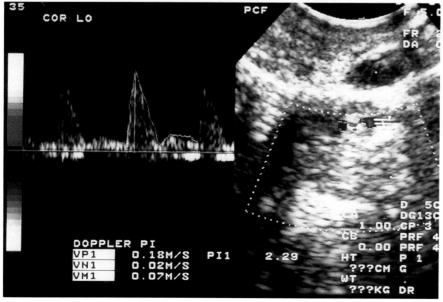

FIG. 2-9. Complex adnexal masses found to be dermoid cysts. **(A)** Transvaginal color Doppler sonogram of a complete pelvic mass with solid area. High impedance peripheral flow is seen. This was a dermoid. **(B)** Solid left adnexal mass with high impedance flow.

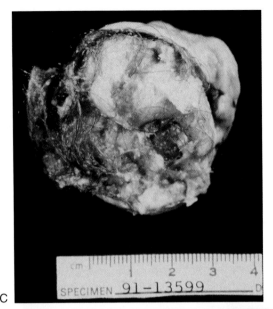

C

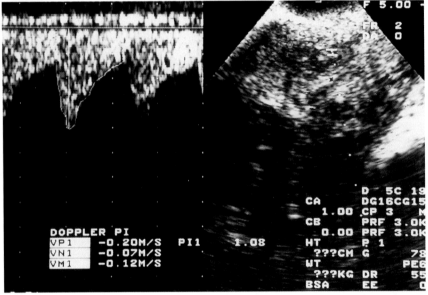

D

DOPPLER PI
VP1   -0.20M/S   PI1   1.08
VN1   -0.07M/S
VM1   -0.12M/S

FIG. 2-9. *Continued.* **(C)** Sectioned specimen of patient shown in **B** showing dermoid elements. **(D)** Relatively low impedance within mass representing a dermoid cyst.

Diverticular abscesses and inflammatory bowel lesions may also have low impedance flow.

ADNEXAL OVARIAN TORSION

One of the major applications of color Doppler sonography is in the diagnosis of ovarian torsion (Figs. 2-12—2-14). Although the ovary has a dual blood supply, torsion typically affects flow from both from the ovarian artery and the adnexal branch of the uterine artery. Typically, there is absent arterial flow within an enlarged ovary that may demonstrate irregular solid areas related to hemorrhage that may precipitate the torsion initially. There may be high resistance flow in the hilar vessels and, in some cases, venous flow in the capsular vessels as well.

The optimal time for diagnosing of ovarian torsion is be-

fore development of gangrenous changes. This challenge may result in some hypoperfused lesions to be overdiagnosed as torsion, but these lesions may be amenable to early surgical intervention anyway.

The topic of adnexal torsion is extensively discussed and illustrated in Chapter 8.

DIAGNOSTIC LIMITATIONS

Because there is a range in sensitivities in commercially available systems and due to operator dependence, the accuracy of transvaginal color Doppler sonography varies from institution to institution.

Certainly there are intrinsic variables such as tumor vascularity that may also affect whether a particular tumor is de-
(*text continued on page 81*)

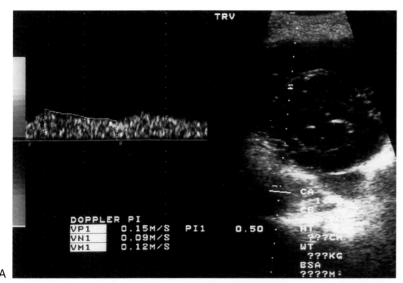

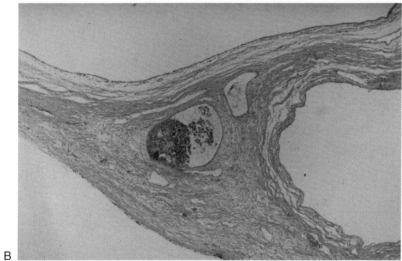

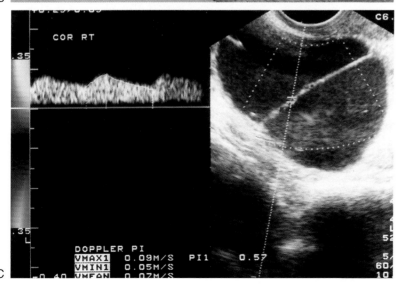

FIG. 2-10. Ovarian tumors. **(A)** Septated cystic mass with low impedance flow within a septation. **(B)** This low power photomicrograph of the area showing low impedance flow in **A** shows a tumor vessel. **(C)** Low impedance flow within the septa of an ovarian mass.

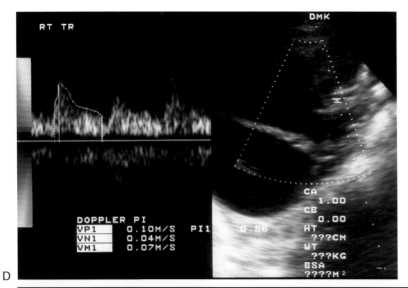

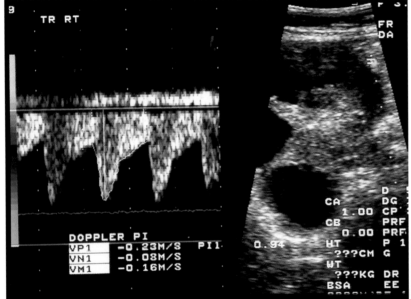

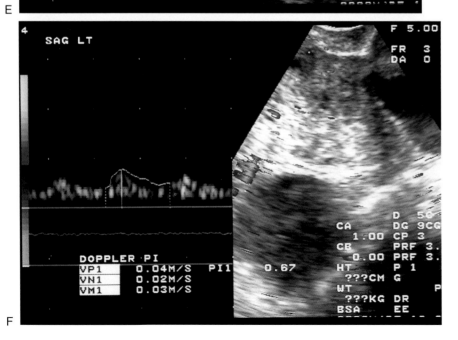

FIG. 2-10. *Continued.* **(D)** Higher impedance flow within the septa of an ovarian mass. This was a borderline ovarian cancer. Transabdominal color Doppler sonogram **(E)** of a right adnexal mass with low impedance flow. Transvaginal color Doppler sonogram **(F)** of a mostly solid mass in the cul-de-sac of the same patient.

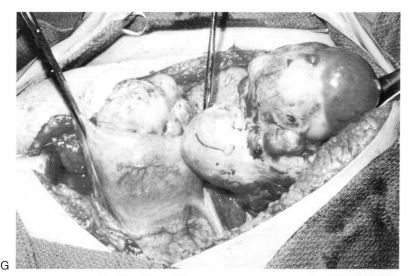

G

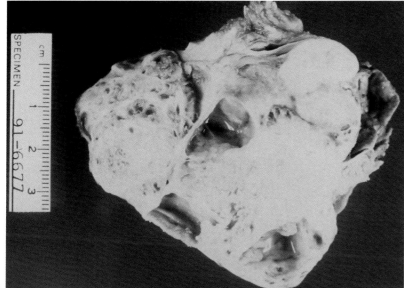

H

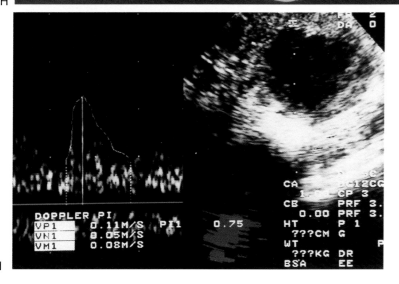

I

FIG. 2-10. *Continued.* **G** and **H** show the endometrioid ovarian cancers, one superior to the uterus **(G)** and the other in the cul-de-sac **(H)**. **(I)** Transvaginal color Doppler sonogram showing an irregular solid area within the left ovary that has low impedance flow.

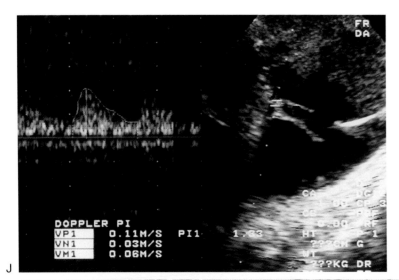

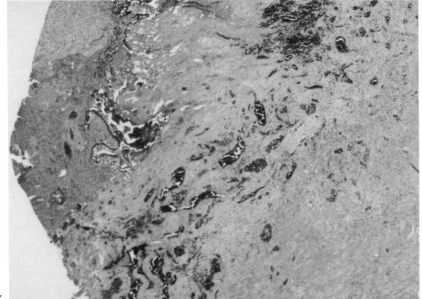

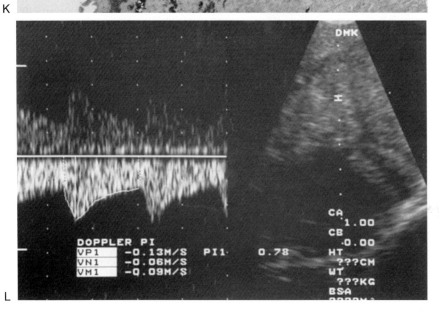

FIG. 2-10. *Continued.* **(J)** The mass extends into the distended left tube. **(K)** Low-power photomicrograph showing abnormal tumor vessels in area of active tumor growth. **(L)** Low impedance flow within irregular solid area of an ovarian cancer.

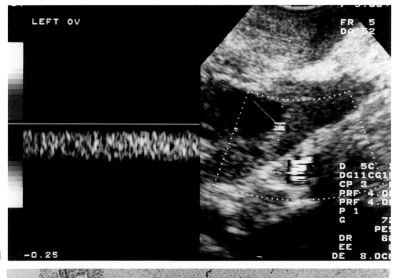

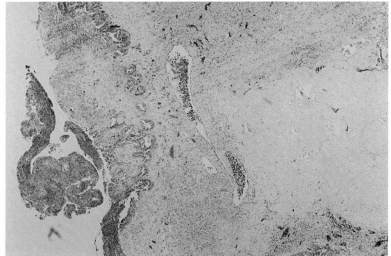

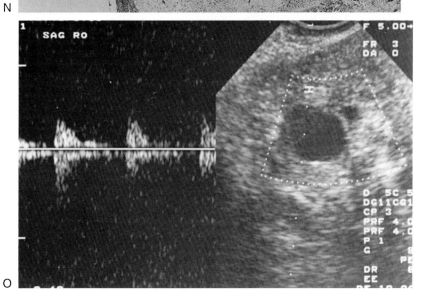

FIG. 2-10. *Continued.* **(M)** Ovarian cancer with venous-like waveform within a solid area. **(N)** Low-power photomicrograph showing sinusoid vessels in area of tissue. **(O)** Normal waveform from within right ovary.

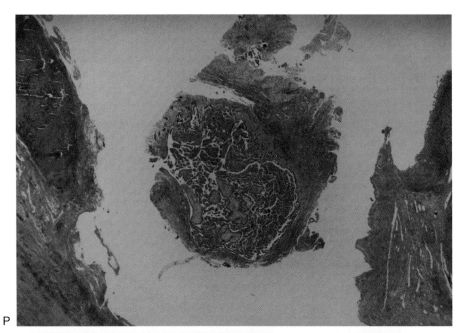

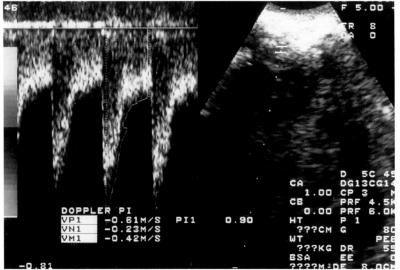

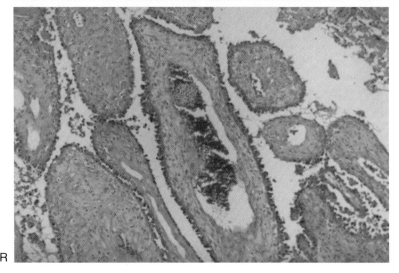

FIG. 2-10. *Continued.* **(P)** On histologic sectioning, a small (2 mm) form of tumor was found that did not initiate tumor neovascularity. **(Q)** Solid ovarian tumor with low impedance, high velocity flow. This was a serous papillary cystadenocarcinoma. **(R)** Low-power photomicrograph showing abnormal tumor vessels.

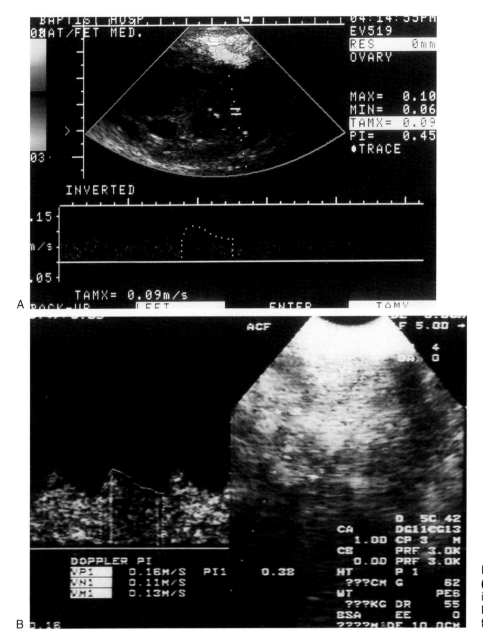

FIG. 2-11. Endocrine active tumors. **(A)** Granulosa cell tumor with low impedance flow in solid area. **(B)** Dysgerminoma with low impedance flow.

tected by transvaginal color Doppler sonography. These include tumor size and initiation of tumor neovascularity, for example. We have encountered some lesions less than 5 mm that did not incite neovascularity whereas some tumors were associated with flow patterns more indicative of venous than arterial signals. Another reason for high impedance flow in tumor is unsuspected torsion or tumor emboli causing obstruction within the arterioles.

On the other end of the spectrum, it is important to realize that some benign lesions associated with vasodilation or high metabolic activity may demonstrate low impedance flow. Such lesions are corpus luteum or inflammatory lesions. Repeat examinations are encouraged particularly in the premenopausal woman with a low impedance pelvic mass because this may be physiologic. If a persistent mass is thought to represent a corpus luteum, a trial of norethindrone (Aygestin) may be indicated. In our experience, this treatment causes physiologic masses to decrease in size and increases flow impedance (see Table 2-6 and Diagram 2-5).[24]

(*text continued on page 86*)

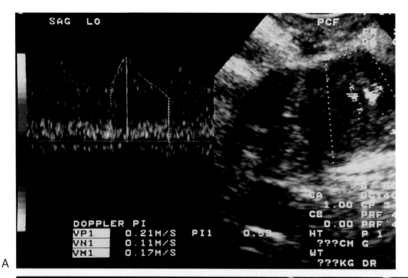

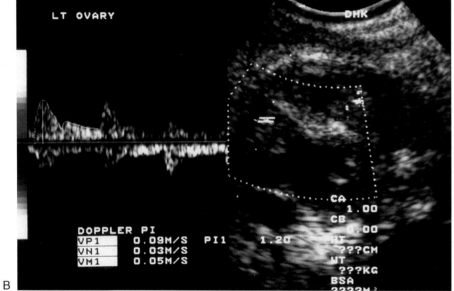

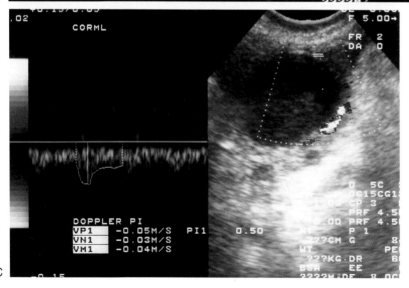

FIG. 2-12. Inflammatory lesions. **(A)** Low impedance flow within an ovarian abscess. **(B)** Intermediate impedance flow with a diastolic notch arising from within ovarian tumor surrounding an intraovarian abscess. **(C)** Localized appendiceal abscess with low impedance flow.

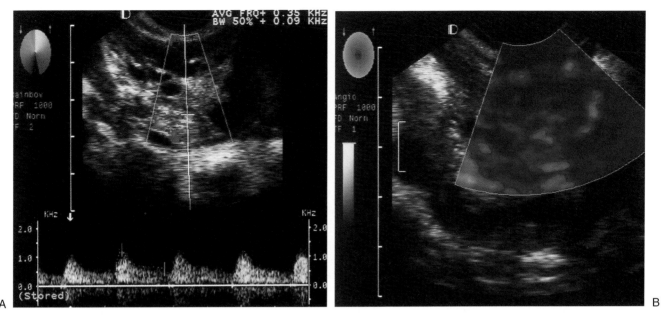

FIG. 2-13. Flow patterns within the ovary as depicted by power or amplitude-mode color Doppler sonography. **(A)** Conventional transvaginal color Doppler sonogram of an enlarged ovary. **(B)** Power color Doppler sonogram showing flow distribution around follicles.

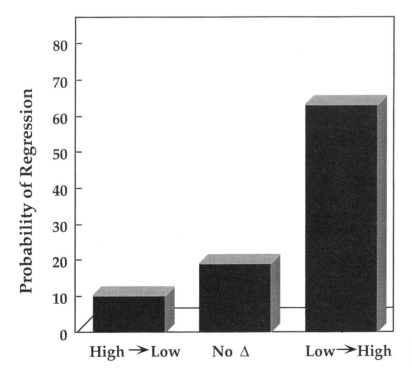

DIAGRAM 2-5. Probability of regression versus change in pulsatility index.

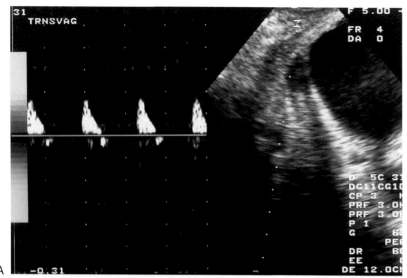

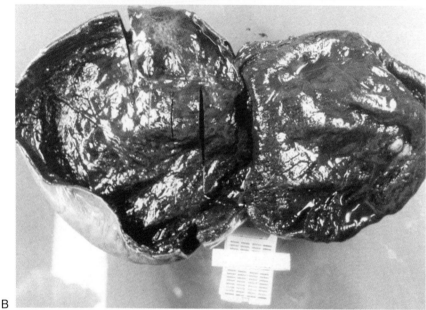

FIG. 2-14. Transvaginal color Doppler sonogram shows ovarian torsion associated with pelvic masses. **(A)** Transvaginal color Doppler sonogram in a woman who had had a hysterectomy and presented with a painful pelvic mass. There is high impedance flow near the capsule. **(B)** Opened specimen of patient shown in **A** demonstrating thick-walled cyst with hemorrhage associated with torsion.

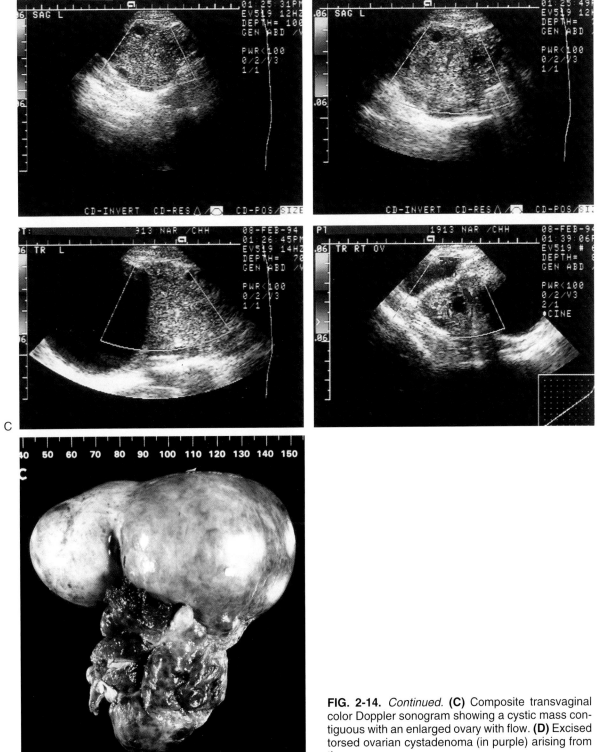

FIG. 2-14. *Continued.* **(C)** Composite transvaginal color Doppler sonogram showing a cystic mass contiguous with an enlarged ovary with flow. **(D)** Excised torsed ovarian cystadenoma (in purple) arising from the ovary.

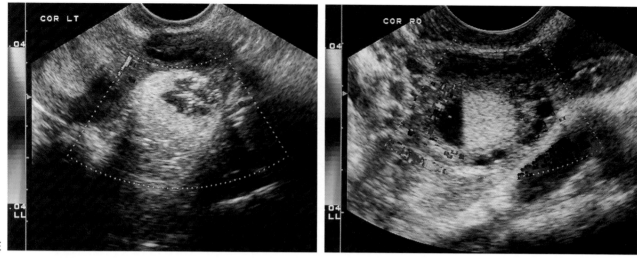

FIG. 2-14. *Continued.* **(E)** Torsed dermoid cyst showing no flow. **(F)** After laparoscopic de-torsion of dermoid cyst in **E,** intraovarian flow is seen. **(D,** courtesy of Mary A. Warner, MD.)

SUMMARY

Color Doppler sonography is most useful in differentiating morphologically similar masses such as hemorrhagic corpora lutea from ovarian neoplasms. It has a primary role in evaluating ovarian torsion. The areas of overlap in benign versus malignant lesions tend to involve masses that contain vasodilated vessels or those that are actively hemorrhaging. The impedance values in tumors depend on several factors, including extent of tumor neovascularization, growth, size, and presence of ascites and other intercurrent disease.[19,22]

REFERENCES

1. Granberg S, Wikland M, Jansson I. Macroscopic characterization of ovarian tumors and the relation to the histological diagnosis: criteria to be used for ultrasound evaluation. Gynecol Oncol 1989;35:139.
2. Bourne T, Campbell S, Steer C, et al. Transvaginal color flow imaging: a possible new screening technique for ovarian cancer. BMJ 1989;299:1367.
3. Kurjak A, Zalud I, Alfirevic Z. Evaluation of adnexal masses with transvaginal color ultrasound. J Ultrasound Med 1991;10:295.
4. Fleischer AC, Rodgers WH, Rao BK, et al.: Assessment of ovarian tumor vascularity with transvaginal color Doppler sonography. J Ultrasound Med 1991;10:563.
5. Weiner Z, Thaler I, Beck D, et al. Differentiating malignant from benign ovarian tumors with transvaginal color flow imaging. Obstet Gynecol 1992;79:159.
6. Kawai M, Kano T, Kikkawa F, et al. Transvaginal Doppler ultrasound with color flow imaging in the diagnosis of ovarian cancer. Obstet Gynecol 1992;79:163.
7. Natori M, Kouno H, Nozawa S. Flow velocity waveform analysis for the detection of ovarian cancer. Med Rev 1992;40:45.
8. Fleischer A, Cullinan J, Kepple D, Williams L. Conventional or color Doppler sonography of pelvic masses: relative specificity. J Ultrasound Med 1993;12:41.
9. Schoenfeld A, Levavi H, Tepper R, et al. Assessment of tumor-induced angiogenesis by three-dimensional display: confusing Doppler signals in ovarian cancer screening? (Letter to the editor) Ultrasound Obstet Gynecol 1994;4:516.
10. Tekay A, Jouppila P. Validity of pulsatility and resistance indices in classification of adnexal tumors with transvaginal color Doppler ultrasound. Ultrasound Obstet Gynecol 1992;2:338.
11. Valentin L, Sladkevicius P, Marsal K. Limited contribution of Doppler velocimetry to the differential diagnosis of extrauterine pelvic tumors. Obstet Gynecol 1994;83:425.
12. Levine D, Feldstein VA, Babcook CJ, Filly RA: Sonography of ovarian masses: poor sensitivity of resistive index for identifying malignant lesions. AJR 1994;162:1355.
13. Brown DL, Frates MC, Laing FC, et al. Ovarian masses: can benign and malignant lesions be differentiated with color and pulsed Doppler US? Radiology 1994;190:333.
14. Kurjak, A, Predanic M. New scoring system for prediction of ovarian malignancy based on transvaginal color Doppler sonography. j Ultrasound Med 1192;11:631.
15. Fleischer AC, Kepple DM, Rodgers W. Color Doppler sonography of ovarian masses: a multiparameter analysis. J Ultrasound Med 1993;12:41.
16. Fleischer AC, McKee MS, Gordon AN, et al. Transvaginal sonography of postmenopausal ovaries with pathologic correlation. J Ultrasound Med 1990;9:637.
17. Timor-Tritsch IE, Lerner JP, Monteagudo A, Santos R. Transvaginal ultrasonographic characterization of ovarian masses by means of color flow-directed Doppler measurements and a morphologic scoring system. Am J Obstet Gynecol 1993;168:909.
18. Lin PY, Lai JI, Wu CC, et al. Color Doppler ultrasound in the assessment of ovarian neoplasms. J Med Ultrasound 1993;1:172.
19. Wu CC, Lee CN, Chen TM, et al. Factors contributing to the accuracy in diagnosing ovarian malignancy by color Doppler ultrasound. Obstet Gynecol 1994;84:1.
20. Schneider VL, Schneider A, Reed KL, Hatch KD. Comparison of Doppler with two-dimensional sonography and CA 125 for prediction of malignancy of pelvic masses. Obstet Gynecol 1993;81:983.
21. Bromley B, Goodman H, Benacerraf BR. Comparison between sonographic morphology and Doppler waveform for the diagnosis of ovarian malignancy. Obstet Gynecol 1994;83:434.
22. Wu CC, Lee CN, Chen TM, et al. Incremental angiogenesis assessed by color Doppler ultrasound in the tumorigenesis of ovarian neoplasms. Cancer 1994;73:1251.
23. Carter J, Saltzman A, Hartenbach E, et al. Flow characteristics in benign and malignant gynecologic tumors using transvaginal color flow Doppler. Cancer 1994;83:125.
24. Fleischer A, Peery C. Serial assessment of ovarian masses with TV-CDS. Ultrasound Med Biol 1995;21:435.

Adnexal Mass: Detection and Evaluation by Magnetic Resonance Imaging

Marcia C. Javitt, MD

Because it is inexpensive, readily available, and usually well tolerated, sonography is the procedure of choice in the initial workup of suspected adnexal masses. Transvaginal sonography has certainly improved the diagnostic accuracy of pelvic sonography beyond transabdominal scans alone. However, sonography is operator dependent and may not be diagnostic in all cases, particularly in patients who are obese. Furthermore, sonography is inaccurate for evaluation of deep pelvic nodal chains, which can be obscured by overlying bowel gas.

CT has lesser soft tissue contrast than MRI, although it provides useful information about extent of disease in the workup of malignancy. Unlike MRI, CT requires exposing the patient to ionizing radiation.

MRI of the pelvis has better soft tissue contrast than either CT or sonography, is directly multiplanar, and shows not only the internal pelvic organs but also the pelvic sidewalls, nodal chains, and bones. Use of tissue-specific techniques such as fat suppression facilitates specific tissue characterization of lesions such as fat-containing dermoid cysts and permits differentiation from blood-containing lesions such as endometriomas. Use of intravenous MRI contrast agents permits identification of solid from cystic elements and improves detection of peritoneal and serosal metastases from ovarian carcinoma. Advances in MRI technology including phased-array multicoils and fast spin-echo techniques have further improved the accuracy of MRI for the diagnosis and characterization of adnexal masses. These newer MRI techniques are probably more accurate than transvaginal sonography.[1–6]

MRI is sufficiently more expensive than sonography that it is unlikely to be cost effective as a screening procedure for adnexal masses, although there have been no comparative cost effectiveness studies to date. MRI is better used as a problem-solving technique when sonography is nondiagnostic or equivocal.

In pregnant patients in whom sonography can be unrewarding for evaluating the adnexa technically, MRI can be used as a noninvasive alternative.[7,8] The risk of MRI in pregnancy is unknown. MRI should be reserved for instances in which the information likely to be gained would alter or influence patient management before parturition or would obviate the need for the use of ionizing radiation from other procedures. In the first trimester, exposure to MRI is considered potentially more risky, owing to organogenesis and a higher spontaneous abortion rate in the absence of MRI.[9]

IMAGING TECHNIQUES

The pelvic phased-array coil yields high-resolution images with improved signal-to-noise ratio and is routinely used for imaging the uterus and adnexa. Both T1-weighted and T2-weighted images are obtained. Fast spin-echo sequences in at least two planes are desirable not only to separate the uterus and adnexa but also to depict the components of complex adnexal masses as well as normal ovarian morphology. Using fat-suppression techniques differentiates fat-containing lesions such as dermoid cysts from blood elements such as those in endometriomas or hemorrhagic cysts. Combined with gadolinium enhancement, fat suppression allows identification of enhancing components of tumor from cystic or necrotic components, surrounding bowel, and pelvic fat.

NORMAL OVARIES

In women of childbearing age, the normal ovary has low to intermediate signal on T1-weighted scans. Ovarian stroma has intermediate to bright signal, whereas the follicular and functional cysts containing fluid appear very bright on T2-weighted images. These cysts are thin walled and contain serous fluid (Fig. 2-15).[6,10] Corpus luteum cysts may have thick walls that are vascular and enhance with gadolinium. They may be hemorrhagic with corresponding bright signal on T1- and T2-weighted scans, owing to the appearance of subacute blood. It may be impossible to differentiate endometriomas from hemorrhagic corpus luteum cysts initially. However, follow-up scans usually reveal resolution of the hemorrhagic corpus luteum cysts in one or two menstrual cycles; this is most efficiently accomplished by sonography. Mural-based clot may mimic solid elements in ovarian carcinomas, but there is no enhancement in the clot of a corpus luteum cyst whereas typically solid elements in malignancies do enhance.[6,10,11]

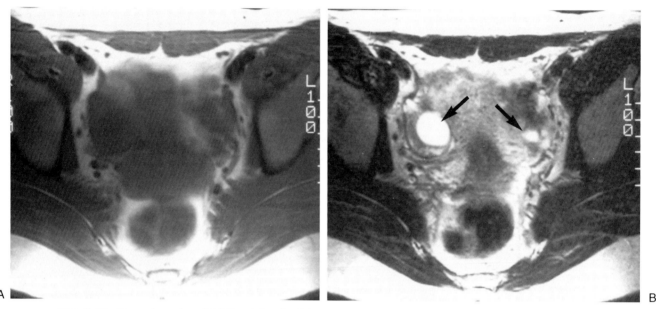

FIG. 2-15. Normal ovaries. **(A)** T1-weighted axial scan shows the normal hypointense signal of fluid in small follicles. **(B)** T2-weighted scan shows the bright signal in the follicles of both ovaries *(arrows).*

BENIGN ADNEXAL ENLARGEMENT

Theca-lutein cysts are caused by excess human chorionic gonadotropin effects on atretic follicles and may result from gestational trophoblastic disease or when infertility patients receive ovarian stimulation agents. These cysts are usually bilateral.[11]

Polycystic ovaries are secondary to absent luteinizing hormone surge in mid cycle in the presence of follicle-stimulating hormone, which is produced by the pituitary gland. Patients usually have resultant amenorrhea and infertility. Obesity and hirsutism are usually present. Scanning can be performed to exclude a masculinizing ovarian stromal tumor. On MRI, the cysts are peripherally located within enlarged ovaries containing prominent central stroma (Fig. 2-16). Sonography may be unrewarding due to obesity. Scanning must be accompanied by laboratory testing to confirm the presence of elevated luteinizing hormone with absent mid-cycle surge.[10,12]

Patients with hemorrhagic cysts often present in acute pain. On sonography, these lesions are often complex, cystic, and indistinguishable from malignancy. Repeat sonography in 4 to 8 weeks is usually advised because most hemorrhagic cysts resolve. MRI can be used to search for blood elements, but it cannot be used to differentiate hemorrhagic cysts from endometriomas, which also contain blood. The appearance of hemorrhagic cysts on MRI depends on the age of the clot.[13,14] Most scans tend to be obtained in the subacute period after 24 to 48 hours and show the typical bright appearance of subacute blood on both T1- and T2-weighted images from methemoglobin (Fig. 2-17). Acute blood containing intact red blood cells can have a bright signal on T1-weighted images but a dark signal on T2-weighted or gradient-echo images, seen both with endometriomas and occasionally with hemorrhagic cysts. A bright signal peripheral ring around the clot in hemorrhagic cysts is not typically seen in endometriomas but can be present in hemorrhagic cysts.[15]

Endometriosis is the presence of endometrial tissue outside the uterus that may respond to hormonal stimuli of menstruation causing bleeding and acute pain. Hemorrhage causing "chocolate cysts" or endometriomas may result. These

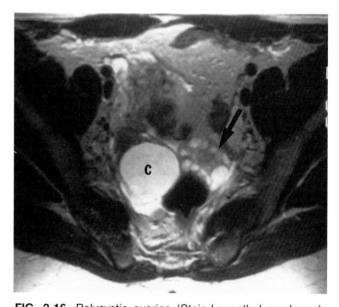

FIG. 2-16. Polycystic ovaries (Stein-Leventhal syndrome). T2-weighted axial scan. Hirsute obese female with amenorrhea. Note the peripheral ring of superficial cysts surrounding the hypointense stroma of the left ovary *(arrow).* The right ovary is enlarged with several large cysts (c).

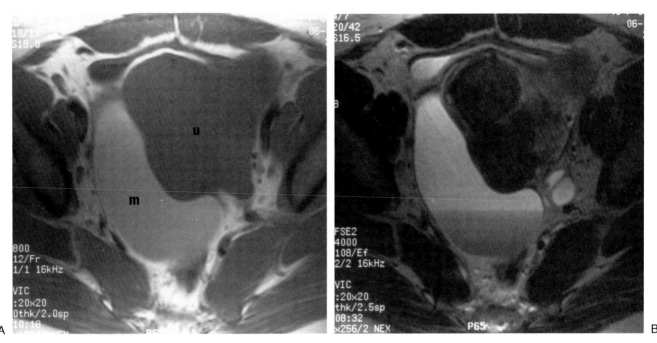

FIG. 2-17. Hemorrhagic cyst. **(A)** T1-weighted axial scan shows a mildly hyperintense right adnexal mass (m) flanking the uterus (u) that has fibroids. **(B)** T2-weighted axial scan. The surgically proved hemorrhagic cyst has a fluid—fluid level. The more dependent area contains more recent hemorrhage and is darker owing to the T2 shortening effect of intracellular methemoglobin. The nondependent layer is subacute blood, which is brighter due to extracellular methemoglobin. This appearance is more common in endometriomas, which are more prone to recurrent hemorrhage.

lesions are most commonly found in the ovaries but also in the cul-de-sac, uterine wall, ligaments, or bladder. If there is resorption of the blood, resultant scarring or adhesions may occur, causing infertility in some cases. However, many women are asymptomatic, with endometriosis noted commonly in women having pelvic surgery for unrelated reasons.[15]

MRI permits identification of blood elements in endometriomas and can locate deep pelvic implants that may be missed on sonography because of overlying gas. On MRI, the bright signal on both T1- and T2-weighted images is commonly seen in endometriomas but is not specific because other blood-containing lesions can have this appearance. If the lesion is bright on T1-weighted scans and has low signal owing to T2 shortening from recurrent bleeding into the lesion, an endometrioma should be suspected because this appearance is less common with hemorrhage into other ovarian cysts or masses.[6] Multiplicity of the lesions should also suggest the diagnosis (Figs. 2-18 and 2-19).

There can be a thick fibrous capsule around endometriomas that enhances after gadolinium administration.[6,11,16] Fat-suppressed images have been useful to locate small implants to bring them out in sharp contrast to surrounding fat.

Small implants typically enhance after gadolinium administration. However, tiny implants and areas with adhesions are not usually detected by MRI. Although MRI has been advocated as a means to follow response to treatment with growth hormone–related analogues for endometriosis, if the

lesions are visible on sonography this method is less expensive and probably better tolerated by patients.[17]

Sonography can fail to detect dermoid cysts because their echogenic texture and attenuation of sound easily mimics the appearance of bowel. CT will permit a specific diagnosis of dermoid cysts by virtue of the fatty content of the adnexal mass. Dermoid cysts can be characterized on MRI also by their fatty contents. The presence of debris or calcifications within the mass suggests a dermoid cyst. Chemical shift artifact from the lipid contents contrasted to water in the mass (ie, a fat–fluid level with chemical shift artifact) is confirmatory. Although hemorrhagic adnexal masses including cysts, endometriosis, and hemorrhagic neoplasms may appear similar to dermoid cysts with bright signal on T1-weighted scans and variably intermediate to bright signal on T2-weighted images, fat-suppressed or chemical shift images are the most reliable to make a definitive diagnosis confirming the lipid contents (Figs. 2-20 and 2-21).[18–22]

Ovarian torsion causes enlargement of the ovary, edema with enlargement, and acute pain with signs and symptoms of an acute abdomen that can be similar to the presentation with acute hemorrhage into an ectopic pregnancy, ovarian cyst, pelvic inflammatory disease, and even appendicitis. There may be an underlying ovarian mass such as a dermoid cyst. Initially the torsion compromises venous flow, causing venostasis, edema, hemorrhage, and infarction. On MRI, ovarian torsion has been reported as showing an enlarged ovary that may contain hemorrhage often with a high inten-

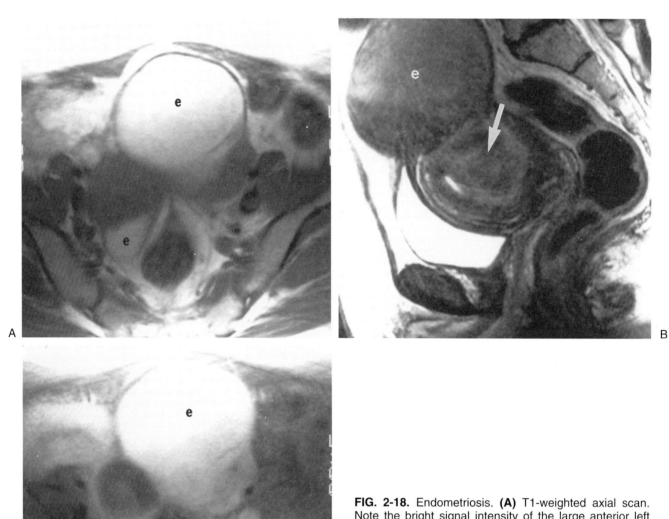

FIG. 2-18. Endometriosis. **(A)** T1-weighted axial scan. Note the bright signal intensity of the large anterior left adnexal mass (e) and the complex bilobed appearance of the right adnexal lesion with bright signal in the posterior loculus (e). **(B)** T2-weighted sagittal scan shows concomitant adenomyosis of the uterus with a lenticular mass thickening the junctional zone in the body of the uterus *(arrow)*. The left-sided complex adnexal mass demonstrates shading typical of endometriomas though not specific due to recurrent bleeding with a T2-shortening effect of intracellular methemoglobin. **(C)** Fat-suppressed T1-weighted axial scan confirms that the lesion remains bright and excludes the possibility of a dermoid cyst.

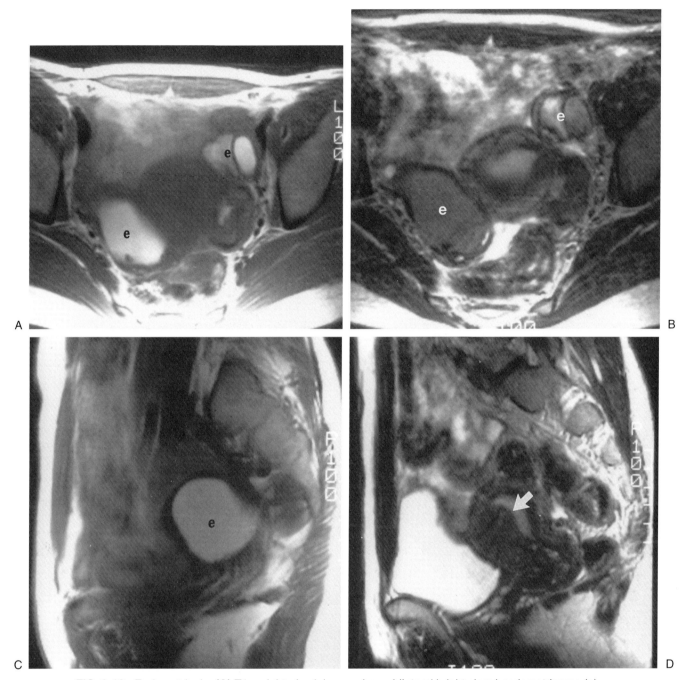

FIG. 2-19. Endometriosis. **(A)** T1-weighted axial scan shows bilateral bright signal endometriomas (e). **(B)** T2-weighted axial scan. Note the shading within the lesions and the low signal fibrous capsule surrounding the right-sided lesion. **(C)** Sagittal T1-weighted image. The capsule is seen to best advantage. **(D)** T2-weighted sagittal scan. There is adenomyosis of the uterus *(arrow)*.

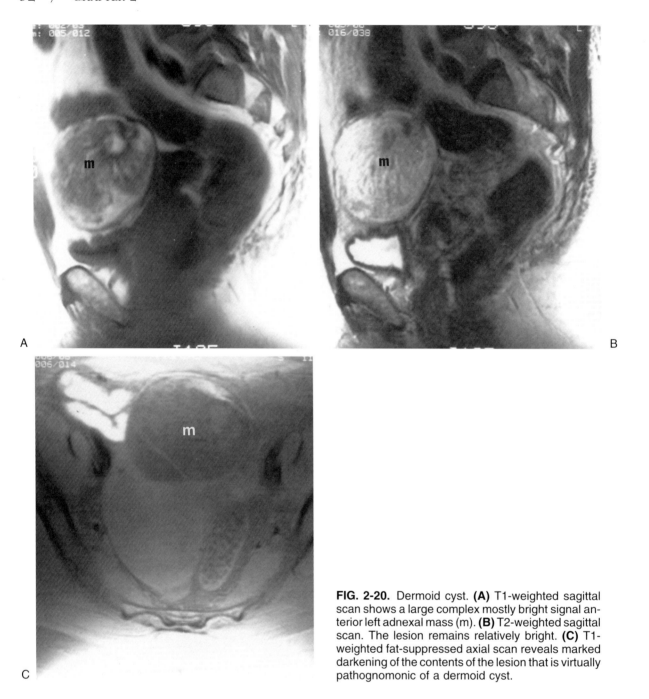

FIG. 2-20. Dermoid cyst. **(A)** T1-weighted sagittal scan shows a large complex mostly bright signal anterior left adnexal mass (m). **(B)** T2-weighted sagittal scan. The lesion remains relatively bright. **(C)** T1-weighted fat-suppressed axial scan reveals marked darkening of the contents of the lesion that is virtually pathognomonic of a dermoid cyst.

sity rim from subacute hemorrhage. There may be a twisted or knotted appearance of the broad ligament with uterine deviation ipsilaterally. If arterial supply is compromised, there will be no inflow and thus gadolinium administration shows no enhancement. On T2-weighted images, the ovary is bright due to edema.[23,24]

Puerperal ovarian vein thrombosis is an important cause of postpartum morbidity usually associated with persistent fever and systemic illness. The ovarian veins are usually clotted and enlarged and show filling defects from clot that

is evident on both T1- and T2-weighted images as well as on flow-sensitive gradient-echo sequences (Fig. 2-22).[25,26]

Pelvic inflammatory disease is a common cause of tender adnexal enlargement and is usually accompanied by fever in a sexually active woman. The findings on sonography may be near normal, or if associated with hydrosalpinx or pyosalpinx they reveal an enlarged fallopian tube with a cystic component to the adnexal mass. The tubular appearance should suggest the diagnosis in the appropriate clinical setting. MRI is usually not indicated for the workup of sus-

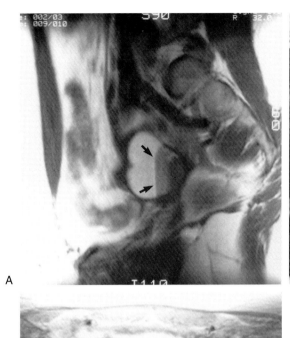

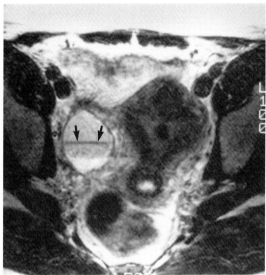

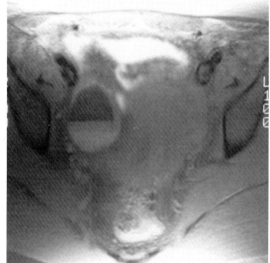

FIG. 2-21. Dermoid cyst with fat—fluid level. **(A)** T1-weighted sagittal scan. The right-sided complex cyst has a multilayered appearance with anterior bright signal and posterior dark signal. Note the chemical shift artifact *(arrows)* in the frequency encoding direction at the fat—fluid interface. This is diagnostic of a dermoid cyst. **(B)** T2-weighted axial scan again shows the fat—fluid level and same chemical shift artifact. The contents overall are brighter. **(C)** T1-weighted axial scan shows darkening of the lesion, which confirms the fatty contents of the lesion.

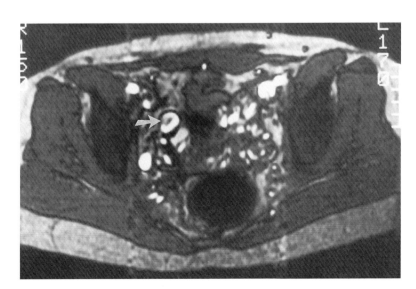

FIG. 2-22. Puerperal ovarian vein thrombosis. Axial flow sensitive multiplanar gradient recalled acquisition in the steady state scan. TR 33.3 ms, TE 17 ms, flip angle 70°. Note the enlarged right ovarian vein contains partially occlusive thrombus with dark signal *(arrow)*. There was propagation of clot into the inferior vena cava in this patient who was 3 weeks status post Caesarian section, with fever and leukocytosis.

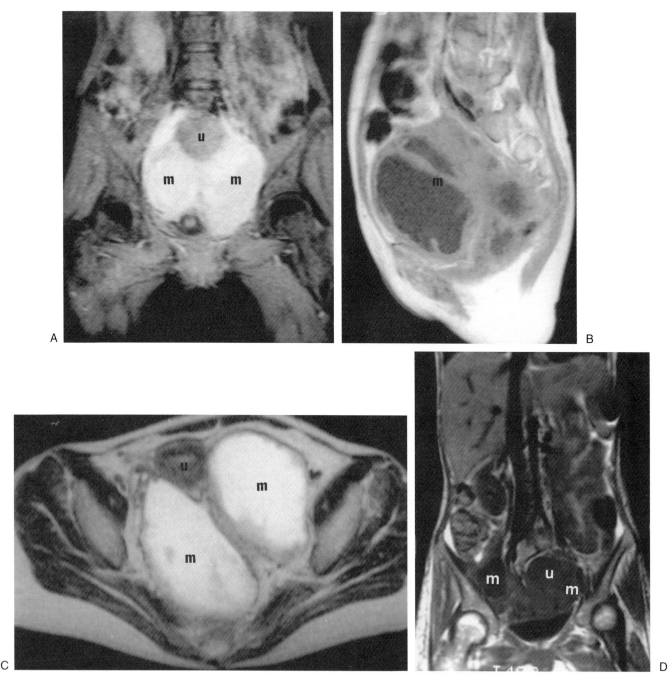

FIG. 2-23. Tuboovarian abscess from pelvic inflammatory disease. **(A)** Coronal inversion recovery scan (TR 1320, TE 20, TI 120 ms) reveals bilateral complex cystic adnexal masses (m) flanking the uterus (u). **(B)** Sagittal T1-weighted scan shows the multiloculated fluid-containing cystic masses that have thick walls. **(C)** Axial T2-weighted scan shows the bright signal of the fluid contents of the adnexal masses. **(D)** Coronal T1-weighted scan 1 month later after antimicrobial therapy, the cystic lesions have decreased in size considerably, but the patient remains symptomatic.

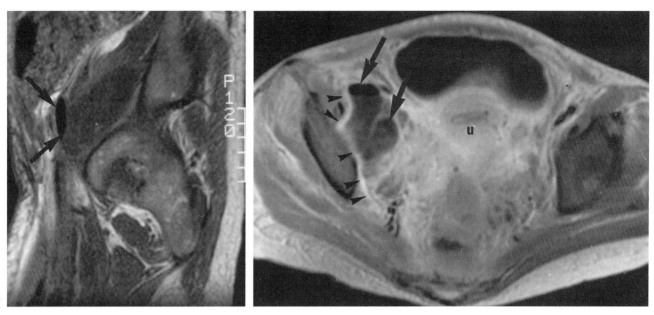

E   F

FIG. 2-23. *Continued.* **(E)** T1-weighted sagittal scan on the right shows the cystic mass has nondependent gas bubbles *(arrows)* from gas-forming organisms. **(F)** Gadolinium-enhanced T1-weighted fat suppressed axial scan shows nondependent gas bubbles *(arrows)* and enhancement in the rim of the right-sided lesion *(arrowheads).* At surgery, bilateral tuboovarian abscesses were found.

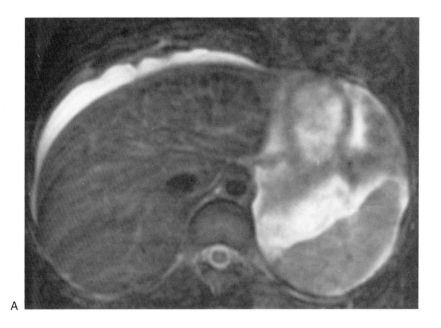

A

FIG. 2-24. Meigs' syndrome. Ovarian fibroma. **(A)** T2-weighted axial scan of the abdomen shows bright signal from ascites.

pected tuboovarian abscess. If performed, MRI shows the dilated tube filled with bright signal fluid on T2-weighted images or filled with hemorrhagic fluid. Sometimes there can be gas visible within the lesion, which usually enhances after gadolinium administration (Fig. 2-23).[12,27]

Solid benign ovarian masses cannot be distinguished from malignancy based on morphology on sonography, CT, or MRI. Fibrous solid ovarian tumors such as fibromas and fibrothecomas may have somewhat decreased signal inten-

sity on both T1-weighted and T2-weighted scans owing to the increased collagen content, but the findings are not specific. Fibromas can be associated with ascites and pleural effusion (ie, Meigs' syndrome) (Fig. 2-24). These findings are suggestive of malignancy and indeed can be seen with Krukenberg tumors and with Brenner tumors.[11,12]

Benign cystic neoplasms are likewise indistinguishable from their malignant counterparts. Serous cystadenomas are common cystic benign ovarian neoplasms and are usually

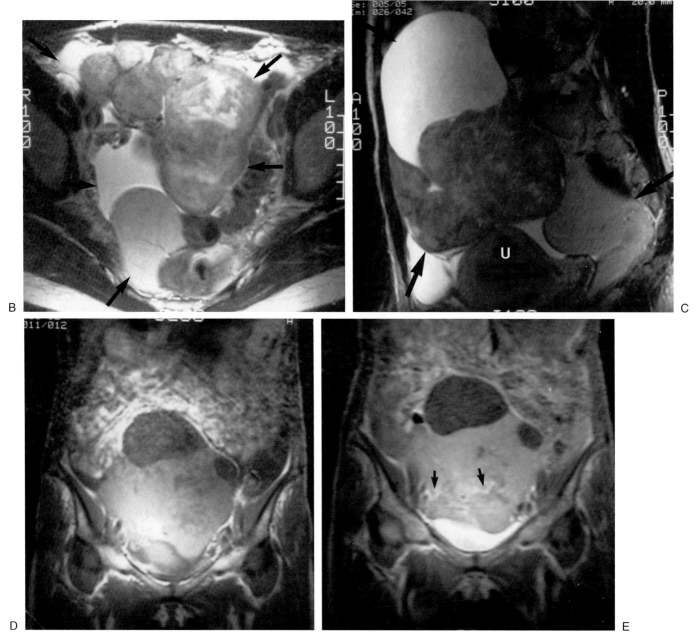

FIG. 2-24. *Continued.* (**B** and **C**) T2-weighted axial and sagittal scans. There is a complex cystic and solid multiloculated mass that fills the true pelvis *(arrows)* and surrounds the uterus (u). (**D**) T1-weighted coronal scan shows the heterogeneous intermediate signal solid elements and the low signal fluid contents of the extensive mass. (**E**) After intravenous administration of gadolinium there are foci of enhancement within the mass *(arrows)*. Preoperatively, malignancy was strongly suspected, but an ovarian fibrothecoma was found at surgery.

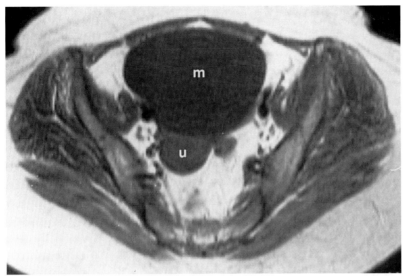

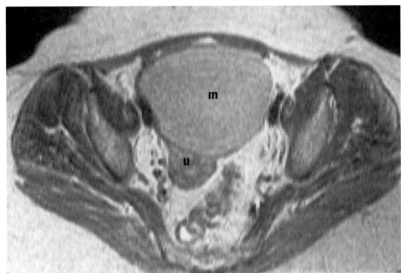

FIG. 2-25. Serous cystadenoma. **(A)** T1-weighted axial scan. A nonspecific cystic mass (m) is noted with low signal intensity anterior to the uterus (u). **(B)** T2-weighted axial scan. The cystic mass (m) is nonspecific and cannot be differentiated from its malignant counterpart based on morphologic findings.

without papillary projections. They have low signal on T1-weighted and high signal on T2-weighted images (Fig. 2-25). Mucinous cystadenomas are usually multilocular with varying signal intensity in the locules owing to various proteinaceous or mucinous contents and to hemorrhage (Fig. 2-26).[28,29]

MRI has accuracy rates of 60% to 84% for characterization of ovarian neoplasms.[30,31] The presence of wall thickness exceeding 3 mm, papillary projections, and solid mural nodules has been reported more frequently in patients with malignancies but is also noted in women with benign lesions. Certainly if ascites, adenopathy, peritoneal or mesenteric implants, or an elevated serum CA 125 level is associated, then the lesion should be considered malignant until proven otherwise. If MRI is performed to characterize the extent of disease, the use of gadolinium is advisable to better identify enhancing papillary projections, implants, and omental disease.[19,32–36]

SUMMARY

MRI can be used as an adjunct to sonography to characterize adnexal masses particularly for cases that are technically inadequate sonographically or for masses that require further characterization for proper management. Specific diagnosis of dermoid cysts, hemorrhagic cysts, and endometriomas and of enlarged fallopian tubes can be made using MRI. For other solid and cystic lesions, no imaging modality can reliably differentiate benign from malignant lesions. The use of gadolinium has been advocated for better characterization of adnexal masses and for extent of disease evaluation of malignancies.

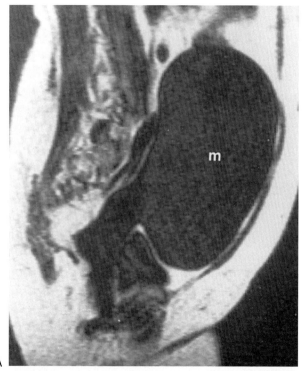

A

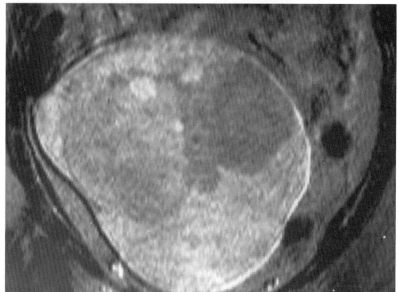

B

FIG. 2-26. Mucinous cystadenoma. **(A)** T1-weighted sagittal scan. A large low signal cystic mass (m) is noted. **(B)** T2-weighted coronal scan. There are mucin-containing and proteinaceous components within the mass that cause the variety of signal intensities in this complex lesion. It is not possible to differentiate this lesion from mucinous cystadenocarcinoma.

REFERENCES

1. Aubel S, Wozney P, Edwards RP. MRI of female uterine and juxta-uterine masses: clinical application in 25 patients. Magn Res Imaging 1991;9:485.
2. DiSantis DJ, Scatarige JC, Kemp G, et al. A prospective evaluation of transvaginal sonography for detection of ovarian disease. AJR 1993; 161:9.
3. Hata K, Hata T, Manabe A, et al. A critical evaluation of transvaginal Doppler studies, transvaginal sonography, magnetic resonance imaging, and CA 125 in detecting ovarian cancer. Obstet Gynecol 1992; 80:922.
4. Schwartz LB, Panageas E, Lange R, et al. Gynecologic MR imaging: utility and net cost analysis. Radiology 1994;192:55.

5. Weinreb JC, Barkoff ND, Megibow A, et al. The value of MR imaging in distinguishing leiomyomas from other solid pelvic masses when sonography is indeterminate. AJR 1990;154:295.
6. Outwater EK, Dunton CJ. Imaging of the ovary and adnexa: clinical issues and applications of MR imaging. Radiology 1995;194:1.
7. Weinreb JC, Brown CE, Lowe TC, et al. Pelvic masses in pregnant patients: MR and US imaging. Radiology 1986;159:717.
8. Kier R, McCarthy SM, Scoutt LM, et al. Pelvic masses in pregnancy: MR imaging. Radiology 1990;176:709.
9. US Food and Drug Administration. Magnetic resonance diagnostic device: panel recommendation and report on petitions for MR reclassification. Fed Register 1988;53:7575.
10. Mitchell DG, Outwater EK. Benign gynecologic disease: applications of magnetic resonance imaging. Topics Magn Res Imaging 1995;7:26.
11. Togashi K. MRI of the female pelvis. New York, Igaku-Shoin, 1993.

12. Fishman-Javitt MC, Stein HL, Lovecchio JL. Imaging of the pelvis: MRI with correlations to CT and ultrasound. Boston, Little, Brown & Co, 1990.

13. Gomori JM, Grossman RI, Goldberg HI, et al. Intracranial hematomas: imaging by high-field MR. Radiology 1985;157:87.

14. Rubin JI, Gomori JM, Grossman RI, et al. High-field MR imaging of extracranial hematomas. AJR 1987;148:813.

15. Togashi K, Nishimura K, Kimura I, et al. Endometrial cysts: diagnosis with MR imaging. Radiology 1991;180:73.

16. Arrive L, Hricak H, Martin MC. Pelvic endometriosis: MR imaging. Radiology 1989;171:687.

17. Zawin M, McCarthy S, Scoutt L, et al. Monitoring therapy with a gonadotropin-releasing hormone analog: utility of MR imaging. Radiology 1990;175:503.

18. Kier R, Smith RC, McCarthy SM. Value of lipid- and water-suppression MR images in distinguishing between blood and lipid within ovarian masses. AJR 1992;158:321.

19. Stevens SK, Hricak H, Campos Z. Teratomas versus cystic hemorrhagic adnexal lesions: differentiation with proton selective fat-saturation MR imaging. Radiology 1993;186:481.

20. Togashi K, Nishimura K, Itoh K, et al. Ovarian cystic teratomas: MR imaging. Radiology 1987;162:669.

21. Yamashita Y, Torashima M, Hatanaka Y, et al. Value of phase-shift gradient echo MR imaging in the differentiation of pelvic lesions with high signal intensity at T1 weighted imaging. Radiology 1994;191:759.

22. Jain KA, Friedman DL, Pettinger TW, et al. Adnexal masses: comparison of specificity of endovaginal US and pelvic MR imaging. Radiology 1993;186:697.

23. Kawakami K, Murata K, Kawaguchi N, et al. Hemorrhagic infarction of the diseased ovary: a common MR finding in two cases. Magn Res Imaging 1993;11:595.

24. Kimura I, Togashi K, Kawakami S, et al. Ovarian torsion: CT and MR imaging appearances. Radiology 1994;190:337.

25. Savader SJ, Otero RR, Savader BL. Puerperal ovarian vein thrombosis: evaluation with CT, US, and MR imaging. Radiology 1988;167:637.

26. Martin B, Mulopulos GP, Bryan PJ. MRI of puerperal ovarian vein thrombosis (case report). AJR 1986;147:291.

27. Mitchell DG, Mintz MC, Spritzer CE, et al. Adnexal masses: MR imaging observations at 1.5 T, with US and CT correlation. Radiology 1987;162:319.

28. Ghossain MA, Buy JN, Ligneres C, et al. Epithelial tumors of the ovary: comparison of MR and CT findings. Radiology 1991;181:863.

29. Cotran RS, Kumar V, Robbins SL. Pathologic basis of disease, ed 4. Philadelphia, WB Saunders, 1989.

30. Hata K, Hata T, Manabe A, et al. A critical evaluation of transvaginal Doppler studies, transvaginal sonography, magnetic resonance imaging, and CA 125 in detecting ovarian cancer. Obstet Gynecol 1992;80:922.

31. Smith FW, Cherryman GR, Bayliss AP, et al. A comparative study of the accuracy of ultrasound imaging, X-ray computerized tomography, and low field MRI diagnosis of ovarian malignancy. Magn Res Imaging 1988;6:225.

32. Stevens SK, Hricak H, Stern JL. Ovarian lesions: detection and characterization with gadolinium enhanced MR imaging at 1.5 T. Radiology 1991;181:481.

33. Hricak H, Kim B. Contrast enhanced MR imaging of the pelvis. J Magn Reson Imaging 1993;3:297.

34. Semelka RC, Lawrence PH, Shoenut JP, et al. Primary ovarian cancer: prospective comparison of contrast enhanced CT and pre- and post-contrast fat suppressed MR imaging with histologic correlation. J Magn Reson Imaging 1993;3:99.

35. Thurner SA. MR imaging of pelvic masses in women: contrast-enhanced versus unenhanced images. AJR 1992;159:1243.

36. Thurner S, Hudler J, Baer S, et al. Gadolinium-DPTA enhanced MR imaging of adnexal tumors. J Comput Assist Tomogr 1990;14:939.

Adnexal Masses: Computed Tomography

R. Brooke Jeffrey, Jr., MD

Sonography and MRI are the primary imaging techniques to evaluate patients with clinically suspected adnexal masses. In selected patients, however, CT may provide valuable diagnostic information and may also be used to guide percutaneous drainage of pelvic abscesses or other fluid collections. CT is often most beneficial in acutely ill patients who may be unsuited for MRI or in whom evaluation with abdominal and transvaginal sonography is limited or equivocal.

ADNEXAL MASSES CAUSING ACUTE PELVIC SYMPTOMS

Pelvic Abscesses

A pelvic abscess may present clinically as a tender adnexal mass. It may be difficult on the basis of clinical evaluation alone to distinguish perforated appendicitis or diverticulitis from a tuboovarian abscess. The results of CT may be valuable in these patients because specific findings that point to either a gastrointestinal or gynecologic origin of the abscess may be demonstrated.[1–4] With periappendiceal abscesses, a calcified appendicolith may be noted and the inflammatory mass is typically localized at the base of the cecum (Fig. 2-27).[1–3] With diverticular abscesses, there is often CT evidence of marked induration and edema of the sigmoid mesentery with ectopic gas and fluid.[4] The presence of gas within a pelvic abscess, particularly if there is a long air–fluid level, strongly suggests the possibility of an underlying enteric source (Fig. 2-28). Gas-forming abscesses are relatively uncommon with tuboovarian abscesses related to salpingitis. CT is also invaluable for diagnosing complications of diverticulitis, such as colovesical fistulas, by demonstrating gas bubbles or an air–fluid level within the bladder.

CT is often the procedure of choice to guide percutaneous drainage of pelvic abscesses. Many patients with periappendiceal or diverticular abscesses can be successfully managed with percutaneous drainage alone using local anesthesia (see Fig. 2-27).[4,5] Surgery and general anesthesia merely to drain the abscess can often be avoided. Indications for percutaneous drainage include a well-localized abscess with a safe

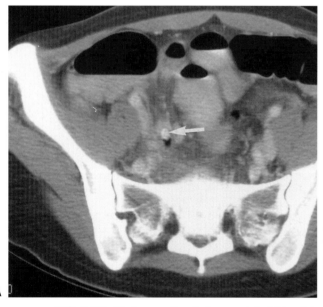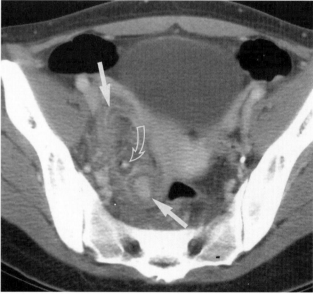

FIG. 2-27. Periappendiceal abscess mimicking tuboovarian abscess. **(A)** Note calcified appendicolith *(arrow)*. **(B)** Note pelvic abscess *(straight arrows)*. A small calcified appendicolith is also noted *(curved arrow)*. The patient was believed to have a tuboovarian abscess but failed to respond to antibiotics.

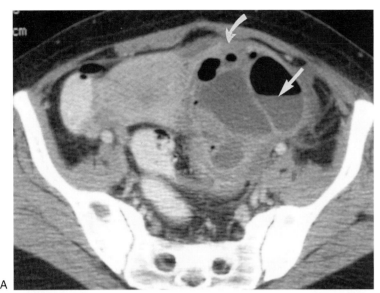

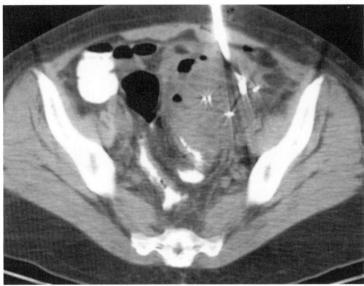

FIG. 2-28. Diverticular abscess mimicking tuboovarian abscess. **(A)** Note complex left adnexal mass with air—fluid level *(straight arrow)*. The mass displaces the left mesosalpinx and, therefore, might mimic a tuboovarian abscess *(curved arrow = mesosalpinx)*. The diverticular abscess was successfully drained percutaneously. **(B)** A scan obtained immediately after catheter insertion. Note complete drainage of the abscess.

access route for catheter insertion. In selected patients, sonography may be used to guide percutaneous drainage of pelvic abscesses using a transabdominal or transvaginal approach. However, the identification of a safe access window for catheter insertion often requires CT. Bowel loops can more readily be identified on CT by use of oral or rectal contrast medium and then safely avoided during catheter insertion.

Tuboovarian Abscesses

On CT, tuboovarian abscesses are typically complex adnexal masses with ill-defined margins (Fig. 2-29).[6,7] Pelvic inflammatory disease typically obscures the normal pelvic fat planes that interface with the uterus (Fig. 2-30). Tuboovarian abscesses may be multiple and bilateral. In the absence of an appropriate history it may be difficult, based on CT imaging criteria alone, to differentiate a tuboovarian abscess from other complex adnexal masses such as an ovarian neoplasm. Not infrequently, there is displacement of the mesosalpinx by the abscess and poor definition of the adjacent uterine contour. Transvaginal sonography is superior to CT in demonstrating the tubular nature of a pyosalpinx that cannot be clearly depicted on axial images alone (Fig. 2-31). In addition, transvaginal sonography may demonstrate a fluid—fluid level indicative of debris and pus within a dilated tube. This finding is virtually pathognomonic for pelvic inflammatory disease in the appropriate clinical setting.

In selected patients, percutaneous drainage of tuboovarian abscess may be a safe and effective alternative to surgery.[8–10] Catheter insertion may be guided by either CT or sonography using a transabdominal, transgluteal, or vaginal approach. Casola and associates[10] reported successful percu-

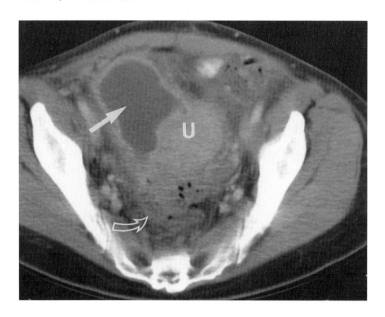

FIG. 2-29. Tuboovarian abscess. Note the low-density right adnexal mass *(straight arrow)* adjacent to the uterus (U). There is surrounding edema and soft tissue infiltration of the pelvic fat *(curved arrow).*

taneous drainage in 15 of 16 patients with 27 tuboovarian abscesses. All 16 patients were refractory to medical therapy with triple antibiotics.

Hemorrhagic Ovarian Cysts

Patients with functional ovarian cysts may present with sudden onset of pelvic pain from acute spontaneous hemorrhage or torsion. In rare cases cyst rupture may lead to life-threatening hemoperitoneum. Although the diagnosis of a hemorrhagic cyst can be readily established with characteristic signal intensity on MRI, CT may suggest the presence of hemorrhage within an ovarian cyst owing to its high attenuation values, which are generally greater than 50 Hounsfield units (Fig. 2-32).[9] If hemorrhage is suspected within

an ovarian mass based on either sonography or clinical findings, CT should be performed with and without the use of intravenous contrast medium enhancement. Hemorrhagic areas are high in attenuation and fail to enhance with contrast medium. The diagnosis of hemorrhage within an ovarian cyst strongly favors a benign process. Serial follow-up with transvaginal sonography can then be performed in 4 to 6 weeks.

Endometriomas

Ectopic endometrial tissue within the ovary may cause recurrent hemorrhage or "chocolate" cysts. The CT features of endometriomas are often variable and nonspecific.[10,11] Unlike hemorrhagic functional cysts, which tend to resolve

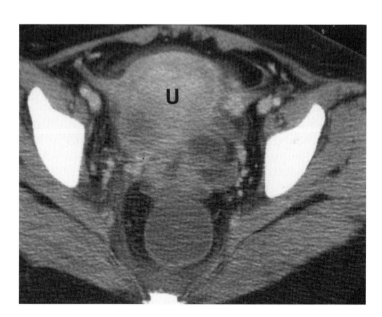

FIG. 2-30. Pelvic inflammatory disease. Note the poor definition of the posterior margin of the uterus (U) that is obscured by fluid and soft tissue infiltration.

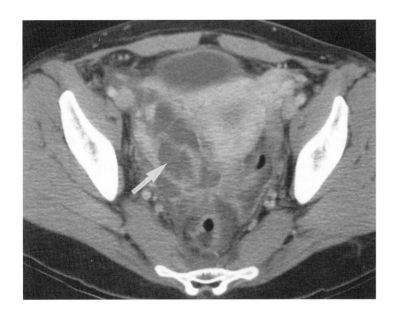

FIG. 2-31. Pyosalpinx. Note a tubular low-density mass in the right adnexa *(arrow)*. Endovaginal sonography demonstrated that this represented a large pyosalpinx. On axial images alone it is often difficult on CT to distinguish a pyosalpinx from a tuboovarian abscess.

quickly, endometriomas are often chronic. One CT feature that suggests the diagnosis of a endometrioma is a crescentic or rounded hyperdense area within a cystic adnexal mass representing acute hemorrhage or clot (Fig. 2-33).[12] Unfortunately, the sensitivity of this finding is low. Buy and associates[12] reported identifying a hyperdense focus in only 9 of 62 surgically proven endometriomas (15%). The specificity of the finding is likely to be high, however, because the vast majority of ovarian neoplasms do not demonstrate macroscopic hemorrhage. Implants from endometriosis may occur anywhere in the peritoneal cavity. Small implants (3–5 mm) commonly involve the cul-de-sac and broad ligaments. These small implants cannot be reliably imaged with CT and thus a "negative" CT does not exclude microscopic involvement of endometriosis.[11]

Ovarian Torsion

Subacute ovarian torsion, with or without an ovarian mass, may be challenging to diagnose clinically. Unlike acute torsion, which typically presents as acute severe pain, the clinical symptoms of a subacute lesion are often vague and nonspecific. Although the diagnosis may be suggested by characteristic gray-scale and color Doppler features, on occasion patients undergo pelvic CT due to diagnostic uncertainty. Kimura and colleagues[13] have described the CT and MRI features of acute and subacute ovarian torsion. The primary findings include deviation of the uterus to the side of involvement, engorgement of adjacent blood vessels on the involved side, ascites, and obliteration of fat planes around an associated mass.[13] In the presence of hemorrhagic infarction a "beaked"

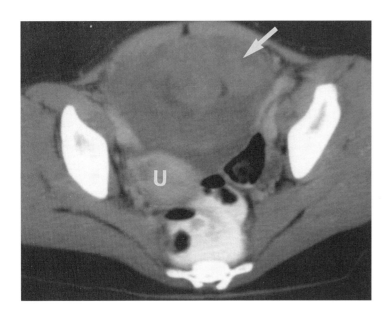

FIG. 2-32. Acute hemorrhage within torsed functional cyst. Note the areas of high attenuation within a complex cystic mass *(arrow)* anterior to the uterus (U). At surgery a torsed hemorrhagic cyst noted with acute internal hemorrhage.

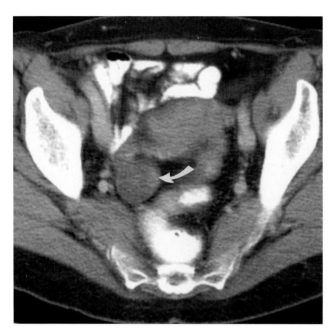

FIG. 2-33. Small endometrioma with hyperdense clot. Note right adnexal complex mass with high-attenuation focus seen along the medial wall. At surgery an endometrioma was noted with adherent clot in this area. If an endometrioma is suspected before CT, scans performed with and without contrast medium enhancement are acquired to distinguish a hyperdense clot that is avascular from an enhancing mural nodule of a neoplasm. With and without contrast medium enhancement, scans in this patient showed that this hyperdense focus had no internal enhancement.

or serpentine protrusion of the mass may be evident. This is typically associated with thickened and engorged blood vessels torsed around the lesion. After contrast medium administration, there is lack of enhancement of the mass on CT, indicating ischemic or nonviable tissue.

OTHER BENIGN ADNEXAL MASSES

Physiologic Ovarian Cysts

Most simple ovarian cysts are either follicular or corpus luteum cysts. These cysts appear on CT as rounded or oval water-density masses (less than 20 Hounsfield units) with a thin or barely perceptible wall (Fig. 2-34).[10] They are rarely larger than 5 cm. The internal morphology of many of these cysts is better depicted with transvaginal sonography than CT. However, if the mass is less than 5 cm and has no mural nodules or septations on CT, a follow-up transvaginal sonogram can be performed in 4 to 6 weeks to ensure stability.

Theca-Lutein Cysts

Theca-lutein cysts typically develop in patients with high serum levels of human chorionic gonadotropin.[14] They are associated with multiple gestations, trophoblastic disease, or the ovarian hyperstimulation syndrome.[14] Theca-lutein cysts are typically large, multiseptated bilateral masses (Fig. 2-35). There are no mural nodules and no evidence of septal thickening to suggest malignancy.[14]

Cystic Teratoma

Cystic teratoma is a commonly encountered ovarian neoplasm in premenopausal women. The fatty elements within a cystic teratoma have a characteristic low CT attenuation value (-20 to -120 Hounsfield units) (see Fig. 2-36; see also Fig. 2-33).[15] Another typical feature is the presence of calcification representing either teeth or abortive bone. Cystic teratomas may be bilateral in 15% of patients. A solid portion of the cyst wall may be evident representing the "dermoid plug." Approximately 90% of cystic teratomas demonstrate pathognomonic CT features.[15] In the absence of fat or calcium, however, a specific diagnosis of cystic teratoma cannot be established by CT, and further characterization of the mass is required with transvaginal sonography or MRI. Although the risk of malignancy is quite low (<2%), most cystic teratomas larger than 3 cm are removed surgically, owing to their potential for torsion and rupture.[10]

Benign Solid Masses

Benign solid masses of the ovary include fibromas, adenofibromas, thecomas, and Brenner tumors. There are no char-

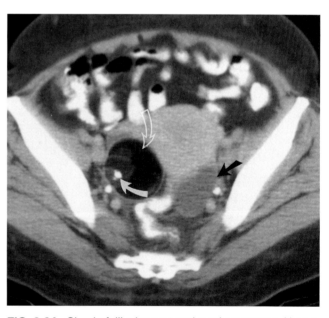

FIG. 2-34. Simple follicular cyst and cystic teratoma. Note a simple follicular cyst in the left adnexa *(straight arrow)*. The wall is imperceptible, and there is no evidence of septations or mural nodularity. In the right adnexa note a cystic teratoma containing fatty elements *(curved open arrow)* and a focal area of calcification *(curved solid arrow)*.

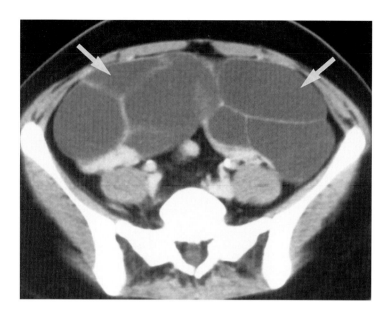

FIG. 2-35. Theca-lutein cysts. Note the large septated bilateral cysts *(arrows)* in a patient with a molar pregnancy.

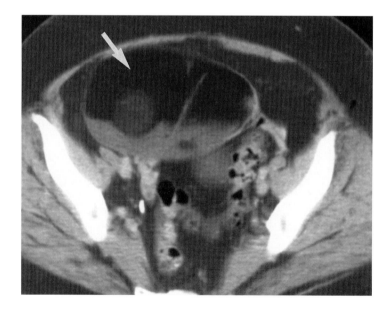

FIG. 2-36. Cystic teratoma. Note large right adnexal mass containing fat *(arrow)* of similar density as subcutaneous fat. At surgery a cystic teratoma was resected.

acteristic CT features to differentiate these lesions from primary or metastatic carcinoma; thus, patients with these lesions are almost always subjected to laparotomy (Fig. 2-36).

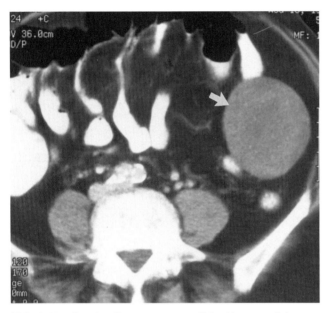

FIG. 2-37. Ovarian fibroma on a pedicle. Note a solid mass in the left hemipelvis *(arrow)*. At surgery a benign ovarian fibroma was noted on the long pedicle from the left ovary.

REFERENCES

1. Jeffrey RBJ, Federle MP, Tolentino CS. Periappendiceal inflammatory masses: CT-directed management and clinical outcome in 70 patients (published erratum appears in Radiology 1988;168:286). Radiology 1988;167:13.
2. Balthazar EJ, Megibow AJ, Siegel SE, Birnbaum BA. Appendicitis: prospective evaluation with high-resolution CT. Radiology 1991;180:21.
3. Balthazar EJ, Megibow AJ, Hulnick D, et al. CT of appendicitis. AJR 1986;147:705.
4. Hulnick DH, Megibow AJ, Balthazar EJ, et al. Computed tomography in the evaluation of diverticulitis. Radiology 1984;152:491.
5. Mueller PR, Saini S, Wittenburg J, et al. Sigmoid diverticular abscesses: percutaneous drainage as an adjunct to surgical resection in 24 cases. Radiology 1987;164:321.
6. Sawyer RW, Walsh JW. CT in gynecologic pelvic diseases. Semin Ultrasound CT MR 1988;9:122.
7. Wilbur A. Computed tomography of tuboovarian abscesses. J Comput Assist Tomogr 1990;14:625.
8. Wilbur AC, Goldstein LD, Prywitch BA. Hemorrhagic ovarian cysts in patients on anticoagulation therapy: CT findings. J Comput Assist Tomogr 1993;17:623.
9. Tyrrel RT, Murphy FB, Bernardino ME. Tubo-ovarian abscesses: CT-guided percutaneous drainage. Radiology 1990;175:87.
10. Casola G, vanSonnenberg E, D'Agostino HB, et al. Percutaneous drainage of tubo-ovarian abscesses. Radiology 1992;182:399.
11. Fishman EK, Scatarige JC, Saksouk FA, et al. Computed tomography of endometriosis. J Comput Assist Tomogr 1983;7:257.
12. Buy JN, Ghossain MA, Mark AS, et al. Focal hyperdense areas in endometriomas: a characteristic finding on CT. AJR 1992;159:769.
13. Kimura I, Togashi K, Kawakami S, et al. Ovarian torsion: CT and MR imaging appearances. Radiology 1994;190:337.
14. Montz FJ, Schlaerth JB, Morrow CP. The natural history of theca lutein cysts. Obstet Gynecol 1988;72:247.
15. Buy JN, Ghossain MA, Moss AA, et al. Cystic teratoma of the ovary: CT detection. Radiology 1989;171:697.

Clinical Gynecologic Imaging, edited
by Arthur C. Fleischer, Marcia C. Javitt,
R. Brooke Jeffrey, Jr., and Howard W. Jones III,
Lippincott-Raven Publishers, Philadelphia © 1997.

CHAPTER 3

Ovarian Cancer

Ovarian Cancer: Clinical Overview

Howard W. Jones, III, MD

Ovarian cancer is the most deadly of gynecologic malignancies. Although it is less common than cancer of the endometrium or cervical cancer, because of an overall survival rate of only about 35%, approximately 13,000 women will die of ovarian cancer in the United States this year. The age-specific incidence rate of ovarian cancer gradually rises, reaching a peak at about age 70, at which time it is 55 per 100,000 white women and somewhat lower among black women. It is estimated that approximately 1 in 70 women will develop ovarian cancer.

The cause of ovarian cancer is unknown. Except for some relatively uncommon familial tendencies and some rare genetic clustering of breast, colon, and ovary cancer, it has not been possible to identify any clinically useful high-risk groups for increased surveillance. Multiple pregnancies and the use of oral contraceptives may be protective because of decreased ovulation and hormonal influences.

DIAGNOSIS

Clinical Presentation

In its earliest stages, ovarian cancer is usually asymptomatic. The natural history of early ovarian cancer is largely unknown. The length of time from the earliest histopathologically recognizable changes in the ovary followed by ovarian enlargement and then diffuse intraabdominal spread is entirely unknown. Occasionally, an enlarged ovary is detected at the time of routine pelvic examination, or cancer may be discovered incidentally at the time of abdominal or pelvic surgery for other indications. In approximately 60% of cases, however, widespread intraabdominal metastases are present by the time the diagnosis is made. Symptoms of abdominal swelling, bloating, and pelvic fullness or pressure are common. It is not unusual for the patient to have had vague abdominal complaints or nonspecific gastrointestinal symptoms for months before the diagnosis. In some cases a workup has been entirely negative. The presenting complaint may be ascites or an abdominopelvic mass, which the patient herself has palpated. The presence of an irregular mass on pelvic examination or cul-de-sac nodularity accompanied by ascites is very suggestive of ovarian cancer. Other patients may present with malignant pleural effusions and shortness of breath.

Screening Tests

Because women with stage I ovarian cancer may have survival rates as high as 90%,[1] early diagnosis of ovarian cancer may offer a significant opportunity to improve survival rates in this deadly disease. Serum levels of the tumor associated antigen CA 125 and other tumor markers and transvaginal sonography have shown promise.[2,3] In the past, simple pelvic examination and cul-de-sac aspiration have been investigated with disappointing results. The relative rarity of ovarian cancer, combined with the nonspecific nature of the currently available screening tests, makes ovarian cancer screening unsatisfactory and not cost effective at the present time.[4]

Differential Diagnosis

A pelvic mass can be caused by either a benign or malignant tumor of the ovary or by inflammatory conditions, physiologic cysts, and malignancies of other pelvic organs and structures that may involve the ovary or may be adjacent to it. Initially, a careful history and physical examination is most helpful. In fertile women a pregnancy test should be done to rule out ectopic pregnancy. A careful contraceptive history is important because functional ovarian cysts, including both follicle cysts and corpus luteum cysts, are common in ovulating women. Inflammatory masses and endometriosis can be confused with ovarian cancer because pelvic examination may show an irregular pelvic mass with nodularity in the cul-de-sac with an elevated CA 125 level and a complex adnexal mass on sonography. In general, pelvic sonography is very helpful in the evaluation of pelvic masses because the dimensions and character of the mass as well as additional findings such as free pelvic fluid may be accurately determined. Smooth-walled, unilocular ovarian cysts are almost always benign, whereas malignancies are most commonly described as ''complex'' with both cystic and solid components. The additional finding of ascites is an ominous sign. Ureteral obstruction can occur but is relatively uncommon with ovarian cancer. In the older age group, diverticular abscesses and carcinoma of the colon must be considered within the differential diagnosis.

Once a complete history and physical examination has been completed and the size and character of the mass confirmed by sonography, several additional studies may be helpful. A barium enema evaluation or colonoscopy is al-most always indicated before surgery to rule out a primary lesion or secondary involvement of the colon. Abdominal and pelvic CT will further characterize the mass and may identify upper abdominal disease, such as omental masses, aortic lymph node involvement, or liver metastases. Renal function and the possibility of ureteral obstruction can also be assessed, and the rare primary carcinoma of the pancreas can be identified.

A chest radiograph to evaluate the possibility of pleural effusion or pulmonary metastasis should also be done, but additional studies such as brain scans, bone scans, and so on should generally be reserved for patients whose symptoms or physical findings suggest involvement of the areas to be studied. Routine preoperative blood tests should be done, and a blood sample for evaluation of CA 125 should be drawn. Tests of additional tumor markers such as carcinoembryonic antigen, α-fetoprotein, β-human chorionic gonadotropin, and others should be considered and obtained when indicated.

PATHOLOGY

Four types of ovarian cancer require separate consideration because of their clinical characteristics and varying prognoses. The common epithelial tumors of the ovary include the serous, mucinous, endometrioid, clear cell, and otherwise unspecified adenocarcinomas. These tumors account for almost 90% of ovarian cancers and are commonly found in postmenopausal women. Germ cell tumors, which arise from the totipotent oocytes, are usually benign. The most common is a benign cystic teratoma (dermoid cyst). These tumors often occur in young woman and are almost always unilateral. When malignant (eg, dysgerminoma, teratoma), they are highly aggressive but very responsive to combination chemotherapy, which is curative in many instances. The ovarian stromal tumors are generally low grade; and because they arise from the granulosa, theca, and Sertoli-Leydig cells of the ovary, they may be hormonally functioning. They are usually unilateral and may occur in any age group but most typically in the fourth and fifth decades. Surgical excision alone may be the only therapy required, but combination chemotherapy is effective for metastatic or recurrent disease. Malignancies of other sites that are metastatic to the ovary must always be considered in the evaluation of patients with a pelvic mass. In some cases a pelvic mass is the first indication of a primary gastrointestinal or endometrial carcinoma. Breast cancer also commonly metastasizes to the ovary.

TREATMENT

Surgery

Surgery for ovarian cancer is both diagnostic and therapeutic. If the pelvic mass in question turns out to be ovarian carcinoma, tumor debulking, including total abdominal hysterectomy and bilateral salpingo-oophorectomy, if possible, should be done. Frozen section pathologic confirmation of the diagnosis is routinely done. Ovarian cancer is surgically staged, and a sample of the ascites or pelvic and abdominal washings is sent for cytologic evaluation.[5] In patients with early disease, biopsy of the omentum, diaphragm, and paraaortic nodes and careful evaluation of the small bowel and mesentery are necessary for accurate staging. When unilateral oophorectomy is being considered in the young woman with stage I disease who wishes to retain her fertility, very careful inspection of the remaining ovary is indicated but biopsy may not be necessary. When metastatic disease is present, aggressive tumor debulking, even when all cancer cannot be removed, improves the length and quality of survival.[6] Occasionally, this surgery will involve bowel resection or procedures involving the urinary tract. If possible, this initial surgery should be done by a gynecologic oncologist whose special training and experience provides optimal surgical and postoperative management.

The goal of the initial operation for ovarian cancer is twofold. First, accurate staging of the tumor and complete histopathologic evaluation is possible only by exploratory laparotomy with multiple biopsies (Table 3-1). Second, the therapeutic goal should be to remove all tumor, if possible, to provide the greatest possibility of cure. In approximately two thirds of patients, however, widespread intraabdominal metastases prevent complete surgical debulking. In addition to the stage of disease, the volume of residual tumor after initial surgery, the histologic type of residual tumor after initial surgery, the histologic type and grade of the tumor, and the age of the patient have important prognostic significance. Women with minimal residual disease and well-differentiated tumors have the most favorable outcome, whereas those younger than age 50 and those with tumors exhibiting mucinous and endometrioid histology also seem to do better. Careful staging evaluation with peritoneal cytology and multiple biopsies of the upper abdomen is especially important in early disease because microscopic metastases often escape clinical detection.

Accurate surgical staging provides the basis for the most appropriate postoperative treatment. Patients with stage IA well-differentiated epithelial ovarian cancers may not require any additional therapy, whereas patients with more advanced disease are routinely treated with combination chemotherapy. In patients with advanced disease, aggressive surgical debulking includes bowel resection or colostomy in as many 25% of patients. It is still controversial as to whether such extensive surgical resection actually improves 5- to 10-year survival rates. It is agreed, however, that optimal tumor debulking (<1 cm residual) results in prolonged, good quality survival.[6] This is where the skills and experienced judgment of the gynecologic oncologist are most important.

TABLE 3-1. *Definitions of the stages in primary carcinoma of the ovary**

Stage	Description
I	Growth limited to the ovaries.
Ia	Growth limited to one ovary; no ascites. No tumor on the external surface; capsule intact.
Ib	Growth limited to both ovaries; no ascites. No tumor on the external surfaces; capsules intact.
Ic	Tumor either stage Ia or Ib, but with tumor on surface of one or both ovaries; or with capsule ruptured; or with ascites present containing malignant cells or with positive peritoneal washings.
II	Growth involving one or both ovaries with pelvic extension.
IIa	Extension and/or metastases to the uterus and/or tubes.
IIb	Extension to other pelvic tissues.
IIc	Tumor either stage IIa or IIb, but with tumor on surface of one or both ovaries; or with capsule(s) ruptured; or with ascites present containing malignant cells or with positive peritoneal washings.
III	Tumor involving one or both ovaries with peritoneal implants outside the pelvis and/or positive retroperitoneal or inguinal nodes. Superficial liver metastasis equals stage III. Tumor is limited to the true pelvis but with histologically proven malignant extension to small bowel or omentum.
IIIa	Tumor grossly limited to the true pelvis with negative nodes but with histologically confirmed microscopic seeding of abdominal peritoneal surfaces.
IIIb	Tumor involving one or both ovaries with histologically confirmed implants of abdominal peritoneal surfaces none exceeding 2 cm in diameter. Nodes are negative.
IIIc	Abdominal implants greater than 2 cm in diameter and/or positive retroperitoneal or inguinal nodes.
IV	Growth involving one or both ovaries with distant metastases. If pleural effusion is present there must be positive cytology to allot a case to stage IV. Parenchymal liver metastasis equals stage IV.

* Nomenclature of the International Federation of Gynecology and Obstetrics (FIGO). Staging is based on findings at clinical examination and surgical exploration.

Chemotherapy

Most patients with ovarian cancer require postoperative chemotherapy. Cisplatin, the cornerstone of most regimens, is usually given in combination with other agents such as cyclophosphamide, doxorubicin, altretamine, or etoposide.[7] Carboplatin, which is an analogue of cisplatin with few renal and neurologic side effects, is being more commonly used, and ifosfamide is another agent with activity in ovarian cancer. Most patients are treated with intermittent intravenous therapy at 3- to 4-week intervals for six treatment cycles, but some centers use intraperitoneal chemotherapy instead.[8] Response rates of 60% to 80% are reported, but only 20% to 30% of this treatment group experiences a complete resolution with normalization of clinical, radiologic, and immunologic testing.

Radiation Therapy

Postoperative external radiation therapy to the whole abdomen is probably equally as effective as chemotherapy for patients with minimal residual tumor.[9] The toxicity of such therapy, especially gastrointestinal effects such as obstruction, has usually been more severe than that associated with chemotherapy, and, for that reason, most oncologists prefer chemotherapy. The definition of "minimal residual" disease is also controversial.

Intraperitoneal radioactive colloidal chromic phosphate has also been used to treat some women with stage I or II disease when no gross residual tumor remains after surgery. Only patients with very early disease are good candidates for this therapy, which requires complete and uniform intraperitoneal distribution of the radioactive suspension.

"Second-Look" Surgery

A planned re-exploration of patients to evaluate the extent of disease after chemotherapy and to resect any residual malignancy has been called "second-look" surgery. This approach allows an excellent opportunity to evaluate the effect of primary therapy and has proven to be an invaluable asset for research, but it has not proven to be of significant clinical benefit to patients with ovarian cancer. Measurement of tumor-associated antigens such as CA 125 used in conjunction with periodic physical examinations and selected radiographic studies has been helpful in monitoring the disease status of treated patients. Until more effective therapy is available, second-look surgery in the asymptomatic patient with a normal physical examination is probably indicated only as a research procedure in patients on specified investigative protocols.

Treatment of Recurrent and Metastatic Disease

Because the overall survival of patients with ovarian cancer is only about 30%, the majority of patients develop progressive recurrent disease despite appropriate primary therapy. Salvage chemotherapy results in a 10% to 15% response rate, which is usually partial and short term. Widespread intraabdominal metastases with bowel obstruction are frequent, but reoperation with resection, bypass, or enterostomy may provide significant palliation. Pleural effusion may require thoracentesis, and pleural sclerosis with the relative effectiveness of prolonged disease-free intervals and relatively long-term survival is not uncommon, but some patients may survive only to develop metastatic cancer to such unusual sites as liver, brain, and meninges. Localized radiation and occasionally surgery have been helpful in some of these patients.

TABLE 3-2. *Carcinoma of the ovary: distribution by stage and 3- and 5-year survival in the different stages*

Stage	Patients treated No.	Patients treated %	3-Year survival (%)	5-Year survival (%)
I	2230	26.1	79.8	72.8
II	1313	15.4	60.5	46.3
III	3330	39.1	27.1	18.6
IV	1391	16.3	10.1	4.8
Unstaged	268	3.1	31.7	21.6
Total	8541	100.0	43.4	34.9

Data from Pettersson F, ed. Annual report on the results of treatment in gynecological cancer, vol 20. Stockholm, Panorama Press, 1988. The annual report is published at regular intervals by the International Federation for Gynecology and Obstetrics and contains vast quantities of statistics generated from institutions that submit their treatment results from throughout the world.

PROGNOSIS

Despite improvements in diagnosis and therapy, the long-term survival rates in patients treated for epithelial ovarian cancer are still disappointing (Table 3-2). Because of the advanced stage of disease at the time of diagnosis, survival is poor. Whereas the majority of women with advanced disease live 2 years with a reasonable quality of life, recurrent cancer eventually becomes symptomatic in most, and by 5 years only 35% still survive. In view of the significantly better survival with early stage disease, efforts to develop methods for early detection of ovarian cancer should be emphasized.

REFERENCES

1. Young RC, Walton LA, Ellenberg SS, et al. Adjuvant therapy in stage I and stage II epithelial ovarian cancer: results of two prospective randomized trials. N Engl J Med 1990;322:1021.
2. Zurawski VR, Sjovall K, Schoenfeld DA, et al. Prospective evaluation of serum CA 125 levels in a normal population: I. The specificities of single and serial determinations in testing for ovarian cancer. Gynecol Oncol 1990;36:299.
3. Bourne TH, Whitehead MI, Campbell S, et al. Ultrasound screening for familial ovarian cancer. Gynecol Oncol 1991;43:92.
4. Creasman WT, DiSaia PJ: Screening in ovarian cancer. Am J Obstet Gynecol 1991;165:7.
5. Buchsbauma HJ, Brady MF, Delgado G, et al. Surgical staging of carcinoma of the ovaries. Surg Gynecol Obstet 1989;169:226.
6. Williams L, Hoskins WJ. Can cytoreductive surgery aid ovarian cancer survival? Contemp Obstet Gynecol 1990;35:13.
7. Sutton GP, Stehman FB, Einhorn LH, et al. Ten-year follow up of patients receiving cisplatin, doxorubicin, and cyclophosphamide chemotherapy for advanced epithelial ovarian carcinoma. J Clin Oncol 1989;7:223.
8. Markman M, Berek JS, Blessing JA, et al. Characteristics of patients with small-volume residual ovarian cancer unresponsive to cisplatin-based ip chemotherapy: Lessons learned from a Gynecologic Oncology Group Phase II trial of ip cisplatin and recombinant α-interferon. Gynecol Oncol 1992;45:1.
9. Sell A, Bertelsen K, Andersen JE, et al. Randomized study of whole abdomen irradiation versus pelvic irradiation plus cyclophosphamide in treatment of early ovarian cancer. Gynecol Oncol 1990;37:369.

Early Detection of Ovarian Cancer With Transvaginal Sonography

Arthur C. Fleischer, MD and Howard W. Jones, III, MD

The increased use of transvaginal sonography with or without color Doppler capabilities affords early detection of ovarian carcinoma when incorporated into a screening program based on identification of women at risk. MRI and spiral CT have an important role in staging and detection of recurrences. This subchapter emphasizes the potentials and limitations of transvaginal sonography with and without color Doppler capabilities for the detection of ovarian cancer. Both practical and theoretical considerations are presented.

EPIDEMIOLOGY AND RISK FACTORS

In 1993 there were some 13,000 deaths from carcinoma of the ovary in the United States, making it the fourth leading cause of death due to cancer in women.[1] This represents a death rate due to ovarian carcinoma that is greater than that of cervical and endometrial malignancies combined. Although transvaginal sonography can detect morphologic abnormality within an ovary, its specificity is limited.[2] The adjunctive use of color Doppler sonography improves the specificity and sensitivity of transvaginal sonography. However, the relatively low incidence and high screening costs seem to limit the efficacy of transvaginal sonography to be used in only those women with risk factors.

Ovarian carcinoma is a "silent" killer and comprises approximately 25% of all gynecologic malignancies.[1] Although there have been several recent advances in the treatment and management of this disease, the overall 5-year survival rate for ovarian carcinoma remains low, at 39%. This is primarily a reflection of the advanced stage of the disease when it is initially detected, because over 75% of newly diagnosed cases are already stage III or IV (spread beyond the ovarian capsule).

The actual incidence of ovarian carcinoma demonstrates significant geographic variability. The incidence is relatively low in Japan, where the rate is 3.1 per 100,000 women, contrasted to Sweden, where it is 21 per 100,000 women. In this country, it is 33 per 100,000 women over the age of 50.[3] Some of these differences may be explained on the basis of a difference in age distribution of women in the various populations. For example, the worldwide peak age of 60 to 70 years for developing ovarian carcinoma contrasts to that in Japan, where the peak is earlier, around age 50. Clearly, the chance of developing ovarian carcinoma is age related. In western countries there is increasing risk after the age of 50, and it continues to rise without a plateau.[4] The average age of initial presentation of women with ovarian carcinoma is 57.

For most patients (approximately 90%) with epithelial ovarian carcinoma, there is no definable genetic predisposition to the development of this neoplasm. However, there are a few families in which the risk of cancer is so high that it appears to be transmitted as an autosomal dominant trait with variable expressivity.[3] These women had a familial history of breast or ovarian cancer or both and tend to get this disease 10 to 15 years earlier than most women with a nonhereditary type. Other tumors that may be associated with increased risk for ovarian carcinoma include carcinoma of the breast, colon, and endometrium. The Lynch type II group of tumors consists of nonpolyposis colonic cancer, endometrial cancer, and ovarian cancer. These may be related to each other through a similar chromosome (17) that disinhibits a particular gene involved in expression of tumor-promoting agents. Identification of this gene locus seems imminent, owing to its proximity to the one associated with breast cancer.

In approximately 10% of women with ovarian carcinoma, a genetic predisposition can be traced. The lifetime risk of ovarian carcinoma for the general population (1 in 70) increases significantly, with one (1 in 20) or two (1 in 14) affected first- or second-degree relatives. Women affected with site-specific ovarian cancer syndrome tend to be affected younger (34–40 years old) than other women with noninheritable ovarian carcinoma.[5] Another established epidemiologic fact is that, when compared with controls, the risk of ovarian carcinoma seems to be highest in single women who have not borne children.[3] However, why pregnancy and oral contraceptives "protect" against developing ovarian carcinoma is unclear. There is significant evidence in animal studies to support the notion that the chance of developing ovarian carcinoma is related to the number of ovulatory events during a woman's childbearing years. Perhaps this is a reflection of a relative increased incidence of ovarian carcinoma with increased frequency of ovulation. This also may indicate that there is a relationship between epithelial (germinal) inclusion cysts, ovulation, and the relative incidence of developing epithelial ovarian neoplasms.[6,7] Indeed, it has been shown that some benign cystic epithelial tumors contain molecular genetic changes seen in ovarian malignancies.[7]

There seems to be an association between ovarian carcinoma and breast carcinoma.[3] Women who have had carcinoma of the breast have twice the expected risk of subsequently developing a separate primary neoplasm in the ovary; women who have had ovarian carcinoma are three to four times as likely as matched controls to develop a separate breast carcinoma. Even though epithelial neoplasms comprise the majority of ovarian tumors (up to 65%), metastases to the ovaries represent up to 20% of all ovarian tumors in some series.[8] Primary lesions are usually from breast and colonic tumors.

There have been several studies that evaluated the possibility that environmental factors play a role in eventual development of ovarian carcinoma. Some theorize that the open peritoneal cavity in the female serves as a passageway for carcinogens and oncogenic viruses.[3] One theory postulates that some cases of ovarian carcinoma arise from totipotential rest cells that line the peritoneum and become malignant by dedifferentiation.[3] This is based on the observation that some patients may have extensive peritoneal disease without evidence of an ovarian tumor.

Studies have indicated a slightly increased risk of ovarian cancer in women with infertility who used fertility medications (eg, clomiphene [Clomid]),[9] whereas tubal ligation and hysterectomy were associated with reduced risk.[10] It is possible that the ovaries of some of the infertility patients harbored undiagnosed cancer before ovulation induction. On the other hand, it can be hypothesized that the induced ovulations might contribute to increased risk of developing ovarian carcinoma.

The risk factors that seem to be most closely associated with ovarian cancer include a family history of ovarian, breast, endometrial, or colonic tumors (Table 3-3).[11] It is thought that these patients should be offered ovarian cancer

screening with CA 125 and transvaginal sonography. Currently, the National Cancer Institute has supported a randomized trial of CA 125 and transvaginal sonography for the detection of ovarian cancer as part of an overall screening test for early detection of lung, colorectal, and ovarian cancer in women.[12]

The recent identification of a breast cancer gene mutation (BRCA1) has enhanced detection in women who are at greater risk for the development of ovarian cancer. The presence of the BRCA1 mutation confers a 30% lifetime risk for the development of ovarian cancer by age 60 years.[12a] Continued refinement of genetic marker identification will improve the efficacy of sonographic early detection schemes, because it can be used to better identify a group of women at greater risk who require more intense evaluation.

NATURAL HISTORY OF OVARIAN CANCER

Unfortunately, ovarian cancer is a "silent" killer. Approximately three fourths of the cases initially present as advanced disease (stages III or IV). Nonspecific symptoms such as moderate discomfort or occasional pelvoabdominal pain are among the most common presenting symptoms. Constipation or urinary frequency are also common presenting complaints. Some patients complain of early satiety. Ascites is a relatively common presenting finding. In addition, affected women may occasionally present with hypercalcemia. It has been proposed that some ovarian carcinomas can produce a parathyroid-like substance causing a paraneoplastic syndrome.[3]

On the other hand, 5-year survival in localized ovarian carcinoma is excellent, in the 70% to 90% range. Furthermore, it has been calculated that mortality for ovarian carcinoma could be halved if the percentage of initial detection of stage I cancers was increased from 20% to 80%.[13]

One theory regarding the development of ovarian carcinoma proposes that it arises from totipotential cells that cover the coelomic peritoneum.[6] For some unknown reason, they can become embedded within the ovarian stroma and undergo malignant transformation.

Metastatic spread to the peritoneal and omental surfaces usually occurs after extension of the tumor beyond the capsule. Ascites may be secondary to the peritoneal implants or due to the effect of the implants on the adjacent normal peritoneum or the result of obstruction of the transdiaphragmatic drainage of lymph. Intraperitoneal fluid can also be secondary to hepatic or cardiorenal disease, as well as to peritonitis secondary to peritoneal metastases. If ascites is present, paracentesis may be necessary to allow for proper palpation of the masses created by ovarian carcinoma. Microscopic examination of the centrifuged ascitic fluid may show malignant cells. Even at the time of surgery, the exact nature of an ovarian tumor may be uncertain and, in some cases, a frozen section may be helpful. Removal of the entire tumor rather than resection of a focal area of the mass facilitates its gross pathologic evaluation and the eventual therapeutic management of the patient. In a large number of cases,

TABLE 3-3. *Ovarian cancer risk*

Risk factors	Lifetime risk (%)
General population	1.4
Family history of ovarian cancer	
Two first-degree relatives*	39.1
One first-degree relative	4.5
One second-degree relative†	2.9
Nulliparity	2.0
Perineal talc exposure	2.0
Infertility	2.0
High-fat diet	2.0
Previous breast cancer	2.0

  * First-degree relative: mother, daughter, sister.
  † Second-degree relative: grandmother, aunt.

Data from Piver MS, Recio FO. Ovarian cancer: who needs screening? Patient Care 1993 (Dec 15):27.

the malignant nature of the ovarian tumor is not suspected before surgery and often not until pathologic examination.[3] In many cases, however, a preoperative diagnosis of ovarian carcinoma is made chiefly on palpation of a pelvic mass in a postmenopausal woman with or without a fluid wave. The vaginal smear may rarely demonstrate exfoliated tumor cells, and other cases may rarely have a shift in the estrogenic maturation index. Infrequently, the patient with ovarian carcinoma may first present with thrombophlebitis due to the proximity of the tumor to the larger pelvic veins.

In some, a mass or fluid wave can be detected on physical examination. In others, no apparent mass can be felt. We have seen large (greater than 10 cm) tumors that were not detected by palpation or suspected clinically before their sonographic demonstration.

Epithelial tumors of the ovary, because of their mode of extension, defy the usual "en bloc" approach that is traditional for the management of cervical and uterine cancer. Once outside the ovary, the tumor is frequently widespread throughout the peritoneal cavity. In fact, at the time of initial diagnosis, approximately 65% of all the epithelial malignancies have progressed to stage III or IV (disease outside the true pelvis). It is presumed that the route of malignant spread of ovarian carcinoma is by peritoneal implantation or subperitoneal lymphatic extension or both. One theory postulates that some form of ovarian carcinoma arises from totipotential cells that dedifferentiate the entire abdomen after being subjected to a "field effect" from some carcinogen-causing multiple primary lesions.[7]

Although the primary means of tumor spread in ovarian carcinoma is mainly along the peritoneal surface, it is noted that in 10% to 20% of stage I and II cases, disease has extended into the paraaortic lymph nodes. In addition, it is not uncommon to find at initial exploration of what was thought to be relatively early disease that there is microscopic and macroscopic disease on the abdominal surface of the hemidiaphragms. At present, there is no established imaging procedure that accurately detects these small miliary-like metastases.[15]

Clearly, the prognosis of ovarian carcinoma is related to the stage of disease at initial presentation. Differences in the behavior of the various histologic grades of ovarian carcinoma may also influence long-term survival. It has been stated that the histologic grade of the tumor and the size of the largest individual mass after primary operation are the only statistically significant factors relative to survivorship.[3]

ROLE OF SONOGRAPHY (BOTH TRANSVESICULAR AND TRANSVAGINAL WITH AND WITHOUT COLOR DOPPLER)

A few large-scale studies have evaluated the role of sonography in early detection of ovarian cancer. In one ongoing study first reported in 1983, which used transabdominal real-time sonography for the study of 1083 women, approximately 3% of the screened population were found to have an adnexal mass and a third of these masses were ovarian carcinoma.[16] A more recent update to this study reported the results of screening more than 5000 women. Nine ovarian carcinomas were detected with transabdominal sonography; five were primary tumors, and four were metastasis. Interestingly enough, all of the primary tumors detected were confined to the ovary (stage I). This shows that transvesicular (scans performed through a fully distended bladder) and transvaginal imaging is capable of detection of even those ovarian neoplasms that are contained in normal to minimally enlarged ovaries.[17] However, for each ovarian tumor found, approximately 60 patients underwent surgery.

A similar study by Andolf and colleagues[18] indicated that sonography could detect ovarian carcinoma in a screened population of asymptomatic women. In this study of over 800 patients who were at risk for ovarian carcinoma due to age, 39 masses (5% of the screened population) were found and 35 of these were abnormal. In 24 patients, ovarian epithelial tumors were found, 8 of which were not palpated before the sonographic study.

In an ongoing study that used transvaginal scanning, van Nagell and co-workers[13] have shown that transvaginal sonography is an accurate means for early detection of ovarian cancer, even though several benign tumors will be detected for every carcinoma found. It has been postulated, however, that up to 15% of benign tumors have the potential for malignant transformation; therefore, their detection and treatment is clinically efficacious.[7] In an update to this study these investigators reported three ovarian carcinomas in 2600 asymptomatic women older than 40.[19]

The small size and location of the typical postmenopausal ovary may make it difficult to image sonographically. The ovary in the postmenopausal woman averages less than 1.5 cm (>3 mL volume) and very frequently is located adjacent to bowel.[19] Factors that may increase the volume of the ovary in postmenopausal women include multiparity, obesity, or hormonal replacement treatment. Transvesical scans may be helpful by identifying the ovary by its surrounding vessels (ie, internal iliac vein and artery). Care should be used if the ovary is not identified by transvaginal sonography because a highly confident diagnosis of normalcy cannot be made based on nonvisualization of the ovary. Transvaginal sonography may be limited in some postmenopausal women owing to the small size of the vagina, hindering sonographic accessibility to the ovary. Transvaginal sonographic depiction of the ovary may be further compromised if the woman has undergone hysterectomy, because the ovaries are not supported by the normal ligaments and are allowed to be located anywhere in the lower pelvis or abdomen.

It is important to attempt to image the ovaries in postmenopausal women with transvesicular approaches if they cannot be seen with transvaginal sonography. In our experience with 33 older postmenopausal (60 to 80 years of age) patients scanned before transabdominal hysterectomy and bilateral salpingo-oophorectomy for endometrial carcinoma, only about 60% of "normal" postmenopausal ovaries can be identified.[20] Some studies have considered the lack of identification of an adnexal mass in proximity to normal pelvic vessels around the expected position of ovaries as evidence of normalcy. We do not consider this "diagnosis of exclusion" an acceptable concept for early detection of ovarian carcinoma because tumors in their earliest stages may only minimally enlarge the ovary.[21] In our study that evaluated the ability to delineate normal postmenopausal ovaries in women undergoing hysterectomy and bilateral salpingo-oophorectomy for endometrial cancer, we found that only about 60% of normal postmenopausal ovaries could be delineated preoperatively. This factor may limit the accuracy of identifying early tumors as textural abnormalities within normal-sized ovaries. In addition, some small solid tumors (0.5 to 2.5 cm) were missed. All of these were benign. In a study that evaluated 150 masses in postmenopausal women without regard to their sonographic features, the authors found that of masses less than 5 cm in size, only 3% were malignant.[22] Several studies have shown that the incidence of malignancy in completely cystic masses in this age group is exceedingly low (less than 1% to 2%).[23–25] Sonographic findings that are highly suggestive of malignancy include demonstration of papillary excrescences, omental or peritoneal masses, liver metastases, ruptured capsules, pseudomyxoma peritonei, and intraperitoneal fluid (Fig. 3-1).[26]

The goal of any attempts to detect ovarian cancer should emphasize its early detection before the development of metastatic disease. This may entail the use of transvaginally guided biopsy or aspiration. However, there remains a healthy reluctance to perform aspiration on a potentially malignant lesion because of the possibility of its later intraperi-

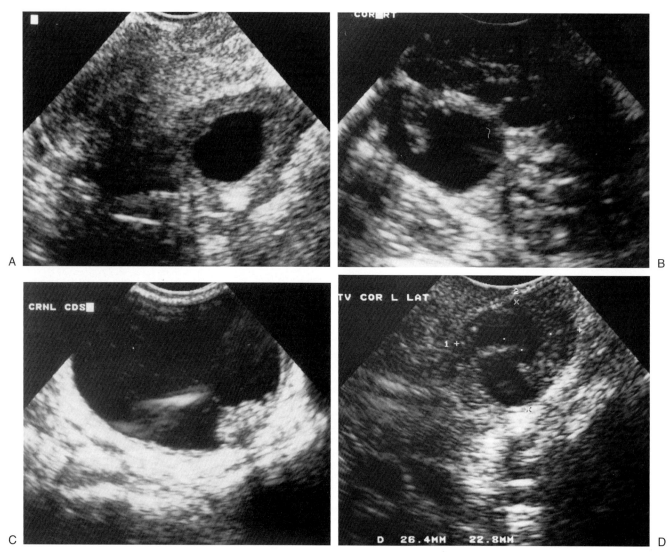

FIG. 3-1. Transvaginal sonographic features suggestive of malignancy. **(A)** A 2-cm cystic mass with a thick and irregular wall within a slightly enlarged ovary was found to represent an ovarian carcinoma. The transvaginal sonographic findings in ovarian carcinoma range from subtle changes to obvious abnormalities. **(B)** A 3-cm cystic mass containing a papillary projection was found on histologic examination to be a cystadenofibroma. **(C)** This 4-cm predominantly cystic mass with a broad-based papillary excrescence is an ovarian carcinoma. **(D)** A normal-sized ovary had two irregularly shaped cystic areas that turned out to be stage I ovarian carcinoma.

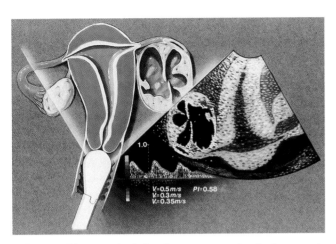

FIG. 3-2. Diagram depicting the components of a transvaginal color Doppler sonogram. The triplex image consists of a transvaginal sonogram with a duplex Doppler interrogation of vessels as depicted on color Doppler sonography.

The rationale of using transvaginal sonography over CA 125 as an entry test to screening was substantiated in published studies of Bourne and Jacobs and their associates.[30,31] Bournes' group studied 1600 women with a familial history of ovarian carcinoma and found a higher percentage of early-stage ovarian carcinomas than Jacobs and co-workers, who used CA 125 as the initial study.[30]

It seems clear that the goal of transvaginal sonography should be identification of ovarian tumors in ovaries that are not significantly enlarged. It is also clear that for every malignancy detected, several benign masses will be found. Several studies have shown that transvaginal color Doppler sonography can be used to distinguish benign from malignant masses (Figs. 3-2 and 3-3).[32,33]

In fact, transvaginal color Doppler sonography seems to be very sensitive in the detection of stage I ovarian carcinoma, possibly owing to the necessity of neovascularity to support tumor growth (Table 3-4).[22,34–50] Transvaginal color Doppler sonography seems to be best used as an adjunct combination of transvaginal sonography. The morphologic features of a pelvic mass with its color Doppler sonographic findings seems to afford the greatest sensitivity and specificity, with combined accuracies reaching 100% in some studies.[33] Problems limiting the use of transvaginal color Doppler imaging include its operator dependence and the lack of standard criteria in distinguishing benign from malignant waveforms. Specifically, a definite cutoff value for impedance of benign versus malignant lesions varies from study to study and equipment utilization. In general, malignancies demonstrate low impedance flow in areas of tumor growth. The improvement of power Doppler may allow characterization of flow patterns between benign and malignant lesions.

toneal spread. There have been no reports of tumor tracking after inadvertent aspiration of an ovarian malignancy. There have been two cases of tumor tracking in the abdominal trocar site in women who underwent laparoscopic resection of unsuspected ovarian malignancies.[27]

A study from England in 41 asymptomatic women reported detection of three ovarian carcinomas as well as a number of unsuspected endometrial disorders.[28] Depending on the inclusion criteria, most studies have found between 250 to 3000, or 0.25% to 0.03%, of the screened population to be abnormal. The incidence of ovarian carcinoma detected in patients studied varies from 1 in 250 in a familial history of ovarian carcinoma to 1 in 3000 in an asymptomatic population of women with risk factors.[13,29]

TABLE 3-4. *Transvaginal color Doppler sonography: reported series*

Source	No. of patients	True positive (% malignancies with low impedance)	False positive (% benign with low impedance)	No. of patients with stage 1 cancer
Bourne et al, 1989[35]	50	88	2	3
Fleischer et al, 1991[36]	63	87	7	7
Weiner et al, 1992[37]	24	94	3	5
Kawai et al, 1992[38]	24	100	0	4
Kurjak and Predanic, 1992[39]	628	100	0.2	16
Natori et al, 1992[40]	30	80	20	2
Tekay and Jouppila, 1993[41]	72	75	23	1
Timor-Tritsch et al, 1993[42]	115	94	62	3
Hamper et al, 1993[43]	67	92	6	?
Schneider et al, 1993[44]	55	87	6	?
Valentin et al, 1993[45]	149	80	20	?
Bromley et al, 1993[46]	33	68	34	7
Brown et al, 1994[47]	14	92	8	?
Levine et al, 1994[48]	34	80	20	?
Carter et al, 1994[49]	80	85	15	?
Jain, 1994[50]	50	80	20	?
Fleischer and Jones, 1994[21]	126	84	16	17

* RI < 0.4; PI < 1.0

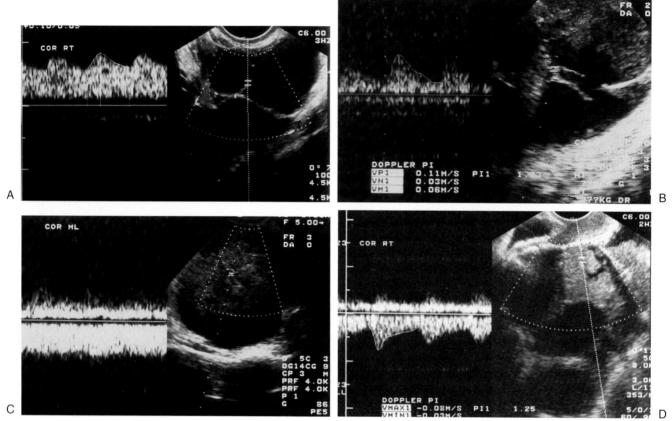

FIG. 3-3. Transvaginal color doppler sonographic features suggestive of malignancy. **(A)** Low impedance (PI = 0.3) flow within a septal vessel. This was a borderline mucinous cystadenocarcinoma. **(B)** Intermediate impedance flow within a tubal vessel surrounding an irregular solid ovarian mass. This ovarian carcinoma extended into the left fallopian tube. **(C)** This 5-cm predominantly solid lesion with low impedance flow is a papillary serous cystadenocarcinoma. **(D)** Intermediate impedance flow (PI = 1.25) within an irregularly solid area of an ovarian mass.

COMBINED SCREENING AND TESTING PROTOCOLS

Transvaginal sonography should be one of several screening tests used for early detection of ovarian carcinoma. In practical terms, a screening test should be more sensitive than it is specific. Transvaginal sonography could be used effectively as a secondary means to differentiate patients with true serum screening tests versus those with false-positive tests.

Today, carcinoma of the cervix is screened effectively by evaluation of exfoliated cells of the cervix taken in a Papanicolaou smear. Not only can noninvasive cervical cancer be detected with this test but the precursors to this neoplasm can also be found. Because the incidence of ovarian carcinoma is higher than carcinoma of the cervix, it seems logical that screening for ovarian carcinoma could be medically indicated. Some practical problems with this include patient reluctance to submit to a transvaginal study and primary physicians who may not be insistent in recommending the study to their patients. However, the transvaginal ultrasound study is clearly less anxiety provoking than sigmoid-oscopy, which is currently a recommended screening procedure for detection of cancer of the rectum.[51] A number of taggable antibodies used in both serum and imaging are under investigation for early detection of CaO. One of these, CA 125, has been shown to be an accurate means for detection of recurrent tumors in women with known ovarian carcinoma.[17] It seems to be most sensitive in nonmucinous tumors.[52] For example, one case report does describe its use in detection of ovarian carcinoma when a sonogram showed a 2 × 3-cm ovary that was nonpalpable.[28] However, its poor sensitivity of only 46% in one series and 50% positive in stage I ovarian carcinoma substantially limits its use as the only screening test for early detection of this tumor.[53]

In a study involving 102 patients, the relative sensitivity and specificity of pelvic examination, CA 125, and routine transabdominal sonography were compared. The relative accuracy of transabdominal sonography and CA 125 were comparable, indicating that when results are abnormal these tests can be additive and complementary.[54] It is clear that an elevated CA 125 level in association with an abnormal sonographic finding is highly indicative of ovarian malignancy.

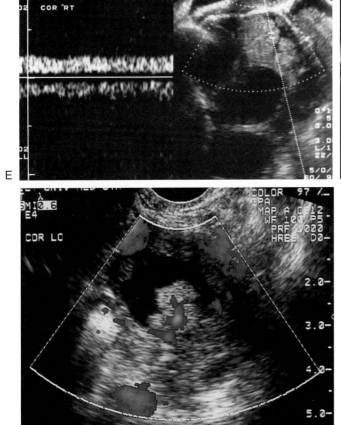

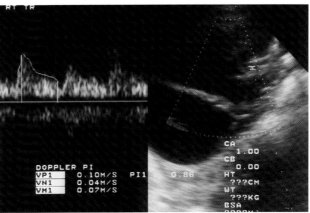

FIG. 3-3. *Continued.* **(E)** Increased venous flow within solid area of same mass as in **D. (F)** Low impedance flow within papillary excrescence. This was a borderline tumor. **(G)** Amplitude transvaginal color Doppler sonogram shows vessel within papillary excrescence of a borderline ovarian carcinoma.

In a study of 1010 postmenopausal women in England, the combination of CA 125, pelvic examination, and transabdominal sonography was found to be nearly 99% specific.[14] These findings indicated that, although no single screening test had an acceptable specificity for ovarian carcinoma, the combination of tests achieved acceptable specificity and is the best hope for a specific and sensitive method for early detection.[14]

Several studies have shown the efficacy of transvaginal sonography in screening for ovarian carcinoma in women with tumor risk factors. One study of 1600 women with a familial history of ovarian carcinoma detected 11 cases, most of which were stage I.[55]

Other studies have used CA 125 as a screen for further evaluation with ultrasound. In one study involving 22,000 women screened with CA 125, seven ovarian carcinomas were found, but most were of an advanced stage.[56] Similarly, in a study involving CA 125 in 5,000 women as a screen, only six ovarian carcinomas were found; and only two were stage I.[57] Some controversy exists as to what the appropriate CA 125 value is that should be make one suspect ovarian carcinoma.[53]

Several institutions continue to examine the efficacy of screening for ovarian carcinoma with transvaginal sonography in populations who are at risk for ovarian carcinoma. Risk factors have been broadened to include women with close relatives with a documented history of breast, colon, or endometrial cancer. In one study in which women with a history of breast cancer were studied, the true positive percentage was increased from 25% to 60% when transvaginal color Doppler sonography was used as an adjunct to transvaginal sonography.[58] The odds ratio of surgery for ovarian carcinoma increased from 9:1 to 2:3, indicating that the addition of transvaginal color Doppler imaging improved the efficacy of surgical exploration for patients with an adnexal mass.

When evaluation for ovarian carcinoma is combined with the detection of endometrial carcinoma, a study involving 5000 asymptomatic women has shown that two cancers may be detected for every 1000 women screened.[59] The majority of tumors were early-stage cancers. This pickup rate is comparable to the role of breast carcinoma detection in asymptomatic women by mammography. It therefore seems logical that a postmenopausal woman desiring a health check-up should undergo transvaginal sonography as well as mammography.

TABLE 3-5. *Screening for gynecologic cancer*

Tissue	Prevalence (1991)	Deaths/Year	Significant disease/1000	Cancer/1000	Screening method
Cervix	13,000	4,500	19	5	Papanicolaou smear
Breast	175,000	44,500	16	5	Mammography
Ovary	20,700	12,500	7	0.4	TVS/TV-CDS
Endometrium	33,000	5,500	20	3–6	TVS/?TV-CDS

TVS, transvaginal sonography; TV-CDS, transvaginal color Doppler sonography.

From Schulman H, Conway C, Zalud I, et al. Prevalence in a volunteer population of pelvic cancer detected with transvaginal ultrasound and color flow Doppler. Ultrasound Obstet Gynecol 1994;4:414.

COST CONSIDERATIONS

Should transvaginal sonography be offered to women in an office setting? One study performed by a private gynecologist in his office suggests that routine screening of postmenopausal women is a valuable addition to the yearly examination. During a 24-month period of offering transvaginal sonography to 478 asymptomatic postmenopausal women, one case of early ovarian carcinoma was diagnosed and one case of superficially invasive endometrial cancer was found.[60] Does the cost and effort justify the detection of cancer in asymptomatic, low-risk women?

The operational cost of screening for either ovarian or endometrial cancer could be reduced significantly if these were combined with mammography. The cost of screening an asymptomatic population of women is greatly affected by the lifetime incidence of the disease. For breast cancer this is 1 in 8, whereas for ovarian cancer it is 1 in 74. Another factor that limits the effectiveness of screening for ovarian carcinoma is the fact that it has a 2-year preclinical phase, much shorter than that for breast cancer.[10] Unfortunately, cost is a major limitation in any scheme to screen for ovarian cancer. However, hope in reducing costs can be envisioned if a more efficacious serum test can be developed to identify those women who need further study.

It has been estimated that $1 million will be needed to detect each case of ovarian cancer, a figure based on the number of surgeries needed to find one cancer and the cost of performing sonography on the remainder of the population. Estimates show that the cost of sonography (per year of life saved) is similar to that for breast ($1200) or colon ($1000) cancer but twice as much as for cervical cancer ($500).[61] The incorporation and use of transvaginal sonography as a part of an annual pelvic examination in a gynecologist office may ultimately result in lowering the cost of this procedure for each carcinoma found.

When compared with the cost of screening other gynecologic cancers, the efficacy of screening for both ovarian and endometrial cancers seems reasonable (Table 3-5). Multiinstitutional studies are needed to assess the lead and length time biases as well as practicality of screening for those two cancers. Initial studies seem to indicate that screening will save five lives per 2000 patients screened.[62]

CONCLUSIONS

The efficacy of a screening program including transvaginal sonography will only be established after a mega-study involving the collection of data from multiple institutions. It has been estimated that such a study would have to involve over 100,000 women, divided into control (pelvic examination only) and experimental (CA 125 plus transvaginal sonography) groups. Such a study will require 15 to 20 years to complete, accounting for adequate follow-up of subjects tested.

However, certain statements involving transvaginal sonography screening for ovarian carcinoma can be made before the completion of such a large study:

1. Transvaginal sonography can detect early-stage ovarian carcinoma.
2. Transvaginal sonography seems to be better than pelvic examination or CA 125.
3. Transvaginal ($\pm$ transvaginal color Doppler sonography) sonography is an integral part of any screening scheme for ovarian carcinoma.

Although it is true that the cost of testing entire populations with such a scheme would be high, it is clear that evaluation of women with risk factors is efficacious and should be offered to any patient at risk.[63] The remaining challenges include further refinement of identifying those women who could be best served by such a screening program.[64] The sonographic technology for the detection of early stage ovarian carcinoma is available and continues to be refined.[65]

REFERENCES

1. Silverberg E, Lubera A. Cancer statistics. CA 1993;38:9.
2. Mendelson EB, Böhm-Velez M, Neiman HL, Russo J. Transvaginal sonography in gynecologic imaging. Semin Ultrasound CT MRI 1988; 9:101.
3. Julian C. General concepts and characteristics of ovarian Ca. In: Jones

H, Jones G, eds. Novak's textbook of gynecology, ed 10. Baltimore, Williams & Wilkins, 1981:543.

4. Heintz AP, Hacker NF, Lagasse LD. Epidemiology and etiology of ovarian cancer: a review. Obstet Gynecol 1985;66:127.

5. Kerlikaske K, Brown JS, Grady DG: Should women with familial ovarian cancer undergo prophylactic oophorectomy? Obstet Gynecol 1992; 80:700.

6. Woodruff JD. History of ovarian neoplasia: facts and fancy. In: Winn RM, ed. Obstetrics and Gynecology Annual, vol 5. New York, Appleton-Century-Crofts, 1976:331.

7. Gallion HH, Powell DE, Morrow JK, et al. Molecular genetic changes in human epithelial ovarian malignancies. Gynecol Oncol 1992;47:137.

8. Bennington JL, Ferguson BR, Haber SL. Incidence and relative frequency of benign and malignant neoplasms. Obstet Gynecol 1968;32: 627.

9. Whittemore AS, Harris R, Itnyre J, and the Collaborative Ovarian Cancer Group: Characteristics relating to ovarian cancer risk: collaborative analysis of 12 US case-control studies. Am J Epidemiol 1992;136: 1184.

10. Hankinson SE, Hunter DJ, Colditz GA, et al: Tubal ligation, hysterectomy, and risk of ovarian cancer: a prospective study. JAMA 1993; 270:2813.

11. Piver MS, Recio FO: Ovarian cancer: Who needs screening? Patient Care 1993(Dec 15):27.

12. Kramer BS, Gohagan J, Prorok PC, Smart C: A National Cancer Institute sponsored screening trial for prostatic, lung, colorectal, and ovarian cancers. Cancer 1993;71:589.

12a. Easton D, Ford D, Bishop DT, and the Breast Cancer Linkage Consortium. Breast and ovarian cancer incidence in BRCA1-mutation. Am J Hum Genet 1995;56:265.

13. Van Nagell JF, DePriest PD, Puls LE, et al. Ovarian cancer screening in asymptomatic postmenopausal women by transvaginal sonography. Cancer 1991;68:458.

14. Jacobs I, Bridges J, Reynolds C, et al. Multimodal approach to screening for ovarian cancer. Lancet 1988;6:268.

15. Megibow AJ, Bosniak MA, Ho AG, et al. Accuracy of CT in detection of persistent or recurrent ovarian carcinoma: correlation with second-look laparotomy. Radiology 1988;166:341.

16. Goswamy RK, Campbell S, Whitehead MI. Screening for ovarian cancer. Clin Obstet Gynecol 1983;10:621.

17. Campbell S, Bham V, Royston P, et al. Transabdominal screening of early ovarian cancer. BMJ 1989;299:1363.

18. Andolf E, Svalenius E, Astedt B. Ultrasonography for early detection of ovarian carcinoma. Br J Obstet Gynaecol 1986;93:1286.

19. van Nagell J. In Fleischer A, Jones H, eds. Early detection of Ovarian Cancer with Transvaginal Sonography: potentials and limitations. New York: Raven Press, 1993.

20. Fleischer A, McKee M, Gordon A, et al. Transvaginal sonography of post-menopausal ovaries with pathologic correlation. J Ultrasound Med 1990;9:637.

21. Fleischer AC, Jones HW: Early detection of ovarian carcinoma with transvaginal color Doppler sonography. Am J Obstet Gynecol, 1996; 174:101–106.

22. Rulin MC, Preson AL. Adnexal masses in postmenopausal women. Obstet Gynecol 1987;70:578.

23. Hall D, McCarthy K. The significance of the postmenopausal simple adnexal cyst. J Ultrasound Med 1986;5:503.

24. Goldstein S, Subvamanyam B, Synder J, et al. The postmenopausal cystic adnexal mass: the potential role of ultrasound in consecutive management. Obstet Gynecol 1989;8:743.

25. Andolf E, Jorgenson C. Cystic lesions in elderly women diagnosed by ultrasound. Br J Obstet Gynaecol 1989;96:1076.

26. Moyle JW, Rochester D, Sider L, et al. Sonography of ovarian tumors: Predictability of tumor type. AJR 1983;141:985.

27. Hsiu JG, Given FT, Kemp GM: Tumor implantation after diagnostic laparoscopic biopsy of serous ovarian tumors of low malignant potential. Obstet Gynecol 1986;68:90S.

28. Smith B. The use of vaginal sonography as the basis of a perimenopausal ovarian and uterine screening program. Presented at the First World Congress on Vaginosonography in Gynecology, Washington, DC, June 1988.

29. Bourne TH, Campbell S, Reynolds KM, et al. Screening for early familial ovarian cancer with transvaginal ultrasonography and colour blood flow imaging. Br J Med 1993;306:1025.

30. Jacobs I, Davies AP, Bridges J, et al. Prevalence screening for ovarian

cancer in postmenopausal women by CA 125 measurement and ultrasonography. BMJ 1993;306:1030.

31. Bourne TH, Campbell S, Reynolds KM, et al. Screening for early familial ovarian cancer with transvaginal ultrasonography and colour blood flow imaging. BMJ 1993;306:1025.

32. Fleischer AC, Rodgers WH, Kepple DM, et al. Color Doppler sonography of ovarian masses: a multiparameter analysis. J Ultrasound Med 1993;12:41.

33. Kurjak A, Zalud I, Alfirevic Z. Evaluation of adnexal masses with transvaginal color ultrasound. J Ultrasound Med 1991;10:295.

34. Kurjak A, Shalan H, Matijevic R, et al: Stage I ovarian cancer by transvaginal color Doppler sonography: a report of 18 cases. Ultrasound Obstet Gynecol 1993;3:195.

35. Bourne T, Campbell S, Steer C. Transvaginal color flow imaging: a possible new screening technique for ovarian cancer. BMJ 1989;299: 1367.

36. Fleischer AC, Rodgers WH, Kepple DM, et al. Color Doppler sonography of benign and malignant ovarian masses. Radiographics 1992;12: 879.

37. Weiner Z, Thaler I, Beck D, et al. Differentiating malignant from benign ovarian tumors with transvaginal color flow imaging. Obstet Gynecol 1992;79:159.

38. Kawai M, Kano T, Kikkawa F, et al. Transvaginal Doppler ultrasound with color flow imaging in the diagnosis of ovarian cancer. Obstet Gynecol 1992;79:163.

39. Kurjak A, Predanic M. New scoring system for prediction of ovarian malignancy based on transvaginal color Doppler sonography. J Ultrasound Med 1992;11:631.

40. Natori M, Kouno H, Nozawa S. Flow velocity waveform analysis for the detection of ovarian cancer. Toshiba Med Rev 1992;40:45.

41. Tekay A, Jouppila P: Validity of pulsatility and resistance indices in classification of adnexal tumors with transvaginal color Doppler ultrasound. Ultrasound Obstet Gynecol 1992;2:338.

42. Timor-Tritsch IE, Lerner JP, et al. Transvaginal ultrasonographic characterization of ovarian masses by means of color flow-directed Doppler measurements and a morphologic scoring system. Am J Obstet Gynecol 1993;168:909.

43. Hamper UM, Sheth S, Abbas FM, et al. Transvaginal color Doppler sonography of adnexal masses: differences in blood flow impedance in benign and malignant lesions. AJR 1993;160:1225.

44. Schneider VL, Schneider A, Reed KL, Hatch KD. Comparison of Doppler with two-dimensional sonography and CA 125 for prediction of malignancy of pelvic masses. Obstet Gynecol 1993;81:983.

45. Valentin L, Sladkevicius P, Marsal K: Limited contribution of Doppler velocimetry to the differential diagnosis of extrauterine pelvic tumors. Obstet Gynecol 1994;83:425.

46. Bromley B, Goodman H, Benacerraf BR: Comparison between sonographic morphology and Doppler waveform for the diagnosis of ovarian malignancy. Obstet Gynecol 1994;83:434.

47. Brown DL, Frates MC, Laing FC, et al. Ovarian masses: can benign and malignant lesions be differentiated with color and pulsed Doppler US? Radiology 1994;190:333.

48. Levine D, Feldstein VA, Babcook CJ, Filly RA: Sonography of ovarian masses: poor sensitivity of resistive index for identifying malignant lesions. AJR 1994;162:1355.

49. Carter JR, Lau M, Fowler JM, et al. Blood flow characteristics of ovarian tumors: implications for ovarian cancer screening. Am J Obstet Gynecol 1995;172:901.

50. Jain KA: Prospective evaluation of adnexal masses with endovaginal gray-scale and duplex and color Doppler US: correlation with pathologic findings. Radiology 1994;191:63.

51. Eddy D. Guidelines for cancer related checkup: recommendations and rationale. CA 1988;30:321.

52. Zurawski VR, Knapp RC, Einhorn N, et al. An initial analysis of preoperative serum CA 125 levels in patients with early stage ovarian carcinoma. Gynecol Oncol 1988;30:7.

53. Helzisouer KJ, Bush TL, Alberg AJ, et al. Prospective study of serum CA-125 levels as markers of ovarian cancer. JAMA 1993;269:1123.

54. Finkler NJ, Benacerraf B, Wojciechowski C, et al. Comparison of serum CA 125, clinical impression, and ultrasound in the preoperative evaluation of ovarian masses. Obstet Gynecol 1988;72:659.

55. Bourne TH, Whitehead MI, Campbell S, et al. Ultrasound screening for familial ovarian cancer. Gynecol Oncol 1991;43:92.

56. Jacobs I, Davies AP, Bridges J, et al. Prevalence screening for ovarian

cancer in postmenopausal women by CA 125 measurement and ultrasonography. BMJ 1993;306:1030.

57. Einhorn N, Sjovall K, Knapp R, et al: Prospective evaluation of serum CA 125 levels for early detection of ovarian cancer. Obstet Gynecol 1992;80:14.

58. Weiner Z, Beck D, Shteiner M, et al. Screening for ovarian cancer in women with breast cancer with transvaginal sonography and color flow imaging. J Ultrasound Med 1993;12:387.

59. Kurjak A, Shalan H, Kupesic S, et al: An attempt to screen asymptomatic women for ovarian and endometrial cancer with transvaginal color and pulsed Doppler sonography. J Ultrasound Med 1994;13:295.

60. Holbert TR: Screening transvaginal ultrasonography of postmenopausal women in a private office setting. Obstet Gynecol 170:1699.

61. Jones-Bey H: Early diagnosis pivotal to ovarian Ca treatment. Diagn Imaging 1992;4:131.

62. Cohen CJ: Screening for ovarian cancer: the role of noninvasive imaging techniques. Obstet Gynecol 1994;94:1088.

63. Crane J. CaO and the role of US. In: Gynecologic ultrasound course syllabus. Presented at the annual meeting of the American Institute of Ultrasound in Medicine, 1993:21.

64. Taylor KJW, Schwartz PE: Screening for early ovarian cancer. Radiology 1994;192:1.

65. Schulman H, Conway C, Zalud I, et al. Prevalence in a volunteer population of pelvic cancer detected with transvaginal ultrasound and color flow Doppler. Ultrasound Obstet Gynecol 1994;4:414.

Magnetic Resonance Imaging of Ovarian Malignancy

Marcia C. Javitt, MD

Sonography remains the study of choice in the initial evaluation of a suspected adnexal mass because it can inexpensively and noninvasively permit characterization of many lesions as benign (eg, simple cysts or broad ligament fibroids), as very suggestive of malignancy, or as indeterminate lesions that require further workup. Sonography is limited by operator dependency and is hampered by large patient body habitus and by intestinal gas. CT certainly allows a careful survey of the solid abdominal organs and nodal chains but is limited by lesser soft tissue contrast as compared to pelvic MRI. The role of MRI has been limited in the evaluation of gynecologic malignancies by its higher cost than sonography and slightly higher expense than CT, by the unfamiliarity of referring physicians with the study, and by the relative inexperience of most radiologists in the community with detailed pelvic MRI.

MRI can show the solid organs and nodal chains like CT but has significant advantages over CT for tissue characterization of ovarian masses with contrast enhancement, including the depiction of internal septations, papillary and other

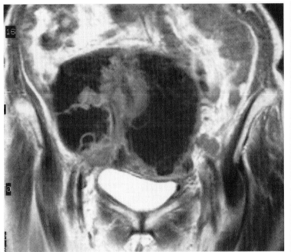

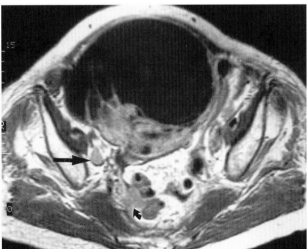

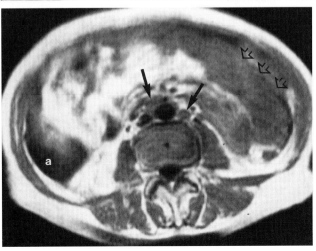

FIG. 3-4. Magnetic resonance imaging features of ovarian malignancy. **(A)** T1-weighted enhanced coronal scan. The large predominantly cystic mass has enhancing solid elements. **(B)** T1-weighted enhanced axial scan. Enhancement is seen in obturator adenopathy *(arrow)*, rectal implant *(curved arrow)*, and the solid elements of the papillary cystadenocarcinoma. **(C)** T1-weighted axial scan. Abdominal carcinomatosis with retroperitoneal adenopathy *(solid arrows)*, ascites (a), and omental cake *(open arrows)*.

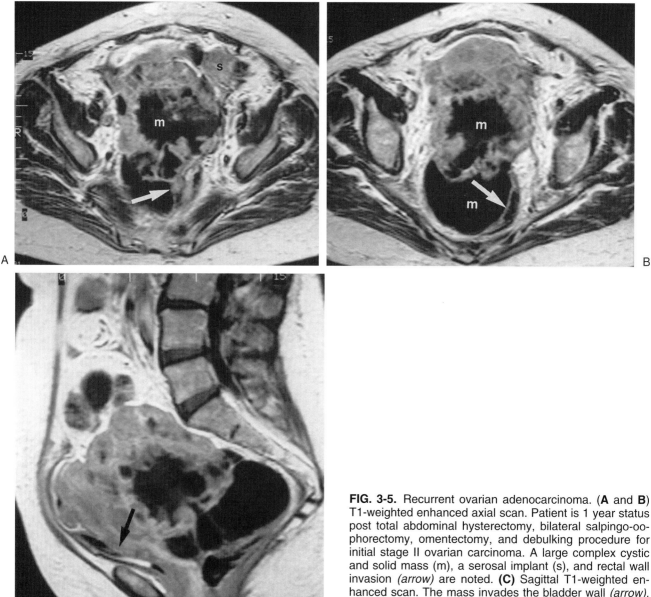

FIG. 3-5. Recurrent ovarian adenocarcinoma. (**A** and **B**) T1-weighted enhanced axial scan. Patient is 1 year status post total abdominal hysterectomy, bilateral salpingo-oophorectomy, omentectomy, and debulking procedure for initial stage II ovarian carcinoma. A large complex cystic and solid mass (m), a serosal implant (s), and rectal wall invasion *(arrow)* are noted. (**C**) Sagittal T1-weighted enhanced scan. The mass invades the bladder wall *(arrow)*. At surgery, a poorly differentiated papillary serous adenocarcinoma with clear cell features with diffuse infiltration of the ovaries, fallopian tubes, uterine serosa, peritoneum, omentum, gastrocolic ligament, bladder, and rectum was found.

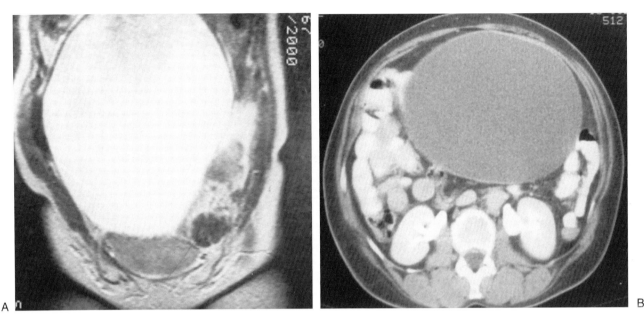

FIG. 3-6. Papillary serous cystadenocarcinoma. **(A)** T2-weighted coronal scan shows a huge unilocular abdominopelvic cystic mass that proved to be stage I papillary serous cystadenocarcinoma. **(B)** CT scan shows the unilocular cystic mass.

solid elements, necrosis, and debris (Fig. 3-4). MRI can show peritoneal and serosal lesions about as well as CT. Like sonography, MRI is multiplanar, but it is not operator dependent. Most importantly, the soft tissue contrast on MRI exceeds that of CT and sonography.

The cost-effectiveness of MRI of the ovary is unknown and may depend on whether the patient came to MRI after sonography or physical examination resulted in plans for surgery. If MRI can obviate the need for surgery, then substantial cost savings can be expected.[1-3] In addition, the potential risks of iodinated contrast materials in patients with renal disease, cardiac disease, and diabetes may make enhanced CT scans more costly than MRI.[3]

As an ancillary technique to sonography, MRI can add significant information to characterize lesions as benign or malignant with an accuracy between 84% and 90%, a sensitivity of 95%, and a specificity of about 97%.[4-8]

The MRI features of ovarian malignancy include solid elements or papillary projections. Both benign and malignant ovarian neoplasms may contain these findings, but they are more likely to be found in malignancies and should be considered suggestive of epithelial neoplasms.[8,9] The increased conspicuousness of enhancing lymphadenopathy, peritoneal implants, omental metastases, and solid elements with ascites has yielded improved ascertainment of the extent of disease (Fig. 3-5).[4,6-11] The accuracy of enhanced MRI to differentiate a benign from a malignant mass has been reported between 60% and 84%.[8-10,12,13]

Whether the tumor is solid, cystic, or both, the appearance of the many cell types of ovarian carcinoma is nonspecific. About 85% of ovarian malignancies are epithelial, of which the most common cell type is serous papillary carcinoma (Figs. 3-6 and 3-7). Mucinous tumors may be large and contain high signal locules owing to proteinaceous or hemorrhagic mucinous material (Figs. 3-8 and 3-9) and can be associated with pseudomyxoma peritonei. Other cell types such as endometrioid and clear cell carcinomas are rare (Fig. 3-10; see also Fig. 3-5).[1,7]

The accuracy of enhanced MRI for staging of ovarian carcinoma (60% to 87%) is probably comparable to that of dynamic enhanced CT (66% to 94%). Tiny implants and local invasion in the peritoneum and omentum escape detection by cross-sectional imaging techniques and limit the accuracy thus far. The entire abdomen and pelvis must be imaged for full evaluation, which is time consuming. Ascites can be easily detected but is not specific for malignancy (Fig. 3-11).[1,6,8,13,14]

Surgical staging (Table 3-6) of ovarian carcinoma is somewhat inaccurate but allows for not only debulking of disease with total abdominal hysterectomy and bilateral salpingo-oophorectomy but also evaluation of extent of disease, including abdominopelvic nodal sampling, excisional biopsies of the omentum and peritoneum, and peritoneal washings. The role of preoperative staging has therefore been limited and is controversial. Surgical staging with cytoreduction and debulking is recommended.[1,15] Selective use of MRI in preoperative staging may be indicated, particularly for patients who are poor operative risks or in cases in which

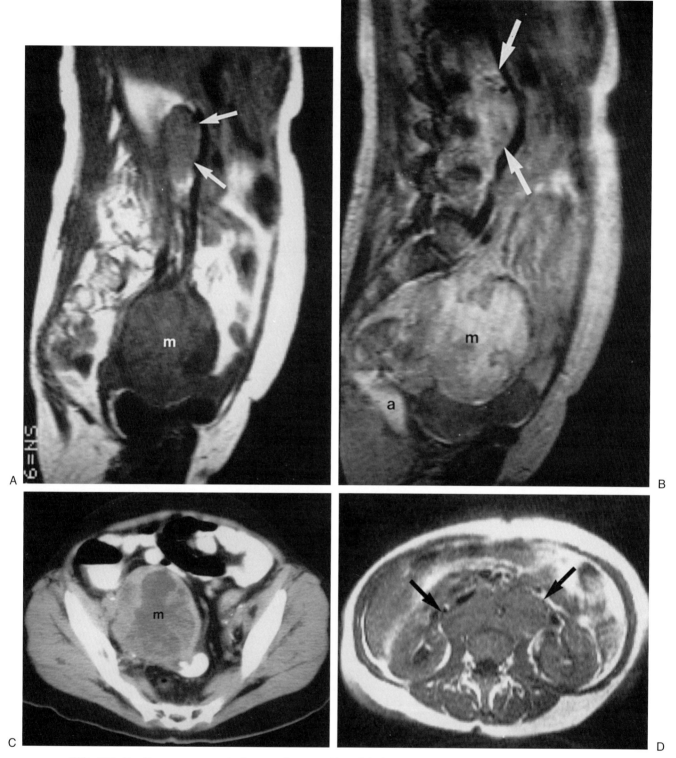

FIG. 3-7. Papillary serous cystadenocarcinoma with solid elements. **(A)** T1-weighted sagittal image shows a nonspecific mostly solid but mixed complex partly cystic pelvic mass (m). There is retroperitoneal lymphadenopathy *(arrow)*. **(B)** T2-weighted sagittal image shows the mass (m) becomes brighter. Adenopathy *(arrows)* and ascites (a) are evident in this case of stage IV ovarian carcinoma. **(C)** The complex nature of the pelvic mass (m) can be appreciated on CT scan but is also nonspecific. **(D)** Axial T1-weighted abdominal scan confirms the large mantle of retroperitoneal nodes *(arrows)*.

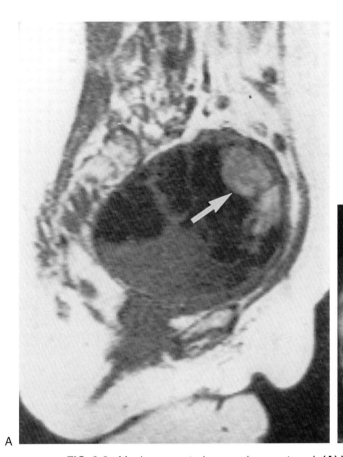

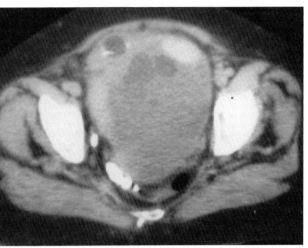

A   B

FIG. 3-8. Mucinous cystadenocarcinoma stage I. **(A)** T1-weighted sagittal scan shows the typical multi-loculated appearance of this lesion. Some of the locules are hyperintense owing to the proteinaceous or hemorrhagic material *(arrow)*. This lesion cannot be differentiated from the benign form, mucinous cystadenoma, if in isolation (in the absence of associated findings such as adenopathy, implants, or ascites). **(B)** Enhanced CT scan shows a nonspecific complex cystic and solid mass.

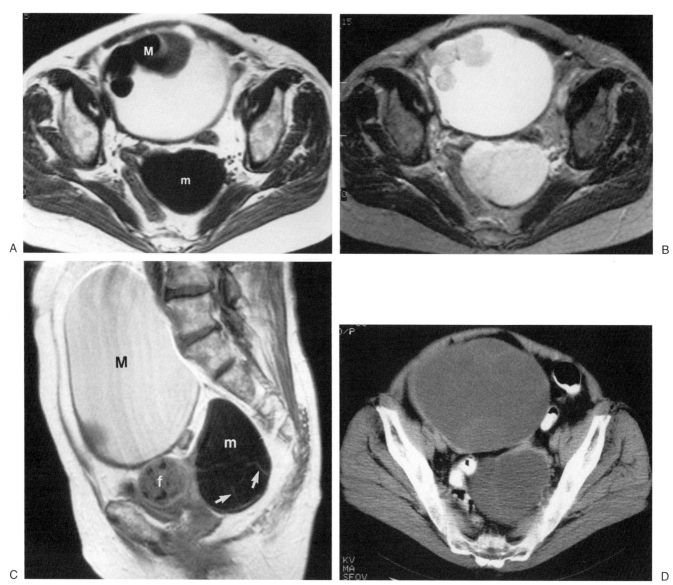

FIG. 3-9. Mucinous cystadenocarcinoma stage IB. **(A)** T1-weighted axial scan shows a large complex predominantly hyperintense cystic anterior mass with low signal loculi (M) and a smaller posterior septated cystic mass (m) of low signal intensity that proved to be bilateral mucinous cystadenocarcinomas. **(B)** T2-weighted axial scan. All portions of both masses become brighter. **(C)** T1-weighted axial enhanced scan shows heterogeneous enhancing fibroid (f) in the uterus, persistent hyperintense signal in the dominant anterior loculus of the larger complex mass (M), and enhancing septations *(arrows)* within the posterior multiloculated mass (m). **(D)** Enhanced computed tomography scan. Complex cystic masses are visible. Neither CT nor MRI showed adenopathy, and no adenopathy was found at surgery.

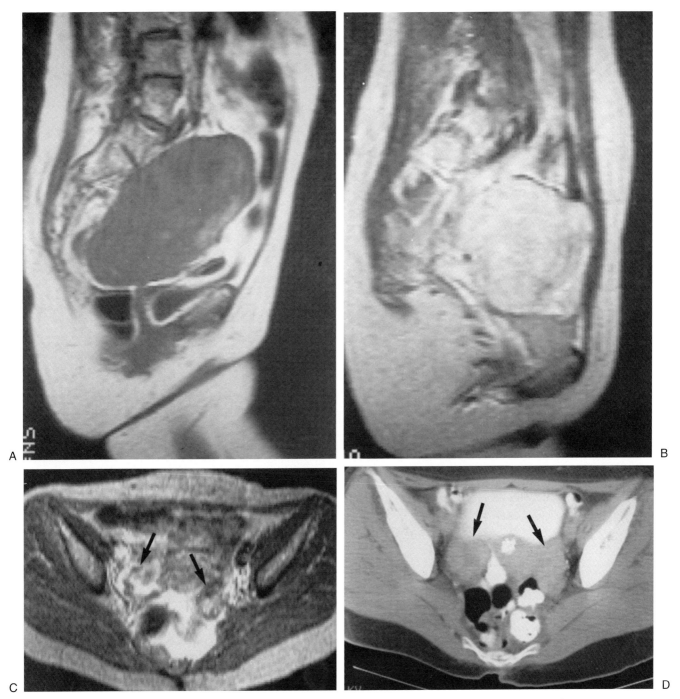

FIG. 3-10. Nonspecific appearance of solid ovarian masses. **(A)** Sagittal T1-weighted image shows a nonspecific predominantly solid ovarian mass that was surgically proved ovarian sarcoma. **(B)** T2-weighted sagittal scan. Ovarian dysgerminoma. The appearance is nonspecific. **(C)** T2-weighted axial scan and **(D)** enhanced CT scan. Metastatic breast carcinoma to both ovaries with malignant ascites. The bilateral masses *(arrows)* are nonspecific.

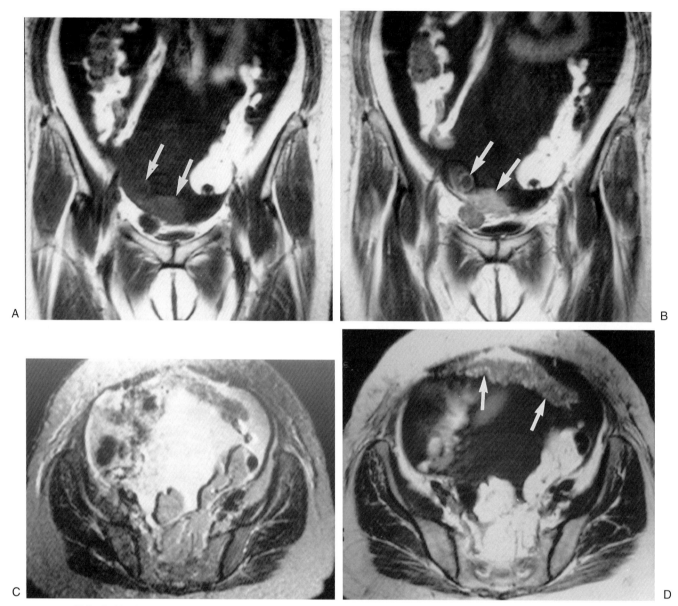

FIG. 3-11. Intraabdominal carcinomatosis. **(A)** T1-weighted coronal scan. Solid peritoneal implants *(arrows)* are present but not conspicuous within the ascites. **(B)** T1-weighted coronal enhanced scan. The enhancing implants *(arrows)* are much more evident. **(C)** T2-weighted axial scan. The omental cake is difficult to differentiate from bowel. **(D)** T1-weighted axial enhanced scan. The omental cake *(arrows)* stands out in sharp contrast from the surrounding ascites and is easily identified as separate from bowel.

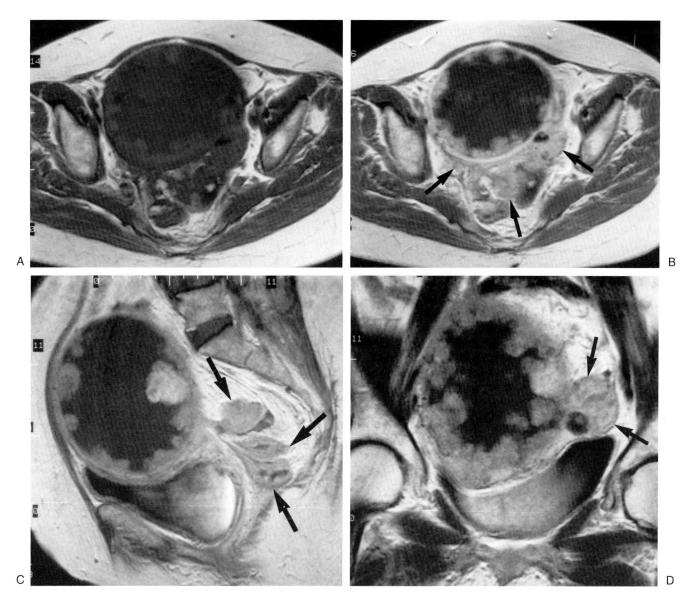

FIG. 3-12. Intraabdominal carcinomatosis involving the rectosigmoid mesentery and tuboovarian ligament. **(A)** Axial T1-weighted scan shows cystic pelvic mass. **(B)** Enhanced T1-weighted axial and **(C)** sagittal scans demonstrate not only enhancing large papillary projections within the cystic papillary serous adenocarcinoma but also enhancing implants in the rectosigmoid mesentery *(arrows).* **(D)** Coronal enhanced T1-weighted scan. There is extension into the left tuboovarian ligament *(arrows)* that was proved at surgery.

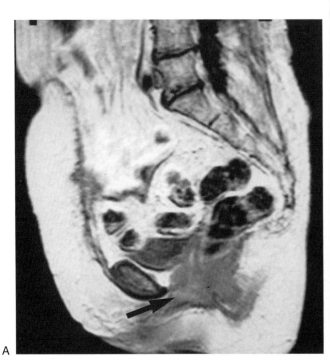
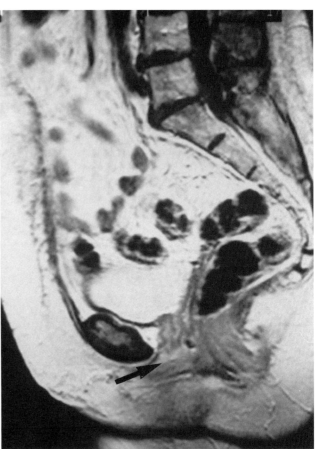

A   B

FIG. 3-13. Recurrent ovarian carcinoma. **(A)** Sagittal T1-weighted scan. A mass with low signal intensity *(arrow)* is present in the lower half of the vaginal canal and has extended posteriorly through the cul-de-sac to the anterior margin of the lower rectum and anus. The patient is 7 months status post optimal debulking for papillary serous adenocarcinoma initial stage III with biopsy-proven recurrence. **(B)** Sagittal T1-weighted enhanced scan. The mass *(arrow)* has a heterogeneous enhancement pattern.

TABLE 3-6. *FIGO staging of ovarian carcinoma*

Stage	Description
I	Limited to the ovaries
Ia	One ovary, no ascites
Ib	Both ovaries, no malignant ascites
Ic	One or both ovaries with malignant ascites
II	Pelvic extension
IIa	Uterine or tubal extension, no malignant ascites
IIb	Further pelvic extension, no malignant ascites
IIc	Pelvic extension with malignant ascites
III	Abdominal extension
IIIa	Microscopic peritoneal metastases
IIIb	Peritoneal metastases <2 cm
IIIc	Peritoneal metaseses >2 cm and/or adenopathy
IV	Distant metastases

Data from Jones HW, Wentz AC, Burnett LS, eds. Novak's textbook of gynecology, ed 11. Baltimore, Williams & Wilkins, 1988; and DiSaia PF, Creasman WT. Clinical gynecologic oncology, ed 3. St. Louis, CV Mosby, 1989.

debulking is suspected to be unsuccessful because of widespread distant metastases (Fig. 3-12).[1,14,15]

Because second-look laparotomy is no longer recommended, noninvasive diagnosis of recurrent ovarian carcinoma is desirable. A strong role for MRI will likely emerge. If recurrence can be reliably detected noninvasively, the need for surgery may be obviated.[16–18] The accuracy of MRI for recurrent lesions less than 2 cm has been reported as 35%, but for lesions greater than 2 cm it is 82%.[16] For CT, the ability to predict unsuccessful debulking has been reported with a sensitivity of 58% and a specificity of 100%.[19] Whether CT or MRI is used, this group of patients can clearly benefit from cross-sectional imaging (Fig. 3-13; see also Fig. 3-5). Because CT is slightly less expensive, and perhaps more accessible, it may be slightly preferable for this purpose, but it may or may not be more accurate. A definitive controlled comparative study has not been performed.

REFERENCES

1. Outwater EK, Dunton CJ. Imaging of the ovary and adnexa: clinical issues and applications of MR imaging. Radiology 1995;194:1.
2. Schwartz LB, Panageas E, OLange R, et al. Female pelvis: impact of MR imaging on treatment decisions and net cost analysis. Radiology 1994;192:55.
3. Lessler DS, Sullivan Sd, Stergachis A. Cost effectiveness of unenhanced MR imaging vs contrast enhanced CT of the abdomen or pelvis. AJR 1994;163:5.
4. Hata K, Hata T, Manabe A, et al. A critical evaluation of transvaginal Doppler studies, transvaginal sonography, magnetic resonance imaging, and CA 125 in detecting ovarian cancer. Obstet Gynecol 1992; 80:922.
5. Scoutt LM, McCarthy SM, Lange R, et al. MR evaluation of clinically suspected adnexal masses. J Comput Assist Tomogr 1994;18:609.
6. Smith FW, Cherryman GR, Bayliss AP, et al. A comparative study of the accuracy of ultrasound imaging, x-ray computerized tomography, and low field MRI diagnosis of ovarian malignancy. Magn Reson Imaging 1988;6:225.
7. Ghossain MA, Buy JN, Ligneres C, et al. Epithelial tumors of the ovary: comparison of MR and CT findings. Radiology 1991;181:863.
8. Stevens SK, Hricak H, Stern JL. Ovarian lesions: detection and characterization with gadolinium enhanced MR imaging at 1.5 T. Radiology 1991;181:481.
9. Thurner SA. MR imaging of pelvic masses in women: contrast-enhanced versus unenhanced images. AJR 1992;159:1243.
10. Thurner S, Hudler J, Baer S, et al. Gadolinium-DPTA enhanced MR imaging of adnexal tumors. J Comput Assist Tomogr 1990;14:939.
11. Yamashita Y, Torashima M, Hatanaka Y, et al. Value of phase-shift gradient-echo MR imaging in the differentiation of pelvic lesions with high signal intensity at T1-weighted imaging. Radiology 1994;191: 759.
12. Hamm B, Laniado M, Saini S. Contrast enhanced magnetic resonance imaging of the abdomen and pelvis. Magn Reson Q 1990;6:108.
13. Semelka RC, Lawrence PH, Shoenut JP, et al. Primary ovarian cancer: prospective comparison of contrast-enhanced CT and pre- and post-contrast, fat-suppressed MR imaging, with histologic correlation. J Magn Reson Imaging 1993;3:99.
14. Forstner R, Hricak H, Occhpinti KA, et al. Ovarian cancer: staging with CT and MR imaging. Radiology 1995;197:619.
15. Outwater EK, Schiebler ML. Magnetic resonance imaging of the ovary. In: Mezrich R, ed. The female pelvis. MRI Clin North Am 1994;2: 245.
16. Forstner R, Hricak H, Powell CB, et al. Ovarian cancer recurrence: value of MR imaging. Radiology 1995;196:715.
17. Miller DS, Spirtos NM, Ballon SC, et al. Critical reassessment of second-look exploratory laparotomy for epithelial ovarian carcinoma. Cancer 1992;69:502.
18. NIH Consensus Development Panel on Ovarian Cancer. Ovarian cancer screening, treatment, and follow-up. JAMA 1995;273:491.
19. Meyer JI, Kennedy AW, Friedman R, et al. Ovarian carcinoma: value of CT in predicting success of debulking surgery. AJR 1995;165:875.

Ovarian Cancer: Computed Tomography

R. Brooke Jeffrey, Jr., MD

Computed tomography may be clinically valuable in both the initial staging of ovarian cancer and in documenting response to therapy and tumor recurrence. On CT, the morphologic features of an ovarian mass that suggest malignancy are similar to the criteria established with transvaginal sonography and MRI. These include either a solid ovarian mass or a complex cystic mass containing mural nodules or thickened septations (Fig. 3-14). Both CT and MRI are clearly limited in demonstrating microscopic metastases involving the mesentery, omentum, and peritoneum. In general, both techniques are not reliable for detecting peritoneal and mesenteric implants less than 5 to 10 mm (Fig. 3-15).

INITIAL TUMOR STAGING FOR CYTOREDUCTIVE SURGERY

The majority of patients presenting with ovarian malignancy unfortunately already have stage III or IV disease with extrapelvic metastases.[1–3] Despite presentation at an advanced stage, prolonged survival is possible with a combination of cytoreductive surgery and postoperative chemotherapy.[4–9] However, the long-term prognosis is relatively poor because most patients ultimately succumb to metastatic disease. Aggressive cytoreductive surgery requires an experienced gynecologic surgeon. It is a prolonged and often arduous surgical procedure that may be associated with significant morbidity. The standard measure of success for cytoreductive surgery for ovarian cancer is near-complete resection of tumor with no residual tumor mass greater than 2 cm.[4]

Preoperative CT may be of value by identifying patients who are likely to benefit from aggressive cytoreductive surgery by identifying the extent of abdominal metastatic disease. Both clinical evaluation and tumor markers such as CA 125 are not reliable in selecting patients for this surgery. Meyer and associates[4] evaluated 28 patients with ovarian carcinoma who underwent preoperative CT. Using a standardized scoring system, they evaluated the omentum, liver, paraaortic lymph nodes, diaphragm, lung base, small bowel mesentery, and degree of ascites to document suitability for cytoreductive surgery.[4] If their scoring system is used to judge successful debulking surgery, CT had a sensitivity of 58% and a specificity of 100%.[4] Similar results were obtained by Nelson and colleagues,[7] who retrospectively reviewed 42 preoperative CT scans and noted that CT accu-

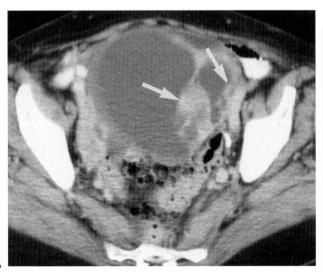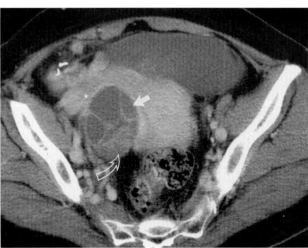

A   B

FIG. 3-14. Typical CT appearance of ovarian carcinoma. **(A)** Note the large complex cystic mass containing both mural and septal nodules *(arrows)*. **(B)** In a second patient note the complex right ovarian mass *(arrow)*. Solid mural nodule is evident *(curved arrow)*.

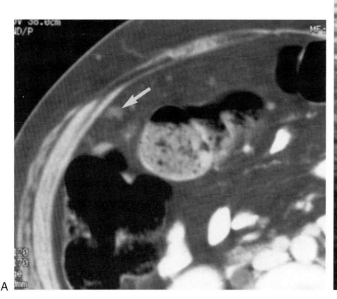
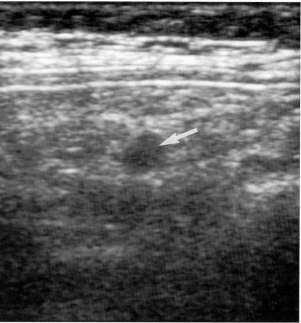

A   B

FIG. 3-15. CT and sonogram of small peritoneal implants secondary to ovarian carcinoma. **(A)** CT scan demonstrating soft tissue nodule *(arrow)* within the fat-containing omentum. **(B)** Sonogram shows the hypoechoic nodule representing the metastatic implant *(arrow)*.

rately predicted surgical outcome with a sensitivity of 92% and a specificity of 79%. Both these studies indicate a role for preoperative CT in assessing both the extent and the site of involvement of disease. Certain specific sites are hazardous for surgical resection, such as upper paraaortic lymph nodes and involvement of the diaphragm and the liver (Fig. 3-16). Patients with involvement in these areas could then be spared needless laparotomy and treated with neoadjuvant chemotherapy.

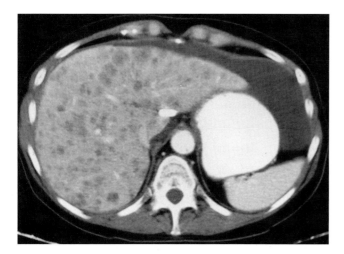

FIG. 3-16. Extensive hepatic metastases from ovarian carcinoma. Note the innumerable low-attenuation metastatic lesions throughout the liver on contrast medium—enhanced CT. Ascites is noted adjacent to the left lobe of the liver.

To optimize detection of ovarian metastases with CT, it is important to give adequate volumes of intravenous and oral contrast agents. Intravenous contrast medium administered as a sustained bolus is essential to detect metastases to solid parenchymal organs such as the liver and spleen. Vascular opacification is critical to differentiate lymph nodes from blood vessels. Complete opacification of the small bowel with dilute oral contrast medium is important to detect mesenteric and serosal implants.

Metastatic disease from carcinoma of the ovary has a varied CT appearance.[8,9] Involvement of the omentum may result in multiple discrete, small soft tissue nodules (see Fig. 3-15) or diffuse soft tissue infiltration, referred to as omental cake (Fig. 3-17). Microscopic omental metastases are commonly not detected with current CT scanning techniques. Mesenteric metastases may also produce soft tissue nodules within the mesenteric fat. Diffuse infiltration of the mesentery may result in tethering of the small bowel and a stellate or radiating appearance of the mesenteric vasculature. Small (<5 mm) serosal implants on the surface of the gastrointestinal tract are common with ovarian carcinoma but are rarely detected by CT. Paraaortic lymph nodes greater than 1 cm in short axis are strongly suggestive of metastases. In addition to hepatic parenchymal metastasis, carcinoma of the ovary has a propensity to metastasize to the spleen, often with a complex cystic appearance (Fig. 3-18). Mucinous adenocarcinoma may result in low-attenuating peritoneal metastases referred to as pseudomyxoma peritonei (see Fig. 3-18). Serous carcinoma of the ovary may result in calcified metastasis, involving the peritoneal surface and mesentery

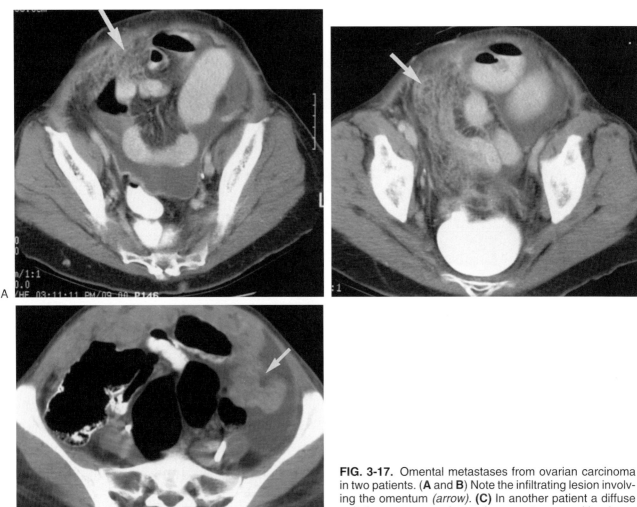

FIG. 3-17. Omental metastases from ovarian carcinoma in two patients. (**A** and **B**) Note the infiltrating lesion involving the omentum *(arrow)*. (**C**) In another patient a diffuse soft tissue mass replaces the omentum, resulting in an omental cake *(arrow)*.

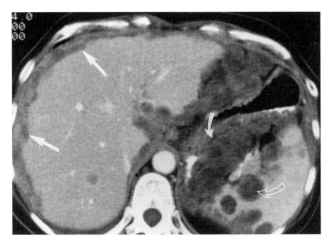

FIG. 3-18. Pseudomyxoma peritonei with hepatic and splenic metastases from ovarian carcinoma. Note the intraperitoneal low-attenuation masses causing scalloping of the liver *(arrows)*. Extensive intraperitoneal tumor is seen adjacent to the spleen *(curved arrow)*. There are cystic intrasplenic metastases *(curved open arrow)*.

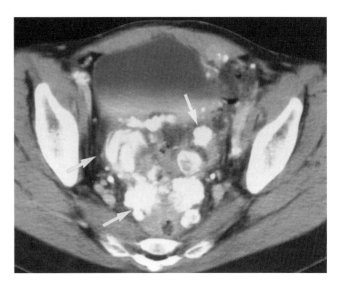

FIG. 3-19. Pelvic metastases from serous cystadenocarcinoma of the ovary. Note extensive calcified pelvic metastases appearing as high-attenuation foci on CT *(arrows)*.

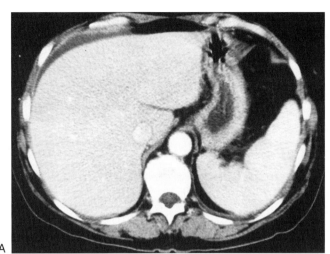 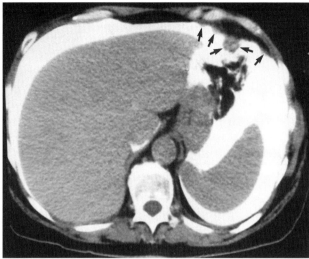

A   B

FIG. 3-20. Value of CT performed with intraperitoneal contrast medium enhancement. **(A)** Conventional CT scan performed with intravenous contrast medium enhancement only. Although there is a small amount of perihepatic ascites, no definite peritoneal implants are demonstrated. After the instillation of intraperitoneal contrast medium **(B)**, multiple soft tissue nodules are clearly visible *(arrows)* on the peritoneal surface, representing metastatic ovarian carcinoma. (From Halvorsen RA et al. Intraperitoneal contrast material improves the CT detection of peritoneal metastasis. AJR 1991;157:37.)

lymph nodes.[9] Because of their high attenuation values, these metastatic lesions are readily detected by CT (Fig. 3-19). It is important not to misconstrue high-attenuation gastrointestinal contrast medium enhancement for calcified metastases, and in selected patients delayed images can be helpful to further clarify this.

Several authors have noted that CT performed with intraperitoneal contrast medium enhancement may improve detection of small peritoneal metastasis from carcinoma of the ovary.[10,11] The technique involves instillation of 1 to 2 L of dilute iodinated contrast agent through a peritoneal catheter. Peritoneal metastases are identified as filling defects within the contrast medium enhancement within the peritoneal compartments (Fig. 3-20). Frasci and colleagues[10] performed CT with intraperitoneal contrast, medium enhancement, in 45 patients with previously normal standard abdominal pelvic CT scans.[10] In 9 of 32 cases, CT with intraperitoneal contrast medium enhancement demonstrated persistence of tumor in 30 of 39 surgically proven cases for a sensitivity of 77%[10] and a specificity of 88%. Intraperitoneal contrast medium was inserted by a temporary indwelling Teflon catheter inserted blindly. The authors concluded that, in patients with previously negative conventional abdominal and pelvic CT and a strong clinical suspicion based on elevated CA 125 levels or other clinical parameters that CT with intraperitoneal contrast medium enhancement may be of clear value in demonstrating subtle peritoneal implants. These results were corroborated by Halvorsen and associates,[11] who evaluated 16 patients with suspected peritoneal metastasis from gynecologic tumors.[11] Conventional CT demonstrated 7 of 11 patients with cervically proven implants. However, CT with intraperitoneal contrast medium enhancement demonstrated peritoneal implants in all 11 pa-

tients.[11] CT with intraperitoneal contrast medium enhancement appears to be most helpful for evaluating the subphrenic spaces and splenic hilum.

COMPUTED TOMOGRAPHIC DIAGNOSIS OF RECURRENT OVARIAN CARCINOMA

After the initial surgical resection and chemotherapy for metastatic ovarian carcinoma, a second-look laparotomy is

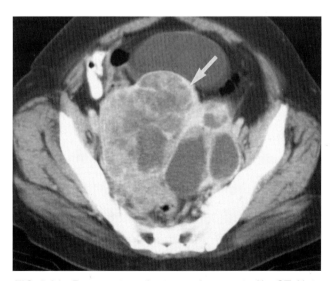

FIG. 3-21. Recurrent ovarian tumor documented by CT. Note the large complex cystic mass representing recurrent ovarian carcinoma *(arrow)*. This was confirmed by CT-guided biopsy. A "second-look" laparotomy was not performed owing to the large recurrent mass.

commonly performed to document the presence of residual disease.[12,13] If CT detects obvious metastatic lesions, the second-look laparotomy may be of limited value (Fig. 3-21). This is particularly true of disease detected in areas not easily resected, such as retroperitoneal lymph nodes, liver, or pleura.[12] Giunta and coworkers[13] combined CT with intraperitoneal contrast and immunocytology to evaluate 45 clinically disease-free patients who were considered to be candidates for second-look laparotomy.[13] CT detected peritoneal recurrences in 22 of the 45 patients. However, the immunocytologic evaluation diagnosed metastases in 8 additional patients who had negative CT scans. Thus, the combination of CT with intraperitoneal contrast medium enhancement plus immunocytology of the peritoneal fluid may be a more accurate means of following patients with ovarian cancer. However, a negative CT scan does not exclude microscopic recurrent disease, which commonly involves the peritoneum. A second-look laparotomy is still valuable in patients with negative CT scans to definitely exclude microscopic disease.

REFERENCES

1. Occhipinti KA, Frankel SD, Hricak H. The ovary: computed tomography and magnetic resonance imaging. Radiol Clin North Am 1993;31:1115.

2. Buist MR, Golding RP, Burger CW, et al. Comparative evaluation of diagnostic methods in ovarian carcinoma with emphasis on CT and MRI. Gynecol Oncol 1994;52:191.

3. Johnson RJ, Blackledge G, Eddleston B, Crowther D. Abdomino-pelvic computed tomography in the management of ovarian carcinoma. Radiology 1983;146:447.

4. Meyer JI, Kennedy AW, Friedman R, et al. Ovarian carcinoma: value of CT in predicting success of debulking surgery. AJR 1995;165:875.

5. Heintz AP, Hacker NF, Berek JS, et al. Cytoreductive surgery in ovarian carcinoma: feasibility and morbidity. Obstet Gynecol 1986;67:783.

6. Wils J, Blijham G, Naus A, et al. Primary or delayed debulking surgery and chemotherapy consisting of cisplatin, doxorubicin, and cyclophosphamide in stage III–IV epithelial ovarian carcinoma. J Clin Oncol 1986;4:1068.

7. Nelson BE, Rosenfield AT, Schwartz PE. Preoperative abdominopelvic computed tomographic prediction of optimal cytoreduction in epithelial ovarian carcinoma. J Clin Oncol 1993;11:166.

8. Megibow AJ, Hulnick DH, Bosniak MA, Balthazar EJ. Ovarian metastases: computed tomographic appearances. Radiology 1985;156:161.

9. Mitchell DG, Hill MC, Hill S, Zaloudek C. Serous carcinoma of the ovary: CT identification of metastatic calcified implants. Radiology 1986;158:649.

10. Frasci G, Contino A, Iaffaioli RV, et al. Computerized tomography of the abdomen and pelvis with peritoneal administration of soluble contrast (IPC-CT) in detection of residual disease for patients with ovarian cancer. Gynecol Oncol 1994;52:154.

11. Halvorsen RJ, Panushka C, Oakley GJ, et al. Intraperitoneal contrast material improves the CT detection of peritoneal metastases. AJR 1991;157:37.

12. Reuter KL, Griffin T, Hunter RE. Comparison of abdominopelvic computed tomography results and findings at second-look laparotomy in ovarian carcinoma patients. Cancer 1989;63:1123.

13. Giunta S, Venturo I, Mottolese M, et al. Noninvasive monitoring of ovarian cancer: improved results using CT with intraperitoneal contrast combined with immunocytology. Gynecol Oncol 1994;53:103.

Clinical Gynecologic Imaging, edited
by Arthur C. Fleischer, Marcia C. Javitt,
R. Brooke Jeffrey, Jr., and Howard W. Jones III,
Lippincott-Raven Publishers, Philadelphia © 1997.

CHAPTER 4

Endometrial Disorders

Clinical Aspects of Postmenopausal Endometrium, Hormone Replacement Therapy, and Tamoxifen Therapy

Murray A. Freedman, MD

After menopause, the endometrium usually becomes atrophic and women normally remain amenorrheic. Stimulation of this typically atrophic endometrium either by endogenous or exogenous hormones may result in bleeding that would otherwise be considered pathologic in a postmenopausal female. Postmenopausal bleeding represents the most common presentation of both endometrial hyperplasia and neoplasia. It becomes critically important to distinguish between normal "physiologic" bleeding commonly induced by hormone replacement therapy and "pathologic" bleeding associated with neoplasia. The characterization of bleeding patterns is especially important, particularly with regard to

TABLE 4-1. *Risk factors associated with endometrial pathology*

Diabetes
Obesity
Low parity
Infertility
History of irregular menses
History of carcinoma of breast or colon
Tamoxifen therapy
"Unopposed" estrogen therapy

the actual timing of the bleeding (ie, progestin withdrawal). Histologic diagnosis still remains the "gold standard" to evaluate suspect cases. The evaluation of abnormal postmenopausal bleeding by endometrial biopsy or dilatation and curettage is covered by Dr. Jones in the next section of this chapter.

Five to 15% of women presenting with postmenopausal bleeding demonstrate neoplasia at endometrial biopsy.[1] Additionally, early diagnosis of endometrial cancer is paramount because the disparity between 5-year survival for stage I versus stage II is so great: 90% versus 50%, respectively.[2] Postmenopausal bleeding, however, is not a prerequisite for endometrial neoplasia. Endometrial cancer has been found in up to 5 patients per 1000 normal, asymptomatic postmenopausal women screened.[3]

This subchapter deals with the role of transvaginal sonography as a diagnostic adjunct in evaluating the postmenopausal endometrium, particularly in patients with atypical bleeding and patients at risk for the development of cancer (Table 4-1).

Thirty years of epidemiologic data demonstrate increased morbidity and mortality in women exposed to prolonged estrogen deficiency compared with women who have received estrogen replacement therapy (ERT). ERT has been shown to be especially beneficial for specific conditions such as hot flushes and osteoporosis. Unfortunately, unopposed estrogen therapy in women with an intact uterus is associated with an alarming increase in the incidence of endometrial hyperplasia and cancer. The addition of a cyclic progestogen to ERT prevents this increased incidence of hyperplasia and neoplasia, but it also typically induces "withdrawal" bleeding in most postmenopausal women younger than 65 years of age. It is imperative that clinicians recognize the "normal" bleeding pattern associated with ERT plus progestogen, which is referred to as hormone replacement therapy (HRT).

Considerable data support the concept that cyclic progestogen administered for 12 or more days per month confers adequate protection against estrogen-induced endometrial hyperplasia or neoplasia.[4–6] In fact, the incidence of endometrial cancer is actually lower in HRT users than in nonusers. Many women, especially the morbidly obese, are exposed to substantial elevations of endogenous estrogen during the climacteric and postmenopausal years, which places them at risk for the development of hyperplasia and possibly neoplasia. The *daily* administration of low-dose progestogen used in combination with estrogen has also been shown to be protective against endometrial neoplasia and hyperplasia. Both cyclic and the "continuous combined" regimens of HRT have been shown to provide the patient protection against any putative risk of endometrial cancer. Figure 4-1 represents the schedule for the two most common forms of HRT.

In addition to inducing withdrawal bleeding, progestogens (especially the synthetic progestins) are occasionally associated with other minor undesirable effects. Progestin therapy and even progesterone on occasion may induce side effects similar to those associated with premenstrual syndrome in some women, but this is usually dose dependent. Progestogen therapy may also blunt but not negate the beneficial lipoprotein changes associated with estrogen therapy; this slightly deleterious effect is also a dose-dependent one. "Negatives" associated with progestogens (especially higher doses of progestins) have led to increased enthusiasm for the low-dose continuous combined forms of HRT.

Experience has demonstrated that the bleeding associated with cyclic administration of progestogen in HRT typically occurs several days after completion of the progestogen therapy, somewhat akin to that seen at the end of a cycle of

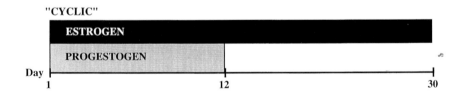

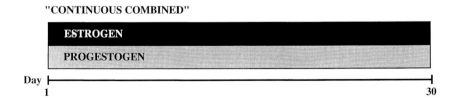

FIG. 4-1. Schedules for "cyclic" and "continuous combined" hormone replacement therapy.

oral contraception. However, bleeding may ensue before the completion of the cyclic progestogen therapy in up to 30% of patients.[7] Bleeding at the completion of cyclic progestogen in HRT is the norm, especially in women younger than 65 years of age.

The goal of low-dose continuous combined HRT is the induction of permanent amenorrhea, as well as the reduction of the dose-dependent, nuisance side effects. The principal drawback to continuous combined HRT has been the occasional unpredictable bleeding associated with the initiation of therapy. The "spotting" or bleeding usually ceases after several months of therapy, and proper counseling usually enhances compliance dramatically. Because of this initial unpredictable bleeding, I prefer to perform a *pretreatment* endometrial biopsy before starting continuous combined therapy, a procedure normally considered unnecessary in patients in whom cyclic HRT is instituted.[8] The reason for this precaution is twofold. First, if no atypicality is detected initially, none will be induced within the first year of therapy. Any bleeding occurring during the 12 months after initiating therapy can be assumed to be "dysfunctional," as opposed to anatomic or pathologic. Second, if bleeding continues for a number of months in a patient not subjected to pretreatment biopsy, physicians may then feel compelled to perform a biopsy. When a biopsy is performed at that time the patient may be convinced that the physician suspects something pathologic and become inordinately apprehensive. Experience dictates that the older the patient, the less likely she is to have bleeding after the initiation of continuous combined HRT. The "older" patient, therefore, is a better candidate for continuous combined therapy.

The majority of patients cease to have bleeding or spotting within 3 to 6 months of the initiation of low-dose continuous combined HRT. The occasional patient, especially "younger" ones, continue to have spotting or bleeding for up to 12 months. This group constitutes patients in whom pretreatment biopsy justifies itself. Patients older than age 65 are less likely to exhibit bleeding after either cyclic HRT or the initiation of continuous combined therapy, and pretreatment biopsy is usually unnecessary in these patients. Counseling is paramount in HRT: "educated" patients usually continue therapy unabated by spotting and other minor side effects.

The role of transvaginal sonography in these situations is covered in detail by Dr. Fleischer in other sections of this chapter. Transvaginal sonography can be a very reliable adjunct in monitoring older patients on HRT because of the reassurance gained when the clinician finds the "endometrial stripe" ≤ 5 mm. Transvaginal sonography is also especially helpful in older patients with cervical stenosis in whom the endometrial cavity is relatively inaccessible.

The occasional patient who experiences bleeding after years of amenorrhea with HRT represents a special situation. These patients frequently present with a truly pathologic cause for the bleeding. As a general rule, the longer the interval of amenorrhea since menopause, the greater the likelihood such "late" bleeding is associated with neoplasia. "Older" patients with episodic bleeding after years of amenorrhea deserve thorough histologic evaluation. In these patients, sonography, sonohysterography, and possibly dilatation and curettage and hysteroscopy may be necessary. On occasion, endometrial hyperplasia and endometrial cancer have remained undetected until the uterus was finally evaluated at hysterectomy.[9]

HORMONES AND CANCER

Despite the existence of overwhelming data documenting that postmenopausal women receiving HRT are not at increased risk for endometrial cancer, the potential oncogenic effect of exogenous hormone therapy continues to concern both physicians and patients. In fact, many women receiving HRT are actually at lower risk of endometrial cancer than untreated women. The data for HRT and breast cancer are far less conclusive, and the definitive answer is not available. In one report it was suggested that even lower-dose ERT and with "natural" conjugated estrogen and 17β-estradiol may be associated with a slight increase in the overall incidence of breast cancer when therapy is given for extended periods of time (ie, longer than 10 to 15 years).[10] This presents a particular dilemma for specific subgroups of women who are at higher risk for the development of breast cancer, such as those with a strong family history of breast cancer or those with biopsy-proven breast atypia. There are also recent data refuting the association of HRT and breast cancer.[11]

Epidemiologic data have failed to demonstrate any consistently elevated statistically significant risk of breast cancer with either ERT or HRT. Considerable concern persists, however, based on several studies that suggest a slight increase with higher-dose therapies among long-term users (ie, those receiving therapy for more than 15 years). From an epidemiologic standpoint, the putative adverse risk is relatively slight: a relative risk of 1.4 in current, long-term users. This "increased risk" is epidemiologically equivalent in magnitude to the effect of either nulliparity or the effect of a high saturated-fat diet. Despite more than 40 observational studies in the literature, there is no definitive answer about the impact of hormone therapy on breast cancer. Although this lack of association is reassuring, a definitive answer concerning the relation between breast cancer and hormone therapy requires experimental rather than observational data, and these data are probably 10 years from publication. In sharp contrast to this lack of association are the consistent, demonstrable, beneficial effects of ERT/HRT with regard to osteoporosis, genital atrophy, and cardiovascular disease. Patients taking ERT or HRT who develop breast cancer demonstrate survival rates that exceed those of nonusers. This provides reassuring evidence, albeit indirect, that estrogen does not adversely effect the biology of breast cancer.

CLINICAL USE OF HORMONE REPLACEMENT THERAPY

Numerous health issues are impacted by estrogen deficiency, and as life expectancy continues to increase in the United States, a woman can now expect to live one third of her life in an ever-increasing estrogen-deficient environment. Although menopause per se is not a disease, the accompanying estrogen deficiency represents an endocrinopathy that is inexorably associated with specific consequences, such as genital atrophy, which are more amenable to prevention than treatment. Estrogen replacement qualifies as a bona fide example of *primary* or preventive therapy, and the majority of the specific pathophysiologic events associated with estrogen deficiency are far easier to prevent than treat (Table 4-2).

CONSEQUENCES OF ESTROGEN DEFICIENCY

Vasomotor Symptoms

The vast majority of women experience hot flushes or ''flushes'' during the climacteric years. Most women demonstrate symptoms for several years, but in some women they may persist for up to 10 years. There are excellent double-blind cross-over studies demonstrating the effectiveness of estrogen replacement for the alleviation of vasomotor symptoms.[12,13] Although ''hot flushes'' are not life threatening, this symptom deserves considerably more attention than it has received, and it is certainly worthy of therapy.

Psychophysiologic Manifestations

There are numerous subjective complaints voiced by postmenopausal women, many of which are difficult to evaluate and quantify. The psychogenic manifestations accompanying estrogen deficiency may in large part represent a secondary or ''domino'' effect of chronic sleep deprivation induced by vasomotor instability. Improved sleep patterns, both in the induction time and rapid eye movement component, occur with ERT.[14] This is a probable mechanism for the improved psychophysiology associated with estrogen therapy. Estrogen deficiency has occasionally been implicated in involutional melancholia, depression, and various other

TABLE 4-2. *Pathophysiologic events associated with estrogen deficiency*

Vasomotor symptoms*
Psycghophysiologic manifestations
Genitourinary atrophy*
Osteoporosis*
Cardiovascular disease

* FDA-approved indications for estrogen replacement therapy.

psychiatric disturbances, but there is literature to the contrary.[15]

There are reports implying improved cerebral circulation and cognitive function in older women treated with estrogen.[16] There are also encouraging data to suggest a significant reduction in the incidence of Alzheimer's disease associated with ERT. This association is strengthened by the linear relationship between duration of treatment and the degree of protection afforded by therapy.[17] If this is substantiated by future studies, ERT's efficacy in reducing Alzheimer's disease would prove extremely valuable since at least one third or more of all women in retirement homes suffer dementia.

Genitourinary Atrophy

Genitourinary atrophy is the most inevitable yet least-publicized aspect of estrogen deficiency. Compared with the extensive literature addressing the life-threatening sequela associated with estrogen deficiency (eg, osteoporosis and cardiovascular disease), there is a paucity of data about two specific events inevitably associated with long-term genital atrophy: sexual dysfunction and pelvic senescence, which is usually manifest as urinary incontinence or pelvic floor relaxation. Not all women will develop osteoporosis and cardiovascular disease, but essentially *every* woman will ultimately develop some form of urinary or sexual dysfunction after prolonged estrogen deficiency. There is a loss of collagen and vasculature in both the dermis and underlying connective tissue in the postmenopausal genital tract, which is very similar to the loss that occurs in bone and skin.[18] This atrophic manifestation of estrogen deficiency develops slowly and is not evident as early as the sexual dysfunction, which usually begins rather rapidly after the decline of estrogen levels. The epithelial change in the genital tract causes sexual dysfunction early on, while the changes in the subcutaneous tissue and dermis require more time before becoming clinically apparent.

Because patients are somewhat reluctant to discuss sexuality and voiding dysfunction during their reproductive years, it is understandable that the consequences of genitourinary atrophy often go unmentioned during the climacteric and after menopause. This is unfortunate because it would be difficult to imagine an estrogen-deficient woman for whom ERT would not provide some benefit regarding genitourinary atrophy. Estrogen is essential in the preservation of a functional genital tract in all females, and this quality-of-life issue warrants far more attention than it currently receives.

Osteoporosis

Osteoporosis is a skeletal disorder in which microarchitectural loss of bone mass occurs without any accompanying abnormality in mineral content. This predisposes individuals

TABLE 4-3. *Osteoporosis and fractures*

Approximately 30 million women older than 65 years old are at risk.

Bone	Fracture rates
Wrist	1 in 6
Hip*	1 in 6
Spine	1 in 4

* One fourth of elderly patients (with hip fractures) die within 6 months.

Modified from Peck W, Barrett-Conner E, Buckwalter J, et al. Consensus conference: osteoporosis. JAMA 1984;252:799. Copyright 1984, American Medical Association.

to atraumatic fracture, especially of the hip and vertebra. Hip fracture in the elderly is associated with significant permanent infirmity and mortality. Up to 50% of patients in the seventh and eighth decades of life never regain the independent lifestyle they enjoyed before the fracture. As longevity increases, osteoporosis has become almost epidemic in older women, as demonstrated in Table 4-3.[19]

The development of sophisticated reproducible bone densitometry, particularly dual-energy radiographic absorptiometry has provided data to substantiate the epidemiology of estrogen deficiency and osteoporosis. Because of the rapidity of bone loss associated with estrogen deficiency, susceptible patients can be identified and monitored accurately with precise measurement of bone mass. Use of such measurements can predict fracture risk using established normograms and help prevent the disease.[20] Reliable quantification of bone has provided data that ERT and HRT are associated with a 50% reduction in the rate of hip fracture. The importance of primary or preventive therapy is equally important for genitourinary atrophy, osteoporosis, and cardiovascular disease. Although prophylaxis is more beneficial than treatment, even in the seventh and eighth decades of life women with established osteoporosis benefit from HRT.[21] The rate of recurrent fractures has been shown to decrease in treated women. Estrogen replacement, exercise, and calcium supplementation (maintaining serum estradiol levels >50 pg/mL combined with 1000 mg of elemental calcium) are known to be associated with a 75% reduction in the number of osteoporotic fractures in older women.[22] Based on the plethora of experimental epidemiologic data substantiating estrogen's role in preventing bone loss, there is current Food and Drug Administration "approval" of ERT for the prevention of osteoporosis, vasomotor symptoms, and genitourinary atrophy.

Cardiovascular Disease

Cardiovascular disease, including coronary heart disease, cerebrovascular disease, and hypertension, is the most common cause of death in the United States. Almost half of the 550,000 deaths in the United States from heart disease occur

in women, and there is considerable epidemiologic evidence as well as a National Institutes of Health consensus meeting opinion that estrogen replacement in menopausal women is associated with a significant decrease in the incidence of coronary heart disease.[23] An interesting population-based study in Minnesota equated ERT to smoking cessation by suggesting that each endeavor conveyed a benefit equal to the daily use of antioxidants, such as aspirin therapy.[24]

There are more than 30 population-based, observational studies in menopausal women demonstrating the cardioprotective benefits of ERT. The only study failing to confirm this beneficial effect was the Framingham Heart Study, which initially used angina as an endpoint for coronary heart disease.[25] A reanalysis of the Framingham data, eliminating angina as the endpoint, confirmed a benefit associated with ERT.[26]

Five cross-sectional studies have involved the use of coronary angiography to compare the extent of coronary occlusion in estrogen users versus nonusers. These studies demonstrated a 50% reduction in the degree of coronary occlusion in estrogen users, and one of the studies showed a relative risk of only 0.3 in women using ERT.[27] In the largest angiographic study, which included over 2200 women, the greatest benefit in survival was seen in patients who demonstrated the most severe degree of coronary occlusion.[28]

A number of prospective, longitudinal studies performed over varying lengths of time have demonstrated a reduced risk of coronary heart disease among estrogen users. The Leisure World Study involved 8807 females, aged 40 to 101 years (average age, 73) living in a retirement community in California.[29] During a 7-year follow-up study, estrogen users had a 20% reduction in "all-cause" mortality and a 40% reduction in fatal myocardial infarction. The Nurse's Health Study was initiated in Boston in 1976 with the registration of 121,700 married female nurses, aged 30 to 50 years.[30] Questionnaires were updated every 2 years, and 48,470 postmenopausal nurses were followed over a 10-year period. The overall age-adjusted risk for major coronary heart disease is reduced by 50% in users (relative risk 0.51 [95% CI 0.37–0.70]). Various individual risk factors have been studied assiduously, including such variables as smoking, diabetes, and obesity, and the overall outcome demonstrated the consistent benefit.

Investigators have done a meta-analysis to evaluate the relationship between ERT and coronary heart disease through 1993.[31] The overall, age-adjusted relative risk for coronary heart disease in the meta-analysis was 0.65. One particularly pertinent facet of these data is the cardioprotective effect associated with "current use" of estrogen, as demonstrated in Figure 4-2. Current users have a combined relative risk of coronary heart disease of 0.49. With regard to benefit associated with estrogen therapy, "recency of use" has been shown to be more important than duration of therapy in other studies as well.[29]

The beneficial effect of estrogen on cardiovascular disease was originally thought to be the result of alterations in the

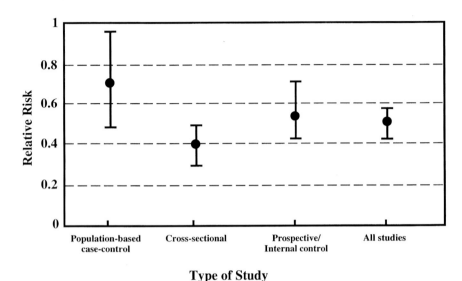

FIG. 4-2. Summary of studies of heart disease among current users of estrogen. (Data from Stampfer M, Colditz G, Willett W, et al. Postmenopausal estrogen therapy and cardiovascular disease: ten-year follow-up from The Nurses' Health Study. N Engl J Med 1991;325:756.)

synthesis and metabolism of lipoproteins. The principal metabolic effect of ERT is a pharmacologic increase in circulating high-density lipoproteins and a decrease in low-density lipoproteins. The additional protection afforded current users strongly suggests that there are other more direct effects on the vascular system. It has now been postulated that the non–lipid-mediated events constitute the major benefit derived from ERT. Evidence for the nonmetabolic or direct vascular effects includes the following:

- Alteration of atherosclerotic plaques (initiation, growth, stabilization, and regression)
- Alteration of blood flow[32,33]
- Endothelium-derived releasing factor formation and release[34,35]
- Alterations in prostacyclin production[36]
- Calcium antagonist activity and effects on sympathetic innervation[23]
- Effects on platelet aggregation and coagulation[37]

There is concern that the beneficial effect of estrogens on the vascular system may be attenuated by the addition of progestogen therapy in women with intact uteri. Route, dose, and duration of progestogen therapy are important because it is recognized that the mildly "androgenic" activity of progestogens has a dose-related deleterious effect on lipoproteins and the vasoactivity of blood vessels. In one study it was demonstrated that while progestogens, especially progestins, may "blunt" the beneficial effect of estrogens, the overall cardioprotective effect of the estrogen persists. For this reason, it is important to remember that use of lower-dose and less androgenic progestogens is associated with proportionately better lipoprotein profiles.[38]

Conclusion

The rationale for estrogen replacement includes a constellation of important clinical conditions often seen in post-menopausal women. In specific situations, such as women at risk for osteoporosis, women predisposed to cardiovascular disease, and women exhibiting genitourinary atrophy and its consequences, there is a compelling reason to consider estrogen replacement therapy. Not only are mortality and morbidity at issue, quality of life can be dramatically enhanced by estrogen replacement therapy for these women.

TAMOXIFEN

Tamoxifen is a synthetic nonsteroidal compound that is structurally very similar to both diethylstilbestrol, a potent estrogen, and clomiphene citrate, a weak estrogen used to induce ovulation. Whereas tamoxifen binds estrogen receptors relatively weakly, in the dose commonly used as an adjunct for breast cancer therapy it suppresses follicle-stimulating hormone in menopausal women as well as the normal doses of estrogen used in ERT, such as 1 to 2 mg of estradiol.[39] As a weak estrogen, it binds with the estrogen receptor; and the specific receptor complex/DNA interaction promotes gene transcription, which then causes either agonistic or antagonistic estrogenic activity, depending on the particular cell involved. Tamoxifen acts as an agonist for most serum proteins and causes changes very similar to those of natural estrogens. Because it increases high-density lipoproteins and sex hormone–binding globulin and lowers low-density lipoproteins, it confers a cardioprotective effect on the cardiovascular system. It also inhibits bone loss so it is protective against osteoporosis as well. Tamoxifen also acts as an agonist on the endometrium and causes proliferation in postmenopausal women in the same manner as other endogenous or exogenous estrogen. Tamoxifen may also potentiate endometriosis and promote vaginal epithelial maturation. The endometrial changes promoted by tamoxifen are similar to the stimulatory changes seen with other estrogens in that duration of therapy is more important than the dose in inducing hyperplastic change. Consequently, long-term tamoxifen therapy as an adjunctive measure in breast cancer therapy has been associated with an increased incidence of both endometrial hyperplasia and polyps.[40] There are also reports in the literature suggesting that tamoxifen therapy increases the incidence of endometrial cancer in patients above the relative risk of 2.4 normally found in patients with a history of breast cancer.[41] More recent studies have questioned this proposed increased incidence of endometrial cancer associated with tamoxifen use.[42,43] Several recent articles have described sonolucencies beneath the endometrium that appear as heterologous, centrally located, benign subepithelial cysts in the myometrium, but a neoplastic potential for such "cysts" has not yet been determined.[44]

Breast cancer patients, especially those treated with tamoxifen adjunctive therapy, are certainly at increased risk for uterine abnormalities. For those patients, increased surveillance seems appropriate. If the endometrium appears thin at sonography (<5 mm) in asymptomatic patients, no further investigation is necessary. If the endometrium appears thickened, sonohysterographic evaluation may prove beneficial in distinguishing truly thickened endometrium from an atrophic endometrium accompanied by benign stromal changes.[45] If a thin endometrium cannot be confirmed sonographically, dilatation and curettage and hysteroscopy may be necessary to rule out hyperplasia or neoplasia.

Monitoring breast cancer patients who are on tamoxifen-adjunctive therapy presents an interesting challenge. The use of "routine endometrial biopsy" as a screening technique would be met with poor patient compliance and, like dilatation and curettage without hysteroscopy, would not provide the necessary information in such high-risk patients. Sonohysterography may prove to be especially helpful in evaluating patients on tamoxifen therapy, and it may help avoid the need for more invasive procedures.

REFERENCES

1. Holst J, Koskela O, von Schoultz B. Endometrial findings following curettage in 2018 women according to age and indications. Ann Chir Gynaecol 1983;72:274.
2. Creasman W, Weed J. Carcinoma of endometrium (FIGO stages I & II): clinical features and management. In: Gynecologic oncology: fundamental principles and clinical practice. New York, Churchill Livingstone, 1981:567.
3. Archer D, McIntyre-Seltman K, Wilborn W, et al. Endometrial morphology in asymptomatic postmenopausal women. Am J Obstet Gynecol 1991;165:317.
4. Gambrell RD Jr. Use of progestogen therapy. Am J Obstet Gynecol 1987;156:1304.
5. Whitehead MI, Hillard TC, Crook D. The role and use of progestogens. Obstet Gynecol 1990;75(suppl):59.
6. Persson I, Adami H-O, Bergkrist L, et al. Risk of endometrial cancer after treatment with oestrogens alone or in conjunction with progestogens: results of a prospective study. BMJ 1989;298:147.
7. Archer DF, Pickar JH, Bottiglioni F, for the Menopause Study Group. Bleeding patterns in postmenopausal women taking continuous combined or sequential regimens of conjugated estrogens with medroxyprogesterone acetate. Obstet Gynecol 1994;83:686.
8. American College of Obstetricians and Gynecologists. Hormone replacement therapy. ACOG technical bulletin No. 166. Washington DC, ACOG, 1992.
9. Stovall T, Solomon S, Ling F. Endometrial sampling prior to hysterectomy. Obstet Gynecol 1989;73:405.
10. Colditz G, Hankinson S, Hunter D, et al. The use of estrogens and progestins and the risk of breast cancer in postmenopausal women. N Engl J Med 1995;332:1589.
11. Stanford J, Weiss N, Voight L, et al. Combined estrogen and progestin hormone replacement therapy in relation to risk of breast cancer in middle-aged women. JAMA 1995;274:137.
12. Coope J. Double-blind cross-over study: estrogen replacement therapy. In: Campbell, S, ed. The management of the menopause and menopausal years. Baltimore, University Park Press, 1976:159.
13. Haas S, Walsh B, Evans S, et al. The effect of transdermal estradiol on hormone and metabolic dynamics over a six-week period. Obstet Gynecol 1988;71:671.
14. Wikland I, Karlberg J, Mattson L. Quality of life of postmenopausal women on a regimen of transdermal estradiol therapy: a double-blind placebo-controlled study. Am J Obstet Gynecol 1993;168:824.
15. Barrett-Conner E, Critz-Silverstein D. Estrogen replacement therapy and cognitive function in older women. JAMA 1993;269:2637.
16. Sherwin B, in press.
17. Henderson B, Paganini-Hill A, Emanuel C, et al. Estrogen replacement therapy in older women. Arch Neurol 1994;51:896.
18. Brincat M, Kabalan S, Studd J, et al. A study of the decrease of skin collagen content, skin thickness, and bone mass in the postmenopausal woman. Obstet Gynecol 1987;70:840.
19. Peck W, Barrett-Conner E, Buckwalter J, et al. Consensus conference: osteoporosis. JAMA 1984;252:799.
20. Johnson G, Melton L, Lindsay R, et al. Clinical indications for bone measurement. J Bone Miner Res 1989;4(suppl 2):1.
21. Felson D, Zhang Y, Hannan M, et al. The effect of postmenopausal estrogen therapy on the bone density in elderly women. N Engl J Med 1993;329:1141.
22. Speroff L, Glass R, Kase N. Clinical gynecologic endocrinology and infertility. Baltimore, Williams & Wilkins, 1994:589.
23. Lobo R, Speroff L. International consensus conference on hormone replacement therapy and the cardiovascular system. Fertil Steril 1994; 62(suppl 2):176S.
24. Beard C, Kottke T, Annegers J, et al. The Rochester Coronary Heart Disease Project, 1960 through 1982. Mayo Clin Proc 1989;64:1471.
25. Wilson P, Garrison R, Costelli W. Postmenopausal estrogen use, cigarette smoking, and cardiovascular morbidity in women over 50: the Framingham study. N Engl J Med 1985;313:1038.
26. Eaker E, Castelli W. Coronary heart disease and its risk factors among women in the Framingham study. In: Coronary Heart Disease in Women. New York, Haymarket Doyma, 1987:122.
27. Hong M, Romm P, Reagen K, et al. Effects of estrogen replacement therapy on serum lipid values and angiographically defined coronary artery disease in postmenopausal women. Am J Cardiol 1992;69:176.
28. Sullivan J, VanderZwaag, Lemp G, et al. Postmenopausal estrogen use and coronary atherosclerosis. Ann Intern Med 1988;108:358.
29. Henderson B, Paganini-Hill A, Ross R. Estrogen replacement therapy and protection from acute myocardial infarction. Am J Obstet Gynecol 1988;159:312.
30. Stampfer M, Colditz G, Willett W, et al. Postmenopausal estrogen therapy and cardiovascular disease: ten-year follow-up from The Nurses' Health Study. N Engl J Med 1991;325:756.
31. Stampfer M, Grodstein F. Estrogen replacement therapy and cardiovascular disease. Menopause Med 1994;2:2.
32. Belfort M, Saade G, Snabes M, et al. Hormonal status affects the reactivity of the cerebral vasculature. Am J Obstet Gynecol 1995;172:1273.
33. Lieberman E, Gerhard M, Uehata A, et al. Estrogen improves endothelium-dependent, flow-mediated vasodilation in postmenopausal women. Ann Intern Med 1994;121:936.
34. Garg U, Hassid A. Nitric oxide-generating vasodilators and 9-bromo-cyclic guanosine monophosphate inhibit mitogenesis and proliferation of cultured rat vascular smooth muscle cells. J Clin Invest 1989;83: 1774.
35. Herrington D, Braden G, Williams K, et al. Endothelial-dependent coronary vasomotor responsiveness in postmenopausal women with and without estrogen replacement therapy. Am J Cardiol 1994;73:951.
36. Foidart J, Dombrowitz N, de Lignieres B. Urinary excretion of prosta-

cyclin and thromboxane metabolites in postmenopausal women treated with percutaneous oestradiol (Oestrogel) or conjugated oestrogens (Premarin). In: Dusitsin N, Notelowitz M, eds. Physiological hormone replacement therapy. Carnforth, England, Parthenon, 1990:99.

37. Bar J, Tepper R, Fuchs J, et al. The effect of estrogen replacement therapy on platelet aggregation and adenosine triphosphate release in postmenopausal women. Obstet Gynecol 1993;81:261.

38. PEPI Trial Writing Group: Effects of estrogen or estrogen/progestin regimens on heart disease risk factors in postmenopausal women. JAMA 1995;273:199.

39. Helgason S, Wilking N, Carlstrom K, et al. A comparative study of the estrogenic effects of tamoxifen and 17β-estradiol in postmenopausal women. J Clin Endocrinol Metab 1982;54:404.

40. Lahti E, Guillermo B, Kauppila A, et al. Endometrial changes in post-menopausal breast cancer patients receiving tamoxifen. Obstet Gynecol 1993;81:660–64.

41. Fornander T, Rutquist L, Sjoberg H, et al. Long-term adjuvant tamoxifen in early breast cancer. J Clin Oncol 1990;8:1019.

42. Gal D, Kopel S, Basherkin M, et al. Oncogenic potential of tamoxifen on endometrium of postmenopausal women with breast cancer. Gynecol Oncol 1991;42:120.

43. Barakat R. The effect of tamoxifen on the endometrium. Oncol 1995;9:129.

44. Goldstein S. Unusual ultrasonographic appearance of the uterus in patients receiving tamoxifen. Am J Obstet Gynecol 1994;170:447.

45. Anteby, E, Yagel S, Hochner-Celnikier D. Letters: Unusual ultrasonographic appearance of uterus in postmenopausal patients receiving tamoxifen. Am J Obstet Gynecol 1995;172:717.

Endometrial Cancer: An Overview

Howard W. Jones, III, MD

CANCER OF THE UTERINE CORPUS

Cancer of the body of the uterus, or uterine corpus, can be subdivided into two major categories. The vast majority of these tumors are adenocarcinomas arising from the endometrium. Approximately 5% of corpus cancers are sarcomas, however; and a still smaller group are mixed tumors that are composed of both sarcomatous and carcinomatous elements. These are generally referred to as mixed müllerian tumors. Because endometrial adenocarcinomas are the most common of all gynecologic malignancies in the United States, the major emphasis here is on these lesions.

Epidemiology and Risk Factors

Endometrial cancer has become the most common type of cancer encountered by gynecologists—about 2.2% of newborn girls, or 1 in 45, develop invasive cancer of the uterine corpus sometime during their lives. Cancer of the endometrium accounts for about 7% of all cancers in women.

Although an increase in the incidence of endometrial carcinoma has been observed in the United States and many other countries throughout the world, in the past few years this trend has appeared to level off. This increased incidence has probably been a result of the increasing longevity of the population, increased surveillance with earlier and more accurate diagnoses, and the increased use of estrogen therapy among menopausal women in the past two decades.

In North America the incidence rates for endometrial cancer vary widely among various locations as well as among different ethnic groups. Among white women in the San Francisco Bay area, there are approximately 40 new cases per 100,000 women, while black women in New Orleans have an incidence rate of only 10.5/100,000 and Native Americans in New Mexico have an incidence rate of only 3.4/100,000. White women in Iowa have a rather intermediate incidence rate of 21/100,000. The reason for these variations is not completely understood but probably relates in great part to the three reasons for the increased frequency of this disease noted earlier. Patients from better socioeconomic classes tend to live longer and receive better medical care and are more likely to be treated with estrogens. The average age of women with endometrial cancer is 59, and the vast majority of patients are in the postmenopausal age group.

The relationship between estrogens and endometrial carcinoma is now well established, and endometrial carcinoma is seen as a result of both exogenous estrogens administered as medication and endogenous estrogens produced in the ovaries or converted from adrenal androstenedione in peripheral adipose tissue.

The increased risk of endometrial carcinoma among women with estrogen-producing ovarian tumors has been observed for many years. The anovulatory patient whose endometrium is exposed to prolonged estrogen stimulation without the modifying effect of progesterone is also at an increased risk of developing endometrial caner. Exogenous estrogen therapy given as menopausal estrogen replacement therapy or prescribed for patients with gonadal dysfunction has been shown to result in a 3- to 20-fold increase in the risk of endometrial carcinoma. This risk varies depending on the dose and duration of the hormonal therapy. In view of these findings, it is advisable to add a progestin such as medroxyprogesterone acetate or hydroxyprogesterone caproate to the hormonal regimen of women who have their uterus and are receiving estrogen replacement therapy.

Several constitutional characteristics are often associated with women who are at high risk for developing endometrial carcinoma. These include obesity, nulliparity or low parity, diabetes, and hypertension. Obese women have a 2- to 3-fold increased risk of developing endometrial carcinoma, and it appears that this is also related to the effect of estrogens. Androstenedione is produced in the adrenal glands and is converted to a weak estrogen, estrone, in peripheral adipose tissue. As a result of this peripheral conversion, the endometrium of obese women is exposed to higher levels of estrogen. Although the mechanism is not well understood, the high progesterone levels that occur in women during pregnancy as well as the use of progestin-dominated combined oral contraceptives during the reproductive years appear to exert a protective effect on the endometrium.

Some types of endometrial hyperplasia represent a transitional or premalignant form of endometrial neoplasia. Many different classification schemes have been suggested for different degrees of hyperplasia. Current terminology favors a description of the degree of typicality of the glandular architecture and nuclear atypia. In one series of 170 patients with all grades of endometrial hyperplasia, 29% of the patients with complex glandular patterns and cytologic atypia developed endometrial carcinoma, while only 1% of those with a simple glandular pattern and no cytologic atypia developed malignancy.

Diagnosis

The most common symptom associated with endometrial carcinoma is abnormal uterine bleeding. Because endometrial carcinoma occurs most frequently in postmenopausal patients, the onset of unexpected spotting or bleeding usually causes the woman to seek prompt gynecologic consultation. A careful history and physical examination may be useful in suggesting possible reasons for the bleeding, but a tissue sample from the endometrium by endometrial biopsy or formal fractional dilation and curettage is absolutely essential in evaluating patients with postmenopausal bleeding. A Papanicolaou test is inadequate because it is an unreliable technique for evaluating the possible cause of uterine bleeding.

In perimenopausal or premenopausal patients, the risk of endometrial cancer is less, and there are many other causes for irregular bleeding. Nevertheless, the prudent clinician will use one of the simple office techniques for obtaining an endometrial sample when the cause of the bleeding is uncertain or symptoms persist.

In regard to endometrial sampling, two points should be emphasized: (1) Before the uterine cavity is instrumented, the endocervix should be sampled separately with a small, sharp curette so that cervical involvement can be evaluated for staging purposes. Hysteroscopy is also being investigated as a staging technique. (2) If office techniques of endometrial biopsy produce tissue insufficient for diagnosis, a formal fractional dilatation and curettage with endocervical and endometrial curettage under general anesthesia should be performed. If endometrial hyperplasia is diagnosed, an appropriate progestational therapy plan should be considered and instituted with the patient's understanding and concurrence. After this hormonal treatment for 2 to 3 months, thorough endometrial sampling should be performed and further management plans developed.

Prognostic Characteristics

Several clinical characteristics are important in defining the prognosis of women with endometrial adenocarcinoma. Tumor cell type and degree of differentiation are most important and are included in the clinical staging system discussed below. Patients with well-differentiated grade 1 adenocarcinomas have a very favorable prognosis, whereas patients with poorly differentiated grade 3 lesions usually have a poor prognosis. Tumors associated with squamous metaplasia are often called adenocanthomas. The adenocarcinoma portion of these tumors is usually well differentiated,

and the prognosis for patients with these tumors is better than average. Conversely, patients with clear cell, serous papillary, and adenosquamous tumors are at high risk for early metastases and have a correspondingly poor prognosis. Measurement of progesterone receptor levels in patients with endometrial cancer may be of some value because low levels of receptor are found in patients with a poor prognosis.

Deep myometrial invasion and extrauterine extension of carcinoma, including lymph node metastases, are also associated with a decreased survival rate. Five to 10% of patients with stage I endometrial carcinoma have evidence of malignant cells in washings obtained by peritoneal lavage with normal saline. Similar to patients with gross evidence of metastatic disease, these women also have an increased risk of recurrence and a decreased 5-year survival rate.

Clinical Staging

Many of the prognostic characteristics noted earlier require exploratory laparotomy or hysterectomy for evaluation. In 1988, the International Federation of Gynecology and Obstetrics (FIGO) approved the long-advocated system of surgical/pathologic staging (Table 4-4). Data derived from careful clinical and surgical staging provide optimal direction for treatment planning. The clinical stage of endometrial carcinoma should be determined for all patients before the start of therapy. Routine intravenous pyelograms, barium enemas, cystoscopy, and proctosigmoidoscopy are not necessary and should be used only when the history or physical findings suggest the possible involvement of the bladder or rectum or to rule out the presence of primary conditions of the urologic or gastrointestinal tract that may complicate therapy or confuse later follow-up. Lymphangiography, CT scans, and MRI may not be considered in the formal clinical staging process

TABLE 4-4. *Surgical/pathologic staging of uterine corpus cancer*

Stage*	Description
Ia	Growth limited to endometrium
Ib	Myometrial invasion of less than one-half full thickness
Ic	Myometrial invasion of greater than one-half full thickness
IIa	Involvement of endocervical glands
IIb	Cervical stromal invasion
IIIa	Involvement of the uterine serosa, adnexa, and/or positive peritoneal cytology
IIIb	Extension to the vagina
IIIc	Positive pelvic or paraaortic nodes
IVa	Invasion into bladder, rectum, or signmoid
IVb	Distant metastasis (out of pelvis)

* FIGO grades 1 to 3 apply to all stages.

Modified from International Federation of Gynecology and Obstetrics. Annual report on the results of treatment in gynecological cancer, vol. 20. Stockholm, FIGO, 1988.

but may provide important information that helps the clinician to plan treatment or evaluate the prognosis.

Therapy

The cornerstone of treatment for endometrial carcinoma is total abdominal hysterectomy and bilateral salpingo-oophorectomy. Although treatment planning must be individualized and stage, histology, and other prognostic characteristics must be weighed in developing a therapeutic plan, surgical removal of the uterus, fallopian tubes, and ovaries continues to be the mainstay of treatment. Hysterectomy and bilateral salpingo-oophorectomy should be done in conjunction with appropriate staging studies, including pelvic peritoneal washings and selective lymph node biopsies. Ten to 12% of patients with clinical stage I endometrial carcinoma have pelvic lymph node metastasis. As many as 35% of patients with clinical stage II disease may have involvement of the pelvic lymph nodes. Although the incidence of aortic lymph node metastases is less well known, in as many as 8% to 10% of women with clinical stage I disease, the disease has already spread to the aortic nodes. One large study suggests that 60% of all patients with stage I endometrial carcinoma who have pelvic lymph node metastases also have involvement of the aortic nodes. The incidence of lymph node metastasis is related to tumor differentiation and depth of myometrial penetration. Pelvic and paraaortic lymph node sampling is suggested for all patients with suspicious nodes encountered at surgery; and in all women with grade 3 tumors, more have superficial invasion or evidence of cervical involvement. Intraoperative histologic evaluation may prove helpful in making decisions regarding indications for lymph node removal.

For patients with clinical stage I disease, primary surgery with a hysterectomy and associated staging studies is favored by most gynecologic oncologists in the United States. Adjunctive irradiation with vaginal cesium, external irradiation, or both may be added selectively, depending on the final surgical-pathologic staging. Although adjunctive irradiation in patients with stage Ia and Ib endometrial carcinomas appears to decrease the risk of recurrence of carcinoma at the vaginal apex, there is no conclusive evidence to suggest that overall survival is improved. Adjunctive irradiation should be used selectively, bearing in mind the potential morbidity. Patients who are unacceptable anesthetic risks or who refuse surgery may be treated for a cure with irradiation alone by both external and intracavitary techniques. The results are not as good as they are with surgery, however.

Patients with clinical stage II endometrial carcinoma have traditionally been treated with whole-pelvis external irradiation followed by intrauterine and vaginal cesium, followed by total abdominal hysterectomy, bilateral salpingo-oophorectomy, and additional surgical staging done 4 to 6 weeks later. However, the trend is now toward primary surgical staging at the time of planned hysterectomy in this group of patients. Many are found not to have true cervical involvement as anticipated (false-positive endocervical curettage), and some have more advanced metastatic disease that was not included in the field of preoperative irradiation, as was done in the past.

Treatment of clinical stage III and clinical stage IV endometrial adenocarcinomas should be individualized, but, when possible, hysterectomy and bilateral salpingo-oophorectomy should be included. Elimination of uterine bleeding and the removal of an infected, necrotic pelvic tumor may provide a significant palliative benefit.

The management of patients with extrauterine disease (stage IV) or positive peritoneal cytology (surgical stage III) is still unsatisfactory. The use of intraperitoneal radioactive colloidal chronic phosphate (^{32}P) has been suggested for those patients with positive peritoneal cytology alone. The treatment consists of instilling 15 mCi of ^{32}P through an indwelling peritoneal catheter with more than 1000 mL of normal saline to provide a uniform distribution throughout the abdominal cavity. Although satisfactory results have been reported with this technique, comparative trials are lacking, and the management of such patients remains controversial.

Both cytotoxic and hormonal chemotherapy has been effective in the treatment of patients with metastatic endometrial carcinoma. Effective cytotoxic agents include doxorubicin, cisplatin, cyclophosphamide, and 5-fluorouracil. When these drugs are used alone or in combination, response rates of 15% to 35% have been reported, but complete responses are uncommon and disease-free intervals are often short.

Hormonal chemotherapy with progestins such as megestrol acetate has minimal morbidity, and response rates of 30% to 35% have been reported. Unlike cytotoxic chemotherapy, hormonal therapy is well tolerated with few serious side effects. Occasionally, patients exhibit long-term responses.

The results of treatment of endometrial carcinoma are shown in Table 4-5. As previously noted, results relate to both stage and grade.

SARCOMAS OF THE UTERUS

Uterine sarcomas arise from the mesenchymal tissue of the uterus and usually occur in postmenopausal women at an average age of 58. An enlarged, irregular uterus is the most common physical finding, and irregular bleeding is the most common symptom, occurring in about 85% of patients. Other less common complaints include abdominal pain (19%), abdominal mass (15%), weight loss (7%), and vaginal discharge (4%). It is rare to find a sarcoma that arises from within a benign leiomyoma, but it is certainly possible for these two lesions to coexist in the same uterus. Therefore, an enlarging fibroid must be treated with suspicion and is

TABLE 4-5. *Treatment results in endometrial carcinoma**

Clinical stage	% of total	Radiation	Surgery ± radiation
I	80	60	80–90
G1	45		88
G2	35		87
G3	20		68
II	8	43	74
III	6	30	
IV	6	7	

G, grade.
* 5-year survival (percent).

generally an indication for hysterectomy. Occasionally, a sarcoma is present as a pedunculated polyp prolapsing through the cervix.

Although there are multiple classifications of uterine sarcomas (Table 4-6), homologous tumors are those that arise from mesenchymal tissues that are usually found in the uterus (endometrial stroma, smooth muscle, blood vessels, fibrous tissue), whereas heterologous tumors arise from mesenchymal elements that are foreign to the uterus (bone, cartilage, striated muscle, fat). The mitotic index, or the number of mitoses per 10 high-power fields, is the chief histologic criterion of malignancy for leiomyosarcomas. Fewer than five mitoses per 10 high-power fields is usually referred to as a cellular myoma and has a good prognosis. With greater than 10 mitoses per 10 high-power fields, the tumor is definitely malignant; with between 5 and 10 mitoses per 10 high-power fields it is usually regarded as an intermediate- or low-grade lesion.

TABLE 4-6. *Classification of uterine sarcomas*

I. Pure Sarcomas
  A. Pure homologous
    1. Leiomyosarcoma
    2. Stromal sarcoma
    3. Angiosarcoma
    4. Fibrosarcoma
  B. Pure heterologous
    1. Rhabdomyosarcoma
    2. Chondrosarcoma
    3. Osteogenic sarcoma
    4. Liposarcoma
II. Mixed Sarcomas
  A. Mixed homologous
  B. Mixed heterologous
  C. Mixed homologous and heterologous
III. Malignant Mixed Müllerian Tumors
  A. Malignant mixed müllerian tumor, homologous type; carcinoma plus one or more of the homologous sarcomas listed under IA above
  B. Malignant mixed müllerian tumor, heterologous type; carcinoma plus one or more of the heterologous sarcomas listed under IB; homologous sarcoma(s) may also be present
IV. Sarcoma, Unclassified
V. Malignant Lymphoma

Extent of disease is the most important prognostic characteristic in patients with uterine sarcoma. When sarcoma has spread beyond the uterus, only rare long-term survivors have been reported. Even when the cancer is confined to the uterus, prognosis is relatively poor, with overall 5-year survival rates of approximately 50%. There does not seem to be any prognostic difference between patients with heterologous tumors and those with homologous tumors. Metastasis to the ovaries is not uncommon, and vascular metastases to lungs and bone are also seen relatively frequently in patients with this disease.

The primary treatment for patients with uterine sarcoma is total abdominal hysterectomy and bilateral salpingo-oophorectomy. Pelvic radiation therapy may reduce the incidence of pelvic recurrence but has not been shown to improve overall survival. Preoperative and postoperative chemotherapy with a variety of agents has also been reported, but response rates are low and the duration of response is short.

ESTROGEN REPLACEMENT THERAPY AFTER ENDOMETRIAL CANCER

There are no definitive data to support specific recommendations regarding the use of estrogen in women with a history of endometrial carcinoma; however, responses from a survey of members of the Society of Gynecologic Oncologists indicate that 83% of the respondents approved the use of estrogen replacement therapy in patients with stage I, grade 1 endometrial cancer; 56% favored the use of estrogen in cases of stage I, grade 2 cancer; and 39% would use estrogen in cases of stage I, grade 3 cancer. The Committee on Gynecologic Practice of the American College of Obstetricians and Gynecologists has concluded that in women with a history of endometrial carcinoma, estrogens can be used for the same indications as they are used for any other woman, except that the selection of appropriate candidates should be based on prognostic indicators and the risk that the patient is willing to assume. If the patient is free of tumor, estrogen replacement therapy cannot result in recurrence. If an estrogen-dependent neoplasm is harbored somewhere in her body, it will eventually recur; however, estrogen replacement therapy may result in an earlier recurrence. Prognostic predictors (depth of invasion, degree of differentiation, and cell type) assist the physician in describing the risks of persistent tumor to the patient.

In the absence of estrogen replacement therapy:

- A well-differentiated neoplasm of the endometrioid cell type with superficial invasion would render a risk of persistent disease of approximately 5%.
- A moderately differentiated neoplasm of the endometroid cell type with up to one-half myometrial invasion would render a 10% to 15% risk of persistent disease. The risk would increase to 20% to 30% for adenosquamous cell-type neoplasms and to approximately 50% for serous papillary tumors.

• A poorly differentiated neoplasm, regardless of cell type, with invasion of over one-half of the myometrium would render a 40% to 50% risk of persistent disease.

Because the metabolic changes associated with estrogen deficiency are significant, the woman should be given complete information, including counseling about alternative therapies, to enable her to make an informed decision. For some women, the sense of well-being afforded by amelioration of menopausal symptoms or the need to treat atrophic vaginitis or prevent osteoporosis and coronary artery disease may outweigh the undetermined risk of stimulating tumor growth.

The need for progestational agents in addition to estrogen in the absence of a uterus is unknown.

Transvaginal Sonography and Sonohysterography of Endometrial Disorders

Arthur C. Fleischer, MD, Jeanne A. Cullinan, MD, and Howard W. Jones, III, MD

Transvaginal sonography is extensively used both in private practitioners' offices and in diagnostic imaging departments as a means to evaluate the endometrium. As a consequence of numerous investigations, the ability of transvaginal sonography to evaluate the thickness and texture of the endometrium has been established.[1,2] Transvaginal sonography has an important impact on the management of patients with endometrial disorders.

Sonohysterography can be used as an adjunct to transvaginal sonography in evaluating thickened or irregular endometrium.[3–5] This procedure involves instillation of saline into the endometrial lumen as a means to delineate endometrial polyps, submucosal fibroids, and synechiae.

In this subchapter we discuss and illustrate the clinical applications of sonographic evaluation of the endometrium by transvaginal scanning or sonohysterography, which include

- Determining which patients should undergo endometrial biopsy
- Detection of submucous fibroids and polyps using sonohysterography
- Sonographic depiction of the extent of myometrial invasion (involvement) by endometrial carcinoma and malignant trophoblastic disease

The use of sonohysterography for detection and evaluation of synechiae and other disorders is also discussed in Chapter 10.

INSTRUMENTATION

There are a variety of configurations of transvaginal transducer/probes. These probes vary according to the number and configuration of transducer elements, overall size and shape of the handle and shaft of the probe, as well as the transducer frequency and beam-focusing characteristics used. In general, transvaginal transducer/probes that afford the highest line density within a sector field of view of 85 to 120 degrees are preferable. The transducer can have a variety of configurations, including a mechanical sector single-element transducer with an oscillating element, an electronically phased-array multielement transducer, a curved linear multielement transducer, or rotating wheel configuration. In general, the curved linear multielement transducers afford the best line density and overall field of view for imaging the endometrium. The frequency of the transducers of these probes ranges from 5 to 10 MHz, and their focal field should be adjustable to the area of the endometrium by the operator.

SCANNING TECHNIQUE

With transvaginal scanning, one can image the endometrium in three different scanning planes:

1. Sagittal or "long-axis" views
2. Semicoronal views
3. Semiaxial or "short axis" views

First, the endometrium should be imaged in its long axis by gently angled (anterior for anteflexed or posterior for retroflexed uterus) sagittal scans through the uterus with the probe head in the region of the uterine cervix. Second, the endometrium can be imaged in its short axis, in a semicoronal or semiaxial plane, by turning the probe approximately 90 degrees. The fundus is imaged by directing the probe in various degrees of anterior or posterior inclinations as it is held next to the cervical lips. One should be aware that images taken oblique to those planes may overestimate endometrial thickness. Because depiction of the endometrium in the semicoronal plane is variable, one should be careful to measure the endometrial bilayer thickness in appropriate true sagittal planes.

In the long axis, one can appreciate the different interfaces arising from the endometrium itself, beginning with the interface at the endocervical canal. This is highly contrasted in the periovulatory period when the cervical mucus has a high fluid content and is relatively anechoic, as compared with the secretory phase when the cervical mucus is thicker, resulting in a more echogenic texture.

TABLE 4-7. *Normal endometrial bilayer thickness as measured on transvaginal sonography*

	Range (mm)
Menstruating	
Menstrual	1–4
Proliferative	3–5
Midcycle	5–8
Secretory	8–12
Postmenopausal	
No hormone replacement therapy	5–8
With hormone replacement therapy*	6–9

* Depends on type of hormone replacement therapy estrogen only, therapy: combined, or sequential, oral vs. patch.

NORMAL ENDOMETRIUM

Transvaginal sonography affords a more complete evaluation of the endometrium than does conventional transabdominal techniques. Specifically, transvaginal sonography allows delineation of the endometrium in three major planes of section: anteroposterior; length, as depicted on long-axis images; and width, as depicted on semiaxial scans (Fig. 4-3). If one is not careful to image the endometrium in its true long axis, it can be depicted in an oblique plane. Measurements of anteroposterior thickness or width would not be accurate if obtained on the obliquely oriented images. Measurements should be reported as the bilayer thickness in the true sagittal plane. If intraluminal fluid is present, one should measure each endometrial layer separately, not including the fluid interface. The hypoechoic inner myometrium should not be included in the measurement of the endometrium.

We established a guideline for normal values of endometrial thicknesses based on our experience with over 100 patients who were scanned transvaginally throughout the cycle for several cycles (Table 4-7).[6] Because estrogens have a trophic effect on the endometrium, patients on these medications may have endometria 2 to 3 mm thicker than other postmenopausal women. Women who have taken combined (estrogen and progesterone) hormone replacement may have a endometrial thickness up to 8 mm,[6] and women on sequential regimens may have less thickening than those on combined hormone replacement.[7]

After menarche, the endometrium undergoes cyclic changes in its thickness and texture that can be related to the relative amount of serum estrogen and progesterone. During the menstrual phase, the endometrium appears as an echogenic interrupted interface of 1 to 4 mm in anteroposterior width.

Sloughing endometrium can appear as an irregular interface, with surrounding hypoechoic areas corresponding to intraluminal hemorrhage. Occasionally formed clots can be identified as echogenic material within the endometrial lumen.

A hypoechoic outer layer can be identified surrounding the endometrium, corresponding to the inner layer of myometrium. This layer is distinct in most premenopausal women but may not be apparent in postmenopausal women or when disrupted in conditions such as adenomyosis or invasive endometrial carcinoma. This hypoechoic appearance of the inner myometrium may be related to the more compact and longitudinal configuration of the myometrial bundles in this area and the relatively smaller amount of connective tissue and smooth muscle in the inner layer as compared with the intermediate and external layers of myometrium. One- to 2-mm vessels can be seen in the outer myometrium representing a venous plexus.[8] In older women, calcification may occur secondary to cystic medial necrosis within the arcuate arteries, which course along the outer myometrium and appear as punctuate echogenicities. Besides calcification, there are other causes of echogenic fluid with the myometrium. Burks and associates recognized echogenic foci along the inner myometrium in 35 of 80 patients with prior dilatation and curettage or biopsy and only 2 of 174 patients who had no prior instrumentation. These foci were identified as linear or punctate nonshadowing and adjacent to the endometrium. It was thought that these foci represent calcification and fibrosis in areas of prior mechanical injury.[9] They should not be confused with leiomyoma, arterial calcification, or air within the endometrial cavity. Arcuate artery calcification disappears as focal punctate echogenicities between the middle and outer myometrium and is seen most commonly in diabetics.[10]

During the proliferative phase, the endometrium thickens between 4 and 8 mm and has an isoechoic or slightly hyperechoic texture relative to the middle and outer myometrium. In the late proliferative or periovulatory phase of endometrial development, a multilayered endometrium can be depicted.[11] The inner hypoechoic area probably represents edema in the compact layer of the endometrium. As imaged in a semiaxial or semicoronal plane, the endometrium has the configuration of a theta (θ).

In the secretory phase, the endometrium achieves a width of between 8 and 14 mm and is echogenic, most likely related to the increased mucus and glycogen within the glands as well as the increased number of interfaces created by tortuous glands in this phase. Stromal edema that begins at the basal layer and extends centrally may also contribute to this pattern of "creeping" echogenicity. The endometrium typically achieves its greatest thickness in the midsecretory phase of a spontaneous cycle, measuring up to 14 mm in width. Refluxed mucus forms the thin median echo. Studies with power transvaginal color Doppler sonography have shown changes in vascularity of the endometrium during the menstrual cycles. Specifically, vessels can be seen extending into the basal and functional layers of endometrium during the secretory phase.[12]

The endometrium in postmenopausal women should be thin (less than 8 mm double-layer thickness) and is histologically atrophic. Mucus trapped within the lumen may give the sonographic impression of a thickened endometrium.[13] A recent series of women comparing body weight and thick-

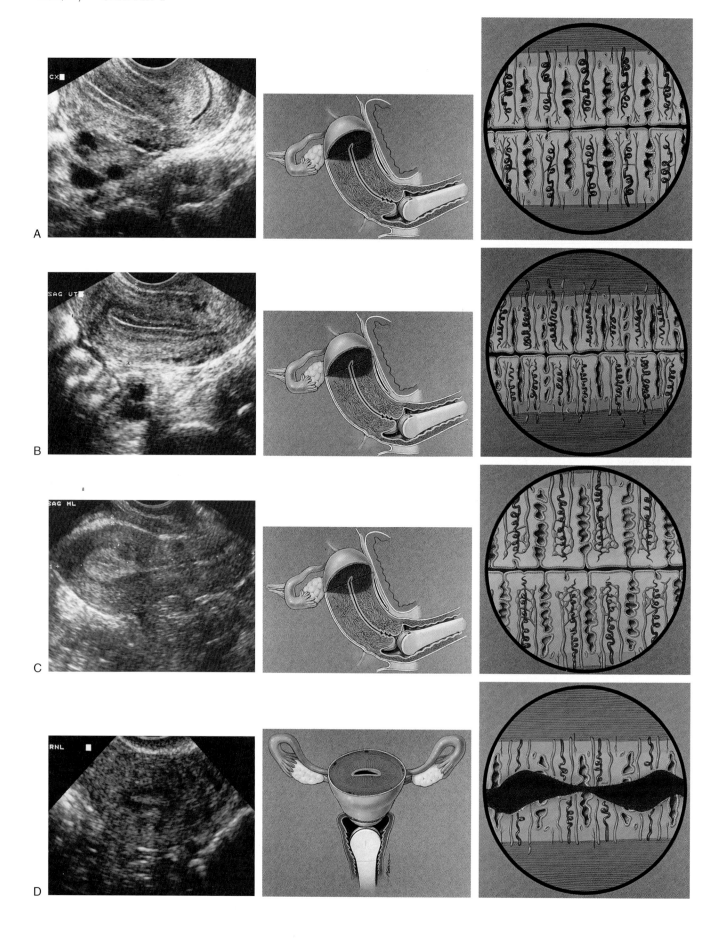

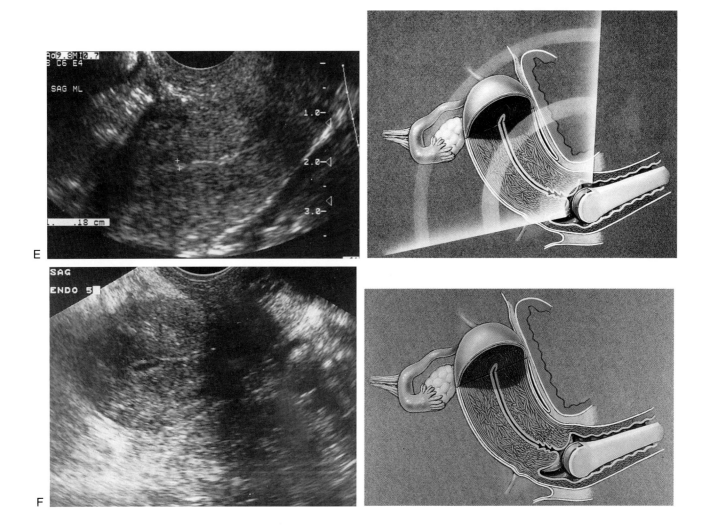

FIG. 4-3. Transvaginal sonography of normal endometrium *(left),* with drawing of scan plane *(middle)* and accompanying line drawings to indicate corresponding microscopic anatomy *(right).* **(A)** At mid cycle the endocervical mucus is hypoechoic and the endometrium displays a multilayered appearance. **(B)** Mid-cycle multilayered endometrium showing centrally located median echoes from refluxed mucus. On either side of this median echo is the hypoechoic functional layer forming the outer layer of endometrium. The hypoechoic subendometrial layer represents the inner, longitudinally oriented layer of myometrium. **(C)** Secretory phase endometrium showing echogenic texture. **(D)** Menstrual phase endometrium is depicted in short-axis image of uterus. **(E)** Thin and regular endometrium in a postmenopausal women with bleeding. Endometrial biopsy specimen showed atrophic endometrium, as could be predicted on transvaginal sonography. **(F)** Normal postmenopausal endometrium separated by intraluminal fluid.

ness of the endometrium in asymptomatic postmenopausal women showed that with increasing weight and body mass index, increasing endometrial thickness was identified. No cancers were seen in this series.[14] Asians may have thinner endometrium than Western women.

Postmenopausal women taking estrogen replacement may have relatively thick endometria (over 8 mm in width) in response to the medication.[7] Women who take combined (estrogen and progesterone) hormone replacement usually have endometria in the expected range (less than 8 mm). Some investigators use transvaginal sonography to monitor the response of the endometrium to estrogen replacement therapy.[15] In some women, the endometrium rapidly thickened in response to estrogen treatment (less than 2 months) whereas in others there was a gradual increase.[15] Progesterone might be withheld in these women whose endometrium does not rapidly thicken in response to estrogen. Transvaginal sonography is being used to monitor endometrial thickening associated with combined estrogen progesterone patches.

BENIGN ENDOMETRIAL DISORDERS

Only 10% to 20% of women with postmenopausal bleeding have cancer; the remainder have a benign cause of the bleeding (Fig. 4-4).[1] Although it is not possible to definitively differentiate benign from malignant endometrial disorders based on sonographic appearance with transvaginal sonography, the imaging technique can distinguish those patients who need endometrial biopsy from those who do not.[2,16,17] In general, endometria greater than 5 mm may be pathologic whereas women with endometria less than 5 mm typically have atrophic endometritis.[18]

Hyperplasia of the endometrium is thought to occur secondary to the trophic influence of unopposed estrogen. The endometrium thickens, and the endometrium itself becomes pseudopolypoid. In mild cases the polyps are microscopic, but in more severe cases the polyps can measure up to 5 cm. In these patients, thickening of the endometrium beyond what is expected for women of comparable age is usually detected on transvaginal sonography. Diffuse polyposis may appear as a

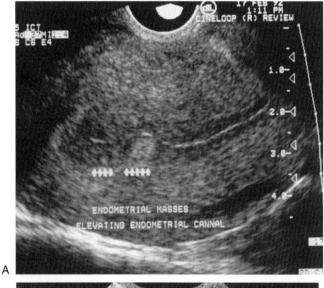

A

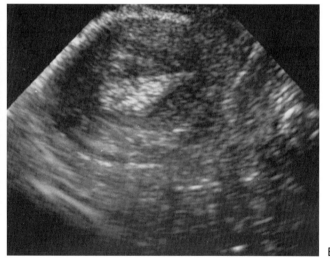

B

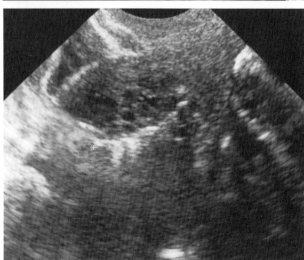

C

FIG. 4-4. Benign endometrial disorders. **(A)** A polyp *(arrow)* is depicted displacing the median echo. **(B)** Adenomatous hyperplasia showing thickening and irregularity of endometrium corresponding to multiple small polyps. **(C)** Large polyp containing punctate hypoechoic areas. The polyp is outlined by air within the endometrial lumen (**A,** courtesy of ATL, Inc.)

relatively homogeneous echogenic endometrial interface; the individual polyps may not be apparent as separate intraluminal structures. In perimenopausal women, endometria of greater than 14 mm in thickness should be considered for further evaluation, whereas in the postmenopausal patient, endometria over 8 mm should be considered abnormal. The sonographic findings must be interpreted in light of the patient's clinical presentation and laboratory findings.

In some patients no tissue will be obtained on dilatation and curettage even though the patient experiences postmenopausal bleeding and transvaginal sonography demonstrates a thickened endometrium. In these cases, fluid distention of the endometrial lumen (sonohysterography) may reveal polyps or submucous fibroids that were not apparent on the initial scan. This is further discussed in Chapter 10.

Women on tamoxifen, which is usually taken after a diagnosis of breast cancer, may be susceptible to endometrial disorders, including hyperplasia and carcinoma.[19,20] These patients may demonstrate an unusually thick endometrial interface, sometimes with punctate hypoechoic areas. Sometimes these represent areas of cystic degeneration within a polyp. Occasionally the hypoechoic areas represent cystic spaces in the inner myometrium.[21]

A study in 103 asymptomatic patients in whom 51 received tamoxifen demonstrated there were atrophic changes in 28% of the women taking tamoxifen versus 87% of the control subjects.[19] Thirty-six percent of the women on tamoxifen demonstrated polyps versus 10% of control subjects, and there was an increase in the endometrial thickness to 10.4 mm versus 4.2 mm in the control population.[20]

One of the most important roles of transvaginal sonography in the evaluation of women who experience postmenopausal bleeding is determining which patients may forego endometrial biopsy. Multiple studies have shown that endometria less than 5 mm are typically associated with atrophic endometritis, and tissue insufficient for diagnosis is usually obtained.[1,2,16,17] It should be remembered that the majority of women who experience post-memopausal bleeding do not have cancer but have either atrophic endometritis or hyperplasia.

Occasionally, unclotted blood within the lumen is hypoechoic whereas clots usually are echogenic. Fluid can also be present within the endometrial lumen in a variety of disorders related to fluid overload or as a reflection of retained secretions related to cervical stenosis from cervical carcinoma or radiation-induced fibrosis with hematometrocolpos. Fluid within the endometrial cavity may also be noted in postmenopausal women.[22] In 20 women with fluid in the uterine cavity five carcinomas were identified (two ovarian, one tubal, one endometrial, and one cervical).[22] Close evaluation of the uterus and ovaries is suggested in the presence of fluid within the endometrial cavity.

MALIGNANT ENDOMETRIAL DISORDERS

The gold standard for the evaluation of the postmenopausal woman with abnormal vaginal bleeding has been dilatation and curettage. However, with the increasing number of women on hormonal replacement therapy this may not be a cost-effective measure. In a series of 76 patients, in 90% of cases the dilatation and curettage correlated with the endometrial biopsy; however, in seven cases hyperplasia was not identified on biopsy sampling.[23] When an endometrial layer of over 5 mm was demonstrated by transvaginal sonography an increased sensitivity and specificity when compared with endometrial sampling was noted. For those women in whom postmenopausal bleeding was identified sonography showed 100% sensitivity and specificity.[24] Shipley and associates[24] noted that the sensitivity of transvaginal sonography in identifying endometrial pathology was 80% whereas that of endometrial biopsy was only 30%, raising a question that biopsy may not be the most appropriate first-line test in asymptomatic women.

Transvaginal sonography appears to be accurate in determining deep versus superficial invasion (defined as less than 50% of myometrial width) (Fig. 4-5). Sonography has an important role in management decisions concerning preoperative radiation therapy in patients with stage I adenocarcinoma of the endometrium.[25–29]

Polypoid tumors (over 3 cm) may cause an apparent distention of the endometrial lumen and extrinsic thinning of the myometrium. In noninvasive tumors the hypoechoic layer of the inner myometrium surrounding the endometrium is usually intact, indicating that the tumor is, at most, superficially invasive. In some cases, it is difficult to delineate the endometrial-myometrial interface. However, the likelihood of invasion is clearly related to the bulk or volume of the endometrial tissue. Problems in estimation of the extent of invasion may also occur if this subendometrial hypoechoic layer, which corresponds to the "junctional zone" on MRI, is not detectable or if the myometrium is extremely attenuated due to muscular atrophy. One should therefore be most cautious in estimating the extent of myometrial invasion when the tumor is bulky or if the myometrium is thin (less than 1 cm).

The accuracy of MRI compared with transvaginal sonography for assessment of myometrial invasion requires a study that uses both modalities on the same patients with similar state-of-the-art equipment. Our feeling, based on preliminary studies, is that transvaginal sonography and MRI have comparable accuracies for determining tumor invasion confined within the uterus but that extrauterine extension and involvement of lymph nodes are better detected by MRI.[30] Certainly, transvaginal sonography is much more operator dependent than MRI, but it is less expensive and more extensively available.

Transvaginal color Doppler sonography may be able to identify some patients who have endometrial carcinoma even though the endometrium is thin.[31] In general, hyperplastic endometria do not exhibit the increased spiral arteriole vascularity seen on transvaginal color Doppler sonography in most viable endometrial cancers. Areas of venous flow can also be observed in areas of tumor.

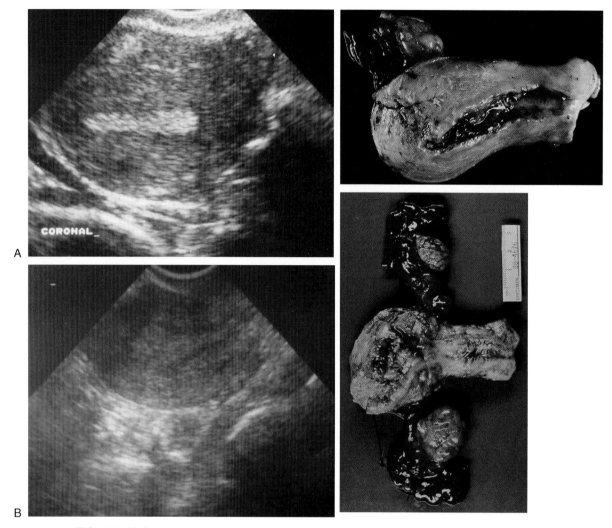

FIG. 4-5. Malignant endometrial disorders. Transvaginal sonograms *(left)* have sectional specimens for comparison *(right)*. **(A)** Noninvasive endometrial carcinoma. The endometrial-myometrial interface is intact. **(B)** Invasive endometrial carcinoma with disruption of endometrial-myometrial interface.

MISCELLANEOUS DISORDERS

Transvaginal sonography shows more textural abnormalities of the transformed endometrium associated with complicated pregnancies (Fig. 4-6). This includes thickening of the endometrium associated with ectopic pregnancy as well as cystic changes that occur with decidual necrosis. The relative amount of retained choriodecidua can also be assessed.

SONOHYSTEROGRAPHY

Sonographic evaluation of the endometrium can be enhanced by instillation of sterile saline into the lumen as observed during transvaginal sonography, a procedure called sonohysterography (Fig. 4-7). For this technique, an intrauterine insemination catheter, 5F pediatric feeding tube, or plastic hysterosalpingogram catheter is inserted through the cervix into the endometrial lumen. Three to 5 mL of sterile saline can be infused during real-time observation with transvaginal sonography.

Sonohysterography affords evaluation of the cavity for endometrial polyps and submucous leiomyomas as well as uterine synechiae.[3,32,33] Endometrial polyps are typically echogenic masses and project into the endometrial lumen.[34] Their stalk can be identified with the infused fluid surrounding it. Submucosal leiomyomas tend to be hypoechoic relative to the endometrium and typically broad-based polyps tend to be hypoechoic.[33] The procedure should be performed in the follicular phase because typically echogenic polyps stand out more relative to the hypoechoic endometrium. Submucosal fibroids tend to be hypoechoic and best delineated against the echogenic secretory-phase endometrium.[35] This type of fibroid usually elevates the overlying endometrium. Sonohysterography may improve assessment of the extent of the fibroid into the myometrium. Extension to the cervix would preclude endoscopic wire-loop resection. Intrauterine

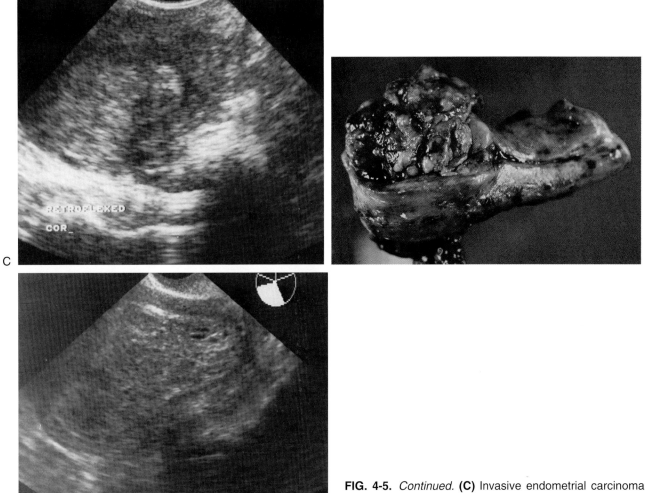

FIG. 4-5. *Continued.* **(C)** Invasive endometrial carcinoma almost to serosa. **(D)** Stage II endometrial carcinoma with extension into cervix.

synechiae are identified as echogenic or hypoechoic bands that extend from one endometrial surface to the other. The hypoechoic synechiae are best depicted against an echogenic secretory endometrium. Polypoid endometrial cancers typically have a more diffusely thickened and irregular appearance compared with benign polyps. However, a definitive distinction between hyperplastic and cancerous polyps cannot be made based on sonographic findings alone. Therefore, focal areas of thickened (over 4 mm single layer thickness) endometrium should be considered suspicious for pathologic changes and might be sampled with directed biopsy if indicated.

Besides identifying intraluminal abnormalities, sonohysterography can be used to locate abnormal areas for further biopsy.[36] The procedure is usually well tolerated and is of particular use in assessment of patients with thickened endometrium on sonography that have scant tissue obtained on dilatation and curettage.[37] This inability to obtain adequate tissue may occur in patients with polypoid lesions because the polyp may impede adequate biopsy.

Sonohysterography can also be used to identify the location and extent of intrauterine synechiae or septa in ruptured uterus. Synechiae typically appear as hypoechoic bands before fluid instillation. After fluid is instilled they are echogenic when compared with the surrounding fluid. The use of sonohysterography for correlation of uterine malformations is covered in Chapter 10.

CONCLUSION

In 1990 it was estimated that 36 million women were older than age 50. This supposes that women will spend approximately a third of their life in the postmenopausal period and many of them will receive hormone replacement therapy.[38] Transvaginal sonography has an important role in the surveillance and management of both symptomatic and asymptomatic women with suspected endometrial disorders.[39,40]

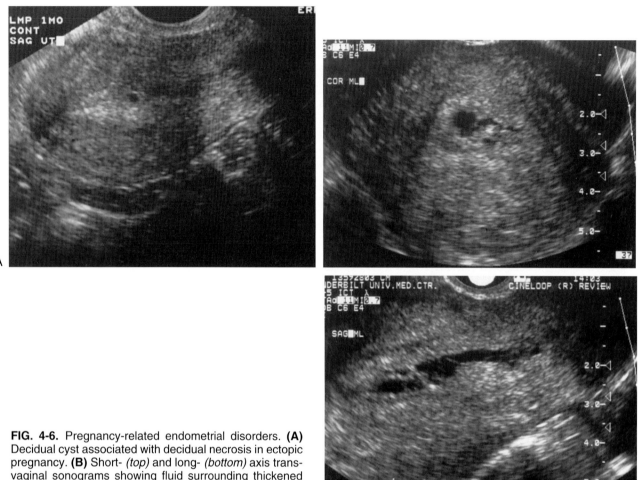

FIG. 4-6. Pregnancy-related endometrial disorders. **(A)** Decidual cyst associated with decidual necrosis in ectopic pregnancy. **(B)** Short- *(top)* and long- *(bottom)* axis transvaginal sonograms showing fluid surrounding thickened and irregular endometrial interface indicates an incomplete abortion.

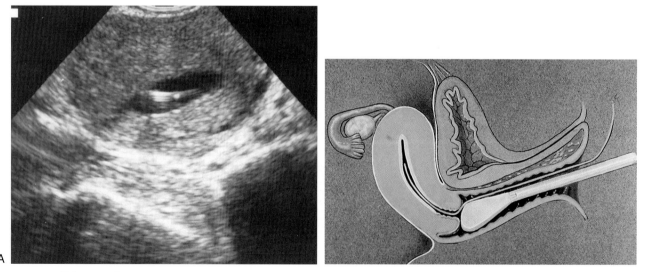

FIG. 4-7. Sonohysterography. **(A)** Normal endometrium surrounding infused intraluminal fluid *(left)*. Diagram showing catheter within lumen *(right)*. Sonohysterogram showing fluid surrounding the catheter and the endometrium that is thin and regular.

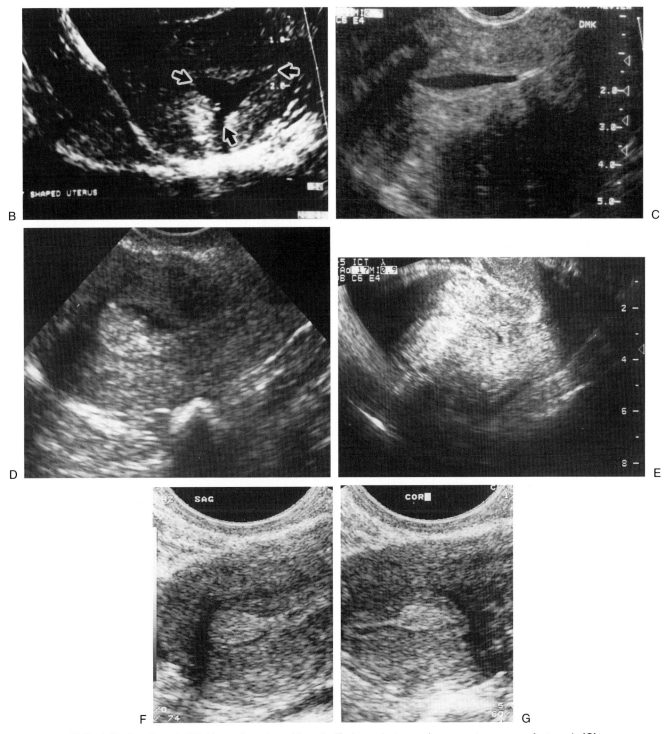

FIG. 4-7. *Continued.* **(B)** Normal endometrium in T-shaped uterus *(arrows at corners of uterus).* **(C)** Normal endometrium adjacent to fundal intramural fibroid. **(D)** Focal thickening of endometrium. There was disordered proliferative endometrium on histologic examination. **(E)** Polyp filling lumen. **(F and G)** Long- *(left)* and short- *(right)* axis of polyp. **(H)** Same patient in **F** and **G**. Sonohysterogram depicts the polyp and its pedicle. **(I)** Endometrial polyp surrounded by fluid *(left)* with hysteroscopic findings *(right).* **(J)** Adhesion shown on sonohysterogram *(left)* and hysteroscopy *(right)* **(B,** courtesy of Anna Parsons, MD; **I** and **J,** courtesy of E. Eisenberg, MD).

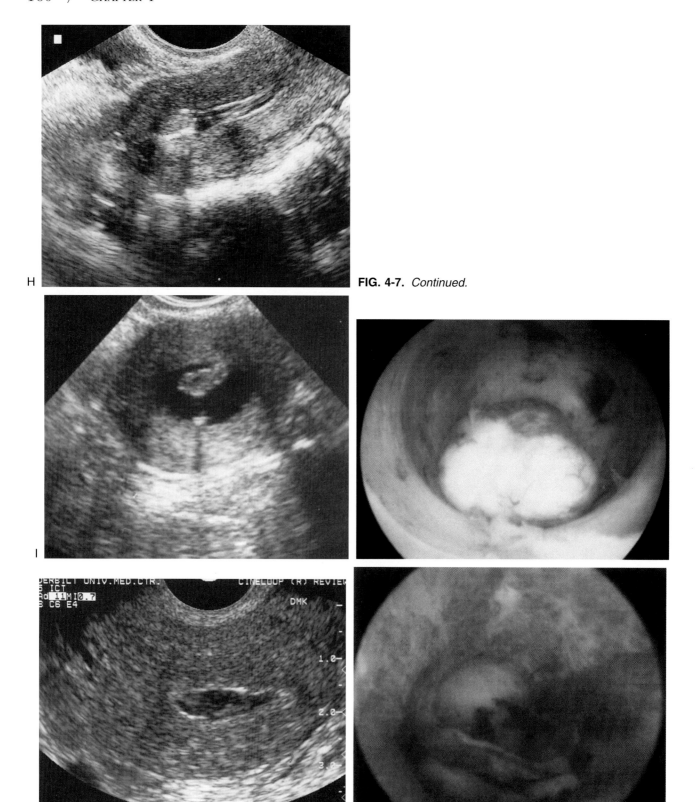

FIG. 4-7. *Continued.*

REFERENCES

1. Granberg S, Wikland M, Karlsson B, et al. Endometrial thickness as measured by endovaginal ultrasonography for identifying endometrial abnormality. Am J Obstet Gynecol 1991;164:47.
2. Goldstein SR, Nachtigall M, Snyder JR, et al. Endometrial assessment by vaginal ultrasonography before endometrial sampling in patients with postmenopausal bleeding. Am J Obstet Gynecol 1990;163:119.
3. Parsons AK, Lense JJ. Sonohysterography for endometrial abnormalities: preliminary results. J Clin Ultrasound 1993;21:87.
4. Dubinsky TJ, Parvey R, Gormaz G, Maklad N. Transvaginal hysterosonography in the evaluation of small endoluminal masses. J Ultrasound Med 1995;14:1.
5. Cullinan JA, Fleischer AF. Color Doppler sonography of pelvic masses. Radiologist 1994;1:225.
6. Fleischer A. Transvaginal sonography of the endometrium. In: Fleischer AC, Romero R, Manning FA, Jeanty P, eds. The principles and practice of ultrasonography in obstetrics and gynecology, ed 4. Norwalk, CT, Appleton & Lange, 1991.
7. Lin MC, Gosink BB, Wolf SI, et al. Endometrial thickness after menopause: effect of hormone replacement. Radiology 1991;180:427.
8. Farrer-Brown, Beilby JOW, Tarbit MH. The blood supply of the uterus. J Obstet Gynaecol Br Commonw 1970;77:673.
9. Burks DD, Stainken BR, Burkhard TK, Balsara ZN. Uterine inner myometrial echogenic foci: relationship to prior dilatation and curettage and endocervical biopsy. J Ultrasound Med 1991;10:487.
10. Occhipinti K, Kutcher R, Rosenblatt R. Sonographic appearance and significance of arcuate artery calcification. J Ultrasound Med 1991;10:97.
11. Forrest TS, Elyaderani MK, Muilenburg MI, et al. Cyclic endometrial changes: US assessment with histologic correlation. Radiology 1988;167:223.
12. Appelbaum M. In: Copel J, Reed K, eds. Doppler Ultrasound in Ob/ Gyn. New York, Raven Press, 1995.6
13. Salm R, Redruth C, Cornwall D. Mucin production of normal and abnormal endometrium. Arch Pathol 1962;73:30.
14. Andolf E, Dahlander K, Aspenberg P. Ultrasonic thickness of the endometrium correlated to body weight in asymptomatic postmenopausal women. Obstet Gynecol 1993;82:936.
15. Menwissen H. Monitoring endometrial thickness during estrogen replacement therapy with vaginosonography. Radiology 1991;180:284.
16. Sheth S, Hamper UM, Kurman RJ. Thickened endometrium in the postmenopausal woman: sonographic-pathologic correlation. Radiology 1993;187:135.
17. Nasri MN, Coast GJ. Correlation of ultrasound findings and endometrial histopathology in postmenopausal women. Br J Obstet Gyn 1989;96:1333.
18. Osmers R, Volksen M, Schauer A. Vaginosonography for early detection of endometrial carcinoma? Lancet 190;335:1560.
19. Hulka CA, Hall DA. Endometrial abnormalities associated with tamoxifen therapy for breast cancer: sonographic and pathologic correlation. AJR 1993;160:809.
20. Lahti E, Blanco G, Kauppila A, et al. Endometrial changes in postmenopausal breast cancer patients receiving tamoxifen. Obstet Gynecol 1993;81:660.
21. Goldstein SR. Unusual ultrasonographic appearance of the uterus in patients receiving tamoxifen. Am J Obstet Gynecol 1994;170:447.
22. Carlson JA, Arger P, Thompson S, Carlson EJ: Clinical and pathologic correlation of endometrial cavity fluid detected by ultrasound in the postmenopausal patient. Obstet Gynecol 1991;77:119.
23. Goldschmit R, Katz Z, Blickstein I et al. The accuracy of endometrial pipelle sampling with and without sonographic measurement of endometrial thickness. Obstet Gynecol 1993;82:727.
24. Shipley CF, Simmons CL, Nelson GH. Comparison of transvaginal sonography with endometrial biopsy in asymptomatic postmenopausal women. J Ultrasound Med 1994;13:99.
25. Fleischer AC, Dudley BS, Entman SS, et al. Myometrial invasion by endometrial carcinoma: sonographic assessment. Radiology 1987;162:307.
26. Gordon AN, Fleischer AC, Dudley BS, et al. Preoperative assessment of myometrial invasion of endometrial adenocarcinoma by sonography (US) and magnetic resonance imaging (MRI). Gynecol Oncol 1989;34:175.
27. DelMaschio A, Vanzulli A, Sironi S, et al. Estimating the depth of myometrial involvement by endometrial carcinoma: efficacy of transvaginal sonography vs MR imaging. AJR 1993;160:533.
28. Yamashita Y, Mizutani H, Torashima M, et al. Assessment of myometrial invasion by endometrial carcinoma: transvaginal sonography vs contrast-enhanced MR imaging. AJR 1993;161:595.
29. Karlson B, Norström, Granberg S, Wikland M. The use of endovaginal ultrasound to diagnose invasion of endometrial carcinoma. Ultrasound Obstet Gynecol 1992;2:35.
30. Hricak HH, Stern JL, Fisher MR, et al. Endometrial carcinoma staging by MR imaging. Radiology 1987;162:297.
31. Bourne THE, Campbell S, Steer CV, et al. Detection of endometrial cancer by transvaginal ultrasonography with color flow imaging and blood flow analysis: a preliminary report. Gynecol Oncol 1991;40:253.
32. Goldstein SR, Nachigall M, Snyder JR, Nachigall L. Myometrial assessment by vaginal ultrasonography before endometrial sampling in patients with postmenopausal bleeding. Am J Obstet Gynecol 1990;163:119.
33. Syrop CH, Sahakian V. Transvaginal sonographic detection of endometrial polyps with fluid contrast augmentation. Obstet Gynecol 1991;79:1041.
34. Stadtmauer L, Grunfeld L. The significance of endometrial filling defects detected on routine transvaginal sonography. J Ultrasound Med 1995;14:169.
35. Fedele L, Bianchi S, Dorta M, et al. Transvaginal ultrasonography versus hysteroscopy in the diagnosis of uterine submucous myomas. Obstet Gynecol 1991;77:745.
36. Cohen JR, Luxman D, Sagi J, et al. Sonohysterography for distinguishing endometrial thickening from endometrial polyps in postmenopausal bleeding. Ultrasound Obstet Gynecol 1994;4:227.
37. Padro J, Kaplan B, Nitke S, et al. Postmenopausal intrauterine fluid collection: correlation between ultrasound and hysteroscopy. Ultrasound Obstet Gynecol 1994;4:224.
38. Judd HL, San Roman GA. Hormone replacement therapy. ACOG technical bulletin 166. Washington, DC, American College of Obstetricians and Gynecologists, 1992:1.
39. Atri M, Nazarnia S, Aldis AE, et al. Transvaginal US appearance of endometrial abnormalities. Radiographics 1994;14:483.
40. Mendelson EB, Bohm-Velez M, Joseph N, Neiman HL: Endometrial abnormalities: evaluation with transvaginal sonography. AJR 1988;150:130.

Magnetic Resonance Imaging of Uterine (Endometrial) Malignancies

Marcia C. Javitt, MD

ENDOMETRIAL CARCINOMA

As the most common gynecologic malignancy, endometrial carcinoma deserves special attention. Most cases present in the sixth decade. About 85% are adenocarcinomas, and 15% contain squamous elements, either adenoacanthomas with histologically benign squamous elements or adenosquamous carcinomas in which more than 10% of the tumor is squamous. Less than 5% are uterine sarcomas.[1]

Risk factors include obesity, diabetes, hypertension, infertility, positive family history, and hyperestrinism. The malignancy may be preceded by endometrial hyperplasia.[1]

The hallmark of endometrial carcinoma clinically is postmenopausal vaginal bleeding. Pain is usually a late finding. Preoperative staging is clinical using the International Federation of Gynecology and Obstetrics (FIGO) system. Preoperative cross-sectional imaging can directly affect patient management but is not included in the FIGO system, presumably because it is not universally available worldwide. FIGO staging alone may understage over 20% of patients.[2]

The prognosis depends on initial staging of the tumor, which is directly related to the depth of myometrial invasion and lymphadenopathy, as well as on the histologic grading (Table 4-8). If the tumor penetrates greater than 50% of the myometrial width, there is a much greater risk of nodal

metastasis (40% for stage Ic compared with 3% for stage Ia), and thus a worse prognosis.[3–6] Preoperative evaluation of myometrial invasion may influence management, prompting alterations in treatment planning with addition of preoperative radiation or surgery to include more extensive nodal dissection.[2,7–10]

Stage Ia and Ib lesions are usually managed surgically with hysterectomy. Stage Ib tumors with high-grade histology may receive preoperative radiation therapy, as do stage Ic and stage II lesions. Advanced stage III and stage IV tumors are usually managed with radiation therapy alone for palliation.

The earliest recognizable finding of endometrial carcinoma on MRI is thickening of the endometrial canal on T2-weighted images. With more advanced disease there can be enlargement of the uterus, enhancing nodules within the endometrium, and hematometrocolpos. Abnormalities can be

TABLE 4-8. *FIGO staging of endometrial carcinoma*

Stage	Description
Ia	Tumor in endometrium only
Ib	Invasion of myometrium less than half thickness
Ic	More than half thickness myometrial invasion
IIa	Invasion of the endocervix
IIb	Invasion beyond the cervical sroma
IIIa	Invasion of the adnexa or through the serosa, and/or positive cytology from peritoneum
IIIb	Vaginal extension
IIIc	Pelvic or paraaortic nodal metastases
IVa	Invasion of bladder or rectum
IVb	Distant metastases or abdominal and or inguinal nodal metastases

Data from Jones HW, Wentz, Burnett LS, eds. Novak's textbook of gynecology, ed 11. Baltimore, Williams & Wilkins, 1988; and DiSaia PF, Creasman WT. Clinical gynecologic oncology, ed 3. St. Louis, CV Mosby, 1989.

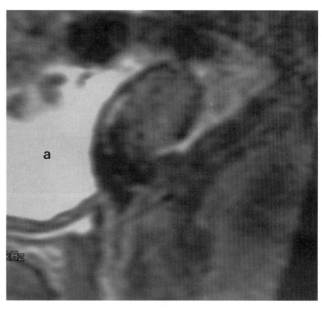

FIG. 4-8. Indistinctness of uterine zonal anatomy. T2-weighted sagittal image shows poor definition of the zonal anatomy of the uterus. This can be normal in postmenopausal females and must be interpreted with caution. There is bright signal pelvic ascites (a) above the bladder from peritoneal dialysis.

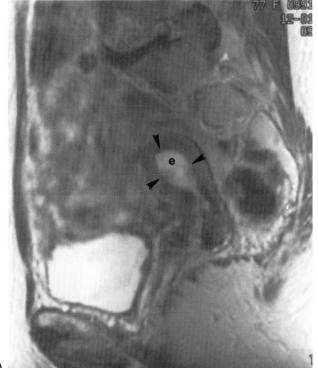

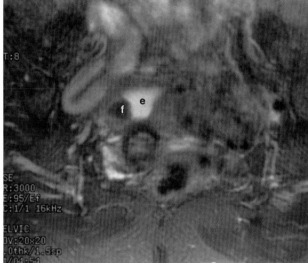

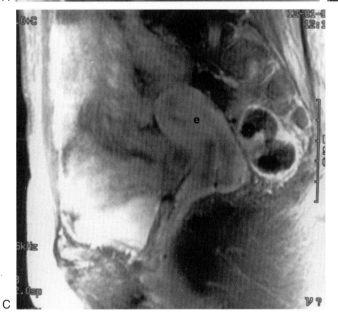

FIG. 4-9. Stage Ia endometrial carcinoma. **(A)** Sagittal T2-weighted scan shows the typical distended endometrial canal (e). The low signal areas are from volume averaging with an intramural fibroid on the right side. The junctional zone is intact *(arrowheads)*. **(B)** Off-axis coronal scan with fat suppression confirms the intact junctional zone and the right uterine body fibroid (f). **(C)** Enhanced sagittal T1-weighted scan with fat suppression shows the endometrial canal (e) is mildly enhanced from tumor but there is no evidence of myometrial invasion through the junctional zone.

detected in about 84% of patients with endometrial carcinoma.[2,7]

Some postmenopausal women have an indistinct junctional zone in the absence of tumor due to aging changes. This finding must be assessed with great caution to prevent overreading (Fig. 4-8). An intact junctional zone on T2-weighted images is seen reliably with stage Ia disease (which is confined to the endometrium) and with stage Ib (Fig. 4-9). If the junctional zone is disrupted particularly with enhancing tumor after administration of intravenous gadolinium, then deep myometrial invasion can be suspected (Fig. 4-10); however, there

can be false-positive results, including older age of the patient with indistinctness of the junctional zone, large polypoid tumors that thin the surrounding myometrium, leiomyomas, congenital anomalies, and small uteri.[4,8,10]

The accuracy of MRI for diagnosis of myometrial invasion has been reported between 71% and 97%.[2,3,5–8,10–16] Viable tumor can be differentiated from necrosis and debris within the endometrial canal on contrast medium–enhanced scans.

It is not possible to differentiate between malignancy within the endometrial canal and benign disorders such as

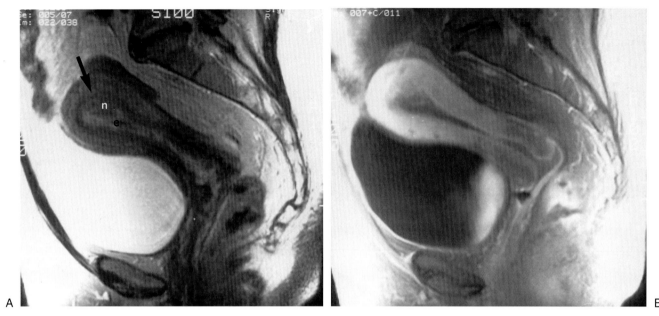

A

B

FIG. 4-10. Stage Ic endometrial carcinoma: myometrial invasion. **(A)** Sagittal T2-weighted scan shows distention of the endometrial canal (e), interruption of the junctional zone in the uterine fundus *(arrow)* indicating deep myometrial invasion, and tumor nodule (n) within the endometrial canal. **(B)** Sagittal T1-weighted fat-suppressed gadolinium-enhanced scan confirms stage Ic disease. Note enhancement of the tumor nodule on a background of low-signal debris and secretions within the endometrial canal.

endometrial hyperplasia (Fig. 4-11), because blood and secretions cause distention with MRI.[7,11,14,15]

The diagnosis of postmenopausal bleeding should be made by endometrial biopsy or dilatation and curettage. MRI should not be used as a screening procedure, not only because it is nonspecific for tissue diagnosis but also because it is probably too expensive. However, MRI is the study of choice for accurate staging of endometrial carcinoma. The staging accuracy of MRI for endometrial carcinoma is between 85% and 92%.[2,7,12]

Addition of contrast material with T1-weighted images provides differentiation of viable tumor from surrounding debris, improved assessment of myometrial invasion, and improved overall staging accuracy (Fig. 4-12).[11,13–15,17]

SARCOMAS OF THE UTERUS

Uterine sarcomas are uncommon gynecologic malignancies usually seen in women older than 40 who present with abnormal vaginal bleeding and pain. The mixed mesodermal sarcoma is probably the most common of these unusual lesions, followed by leiomyosarcomas. The mixed mesodermal sarcomas may contain elements of both sarcomatous and carcinomatous tissues. These tumors are often aggressive and present as large heterogeneous uterine masses that often have metastasized hematogenously or lymphogenously by the time of diagnosis.[18,19]

Leiomyomas often coexist in the same uterus, but in patients who undergo surgery for fibroids the incidence of sar-

comas is rare, less than 1%. If invasive, this tumor often spreads hematogenously.[18–20]

Imaging characteristics of these typically large heterogeneous masses are nonspecific, and the lesion may resemble its benign counterpart, the leiomyoma, especially if the heterogeneous appearance of necrosis and the degeneration of large benign leiomyomas are considered. For extent of disease evaluation, MRI may reveal an enlarged heterogenous uterus on T2-weighted scans, may define mural invasion by the lesion in some cases if the zonal anatomy is at all visible, and may show local tumor extension as well as nodal and hematogeneous metastases (Fig. 4-13).[21,22]

GESTATIONAL TROPHOBLASTIC DISEASE

Gestational trophoblastic disease encompasses a spectrum of tumors that arise from placental villous tissue and range from the more common and benign form, the hydatidiform mole, to the most malignant choriocarcinoma. The incidence is about 1 in 2000 pregnancies.[18–20,23]

The hallmark of gestational trophoblastic disease is elevation of the serum human chorionic gonadotropin (hCG) level, which is a useful serologic marker not only for diagnosis but also for assessing response to treatment and surveillance for recurrence. Symptoms mimic early pregnancy with hyperemesis, uterine enlargement, pain, and vaginal bleeding in the presence of markedly elevated hCG. There may be expulsion of the grapelike vesicles of the tumor or preeclampsia. There may be theca-lutein cysts of the ovaries.

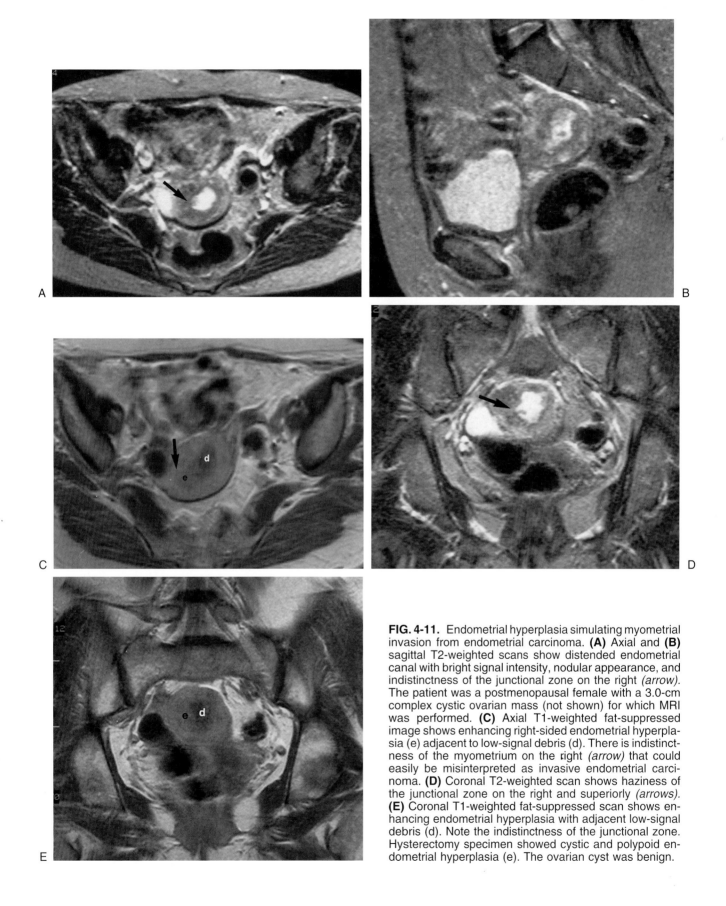

FIG. 4-11. Endometrial hyperplasia simulating myometrial invasion from endometrial carcinoma. **(A)** Axial and **(B)** sagittal T2-weighted scans show distended endometrial canal with bright signal intensity, nodular appearance, and indistinctness of the junctional zone on the right *(arrow)*. The patient was a postmenopausal female with a 3.0-cm complex cystic ovarian mass (not shown) for which MRI was performed. **(C)** Axial T1-weighted fat-suppressed image shows enhancing right-sided endometrial hyperplasia (e) adjacent to low-signal debris (d). There is indistinctness of the myometrium on the right *(arrow)* that could easily be misinterpreted as invasive endometrial carcinoma. **(D)** Coronal T2-weighted scan shows haziness of the junctional zone on the right and superiorly *(arrows)*. **(E)** Coronal T1-weighted fat-suppressed scan shows enhancing endometrial hyperplasia with adjacent low-signal debris (d). Note the indistinctness of the junctional zone. Hysterectomy specimen showed cystic and polypoid endometrial hyperplasia (e). The ovarian cyst was benign.

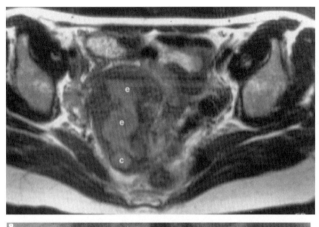

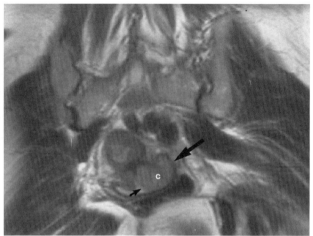

A

B

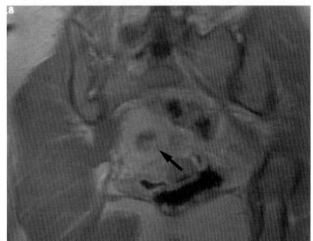

C

FIG. 4-12. Endometrial carcinoma stage IIa with extension to the cervix. **(A)** T2-weighted axial and **(B)** coronal images. The high signal endometrial canal (e) has a multinodular appearance with distention from tumor. There is a cervical mass (c). Note that the fibrous stroma is intact about the cervical mass *(large arrow)*. There was concern for extension into the left vaginal vault *(small arrow)*, but at surgery this was only mass effect without invasion of tissue planes or the muscular wall of the vaginal canal. The lesion was stage IIa. **(C)** T1-weighted coronal scan shows enhancing endometrial and cervical tumor with invasion of the junctional zone inferiorly *(arrow)*.

Rarely, a coexistent intrauterine pregnancy may be present.[18–20,23]

About 80% of molar pregnancies are hydatidiform moles that are benign and resolve after dilatation and curettage. About 15% are locally invasive into the myometrium and may metastasize. About 5% may be due to choriocarcinoma, which can arise in a prior hydatidiform mole or after any pregnancy. Treatment of the malignant forms is by chemotherapy with methotrexate.[18–20,23]

Usually the initial imaging study ordered is sonography. MRI may be used in cases that are malignant to assess extent of disease; however, CT of the chest, abdomen, and pelvis has been successfully used for this purpose. If the sonographic findings are equivocal or technically limited, or if the tumor is intramural and does not extend to the endometrium thus remaining undetected with curettage, MRI is a useful adjunct.[24] MRI typically shows an enlarged heterogeneous uterus with loss of the normal zonal anatomy on T2-weighted images, some with foci of hemorrhage. After treatment, there is usually a return toward more normal size and zonal anatomy (Fig. 4-14). Recurrent tumor after curettage

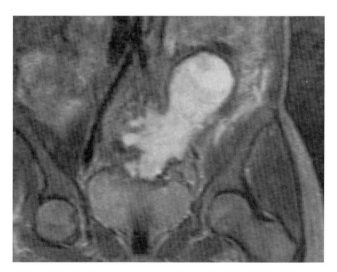

FIG. 4-13. Leiomyosarcoma. Coronal T2-weighted image shows a heterogeneous predominantly bright signal mass with very irregular margins that proved to be malignant. The appearance is not specific and may resemble benign and degenerated leiomyomas.

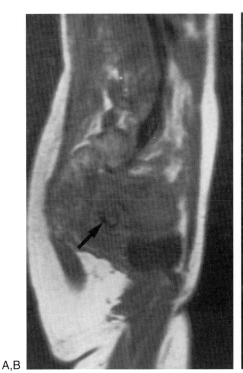
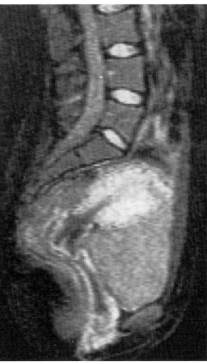
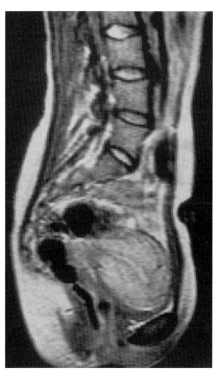

A,B

C

FIG. 4-14. Choriocarcinoma. **(A)** Sagittal T1-weighted scan shows flow void in prominent tumor vessels *(arrow)* typical of gestational trophoblastic disease. **(B)** Sagittal T2-weighted scan shows heterogeneous signal intensity in the body and fundus of the uterus from tumor that obscures the normally obvious zonal anatomy of the uterus. **(C)** Sagittal T2-weighted scan performed 1 month later after chemotherapy with methotrexate shows improved differentiation of the endometrial canal from the junctional zone and myometrium. There was also a decrease in abnormal vascularity. The serum human chorionic gonadotropin levels had decreased, indicating response to treatment.

usually appears heterogeneous on T2-weighted images and may have prominent blood vessels with flow void.[23–25] MRI can be used to perform surveillance on these patients after treatment.

REFERENCES

1. Cotran RS, Kumar V, Robbins SL. Pathologic basis of disease, ed 4. Philadelphia, WB Saunders, 1989.
2. Hricak H, Rubinstein LV, Gherman GM, et al. MR imaging evaluation of endometrial carcinoma: results of an NCI cooperative study. Radiology 1991;179:829.
3. Chen SS, Rumancik WM, Spiegel G. Magnetic resonance imaging in Stage I endometrial carcinoma. Obstet Gynecol 1990;75:274.
4. Gordon AN, Fleischer AC, Dudley BS, et al. Preoperative assessment of myometrial invasion of endometrial carcinoma by sonography (US) and magnetic resonance imaging (MRI). Gynecol Oncol 1989;34:175.
5. DelMaschio A, Vanzulli A, Sironi S, et al. Estimating the depth of myometrial involvement by endometrial carcinoma: efficacy of transvaginal sonography vs MR imaging. AJR 1993;160:533.
6. Lien HH, Blomlie V, Trope C, et al. Cancer of the endometrium: value of MR imaging in determining depth of invasion into the myometrium. AJR 1991;175:1221.
7. Hricak H, Stern JL, Fisher MR et al. Endometrial carcinoma staging by MR imaging. Radiology 1987;162:297.
8. Scoutt LM, McCarthy SM, Flynn SD. Clinical stage I endometrial carcinoma: pitfalls in preoperative assessment with MR imaging: work in progress. Radiology 1995;194:567.
9. Hricak K, Tscholakoff D, Heinrichs L, et al. Uterine leiomyomas: correlation of MR, histopathologic findings, and symptoms. Radiology 1986;158:385.
10. Sironi S, Taccagni G, Garancini P, et al. Myometrial invasion by endometrial carcinoma: assessment by MR imaging. AJR 1992;158:565.
11. Hricak H, Hamm B, Semelka RC, et al. Carcinoma of the uterus: use of gadopentetate dimeglumine in MR imaging. Radiology 1991;181:95.
12. Posniak HV, Olson MC, Dudiak CM, et al. MR imaging of uterine carcinoma: correlation with clinical and pathologic findings. Radiographics 1990;10:15.
13. Sironi S, Colombo E, Villa G, et al. Myometrial invasion by endometrial carcinoma: assessment with plain and gadolinium-enhanced MR imaging. Radiology 1992;185:207.
14. Yamashita Y, Hirada M, Sawada T, et al. Normal uterus and FIGO stage I endometrial carcinoma: dynamic gadofinium enhanced MR imaging. Radiology 1993;186:495.
15. Yamashita Y, Mizutani H, Torashima M, et al. Assessment of myometrial invasion by endometrial carcinoma: transvaginal sonography vs contrast enhanced MR imaging. AJR 1993;161:595.
16. Yazigi R, Cohen J, Munoz AK, et al. Magnetic resonance imaging determination of myometrial invasion in endometrial carcinoma. Gynecol Oncol 19889;34:94.
17. Hirano Y, Kubo K, Hirai Y, et al. Preliminary experience with gadolinium-enhanced dynamic MR imaging for uterine neoplasms. Radiographics 1993;12:243.
18. Jones HW, Wentz AC, Burnett LS, eds. Novak's Textbook of Gynecology, ed 11. Baltimore, Williams & Wilkins, 1988.

19. DiSaia, PF, Creasman WT. Clinical gynecologic oncology, ed 3. St. Louis, CV Mosby, 1989.
20. Cotran RS, Kumar V, Robbins SL. Pathologic basis of disease, ed 4. Philadelphia, WB Saunders, 1989.
21. Shapeero LG, Hricak H. Mixed müllerian sarcoma of the uterus: MR imaging findings. AJR 1989;153:317.
22. Janus C, White M, Dottino P, et al. Uterine leiomyosarcoma-magnetic resonance imaging. Gynecol Oncol 1989;32:79.
23. Mirich DR, Hall JT, Kraft WL, et al. Metastatic adnexal trophoblastic neoplasm: contribution of MR imaging. J Comput Assist Tomogr 1988; 12:1061.
24. Hricak H, Demas BE, Braga CA, et al. Gestational trophoblastic neoplasm of the uterus: MR assessment. Radiology 1986;161:11.
25. Barton JW, McCarthy SM, Kohorn EI, et al. Pelvic MR imaging findings in gestational trophoblastic disease, incomplete abortion, and ectopic pregnancy: are they specific? Radiology 1993;186:163.

Computed Tomography of Endometrial Malignancy

James W. Walsh, MD

Computed tomography has been a widely used imaging modality for staging endometrial carcinoma or sarcoma.[1-5] The overall accuracy of CT staging is 84% to 88%, with a correct diagnosis of stage I or II disease in 83% to 92% of patients, and for stage III or IV disease it is 83% to 86%.[3-4] Thus, CT is a useful noninvasive screening test to differentiate disease confined to the uterus from extrauterine pelvic and abdominal spread. Although one center reported a CT accuracy of 77% in determining the depth of myometrial invasion,[5] clinical experience has shown that CT is inferior to sonography and MRI for detecting myometrial tumor penetration.

Over the past decade, MRI has gradually replaced CT as the imaging procedure of choice for staging endometrial malignancy. MRI is uniquely suited to differentiate International Federation of Gynecology and Obstetrics (FIGO) stages IA, IB, IC, IIB, and IIIA (serosal invasion) because of its superior contrast resolution and multiplanar display. However, one report showed that MRI was suboptimal for adnexal or peritoneal metastases,[6] and further MRI studies of advanced stage III and stage IV tumors are necessary. Thus, CT still has a role in evaluating unsuspected lymphatic, peritoneal, and parenchymal organ metastases in the abdomen, an area where CT excels as an imaging modality.

INDICATIONS

The basic indications for CT staging of endometrial malignancy are (1) advanced local disease and (2) potential stage III or stage IV tumors. Advanced pelvic tumor is documented when a large bulky uterus with possible parametrial or pelvic sidewall spread or adnexal mass is palpated on bimanual pelvic examination. Advanced stage III or IV disease is possible when unfavorable histologic findings are evident on a biopsy specimen; these may include poorly differentiated carcinoma; clear cell, papillary serous, or adenosquamous carcinoma; sarcoma; or lymphoma (Fig. 4-15). Advanced disease is also suspected when results of liver function tests are abnormal; ascites, hepatomegaly, or a palpable abdominal mass is present (see Fig. 4-15B); or the chest radiograph shows pulmonary nodules. CT is also indicated when MRI is not available.

TECHNIQUE

Intravenous contrast medium enhancement during a dedicated dynamic or spiral pelvic CT study is necessary to maximize uterine parenchymal and vascular enhancement and optimize the images for staging information. Intense myometrial enhancement permits detection of mural tumor and helps delineate the endometrial cavity containing fluid and tumor. Pelvic vascular enhancement helps to detect lymph node metastases, differentiate parametrial vessels from parametrial tumor extension, and detect hypervascular tumors such as gestational trophoblastic disease (Fig. 4-16). Thin 3- to 5-mm sections through the tumor may better delineate an endometrial mass or confirm subtle parametrial invasion.

COMPUTED TOMOGRAPHIC FEATURES

Carcinoma

Contrast medium–enhanced CT typically shows endometrial cancer as a hypodense mass in a dilated endometrial cavity or in the uterine wall (Figs. 4-17 and 4-18; see also Fig. 4-15A). Occasionally, a fluid-filled uterus due to tumor obstruction of the endocervical canal may be detected (see Fig. 4-18).[7] Endometrial or myometrial tumor is usually intermediate in density between less dense endometrial fluid and normal enhancing myometrium (see Figs. 4-15A, 4-17, and 4-18). Although endometrial cancer has been reported as a contrast medium–enhancing lesion in the myometrium,[1] we have not observed this pattern. When focal invasion of the myometrium is detected on CT, this finding usually corresponds to invasion of greater than one third to one half of the myometrium (see Fig. 4-18).[1-2] However, CT usually cannot differentiate FIGO stage I and II lesions.[3]

CT staging criteria for endometrial cancer are based on the FIGO staging classification. Endometrial cancer involvement of the cervix (stage IIB) is characterized on CT as cervical enlargement greater than 3.5 cm in diameter and a heterogeneous hypodense mass in the cervical stroma (Fig. 4-19).[2,4] Stage IIIA is characterized by parametrial (Fig. 4-20) and pelvic sidewall extension or metastatic disease to the ovary (Fig. 4-21). When a solid ovarian mass is detected

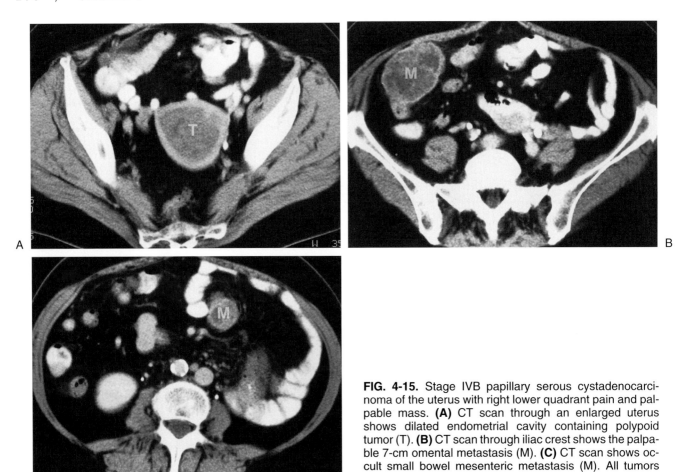

FIG. 4-15. Stage IVB papillary serous cystadenocarcinoma of the uterus with right lower quadrant pain and palpable mass. **(A)** CT scan through an enlarged uterus shows dilated endometrial cavity containing polypoid tumor (T). **(B)** CT scan through iliac crest shows the palpable 7-cm omental metastasis (M). **(C)** CT scan shows occult small bowel mesenteric metastasis (M). All tumors were resected at staging laparotomy.

FIG. 4-16. (A) Dynamic CT scan shows persistent gestational trophoblastic disease in uterine corpus *(curved black arrows)* after prior evacuation of molar pregnancy. The curvilinear right uterine artery *(white arrows)* supplies the tumor, and the right ovary is normal (O). **(B)** Delayed scan through uterus (U) 15 minutes later shows no diagnostic information.

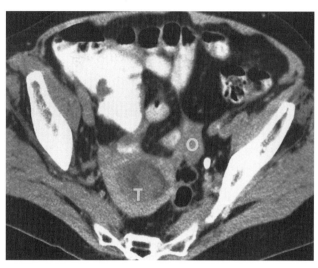

FIG. 4-17. Stage II adenocarcinoma. CT scan through uterus and left ovary (O) shows polypoid tumor (T) surrounded by fluid in dilated endometrial cavity. Myometrium and extrauterine structures are normal.

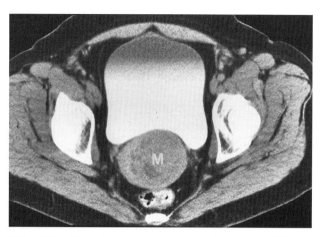

FIG. 4-19. Stage II endometrial stromal sarcoma. CT scan shows eccentric 5-cm heterogeneous mass (M) in enlarged 8-cm cervix. Hysterectomy specimen showed full-thickness tumor involvement of left cervical stroma. Tumor was not palpable, even under anesthesia.

with the uterine cancer, the differential diagnosis includes an ovarian metastasis, an ovarian thecoma associated with hyperestrinism and a coexisting uterine cancer, and other incidental solid benign ovarian neoplasms (Fig. 4-22; see also Fig. 4-21). When the ovarian mass is a metastasis, it often has the same CT enhancement characteristics as uterine tumor (see Fig. 4-21).

Uterine fluid collections are usually due to occlusion of the endocervical canal or proximal vagina from carcinoma of endometrium or cervix. CT demonstrates an obstructed uterus as an enlarged uterine corpus with a distended, fluid-density endometrial cavity surrounded by a myometrial wall of varying thickness (see Fig. 4-18).[7] Pus, blood, or serous fluid may fill the obstructed uterine cavity (Fig. 4-23A). CT

detection of intrauterine gas may be due to a pyometra, but it is more commonly associated with an underlying necrotic tumor.[8] The differential diagnosis of uterine fluid collections includes a uterine sarcoma (see Figs. 4-18 and 4-23A), radiation therapy, and postsurgical scarring.

Sarcoma—Lymphoma—Metastasis

The characteristic patterns of uterine sarcoma are a large polypoid mass filling the endometrial cavity (see Fig. 4-21) or a huge heterogeneous lobulated uterine mass extending from the pelvic sidewalls to the iliac crest (see Fig. 4-23A). Uterine sarcomas are frequently associated with multiple

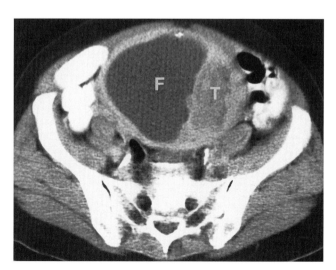

FIG. 4-18. Uterine sarcoma after prior radiation therapy. CT through enlarged uterus shows hypodense tumor (T) in left myometrial wall and large endometrial fluid collection (F).

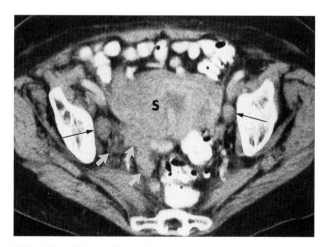

FIG. 4-20. CT scan through large uterine mixed mesodermal sarcoma (S) shows bilateral 1.5-cm obturator lymph node metastases *(black arrows)* and extensive right parametrial tumor extension *(white arrows)*. Tumor was not resectable at laparotomy.

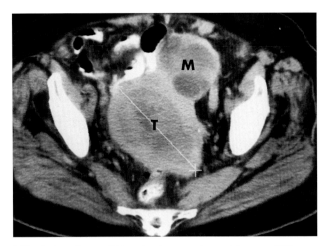

FIG. 4-21. Stage IIIA mixed mesodermal tumor. CT scan through central uterine tumor (T) with left ovarian metastasis (M) confirmed at laparotomy. Both lesions have a similar heterogeneous contrast medium enhancement.

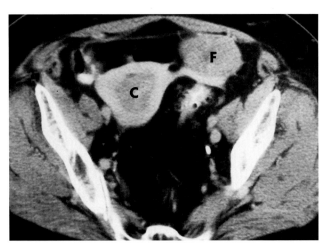

FIG. 4-22. CT scan through endometrial cavity adenosquamous cancer (C) and incidental homogeneous left ovarian fibroma (F) confirmed at laparotomy.

paraaortic lymph node metastases and hematogenous metastases to the liver, spleen, kidneys, or lungs (see Fig. 4-23B). Uterine non-Hodgkin's lymphoma has a similar CT appearance to uterine carcinoma, and it may be associated with ascites and bilateral ovarian involvement. Uterine metastases have the same appearance as uterine cancer (Fig. 4-24).

Gestational Trophoblastic Disease

Widely used for the initial assessment of persistent pelvic and metastatic gestational trophoblastic disease, CT has the ability to screen the pelvis, abdomen, chest, and brain with one imaging modality.[9–12] Also, CT findings are easily integrated into the FIGO staging system for gestational tropho-

blastic disease. MRI is an alternate imaging technique if use of intravenous contrast medium is contraindicated.[13] MRI, like CT, can detect both uterine and extrauterine gestational trophoblastic disease involving the parametria, adnexa, broad ligament, and pelvic fascia and muscle (stage II).

The classic CT findings of uterine invasive mole or choriocarcinoma are irregular, eccentric hypodense foci in the myometrium or endometrial cavity.[9,10,12] Disease foci in these reports may have appeared hypodense if rapid intravenous contrast enhancement was not used during pelvic image acquisition. Two reports show peripheral ring enhancement or adjacent hypervascular areas associated with some hypodense foci.[9–10] Dynamic or spiral CT is necessary to show the characteristic hypervascular endometrial (Fig. 4-25) or myometrial lesions (see Fig. 4-16) and associated enlarged

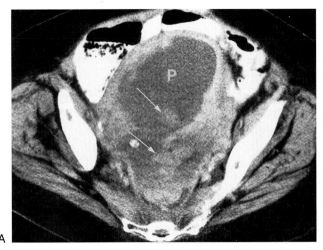

A

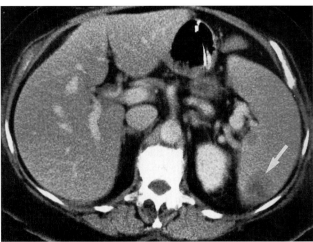

B

FIG. 4-23. Stage IVB mixed mesodermal tumor. **(A)** CT scan shows enlarged uterus filling entire pelvis with central polypoid tumor *(arrows)* and large fluid collection shown to be a pyometra (P). **(B)** CT scan shows a splenic metastasis *(arrow)*. Other images showed paraaortic lymph node and pulmonary metastases.

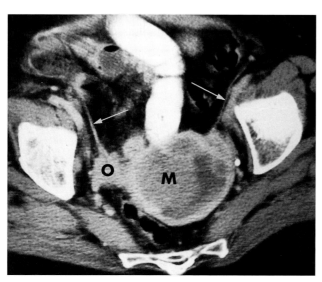

FIG. 4-24. CT scan through the round ligaments and ovary (O) shows metastasis to the uterus (M) from previously treated malignant melanoma of the urethra.

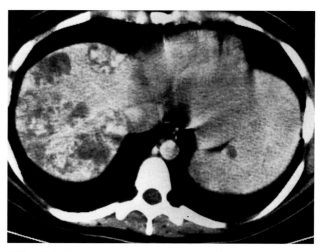

FIG. 4-26. Metastatic choriocarcinoma. CT scan through the dome of the liver shows the classic hypervascular metastases of this tumor.

uterine arteries in the broad ligament.[10] Chest CT can identify unsuspected pulmonary micrometastases (stage III) not detected by chest radiography.[11] Dynamic or spiral CT can also detect the characteristic hypervascular liver metastases (stage IV) of choriocarcinoma (Fig. 4-26).

LIMITATIONS

Limitations of CT staging include (1) differentiating a submucosal or intramural leiomyoma from uterine cancer (Fig. 4-27), (2) determining the depth of myometrial invasion and differentiating stage I and II tumors, and (3) detecting rectosigmoid invasion (stage IVA). MRI is superior to

CT for distinguishing a leiomyoma from tumor because of different MRI signal characteristics. Because the uterine corpus (often anteflexed) and sigmoid colon are frequently oblique to the axial plane, rectosigmoid invasion may be difficult to diagnose. Rectal contrast may be very helpful when there is no plane of separation between the uterine tumor and the colon.

RECURRENT ENDOMETRIAL MALIGNANCY

CT has been the imaging modality of choice for detecting recurrent endometrial malignancy because of its ability to rapidly screen the pelvis, abdomen, and chest for metastatic

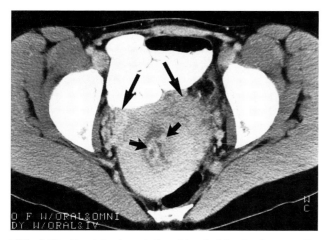

FIG. 4-25. Persistent gestational trophoblastic disease. Dynamic CT scan shows prominent uterine vasculature *(long arrows),* enlarged uterus, and central hypervascular endometrial tumor *(short arrows)* that was an invasive mole at hysterectomy.

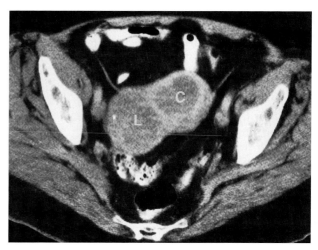

FIG. 4-27. CT scan at the level of the round ligaments shows the similar appearance of a stage I adenocarcinoma (C) and a subserosal leiomyoma (L).

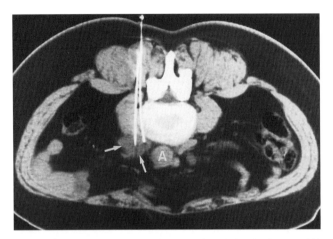

FIG. 4-28. Prone CT scan through the abdominal aorta (A) shows the tips of two 22-gauge needles, which confirmed recurrent endometrial adenocarcinoma in this retroperitoneal lymph node metastasis *(arrows).*

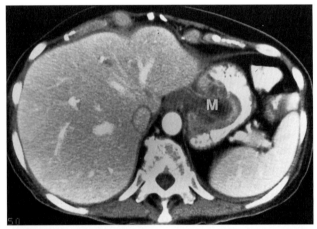

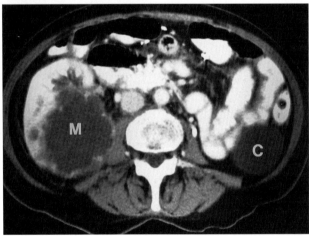

FIG. 4-29. Recurrent mixed mesodermal tumor. **(A)** CT scan shows large metastasis (M) to medial gastric wall confirmed by endoscopy. **(B)** CT scan shows large right renal metastases (M) and left renal cyst (C).

disease and guide a percutaneous biopsy to confirm persistent or recurrent tumor (Fig. 4-28). These data are used to supplement the clinical evaluation and facilitate decisions for further therapy. CT features of recurrent carcinoma include a central pelvic mass, pelvic and paraaortic lymph node metastases, and mesenteric, peritoneal, omental, and liver metastases.[3–4] The CT findings of recurrent uterine sarcoma are similar to those of endometrial carcinoma except that widespread hematogenous metastases to the spleen, kidney, and bowel and abdominal walls are also frequently detected (Fig. 4-29).

CONCLUSION

CT is indicated for staging endometrial malignancy when there is advanced pelvic disease or when abdominal metastases are suspected because of unfavorable histology or abdominal symptoms or physical findings. CT is also appropriate for evaluating recurrent endometrial malignancy because multiple anatomic areas can be rapidly assessed with one imaging technique and metastases can be confirmed by CT-guided biopsy.

REFERENCES

1. Hamlin DJ, Burgener FA, Beecham JB. CT of intramural endometrial carcinoma: contrast enhancement is essential. AJR 1981;137:551.
2. Hasumi K, Matsuzawa M, Chen HF, et al. Computed tomography in the diagnosis and treatment of endometrial carcinoma. Cancer 1982; 50:904.
3. Walsh JW, Goplerud DR. Computed tomography of primary, persistent, and recurrent endometrial malignancy. AJR 1982;139:1149.
4. Balfe DM, Van Dyke J, Lee JKT, et al. Computed tomography in malignant endometrial neoplasms. J Comput Assist Tomogr 1983;7:677.
5. Dore R, Moro G, D'Andrea F, et al. CT evaluation of myometrium invasion in endometrial carcinoma. J Comput Assist Tomogr 1987;11:282.
6. Hricak H, Stern JL, Fisher MR, et al. Endometrial carcinoma staging by MR imaging. Radiology 1987;162:297.
7. Scott WW, Rosenshein NB, Siegelman SS, et al. The obstructed uterus. Radiology 1981;141:767.
8. Gross BH, Jafri SZH, Glazer GM. Significance of intrauterine gas demonstrated by computed tomography. J Comput Assist Tomogr 1983;7:842.
9. Davis WK, McCarthy S, Moss AA, et al. Computed tomography of gestational trophoblastic disease. J Comput Assist Tomogr 1984;8:1136.
10. Miyasaka Y, Hachiya J, Furuya Y, et al. CT evaluation of invasive trophoblastic disease. J Comput Assist Tomogr 1985;9:459.
11. Mutch DG, Soper JT, Baker ME, et al. Role of computed axial tomography of the chest in staging patients with nonmetastatic gestational trophoblastic disease. Obstet Gynecol 1986;68:348.
12. Sanders C, Rubin E. Malignant gestational trophoblastic disease: CT findings. AJR 1987;148:165.
13. Hricak H, Demas BE, Braga CA. Gestational trophoblastic neoplasm of the uterus: MR assessment. Radiology 1986;161:11.

Clinical Gynecologic Imaging, edited
by Arthur C. Fleischer, Marcia C. Javitt,
R. Brooke Jeffrey, Jr., and Howard W. Jones III,
Lippincott-Raven Publishers, Philadelphia © 1997.

CHAPTER 5

Myometrial Disorders

Clinical Overview

Stephen S. Entman, MD

In this subchapter the clinical aspects of two common non-malignant conditions of the uterus are considered: myoma and adenomyosis. These conditions often coexist and share many common clinical features. In a review of 1851 hysterectomies listed in the Collaborative Review of Sterilization (CREST),[1] 7% of all pathologic specimens demonstrated both lesions, ranging from 2% for uteri removed for cervical neoplasia to 14% for uteri removed for myomas. Each of the abnormalities is noted most frequently in late reproductive years. Each may be asymptomatic, may be detected as an incidental pathologic finding, or may cause abnormal uterine bleeding, uterine enlargement, or pelvic pain. Finally, the most common therapy offered to symptomatic patients is simple hysterectomy.

UTERINE MYOMA

This benign neoplasm of the myometrium, also commonly referred to as a fibroid tumor of the uterus, should most accurately be described as a leiomyoma because of its origin from smooth muscle. For simplicity and because of common usage, the term *myoma* is used in this text.

The incidence of occurrence has been estimated to be as high as 50% in autopsy series. In the CREST surveillance, uterine myoma was the preoperative diagnosis in 30% of hysterectomies performed for nonmalignant indications and myomas were identified in 42% of all pathology specimens examined. In a case-control study, Parazzini and colleagues[2] found nulliparity, early menarche, and early last birth to be associated with having had a hysterectomy for myomas. Lindegard,[3] in a population-based study in Sweden, found significant coexistence between myomas and nonfatal breast cancer.

Pathology

The myomatous uterus may have a solitary nodule or multiple nodules ranging from microscopic proportions to mammoth tumors weighing over 100 pounds. The nodules may originate from the cervix or corpus. They may be confined to the myometrium (interstitial or intramural), project into the uterine cavity, distorting the endometrium and the contour of the cavity (submucous), or project off the peritoneal surface of the uterus (subserous) (Fig. 5-1). Either the submucous or subserous configurations may be sessile or pedunculated (Fig. 5-2). The pedunculated submucous myoma can become prolapsed through the cervix; the projection of the subserous lesion between the leaves of the broad ligament is an intraligamentous myoma.

Myomas may undergo secondary changes of pathologic or clinical importance (Fig. 5-3). Hyaline degeneration may be focal or involve broad areas of the tumor (Figs. 5-4 and 5-5; see also Fig. 5-3). Coalescence of hyalinized areas with liquefaction may result in cystic degeneration, thereby softening the lesion and creating a clinical or sonographic misdiagnosis of pregnancy or an ovarian cyst (Fig. 5-6). Calcification may occur in lesions with poor vascular supply,

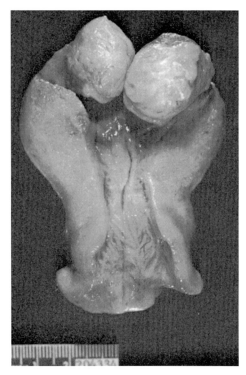

FIG. 5-2. Solitary submucous myoma.

especially in older women. Necrotic changes, carneous or red degeneration, may be caused by aseptic necrosis from tissue ischemia or hemolysis and are most often found in association with pregnancy (Fig. 5-7). Sarcomatous changes in myomas are rare, and the risk of malignant degeneration should not influence the management of most patients. Myomas may become infected, causing symptoms of pelvic inflammatory disease.

Clinical Features

Patients with uterine myomas may be free of symptoms. This can be true even in the presence of very large tumors, based on slow growth with gradual accommodation of the abdominal viscera to the expanding mass. Symptomatic patients may complain of a self-detected mass, abnormal uterine bleeding, acute or chronic pelvic pain, or pressure symptoms.

The mechanism of abnormal uterine bleeding, generally excessive or prolonged menses, is not entirely clear. With large myomas, the endometrial cavity is expanded, creating a larger surface from which menstrual shedding can occur.[5] With intramural myomas, impedance of venous return from the endometrium may produce heavier flow. Deligish and Loewenthal[6] described endometrial atrophy overlying submucous myomas and on the wall opposite the myomas with distortion, dilation, and elongation of endometrial glands at the margins of the myoma. In these areas, normal endometrial cyclic changes could not be identified and stromal hemorrhage was noted. These researchers propose that mechani-

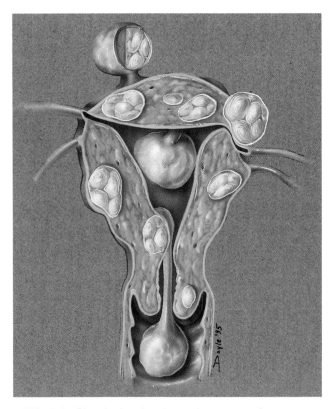

FIG. 5-1. Sketch showing the various types of myomas.

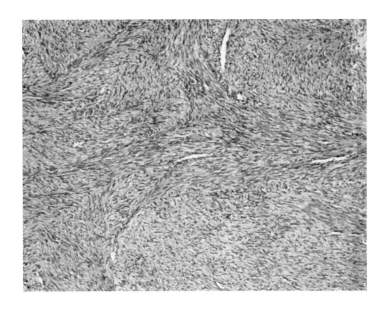

FIG. 5-3. Microscopic appearance of myoma.

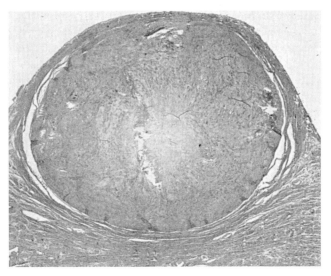

FIG. 5-4. Hyaline change in small myoma.

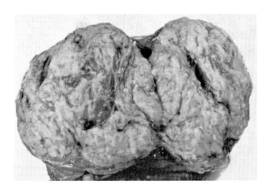

FIG. 5-6. Extensive degeneration with early cystic changes.

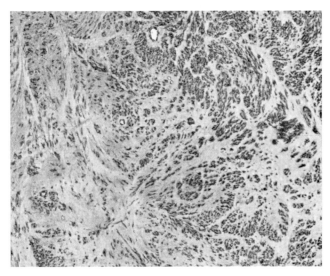

FIG. 5-5. Hyaline degeneration of myoma (microscopic).

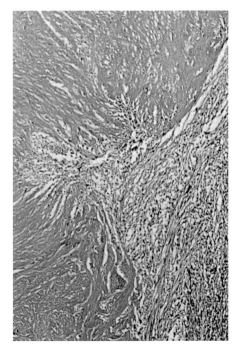

FIG. 5-7. Margin of myoma undergoing necrosis.

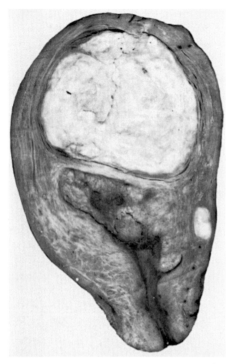

FIG. 5-8. Myoma with associated endometrial cancer. (Courtesy of Professor Robert J. Kellar, Edinburgh.)

cal alterations of the endometrium contribute to the menorrhagia often noted in patients with submucous myomas. In addition, however, they noted some degree of endometrial hyperplasia in half of the specimens evaluated, which is consistent with hyperestrogenism. This raises the serious clinical consideration that abnormal bleeding, especially intermenstrual in pattern, should not be automatically attributed to the presence of myomas (Fig. 5-8).

Pain, when present, is generally described as sensation of weight or dysmenorrhea. Acute onset of pain in previously asymptomatic myomas raises the possibility of necrosis, inflammation with visceral adhesions, or torsion of a pedunculated subserous myoma. Prolapse of a submucous myoma may present as intense cramping pain, often accompanied by discharge or bleeding. Pain in the low back or legs may reflect alterations in body posture or pressure on lumbosacral nerve trunks.

Large myomas may produce extrinsic pressure on pelvic viscera. Urinary frequency or urgency occurs because of diminished bladder capacity. Compression of the ureters may result in hydroureteronephrosis. A mass in the cul-de-sac may produce obstipation, constipation, or hemorrhoids because of rectal pressure.

Myomas in Menopause

The menopausal woman with myomas should demonstrate regression in uterine size. Calcified tumors will remain stable. Any increase in size should prompt immediate action because of the increased risk of sarcomatous degeneration or the possibility of misdiagnosis of an evolving ovarian neoplasm. Consideration of hysterectomy should be given if the uterus, although not excessively enlarged, has multiple subserous nodules masking the position and size of the ovaries.

Diagnosis

Presumptive diagnosis of myomas is made by abdominal and bimanual palpation with the finding of an enlarged irregularly shaped uterus. The word "presumptive" is used advisedly. In the CREST surveillance, pathologic examination of the uterus confirmed the preoperative diagnosis of myoma only 84% of the time and 30% of pathologically identified tumors were not diagnosed preoperatively.[1] Thus, there is potential for errors of diagnosis. Among these errors are several of clinical importance. A normal but retroflexed uterus may be erroneously considered to be a posterior wall myoma projecting into the cul-de-sac. An inflammatory or neoplastic mass of the ovary or bowel may become adherent to the uterus with spurious enlargement of that organ. A pedunculated myoma may be confused with a solid ovarian tumor. Early pregnancy, with or without known preexisting myomas, can be missed. The enhanced diagnostic imaging afforded by sonography, CT, and MRI has simplified these diagnoses in most cases but may introduce other errors. There are reports of the erroneous diagnosis of hydatidiform mole by sonologists who identify multiple echogenic foci in a solitary spherical, edematous myoma and miss an early gestational sac.[7]

Surgery

The mere presence of myomas does not mandate intervention. The introduction of gonadotropin-releasing hormone analogues that effectively reduce estrogen function and result in shrinkage of many myomas has provided an alternative or, in many cases, an adjunct to surgery. The asymptomatic patient may be managed expectantly with examination every 6 months to rule out rapid enlargement. This is especially true in women who are planning pregnancies or who are approaching menopause with the expectation of subsequent regression. The rapidly enlarging myoma warrants intervention because of the potential of malignant degeneration. The patient with pelvic pain or pressure from uterine myomas should also be considered for hysterectomy. A uterus that is larger than 12 to 14 weeks' gestational size in a woman with at least several years of potential growth before menopause and who is planning no further pregnancies should be considered for removal before there is further growth, resulting in increased technical difficulty and consequent operative complications. The uterus with subserous pedunculated myomas that obscure the examination of the ovaries or present as an undiagnosed adnexal mass may warrant hysterectomy.

The young woman who has asymptomatic myomas who is prepared to attempt pregnancy should be encouraged to do so. The role of myomas and myomectomy in infertility is highly questionable. There is controversy about the management of the young woman who has myomas but is not ready for a pregnancy.

The role of gonadotropin-releasing hormone agonist medications that induce a hypoestrogenic state in the clinical management of patients with uterine myomas is still to be defined, but three clear roles exist. The first is the perimenopausal woman who wants to temporize until menopause relieves her symptoms. The second is the woman wishing to preserve fertility with a myomectomy, for whom preoperative shrinkage of lesions would facilitate the procedure. Finally, Stovall and colleagues[8] have described the salutary effect of leuprolide on uterine size before attempting vaginal hysterectomy.

Intraoperative use of transrectal sonography can afford continuous visualization of myoma resection by wire-loop or laser. Linear-array transducers mounted on a laparoscopic probe may also provide a means to monitor and assess myomatous involvement of the myometrium.

ADENOMYOSIS OF THE UTERUS

Adenomyosis is characterized by the ectopic presence of endometrial tissue within the myometrium. It is sometimes referred to as endometriosis interna to distinguish it from endometriosis externa, which is ectopic endometrium beyond the uterine serosal layer. Adenomyosis spontaneously evolves from a downward growth of surface endometrium,[9] but association has been suggested with cesarean section scars[10] and prior intrauterine instrumentation. Adenomyosis

has been reported to occur in 10% to 47% of hysterectomy specimens, with the higher figure being associated with hysterectomies performed for ovarian endometriosis.[11] In the CREST surveillance of hysterectomies performed for benign disease, the incidence was 19%.[1]

Clinical Features

Adenomyosis, when it becomes symptomatic, is characterized by either menorrhagia or dysmenorrhea in the late reproductive years. The lack of specificity of these symptoms is demonstrated by Kilkku and coworkers,[12] who prospectively interviewed patients undergoing hysterectomy for benign pelvic disease.[12] They found no differences in the frequency of symptoms or the anatomic location of pelvic pain between the group with histologically confirmed adenomyosis and those without the lesion.

The mechanisms by which these symptoms could be attributed to the presence of adenomyosis are not clear. Nishida[13] correlated dysmenorrhea with histology and noted that severity was linked to the number of islands and glands and the depth of invasion (Figs. 5-9 through 5-12).[13] Mechanistically, intramural masses may impede venous return from the endometrium, causing increased menstrual flow. Similarly, intramyometrial bleeding may cause menstrual cramps, but the frequent association with endometriosis offers an alternate explanation for this symptom.

Diagnosis

Presumptive diagnosis of adenomyosis is made by eliciting a typical history and the identification of a diffusely enlarged, soft uterus with a proven absence of pregnancy. The pitfalls of this process are pointed out in the CREST

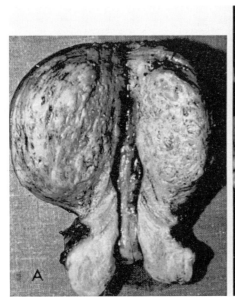
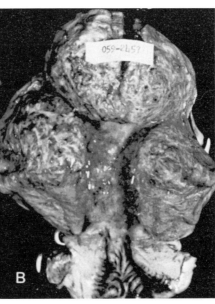

FIG. 5-9. Adenomyosis. **(A)** Extensive adenomyosis of posterior wall. **(B)** Extensive diffuse adenomyosis extending into cervix. (**B** from Emge L. Elusive adenomyosis of the uterus: its historic past and its present state of recognition. Am J Obstet Gynecol 1962;83:1541.)

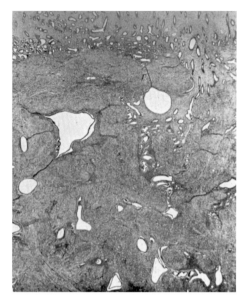

FIG. 5-10. Photomicrograph showing how glands of basal endometrium push down into uterine muscle in adenomyosis.

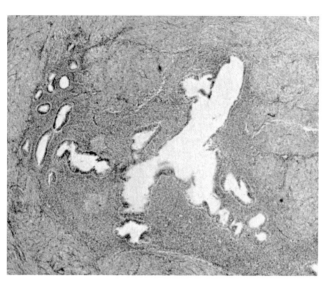

FIG. 5-12. Microscopic appearance of adenomyosis in which the invading endometrium is of the functioning (secretory) type.

study, in which fewer than 2% of patients had a preoperative diagnosis of adenomyosis but pathologic evaluation of the specimens identified the lesion in 19%.[1] The figure was fairly constant regardless of the clinical indication for surgery (13% for cervical neoplasia; 22% for menstrual disorders; 15% for pelvic pain). Conversely, pathologic confirmation of preoperatively diagnosed adenomyosis was possible only 48% of the time.

Increased accuracy of diagnosis may be offered by imaging studies. Hysterography may demonstrate filling of small myometrial cavities with contrast material. Sonography may identify hypoechoic islands in the myometrium caused by adenomyotic implants. MRI can detect ill-defined, homogeneous low intensity areas in the myometrium embedded with high intensity spots.[14] These studies would be only rarely indicated to direct the course of management, but observation of these findings in images obtained for other possible diagnoses may help clarify the clinical presentation.

Treatment

Management of patients should be based on symptoms and age. If symptomatic relief can be obtained with nonste-

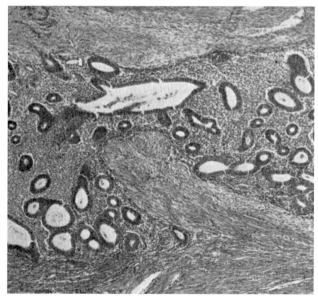

FIG. 5-11. Adenomyosis showing a nonfunctioning hyperplasia-like endometrial island.

roidal antiinflammatory drugs, or if the patient is perimenopausal with anticipated cessation of ovarian function, conservative management is warranted. The patient who faces unacceptable symptoms for a prolonged interval will benefit from hysterectomy. The surgical management of the ovaries is governed by patient age and adnexal pathology.

Medical alternatives are not readily available. These patients are generally at an age for which oral contraceptives are relatively contraindicated, and, besides, anecdotal reports suggest worsening dysmenorrhea with this regimen. Danazol has been anecdotally reported to be of no benefit. Artificial menopause induced by luteinizing hormone–releasing hormone agonists has been suggested as a temporizing measure,[15] but whether the benefits will outweigh cost and side effects remains to be seen.

REFERENCES

1. Lee NC, Dicker RC, Rubin GL, Ory HW. Confirmation of preoperative diagnoses for hysterectomy. Am J Obstet Gynecol 1984;150:283.
2. Parazzini F, La Vecchia C, Negri E, et al. Epidemiologic characteristics of women with uterine fibroids: a case-control study. Obstet Gynecol 1988;72:853.
3. Lindegard B. Breast cancer among women from Gothenburg with regard to age, mortality and coexisting benign breast disease of leiomyoma uteri. Oncology 1990;47:369.
4. Summers WE, Watson RL, Woolridge WH, Langford HG. Hypertension, obesity and fibromyomata uteri as a syndrome. Arch Intern Med 1971;128:750.
5. Sehgal N, Haskins AL. The mechanism of uterine bleeding in the presence of fibromyomas. Am Surg 1960;26:21.
6. Deligish L, Loewenthal M. Endometrial changes associated with myomata of the uterus. J Clin Pathol 1970;23:676.
7. Reid MH, McGehan JP, Oi R. Sonographic evaluation of hydatidiform moles and its look-alikes. AJR 1983;140:307.
8. Stovall TG, Ling FW, Henry LC, Woodruff MR. A randomized trial evaluating leuprolide acetate before hysterectomy as treatment for leiomyomas. Am J Obstet Gynecol 1991;164:1420.
9. Cullen TS: Adenomyoma of uterus. Philadelphia, WB Saunders, 1908.
10. Harris WJ, Daniell JF, Baxter JW. Prior cesarean section, a risk factor for adenomyosis? J Reprod Med 1985;30:173.
11. Henderson DN. Endolymphatic stromal myosis. Am J Obstet Gynecol 1946;52:1000.
12. Kilkku P, Erkkola R, Gronroos M. Nonspecificity of symptoms related to adenomyosis. Acta Obstet Gynecol Scand 1984;63:229.
13. Nishida M. Relationship between the onset of dysmenorrhea and histologic findings in adenomyosis. Am J Obstet Gynecol 1991;165:229.
14. Togashi K, Ozasa H, Konishi I, et al: Enlarged uterus: differentiation between adenomyosis and leiomyoma with MR imaging. Radiology 1989;171:531.
15. Grow DR, Filer RB. Treatment of adenomyosis with long-term GnRH analogues: a case report. Obstet Gynecol 1991;783(pt 2):538.

Transvaginal Sonography of Myometrial Disorders

Arthur C. Fleischer, MD and Jeanne A. Cullinan, MD

Transvaginal sonography depicts the texture of the myometrium in exquisite detail. This information can be used clinically to assess the integrity of the myometrium as well as the location and extent of masses within the myometrium such as leiomyomas. Transvaginal color Doppler sonography can be used to assess the relative flow to leiomyomas as a means of determining which patients might benefit from treatment with gonadotropin releasing hormone. Certain disorders that affect the myometrium in a diffuse manner such as adenomyosis may be difficult to detect by transvaginal sonography, however. In this subchapter the sonographic findings of a variety of myometrial disorders are presented and should be assimilated with the subchapter on transvaginal sonography of endometrial disorders in Chapter 4 for the reader to appreciate the full range of applications of transvaginal sonography of uterine abnormalities.

NORMAL ANATOMY

The first feature that is evident on transvaginal sonography of the myometrium is that this structure consists of muscle bundles that course in a variety of circular, longitudinal, and oblique patterns (Fig. 5-13). The myometrium consists of three major layers (Fig. 5-14). The inner layer of myometrium immediately beneath the endometrium is typically hypoechoic. Its thickness varies from 1 to 5 mm, possibly depending on the day of the cycle it is imaged and whether endometrial peristalsis is present. The hypoechoic texture is probably related to the relatively compact configuration of the myometrial cells and orientation of the long muscle bundles parallel to the endometrium. In the middle layer, which lies between the inner myometrial layer and the zone where the arcuate vessels lie, the muscle bundle layers course in a somewhat oblique and circular fashion. These circular muscle fibers sweep around the uterus in both clockwise and counterclockwise directions. Interestingly, each muscle bundle is innervated independently by contractions that originate in each of the tubes. It seems that peristaltic waves initiate in the tubal walls and these pacemakers seem to regulate the uterine contractions that are particularly evident during the periovulatory phase when the uterine contractions sweep from the cervix to the fundus and in the opposite direction during menses. The outer muscle bundle or myometrium contains smooth muscle bundles that interdigitate with the supporting ligaments (see Fig. 5-13).

Myometrial contractions are best visualized when recorded on videotape and played back at fast forward. There have been several studies that quantitate the force and direction of these myometrial contractions.[1] In general, oral contraceptives seem to dampen the myometrial contractions. They are discoordinated during the latter half of the cycle, during which time implantation might occur if egg and sperm cause fertilization. These contractions most likely have an important role between the time of fertilization in the tube and implantation. These contractions account for enhanced sperm transport, as evidenced by the difference between the rate of unassisted sperm mobility and time between coitus and fertilization in the tube.

The vascularity of the myometrium is derived from the uterine artery, which is a branch of the internal iliac artery.[2] At the level of the internal cervical os, the uterine artery courses along the lateral aspect of the uterine corpus, sending small branches into the myometrium representing the arcuate arteries. These arteries are configured in a spoke wheel configuration with radial branches coursing within the myometrium followed by spiral arterioles within the endometrium (Fig. 5-15). The venous circulation courses in a similar pat-

FIG. 5-14. Transvaginal sonography of normal myometrium. **(A)** In long axis the layers of the endometrium and myometrium are clearly seen. The inner myometrium appears hypoechoic, owing to the arrangement of muscular fibers and the presence of periodic contractions. The middle layer is more echogenic with the muscle fibers imaged in short axis. The boundary between the middle and outer layer is delineated by the arcuate vascular network. **(B)** In short axis the concentric orientation of the inner and middle layers is seen.

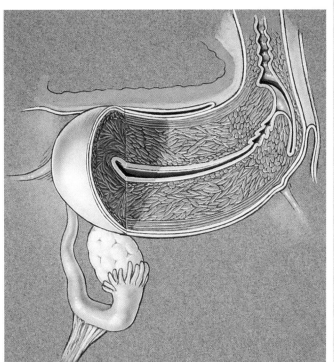

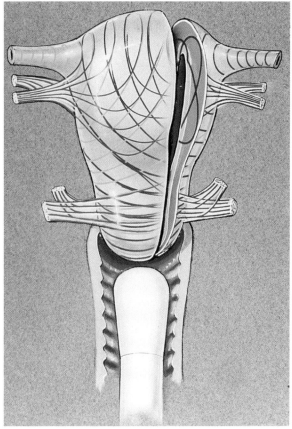

A

B

FIG. 5-13. Myometrial layers. **(A)** Diagram showing arrangement of myometrial fibers with outer myometrial layer surrounding the middle and inner layers of myometrium. The middle myometrium is arranged in a more circular or concentric pattern whereas the inner myometrium is more or less in the longitudinal plane. Appreciation of the orientation of the muscle groups allows for detection of disruptions in the layers of myometrium. The demarcation between middle and outer zones is the boundary created by the arcuate arteries and veins. **(B)** Myometrial fiber arrangement as depicted in various colors. The outer fibers are continuous with the tubal muscle whereas the middle layer is concentric around the lumen. The inner layer surrounds the endometrium and provides endometrial peristalsis (Adapted from Netter; drawings by Paul Gross, MS).

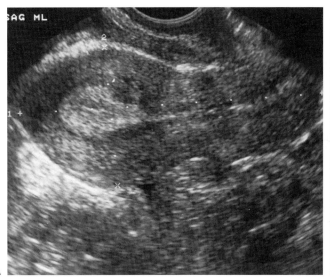

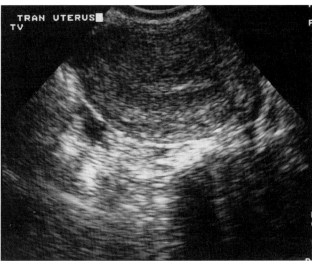

A

B

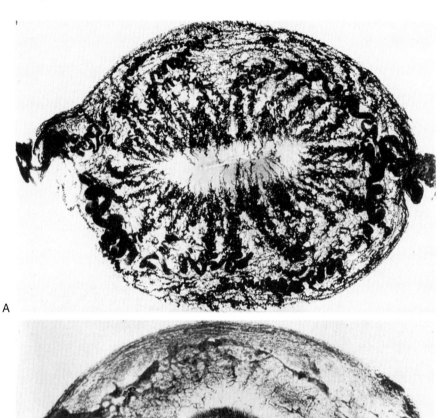

A

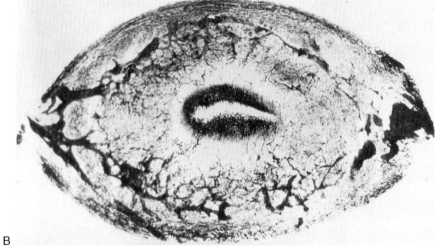

B

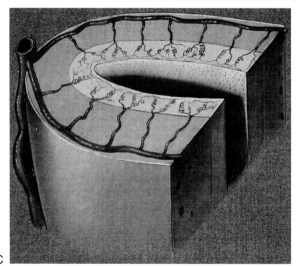

C

FIG. 5-15. Normal uterine arterial and venous network. **(A)** The uterine artery courses along the lateral aspect of the uterus, giving off the arcuate vessels. These further divide into the radial branches, which traverse the myometrium, giving off the spiral branches that course within the endometrium. **(B)** Venous flow shows high vascular density within the endometrium during the secretory phase. **(C)** Diagram showing uterine arterial vessels. The main uterine artery branches into the arcuate vessels, which further divide into the radial vessels that traverse the myometrium. The spiral arterioles supply the endometrium. The relative density of vessels is greater in vivo than displayed in this schematic drawing. (Image in **A** was prepared after thin sections of barium injection within uterine artery as described in Farrer-Brown G, Beilby JOW, Tarbit MH. The blood supply of the uterus. J Obstet Gynaecol Br Commonw 1970 :673; **B** is from same source; **C,** drawn by Paul Gross, MS.)

tern. In fact, the arcuate veins can be distended, particularly in uteri that are retroflexed and in patients with "pelvic congestion syndrome" (Fig. 5-16).[3] In these patients, the arcuate veins may measure 2 to 3 mm in diameter and appear as anechoic tubular structures in the layer between the intermediate or middle and outer myometrium. The correlation between symptoms and the presence of distended veins is not straightforward because many women with distended veins do not suffer from the typical symptoms of pelvic congestion syndrome.

Depending on the sensitivity of the scanner, these myometrial vessels can be depicted with most transvaginal color Doppler sonography systems (see Fig. 5-17). The radial vessels are only inconsistently seen, and the spiral vessels are usually not depicted when the endometrium is normal.[4] One

can have an overall sense of uterine perfusion using the color data from transvaginal color Doppler sonography, especially using the power or amplitude mode. The "warm" pattern is seen particularly during pregnancy as opposed to the "cold" pattern consisting of only scattered color within the myometrium seen in the nongravid state or in patients with ectopic pregnancies.[5]

Calcification can be seen in the arcuate vessels in elderly patients, particularly diabetics (Fig. 5-18).[6] Other normal variants within the myometrium include echogenic foci from previous dilatation and curettage, probably related to focal areas of fibrosis, and various forms of myometrial septa in patients with septated uteri. The myometrial septa are hypoechoic relative to the echogenic endometrium, and therefore evaluation of congenital anomalies should be scheduled dur-

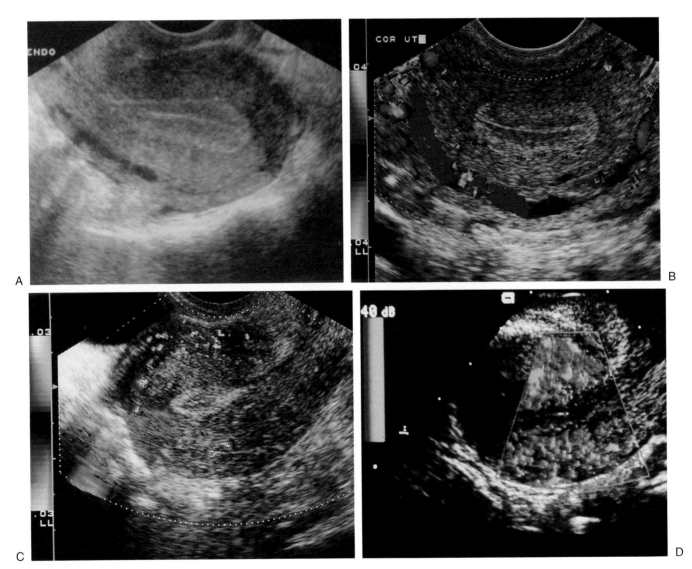

FIG. 5-16. Uterine vascularity as depicted by transvaginal sonography and transvaginal color Doppler sonography. **(A)** Transvaginal sonogram of retroflexed uterus containing distended arcuate veins. **(B)** Transvaginal color Doppler sonogram showing distended arcuate veins. **(C)** Frequency-based transvaginal color Doppler sonogram of gravid uterus showing myometrial vascularity. **(D)** Amplitude-based transvaginal color Doppler sonogram showing numerous myometrial vessels in a patient who is multiparous. **(B** and **D,** courtesy of Acuson, Inc., Mountainview, CA).

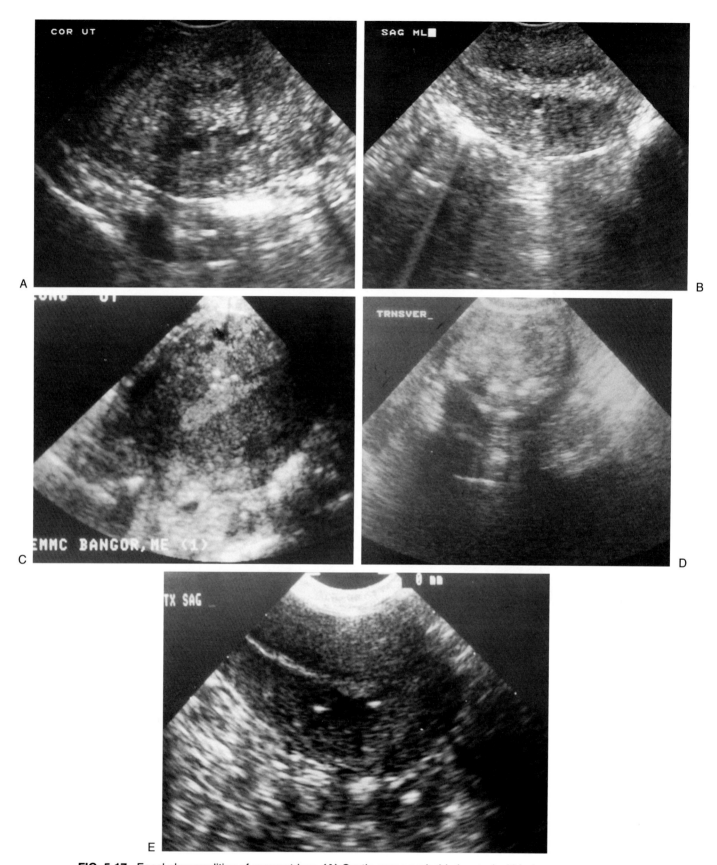

FIG. 5-17. Focal abnormalities of myometrium. **(A)** Cystic areas probably located within inner myometrium in a patient on tamoxifen. **(B)** Similar cystic areas in a patient status post endometrial ablation. **(C)** Echogenic foci probably representing areas of fibrosis from prior dilatation and curettage. **(D)** Echogenic foci representing calcification of arcuate arteries. **(E)** Echogenic foci within inner myometrium in a woman status post dilatation & curettage. (**C,** courtesy of Mary Warner, MD, **E,** courtesy of Deland Burks, MD)

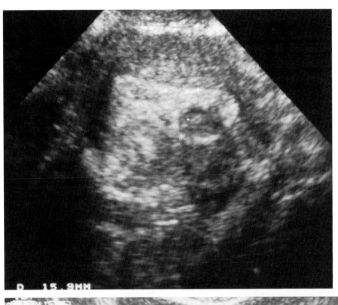

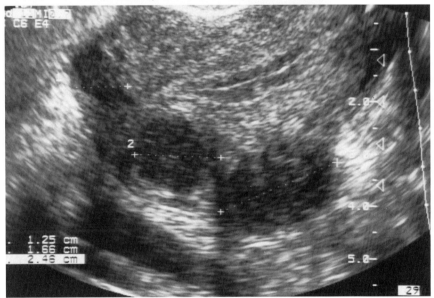

FIG. 5-18. Transvaginal sonography of fibroids. **(A)** Submucosal fibroid causing extrinsic displacement of the endometrium. **(B)** Three intramural fibroids not displacing the endometrium.

ing the luteal phase of the cycle. The thickness of the myometrium varies with age. It measures 1.0 to 1.5 cm in thickness but thins as the uterus decreases in thickness after menopause.

LEIOMYOMAS

Clinical Aspects

Uterine leiomyomas are benign tumors that consist of smooth muscle and connective tissue. They are the most common tumors encountered in gynecologic practice and are commonly referred to as fibroids or myomas. It is estimated that leiomyomas are present in 20% of women older than 35 years of age.[7] Such tumors are estrogen dependent and usually regress after menopause. Leiomyomas are most prevalent in black women and other dark-skinned groups. The usual clinical picture is a palpable mass in a middle-aged woman, but leiomyomas may be associated with excessive menstrual bleeding and pelvic pain. They may cause infertility owing to distortion of the isthmic portion of the tube. In addition, fibroids can contribute to uterine dystocia or to pelvic obstruction in the laboring patient.

The fibroid is important to the sonologist for two reasons. First, as a neoplasm, fibroids do have a small malignant potential. More commonly, however, the clinician needs to differentiate a palpable mass of uterine origin from an adnexal mass. For these reasons, detailed sonographic examination of fibroid tumors is warranted.

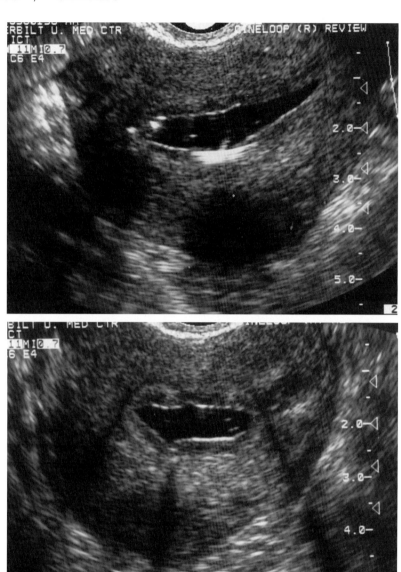

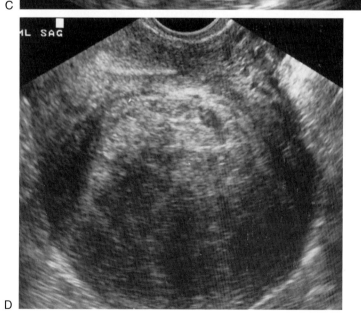

FIG. 5-18. *Continued* **(C)** Sonohysterogram of patient in **C** showing normal endometrium and relationship of endometrium to submucosal fibroids in long *(top)* and short *(bottom)* axes. **(D)** Large intramural fibroid extending to the serosa but not displacing the endometrium. **(E)** Sonohysterogram of patient in **D** showing normal endometrium as depicted in long axis. **(F)** Initial transvaginal sonogram showing possible submucosal fibroid *(between cursors)*. **(G)** After saline instillation, the protrusion of the fibroid into the lumen is better delineated. **(H)** Pedunculated subserosal fibroid mimicking a solid left ovarian mass. **(I)** Pedunculated subserosal fibroid extending from right fundal region.

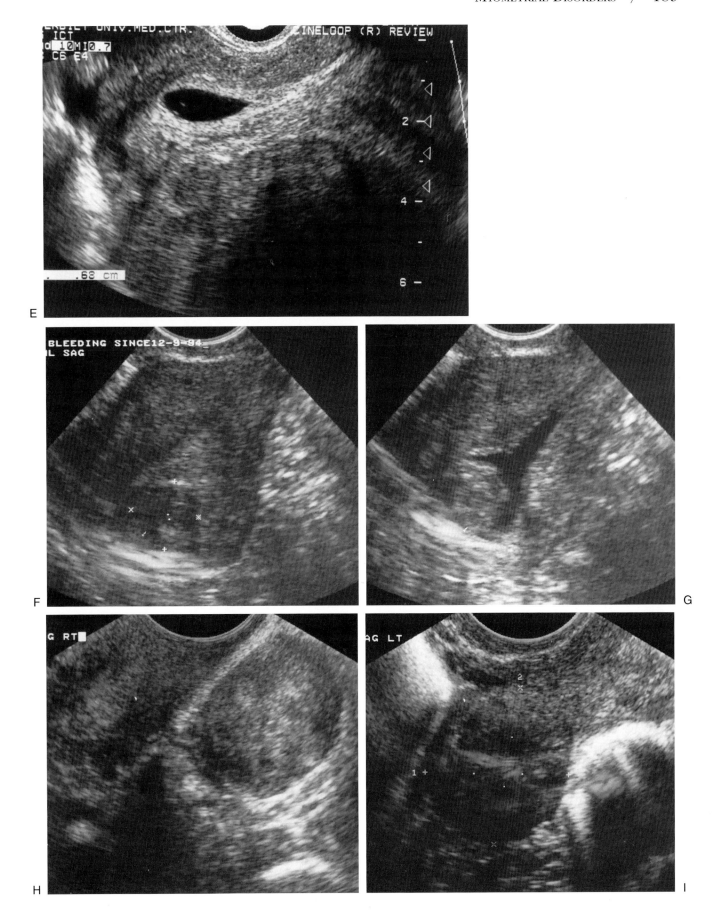

Leiomyomas usually develop in the myometrium of the upper contractile fundal and corporeal portions of the uterus. Only 3% of the leiomyomas are of cervical origin. Microscopically, these tumors arise from the smooth muscle and connective tissue that surround the smaller vessels coursing within the outer layers of the myometrium. Intramural leiomyomas cause the uterus to contract, and the resultant compression of these tumors is believed to displace them either toward the peritoneal surface to form subserous nodules or toward the endometrial cavity to produce submucous nodules. Intraligamentary nodules can arise by extrusion of the intramural nodule retroperitoneally into the areolar tissue between the leaves of the broad ligament. Also, rarely, leiomyomas can develop from fibromuscular structures in the round ligament or from those surrounding the vessels.

Leiomyomas of the uterus are usually multiple and of various sizes. A solitary nodule is found in only 2% of patients; the number of tumors in a uterus may reach hundreds. The size ranges from microscopic to massive, with 100 pounds being the largest single fibroid reported. Microscopically, each nodule is delineated by a pseudocapsule through which vascular channels enter and arborize within the tumor. As the tumor increases in size, it may eventually outgrow the blood supply and central ischemia is followed by various stages of degeneration.

Degenerative processes may be benign or malignant and asymptomatic or symptomatic. Asymptomatic benign degenerative processes include atrophic, hyaline, cystic, myxomatous, lipomatous, and carneous degeneration.

The symptomatic group includes carneous degeneration, infarction, and infection. Under the effect of strong uterine contractions, rotation of nodules within the pseudocapsule may shear supplying vessels and result in necrobiosis of the tumor. This process is most frequently found during pregnancy.

Both subserous and submucous nodules may become pedunculated and undergo torsion of the pedicle, with subsequent infarction, degeneration, necrosis, and potential infection. For some pedunculated nodules whose circulation is occluded, attachment to the omentum or intestine allows the entry of new vessels and a revitalized blood supply. Under such circumstances, the pedicle may atrophy and the nodule become completely detached from the uterus, giving rise to a so-called parasitic fibroid.

Submucous fibroids are prone to necrosis because their blood supply is frequently insufficient to support the tumor mass. More importantly, their exposed position subjacent to the uterine lumen predisposes them to ascending infection. Pelvic inflammatory diseases may involve adjacent fibroids by direct extension or through the lymphatics; curettage can injure submucous nodules and introduce bacteria. Occasionally, when the fibroid is infected, the central core may be filled with purulent material.

Malignant change in the tumor is a generative process. Although the occurrence of leiomyosarcoma in a preexisting leiomyoma is 0.2% or less, the prevalence of leiomyomas results in this form of sarcoma being the most common malignant stromal uterine tumor (25%). Malignancy in a fibroid is seldom diagnosed preoperatively because there are no characteristic symptoms to distinguish this entity from preexisting fibroid nodules. Sudden accelerated growth in a previously static tumor and postmenopausal enlargement should suggest the possibility of a superimposed malignant process.

The clinical manifestations of fibroids are variable and depend on the size and number of the tumors, age of the patient, proximity of the tumor to the endometrial cavity, mobility of the fibroid (sessile or pedunculated), and presence or absence of degenerative processes. Submucous tumors typically encroach on the endometrium and distort the endometrial cavity. Owing to pressure necrosis, alteration in the vascular architecture of the endometrium may occur and cause excessive menstrual bleeding to be the presenting symptom. When submucous fibroids outgrow their blood supply, surface necrosis, slough, and bloody discharge may result. Pain is not a common symptom except in the presence of degenerative changes or torsion of the pedicle of a subserous nodule. Pelvic discomfort due to pressure on the surrounding organs may be present with large tumors, but often the only symptoms are abdominal enlargement and a palpable mass. Pedunculated submucous leiomyomas ("fibroid polyps") can be partially or completely extruded through the cervical canal and can cause infection, necrosis, and ascending endometritis. This event may also be associated with inversion of the uterus. Larger fibroids, particularly of the intraligamentous type, may compress the ureter, with resultant hydroureter and hydronephrosis.

Sonographic Features

The typical sonographic appearance of a leiomyoma consists of a mildly to moderately echogenic intrauterine mass that causes nodular distortion of the uterine outline. Small intramural or submucous leiomyomas may be recognized by their distortion of the normally linear central endometrial echoes (Fig. 5-19). The solid nature of a fibroid often may cause an indentation on the bladder or rectum.

The echogenicity of a fibroid depends on the relative ratio of fibrous tissue to smooth muscle. With a more fibrous component, there is increased echogenicity of the nodule. The sonographic texture of fibroids also depends on the type and presence of degeneration and on the vascular supply. Interfaces between the normal myometrium and the pseudocapsule of the mass can sometimes be demonstrated. With transvaginal sonography, the distortion of the endometrial lumen associated with the fibroid can be demonstrated. In some fibroids, the whorled internal architecture can be appreciated. The whorled appearance corresponds to bundles of smooth muscle and connective tissue that are arranged in a concentric pattern. In some cases, leiomyomas are only minimally echogenic and appear as cystic masses, except

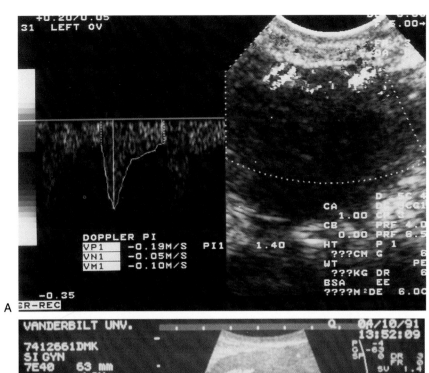

A

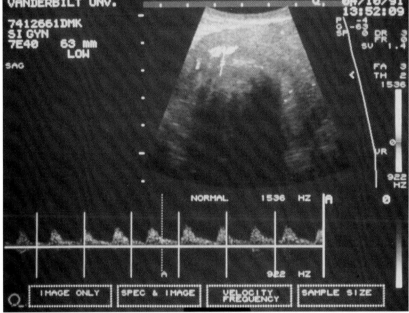

B

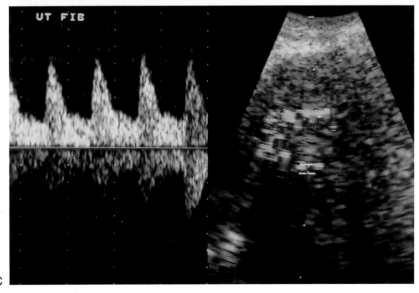

C

FIG. 5-19. Transvaginal color Doppler sonography of fibroids. **(A)** Sonogram of a pedunculated subserosal fibroid showing extensive vascularity along the periphery of the mass. **(B)** Relatively hypovascular intramural fibroid. **(C)** Relatively vascular pedunculated submucosal fibroid. The sample volume is on an artery within the pedicle of the submucosal fibroid.

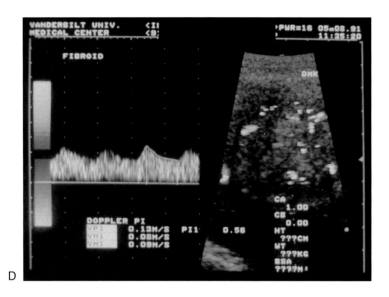

FIG. 5-19. *Continued.* **(D)** Relatively vascular intramural fibroid with low impedance flow.

that their posterior wall is not as prominent as expected. Irregular anechoic areas may be seen within leiomyomas if cystic degeneration has occurred. Calcific degeneration within a leiomyoma is common and can be recognized as clusters of high-level echoes that are associated with distal acoustical shadowing.

The most common cause of calcification within the uterus is calcific degeneration within a fibroid. Twenty-five percent of one series of 75 patients with fibroids had calcifications.[7] The pattern of calcification varied from a few small foci to a large rim of globular calcification. If the calcification is extensive and located along the anterior portion of the fibroid, it may prohibit complete sonographic delineation of the mass. Intrauterine calcifications can also be encountered in uterine sarcomas, but this condition is much less common than in leiomyomas.

Other types of degeneration within leiomyomas that produce sonographically recognizable changes in uterine texture include cystic, myxomatous, and hyaline degeneration. Among these, hyaline degeneration is the most common and appears as anechoic areas within a fibroid. Areas of hyaline degeneration can be distinguished from areas of cystic degeneration in that areas of cystic degeneration usually demonstrate distal wall enhancement. Accelerated enlargement of a fibroid after menopause may indicate sarcomatous degeneration. There do not appear to be any sonographic signs that distinguish benign from malignant changes, however.

Leiomyomas that are pedunculated can be confused with other adnexal masses if their pedicle is not visualized. The most common location of pedunculated leiomyomas is superior to the uterine fundus. In most cases, an echogenic interface corresponding to the tissue plane connecting the fibroid and the fundus can be delineated. Pedunculated subserosal fibroids can also extend into the broad ligament, and thus appear as an extrauterine mass. However, the typical whorled configuration of the fibroid usually can be recognized. To ascertain whether a mass is connected to the uterus by a pedicle, applying slight pressure with the examiner's hand or the transvaginal sonographic probe to the mass while scanning has been suggested. The mass moves with the uterus if the two are connected. This procedure should be performed by an experienced sonographer or sonologist and monitored with real-time sonography.

Submucous leiomyomas may be difficult to differentiate from intramural leiomyomas. Both may produce distortion of the endometrial interfaces. Submucosal fibroids are best documented by transvaginal sonography or by sonohysterography. Submucosal leiomyomas tend to more echogenic than endometrial polyps. This topic is covered in more detail in Chapter 4.

Fibroids can be particularly difficult to detect with transabdominal sonography in the retroflexed uterus. Because the uterine fundus curves posteriorly in the retroflexed uterus, this area may be relatively hypoechoic. Appropriate gain settings and time compensation gain curves should be used; a hypoechoic area within the fundus of a retroflexed uterus could be technical in origin rather than a fibroid.

Serial sonographic evaluation of leiomyomas can be of significant clinical value. Follow-up scans of the fibroid uterus of a pregnant woman can help assess the growth and accelerated degeneration of this mass. In one study of fibroids during pregnancy it was revealed that the size of most fibroids remains stable during pregnancy.[8] Fibroids can be differentiated from focal contractions by more distinct borders within the myometrium and lack of change on follow-up studies within 1 hour of initial examination. Because fibroids should regress after menopause, serial sonograms can objectively document enlargement or regression of leiomyomas in the older woman. Because of its ability to portray larger areas of interest, transabdominal sonography is needed in fibroids that enlarge the uterus to over 8 to 10 weeks in size. When the uterus is smaller than this, transvaginal sonography is recommended. Depiction of the endometrial interfaces by transvaginal sonography is particularly helpful in identifying myometrial masses by their displacement of this interface. Transvaginal sonography can reveal differences in echogenicity of the fibroid and surrounding myometrium to ascertain the true size of the lesion.

Color Doppler sonography may be used to assess flow within the fibroid and its response to medical treatment.[9] In general, well-vascularized fibroids tend to be more responsive to medical treatment than hypovascular ones. Fibroids that parasitize major vessels for their blood supply may have low impedance, high diastolic flow similar to that seen in some malignant pelvic masses (Fig. 5-20). Color Doppler imaging may also diminish displacement of intrauterine vascularity resulting from leiomyomas.

Sonographic Mimics

Occasionally, solid masses that are adjacent to the uterus appear as masses within the uterine contour. This finding has been referred to as ''the indefinite uterus sign.''[10] In such a setting, a retrouterine mass may be misdiagnosed as an enlarged uterus. The most common solid masses to simulate the sonographic appearance of a fibroid are the solid ovarian tumors. In particular, cystadenofibromas can calcify, simulating the appearance of a fibroid. Metastases that settle and enlarge in the cul-de-sac, such as those associated with breast tumors, can also produce apparent enlargement of the uterine contour.

Transvaginal sonography can be helpful in distinguishing fibroids from other adnexal or ovarian masses. In particular, transvaginal sonography is helpful in identifying the ovaries in patients with fibroids because it usually is difficult to distinguish a fibroid from the ovary by palpation. We have also been able to distinguish a mass, representing a tubal carcinoma, from a fibroid by using transvaginal sonography.

Adenomyomas may coexist with leiomyomas. Adenomyomatosis is a condition in which the basal layer of the endometrium burrows into the myometrium and is frequently associated with endometriosis. On transvaginal sonography, adenomyomas may appear as echogenic myometrium with punctate hypoechoic areas (Fig. 5-21). The boundary between adenomyosis and normal myometrium may be difficult to ascertain in some cases, however.[11,12] A similar condition can be observed in patients who take tamoxifen or have had endometrial ablation. The cystic areas may represent degenerative changes in the inner myometrium.[13] MRI may be helpful in distinguishing leiomyomas from adenomyosis.[14]

MRI may be more accurate than sonography in delineation of the number, extent, and location of multiple leiomyomas. MRI may also be useful in distinguishing adenomyosis from multiple leiomyoma, an important distinction in management decisions because focal excision might be used for leiomyoma but adenomyosis is typically a diffuse nonresectable disorder.

LEIOMYOSARCOMA

Leiomyosarcomas are typically considered degenerative leiomyomas that exhibit sarcomatous changes. They range from large bulky echogenic masses to cystic septated intrauterine lesions. In general, these tumors have low impedance blood flow but there is significant overlap in leiomyomas that have low impedance (see Fig. 5-21).[15]

CHORIOCARCINOMA

Choriocarcinoma is really a malignant process but is included here because it can mimic the transvaginal sonographic finding in adenomyosis. However, these tumors are typically highly vascular with high velocity, low impedance flow (Fig. 5-22).

ADENOMYOSIS

Adenomyosis is a condition in which endometrial implants are present within the myometrium. Histologically, this disorder is found in approximately 30% of patients with endometriosis. This condition may not be detectable by sonography in its very subtle forms but only appreciated when the myometrium is examined histologically. In more severe and extensive forms of adenomyosis, however, the myometrium becomes course and irregular (see Fig. 5-20).[11,14–17] This diagnosis may be better made with MRI because the extent of disease may not be as readily apparent on transvaginal sonography.[14]

A variant of adenomyosis may be encountered in some patients taking tamoxifen evident as the development of cystic areas in the inner myometrium (see Fig. 5-17).[18] It is not clear what these cystic areas actually represent histologically. They may represent cystic spaces within the myometrium associated with breaks in the myometrium encountered with aging. Alternatively, they may represent obstructed and dilated glands within remnants of endometrium.

Differentiation of adenomyomas from fibroids has clinical importance when local resection is considered. Because adenomyosis is usually a diffuse process, it may be difficult to surgically remove the affected area whereas a leiomyoma can be excised by wire-loop resection. Some researchers advocate performing myometrial biopsy to differentiate these two entities.[19] Transvaginal color Doppler sonography may also show more flow to areas of adenomyosis.[20] MRI may be helpful in equivocal cases.

Transvaginal color Doppler sonography can be used to differentiate cystic areas within the inner myometrium from cystic degeneration within polyps because polyps tend to be vascular and cystic areas within the myometrium are usually hypovascular.

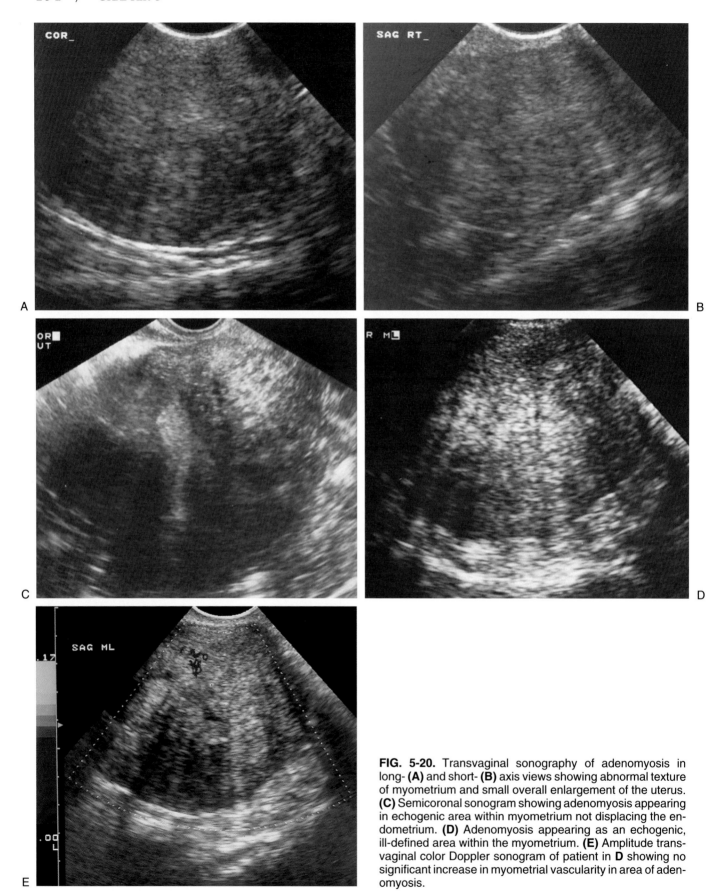

FIG. 5-20. Transvaginal sonography of adenomyosis in long- **(A)** and short- **(B)** axis views showing abnormal texture of myometrium and small overall enlargement of the uterus. **(C)** Semicoronal sonogram showing adenomyosis appearing in echogenic area within myometrium not displacing the endometrium. **(D)** Adenomyosis appearing as an echogenic, ill-defined area within the myometrium. **(E)** Amplitude transvaginal color Doppler sonogram of patient in **D** showing no significant increase in myometrial vascularity in area of adenomyosis.

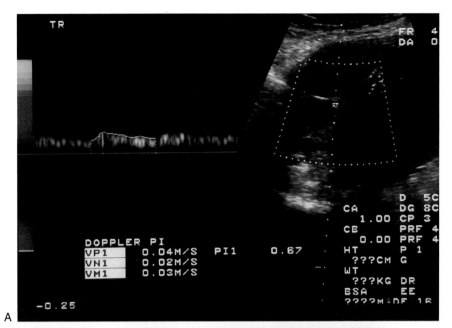

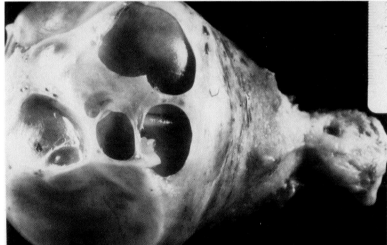

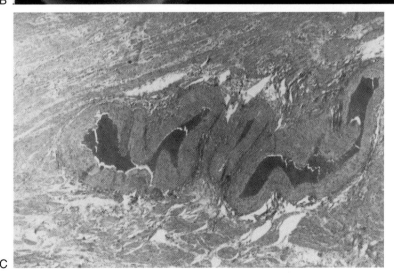

FIG. 5-21. Transvaginal color Doppler sonography of leiomyosarcoma. **(A)** Sonogram showing a multiloculated cystic uterine mass with velocity, low impedance flow. **(B)** Opened uterus shown in **A** demonstrating several cystic areas. **(C)** Low-power photomicrograph showing dilated vessels.

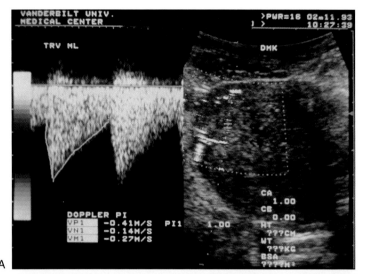

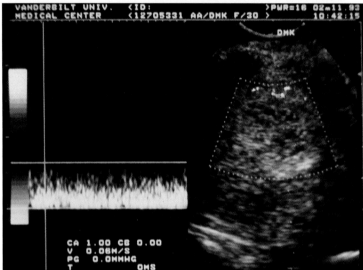

FIG. 5-22. Transvaginal color Doppler sonography of choriocarcinoma. **(A)** Hypervascularity of invasive trophoblastic tumor showing high velocity, low impedance flow. **(B)** Same mass as in Figure 5-22**A** showing increased venous flow.

CONCLUSION

The main applications of both conventional and color Doppler transvaginal sonography in diagnosing myometrial disease include the evaluation of uterine leiomyomas as to size, location, and any change during treatment. Adenomyosis may be difficult to depict on sonography, and MRI may be recommended in these cases.

REFERENCES

1. de Vries K, Lyons EA, Ballard G, et al. Contractions of the inner third of the myometrium. Am J Obstet Gynecol 1990;162:679.
2. Farrer-Brown, Beilby JOW, Tarbit MH. The blood supply of the uterus. J Obstet Gynaecol Br Commonw 1970;77:673.
3. Bouillas-Musoles F, Ballester M. Transvaginal color Doppler in the diagnosis of pelvic congestion syndrome In: Kurjak A, ed. Transvaginal color Doppler, ed 2. London, Parthenon, 1993:207.
4. Bourne THE, Campbell S, Steer CV, et al. Detection of endometrial cancer by transvaginal ultrasonography with color flow imaging and blood flow analysis: a preliminary report. Gynecol Oncol 1991;40:253.
5. Emerson D. Early pregnancy. In: Fleischer A, Emerson D, eds. Color Doppler sonography in obstetrics and gynecology. New York, Churchill-Livingstone, 1993.
6. Occhipinti K, Kutcher R, Rosenblatt R. Sonographic appearance and significance of arcuate artery calcification. J Ultrasound Med 1991;10: 97.
7. von Micsky L. Sonographic study of uterine fibromyomas. In: Sanders R, James AE Jr, eds. Ultrasonography in obstetrics and gynecology. New York, Appleton-Century-Crofts, 1977.
8. Lev-Toaff A, Coleman B, Arger P. Leiomyomas in pregnancy: sonographic study. Radiology 1987;164:683.
9. Matta WHM, Stabile I, Shaw RW, Campbell S. Doppler assessment of uterine blood flow changes in patients with fibroids receiving the gonadotropin-releasing hormone agonist Buserelin. Fertil Steril 1988; 49:1083.
10. Bowie J. Ultrasound of gynecologic pelvic masses: the indefinite uterus

sizes and other patterns associated with diagnostic error. J Clin Ultrasound 1977;5:323.

11. Fedele L, Bianchi S, Dorta M, et al. Transvaginal ultrasonography in the differential diagnosis of adenomyoma versus leiomyoma. Am J Obstet Gynecol 1992;167:603.

12. Hirai M, Sagai H, Shibatu F. Transvaginal pulsed and color Doppler for diagnosis of adenomyosis. Ultrasound OB/Gyn Suppl 1994.

13. Huang RT, Chou CY, Chang CH, et al. Differentiation between adenomyoma and leiomyoma with transvaginal ultrasonography. Ultrasound Obstet Gynecol 5:47, 1995.

14. Ascher SM, Arnold LL, Patt RH, et al. Adenomyosis: prospective comparison of MR imaging and transvaginal sonography. Radiology 1994; 190:803.

15. Kurjak A. Malignant uterine tumors. In: Transvaginal color Doppler, ed 2. London, Parthenon, 1993.

16. Bohlman ME, Ensor RE, Sanders RC. Sonographic findings in adenomyosis of the uterus. AJR 1987;148:765.

17. Siedler D, Laing FC, Jeffrey RB, Wing VW. Uterine adenomyosis: a difficult sonographic diagnosis. J Ultrasound Med 1987;6:345.

18. Goldstein SR. Unusual ultrasonographic appearance of the uterus in patients receiving tamoxifen. Am J Obstet Gynecol 1994;170:447.

19. Perrot N, Guyst B, Antoline M, Uzan S. The effect of tamoxifen on the endometrium. Letter to editor. Ultrasound OB/Gyn 1994;4:83.

20. Popp LW, Schwiedessen JP, Gaetje R. Myometrial biopsy in the diagnosis of adenomyosis uteri. Am J Obstet Gynecol 1993;169:546.

Magnetic Resonance Imaging of Myometrial Disorders

Marcia C. Javitt, MD

UTERINE LEIOMYOMAS

Uterine leiomyomas (fibroids) are seen in about 25% of women in the childbearing age group.[1] These lesions are made of fibrous tissue and smooth muscle and may be single or multiple. Most commonly involving the body of the uterus, fibroids can be in the lower uterine segment or cervix infrequently where they can be problematic in pregnancy during vaginal delivery (Fig. 5-23).[2,3] Although they are benign histologically, leiomyomas can cause significant abnormal bleeding, pain, and even infertility. It is the submucosal myomas that are often the most symptomatic because they may protrude into the endometrial canal, thereby causing bleeding (Fig. 5-24). Pedunculated subserosal lesions are subject to torsion and may simulate an adnexal mass (Fig. 5-25).

Because they can degenerate, the appearance of leiomyomas can be quite variable. Not only necrosis from outgrowing the blood supply, which is characteristic of submucous lesions, but also hyaline degeneration, myxomatous degeneration, and fatty necrosis and calcification have been described.[1–4]

Sonography remains the most cost-effective screening technique for detecting fibroids. However, MRI is the most sensitive cross-sectional imaging modality for detection of fibroids.[3,5] The use of MRI should be reserved for cases in which the sonographic findings are equivocal or if precise anatomic localization preoperatively is required, such as in patients undergoing myomectomy for infertility. MRI is particularly helpful in patients who are obese or in those with a retroverted uterus because sonography can be unrewarding in these cases.

Most commonly, leiomyomas have a decreased signal intensity on T1- and T2-weighted images (Fig. 5-26). Lesions that have degenerated can contain foci of bright signal (Figs. 5-27 and 5-28).[2,4,6,7] A peripheral bright rim has been reported due to dilated vessels, lymphatics, or edema.[8] After gadolinium administration, there is a variable amount of enhancement in myomas depending on the degree of cellularity of the lesion.[9]

Gonadotropin-releasing hormone analogues have been used to treat leiomyomas and act on nondegenerated cells by inducing hypoestrogenemia. Degenerating fibroids en-

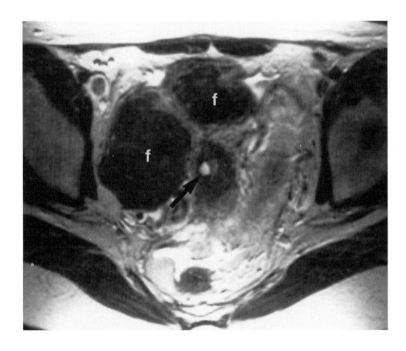

FIG. 5-23. Cervical leiomyomas. Probably seen in only 1% of cases, cervical fibroids can be problematic at the time of vaginal delivery. T2-weighted fast spin-echo scan shows two large anterior cervical fibroids (f). Note the small nabothian cyst *(arrow).*

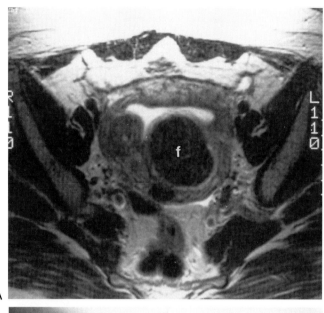

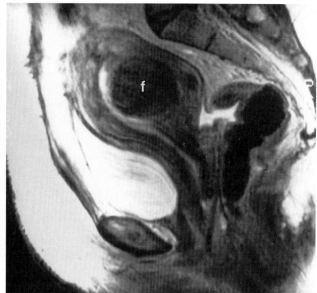

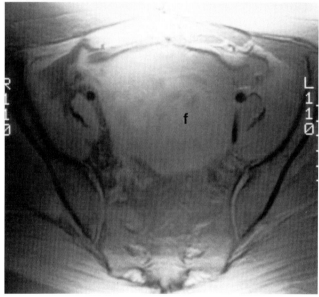

FIG. 5-24. Enhancing submucous fibroids. **(A)** T2-weighted axial and **(B)** sagittal scans show several submucous fibroids. The dominant lesion (f) distorts the contour of the endometrial canal in this patient, who presented with severe menometrorrhagia. **(C)** T1-weighted and gadolinium-enhanced T1-weighted scans with fat saturation show enhancement in the submucous fibroid.

hanced less in one series of patients. Thus, contrast medium–enhanced MRI may be a way of evaluating the candidacy of patients for treatment with these agents (see Fig. 5-24).[10,11] MRI cannot reliably differentiate between leiomyomas and leiomyosarcomas because both lesions can be bulky, inhomogeneous masses[12]; however, leiomyosarcomas are rare lesions. Their possible origination in preexisting leiomyomas remains controversial.[1] Unlike adenomyosis, leiomyomas, even when multilobular, are typically spherical and well demarcated from the myometrium.

ADENOMYOSIS

Adenomyosis is a common benign but troublesome condition that is caused by invasion of the basal zone of the endometrium into the myometrium with reactive proliferation of the adjacent myometrium. The incidence has been variably reported in hysterectomy specimens between 15% and 60% and is probably about 20%.[1,13] It occurs most commonly in multiparous women in the fifth decade of life. The uterus is often but not universally enlarged with mural thickening. The invaginated endometrium may function with hormonal cycle, producing hemorrhagic reddish brown pigmented cysts in the uterine wall.[1] Symptoms include dysmenorrhea and menorrhagia, both of which can progress and become severe and debilitating.

Sonography and CT have not permitted the specific diagnosis of adenomyosis, both showing nonspecific uterine enlargement. Only MRI has been useful for this purpose. Clinically, the diagnosis of this condition has been problematic, because the signs and symptoms are nonspecific and may be simulated by several other processes, such as leiomyomas,

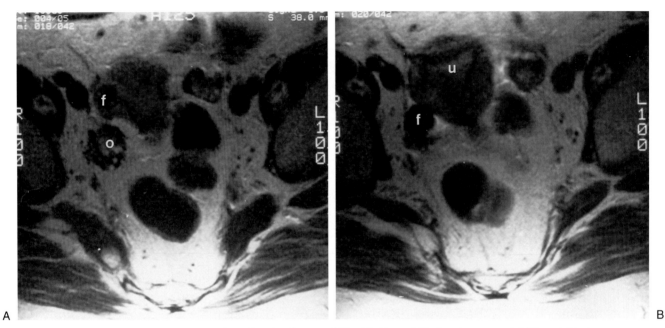

FIG. 5-25. Broad ligament pedunculated subserosal fibroid. (**A** and **B**) Contiguous axial T2-weighted fast spin-echo scans show the contiguity of the fibroid (f) with the right uterine body (u) and its extension into the right broad ligament, which simulated an adnexal mass clinically. Ovary (o) containing bright signal follicles is immediately superior to the fibroid.

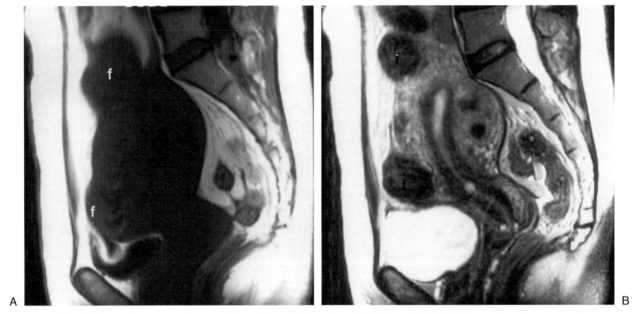

FIG. 5-26. Leiomyomas. Sagittal T1-weighted (**A**) and sagittal T2-weighted (**B**) fast spin-echo scans of myomatous uterus demonstrate the typical low signal intensity of the focal subserous contour distorting fibroids (f).

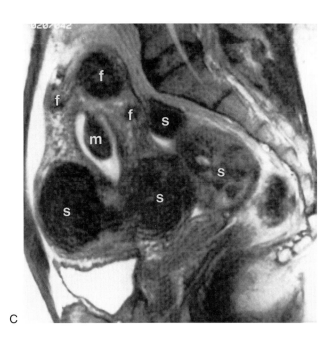

C

FIG. 5-26. *Continued* (C) Another patient's T2-weighted sagittal scan shows submucous fibroids protruding into the endometrial canal (m), multiple intramural fibroids (f), and subserous fibroids (s).

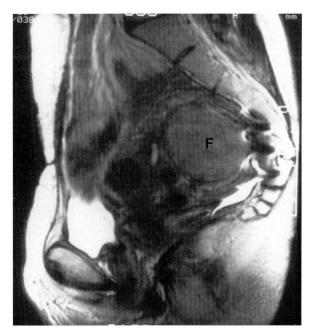

FIG. 5-27. Degenerated leiomyoma. Sagittal T2-weighted fast spin-echo scan shows a large posterior uterine body fibroid (F) with inhomogeneous increased signal intensity that stands out in sharp contrast from the typical low signal intensity of the lower uterine segment fibroids. This patient is not an optimal candidate for gonadotropin-releasing hormone analogues. Presacral clips are from proctocolectomy for ulcerative colitis.

endometrial carcinoma, pregnancy, and pelvic endometriosis. Unlike leiomyomas, which can be treated by myomectomy, thereby preserving fertility, adenomyosis has been treated by hysterectomy, making differentiation between these two abnormalities of paramount importance in women of childbearing age. Even more confounding is the fact that the leiomyomas and adenomyosis can coexist (see Fig. 5-28). Adenomyosis can be focal or diffuse.[13–15]

The diagnosis on MRI is made using T2-weighted images. The junctional zone of the uterus should not exceed 6 mm in normal patients.[16] The hallmark of adenomyosis is thickening of the junctional zone with an ill-defined mass that is isointense to the junctional zone (Fig. 5-29; see also Fig. 5-28). The mass is poorly circumscribed, is often elliptical with ill-defined border with the myometrium, and may contain small hemorrhagic foci of bright signal intensity. Adenomyosis does not enhance appreciably after gadolinium administration.[13–16] Coincident endometriomas are often present (Figs. 5-30 and 5-31).[13]

MRI is the only imaging modality that can noninvasively provide a means of detecting adenomyosis. Because differentiation of adenomyosis from other treatable causes of pelvic pain and bleeding, such as leiomyomas and pelvic endometriosis, is of paramount importance for proper and cost-effective patient management and to preserve fertility, MRI is the preferred imaging modality after sonographic screening for obvious leiomyomas in this clinical setting.

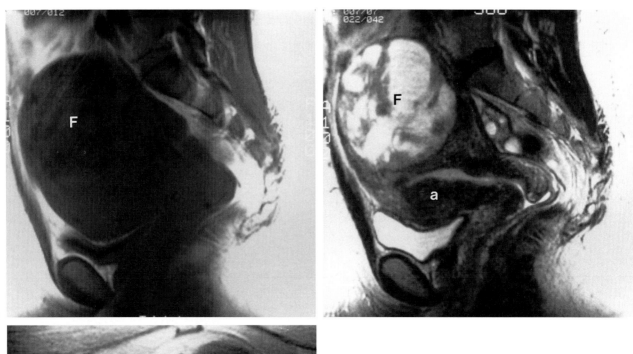

A

B

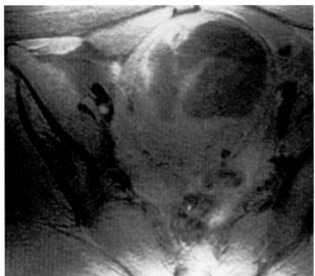

C

FIG. 5-28. Necrotic degenerated leiomyoma and adenomyosis. Sagittal T1-weighted scan **(A)** and T2-weighted fast spin-echo scan **(B)** show a large necrotic fundal fibroid (F) with liquefaction. Note the thickened junctional zone and lenticular mass at the anterior uterine body (a) that are characteristic of adenomyosis. **(C)** Gadolinium-enhanced T1-weighted axial scan with fat suppression shows unenhanced necrotic portions of the fibroid.

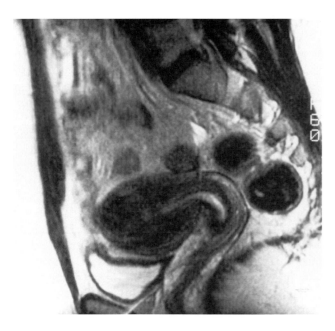

FIG. 5-29. Diffuse adenomyosis. Sagittal T2-weighted fast spin-echo scan shows thickening of the junctional zone with an ill-defined mass that is isointense to the junctional zone.

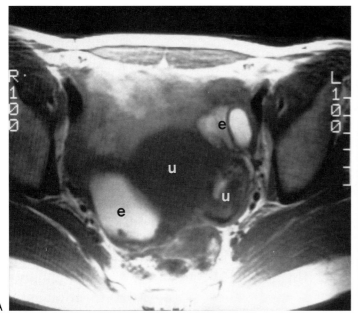

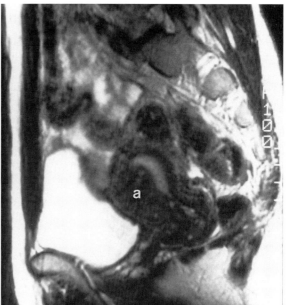

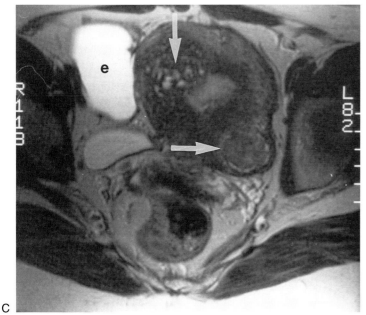

FIG. 5-30. Focal adenomyosis with bilateral endometriomas. **(A)** Axial T1-weighted scan shows enlargement of uterine contour (u) with bilateral bright signal adnexal cystic masses (e) characteristic of hemorrhagic elements within endometriomas. **(B)** T2-weighted fast spin-echo scan demonstrates the poorly circumscribed elliptical mass (a) in the anterior uterine body that is inseparable from the diffusely thickened junctional zone. Small hemorrhagic foci of bright signal intensity were visible. **(C)** Another patient with diffusely thickened junctional zone, focal adenomyosis in the right upper uterine body, and bilateral endometriomas (e, only right side shown) has much more obvious hemorrhagic foci (arrows).

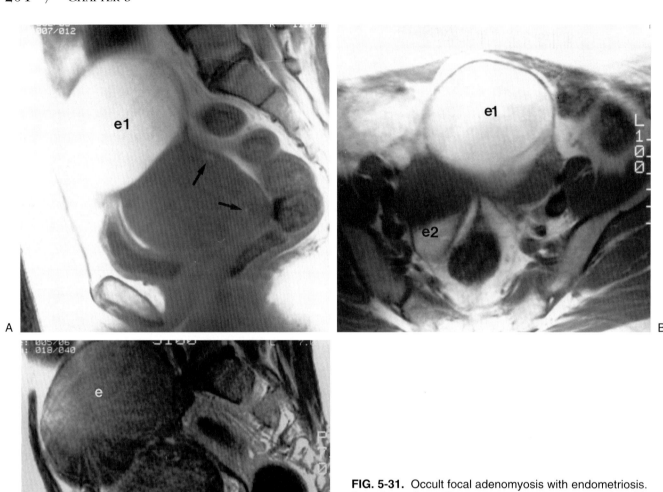

FIG. 5-31. Occult focal adenomyosis with endometriosis. An echogenic cystic mass was seen on sonography with an inhomogeneous enlarged uterus. MRI was performed to differentiate between dermoid cyst and endometrioma. **(A)** T1-weighted sagittal scan. The large cystic septated bright signal mass cephalad to the fundus had the typical bright signal of blood elements seen with endometriosis (e1). Note the tiny hemorrhagic foci in the enlarged uterine body *(arrows)*. **(B)** T1-weighted axial scan reveals a second lesion in the right adnexa (e2). **(C)** Sagittal MRI showed unexpected adenomyosis of the uterus with focal mass in the posterior uterine body with thickened junctional zone.

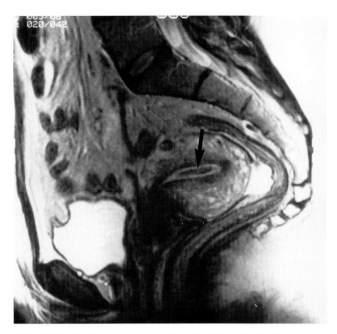

FIG. 5-32. Endometrial polyp. Sagittal T2-weighted fast spin-echo scan shows a nonspecific linear endometrial filling defect *(arrow)* of somewhat decreased signal intensity. It is not possible to differentiate benign from malignant polyps based on their morphology or signal characteristics.

ENDOMETRIAL POLYPS

These benign endometrial filling defects appear bright or inhomogeneous and are commonly visualized on MRI (Fig. 5-32). Even though they may enhance less than the normal endometrial lining, these lesions cannot be differentiated from pedunculated fibroids nor from polypoid endometrial carcinoma.[13,17]

REFERENCES

1. Cotran RS, Kumar V, Robbins SL. Pathologic basis of disease, ed 4. Philadelphia, WB Saunders, 1989.
2. Hricak H, Tscholakoff D, Heinrichs L, et al. Uterine leiomyomas: correlation of MR, histopathologic findings, and symptoms. Radiology 1986;158:385.
3. Zawin M, McCarthy S, Scoutt L, et al. High field MRI and US evaluation of the pelvis in women with leiomyomas. Magn Reson Imaging 1990;8:371.
4. Weinreb JC, Barkoff ND, Megibow A, et al. The value of MR in distinguishing leiomyomas from other solid pelvic masses when sonography is indeterminate. AJR 1990;154:295.
5. Dudiak CM, Turner DA, Patel SK, et al. Uterine leiomyomas in the infertile patient: preoperative localization with MR imaging versus US and hysterosalpingography. Radiology 1988;167:627.
6. Lee JKT, Gersell DJ, Balfe DM et al. The uterus: in vitro MR anatomic correlation of normal and abnormal specimens. Radiology 1985;157:175.
7. Worthington JK, Balfe DM, Lee JKT, et al. Uterine neoplasms: MR imaging. Radiology 1986;159:725.
8. Mittl RL, Yeh IT, Kressel HY. High signal intensity rim surrounding uterine leiomyomas on MR images: pathologic correlation. Radiology 1991;180:81.
9. Yamashita Y, Harada M, Hatanaka Y, et al. MR signal intensity of uterine leiomyoma: correlation with pathologic findings and clinical implications. Radiology 1994;190:337.
10. Zawin M, McCarthy S, Scoutt L, et al. Monitoring therapy with a gonadotropin-releasing hormone analogue: utility of MR imaging. Radiology 1990;175:503.
11. Okizuka H, Sugimura K, Takemori M, et al. MR detection of degenerating uterine leiomyomas. J Comput Assist Tomogr 1993;17:760.
12. Fishman-Javitt MC, Stein HL, Lovecchio JL, Imaging of the pelvis: MRI with correlations to CT and ultrasound. Boston, Little, Brown & Co, 1990.
13. Togashi K. MRI of the female pelvis. New York, Igaku-Shoin, 1993.
14. Mark AS, Hricak H, Heinrichs LW, et al. Adenomyosis and leiomyoma: differential diagnosis with MR imaging. Radiology 1987;163:527.
15. Togashi K, Ozasa H, Konishi I, et al. Enlarged uterus: differentiation between adenomyosis and leiomyoma with MR imaging. Radiology 1989;171:531.
16. Ascher S, Arnold L, Patt R, et al. Adenomyosis: prospective comparison of MR imaging and transvaginal sonography. Radiology 1994;190:803.
17. Hricak H, Finck S, Honda G, et al. MR imaging in the evaluation of benign uterine masses: value of gadopentetate dimeglumine-enhanced T1 weighted images. AJR 1992;158:1043.

Computed Tomography of Myometrial Disorders

James W. Walsh, MD

Computed tomography is not considered the primary imaging modality for diagnosis of uterine leiomyomas. However, knowledge of the appearance of leiomyomas on CT is essential for the differential diagnosis of large abdominopelvic masses, especially in older nonchildbearing women suspected of having ovarian carcinoma. Also, familiarity with their CT features is necessary when leiomyomas are found incidentally during CT studies performed for other indications. Adult women of all ages may also be referred for CT evaluation because of symptomatic leiomyomas accompanied by bleeding, pain, or compression of the renal collecting system, bladder, or rectum.

UTERINE LEIOMYOMAS

The CT features of uterine leiomyomas are diverse, and their typical appearance may be altered either by various types of degeneration or by complications such as infarction, necrosis, infection, and hemorrhage.[1,2] The typical CT findings in uterine leiomyomas include uterine enlargement with a lobulated outer contour, focal myometrial wall thickening, deformity of the endometrial cavity, focal calcifications, and an abnormal density within the uterine soft tissue mass (Fig. 5-33).[1,3–5] Pedunculated subserosal leiomyomas may lie in the adnexa, in the iliac fossa, anterior to the aortic bifurcation, or in the upper abdomen. Recognition of the uterine artery blood supply to the tumor and focal attachment to the uterus are crucial to the correct diagnosis (Fig. 5-34). The presence of coarse dystrophic calcification is the most specific CT sign of a leiomyoma, and it may have an amorphous, mottled, popcorn, or rare rimlike appearance (Fig. 5-35).[1] Calcification, however, is not noted in the majority of leiomyomas. Helpful CT signs for identifying the uterus as the site of origin of an adjacent leiomyoma include myometrial contrast enhancement, a characteristic pear shape and midline location of the enlarged uterus, uterine arteries lateral to the uterine corpus, and attachments of the round, cardinal, and uterosacral ligaments (see Figs. 5-33 and 5-34).[6] Coronal and sagittal reformatted CT scans may better show the attachment of pedunculated leiomyomas to the uterus (see Fig 5-33B). Submucosal leiomyomas are the most difficult tumors to image on CT because of the lack of inherent contrast in this location.

Leiomyomas may be hypodense (see Figs. 5-33 and 5-34A), isodense (Fig. 5-34B), or hyperdense (Fig. 5-36) relative to normal contrast medium–enhanced myometrium, and this density may be homogeneous (see Fig. 5-31) or, more commonly, heterogeneous (see Figs. 5-33A and 5-36). The enhancement pattern of leiomyomas probably relates most to the proximity of intravenous contrast medium administration to acquisition of pelvic images. Thus, a dedicated dynamic or spiral pelvic CT scan would more likely image a hyperdense leiomyoma, whereas delayed uterine scans performed after a dedicated abdominal CT scan would more likely show an isodense or hypodense leiomyoma. Hyperdense leiomyomas are probably due to their enhanced blood supply from parasitized uterine artery branches. High attenuation areas may also be present in a fibroid uterus from hemorrhage (Fig. 5-37).

Low-attenuation areas may be present in a leiomyoma from hyaline or cystic degeneration, necrosis, or infection.[1,2] Hyaline degeneration is seen in almost all leiomyomas, and it probably accounts for the characteristic bands of hypodense tissue in large leiomyomas after bolus intravenous contrast medium instillation (see Fig. 5-33A). Cystic degeneration rarely can cause unusual CT manifestations in large pedunculated leiomyomas, which grow rapidly and simulate ovarian carcinoma.[7] These rare leiomyomas may have a multiloculated cystic appearance with thin septations. Careful CT density measurements are important to differentiate the hypodense solid or intermediate density elements of hyaline degeneration or necrosis or infection from the true water-density elements of ovarian neoplasms or leiomyomas with cystic degeneration.

Lipomatous uterine tumors are rare benign neoplasms that can be differentiated from benign ovarian teratomas on CT, and asymptomatic uterine tumors require no treatment.[8] The presence of fat within the uterine mass on CT is virtually diagnostic of a lipomatous uterine tumor (Fig. 5-38). Although pure uterine lipomas have been reported, most tumors are either lipoleiomyomas or fibromyolipomas.[8]

Uterine leiomyomas may coexist with a cancer of the cervix or endometrium, and this presents problems in tumor

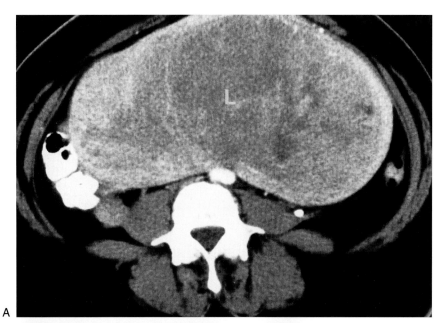

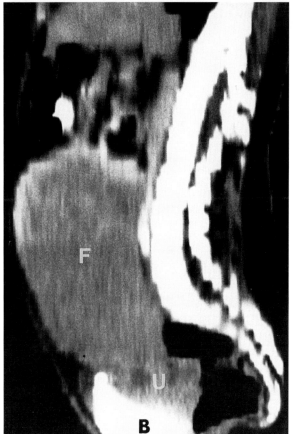

FIG. 5-33. (A) CT scan at the aortic bifurcation shows a large heterogeneous hypodense leiomyoma (L) filling the lower abdomen. (B) A midline sagittal reconstruction shows the pear-shaped myomatous uterine fundus (F) related to the lower uterine segment (U) and bladder (B).

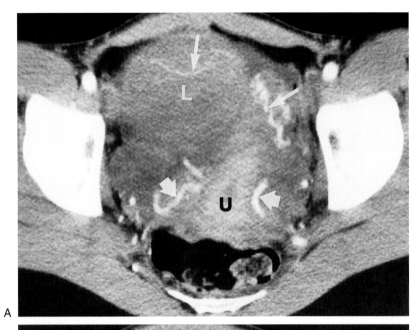

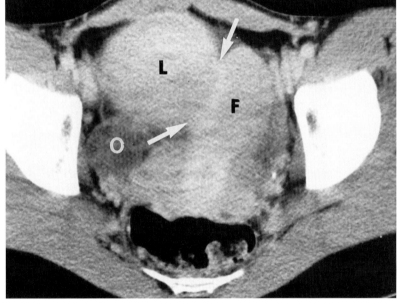

FIG. 5-34. (A) Dynamic CT during arterial phase shows normal uterine arteries in broad ligaments *(wide arrows),* normal lower uterine segment (U), and enlarged uterine artery branches *(narrow arrows)* to hypodense pedunculated leiomyoma (L). **(B)** Delayed images 5 minutes later show normal right ovary (O) and uterine fundus (F) with point of attachment *(arrows)* of the leiomyoma (L), which is now isodense to uterus.

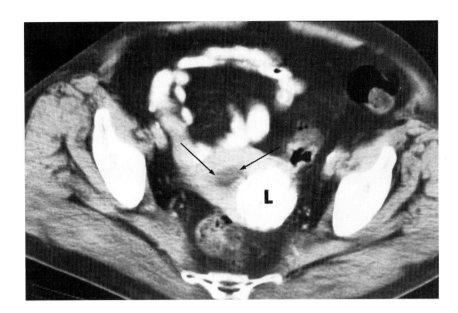

FIG. 5-35. CT scan through body of uterus shows normal endometrial cavity *(arrows)* and popcorn-type calcification in an intramural leiomyoma (L).

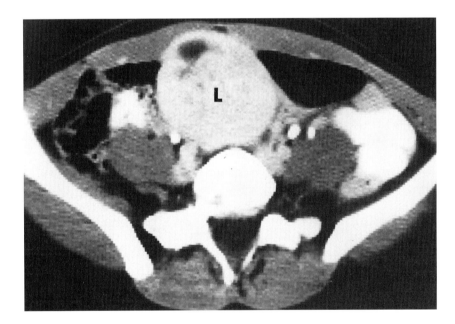

FIG. 5-36. CT scan through sacral promontory shows slightly heterogeneous hyperdense fundal leiomyoma (L).

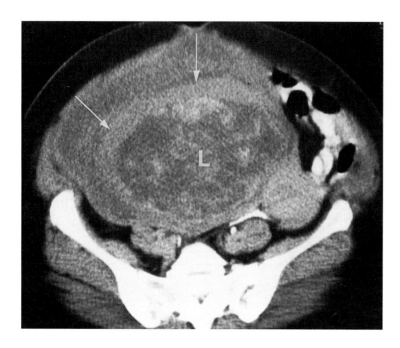

FIG. 5-37. CT scan through the iliac fossae shows large leiomyoma (L) surrounded by high-density intramural hemorrhage *(arrows)* in an enlarged uterus.

localization on CT because both benign and malignant uterine tumors are often heterogeneous and hypodense (see Fig. 5-33).[2] Also, a subserosal leiomyoma may protrude out of the cervical os and mimic the CT appearance of cervical cancer.[4]

LIMITATIONS OF COMPUTED TOMOGRAPHY

Extrauterine masses, in particular cystic or solid ovarian tumors, may be misdiagnosed as subserous or pedunculated uterine myomas (Fig. 5-39).[3] Cystic pedunculated leiomyomas can likewise be misinterpreted as ovarian carcinoma.[6] Intraligamentous leiomyomas, although rare, also present a problem in differentiating an adnexal from a uterine mass (Fig. 5-40).

Unless they have characteristic CT features, leiomyomas cannot be reliably distinguished from uterine carcinoma, sarcoma, or lymphoma on the basis of their CT appearance alone.[4] Also, it is impossible on CT to differentiate adenomyosis from a myoma of the uterus.[3] Finally, CT has limitations in imaging submucosal leiomyomas.

CONCLUSION

Although CT is not the primary imaging procedure for diagnosis of uterine leiomyomas, knowledge of the CT fea-

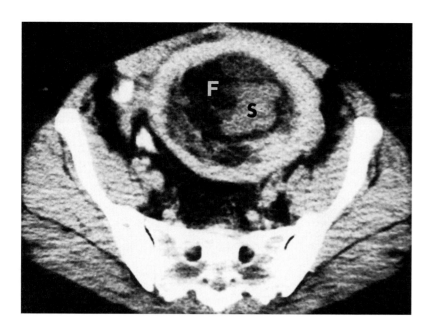

FIG. 5-38. CT scan through an enlarged uterus with central mass shows soft tissue (S) components and fat (F) elements, which match the density of presacral and subcutaneous fat. Lipoleiomyoma was confirmed at hysterectomy.

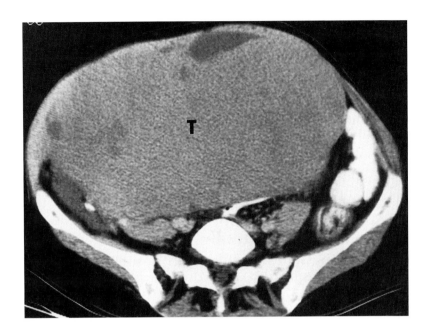

FIG. 5-39. CT scan through a proven, predominantly solid, ovarian fibrothecoma (T) shows imaging findings similar to a giant leiomyoma with some degenerative changes.

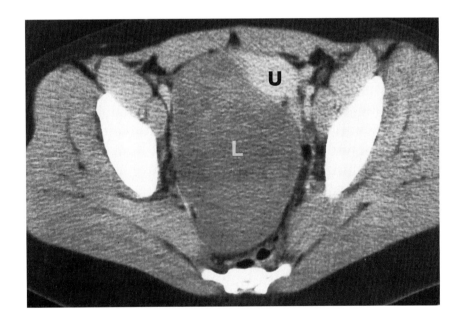

FIG. 5-40. CT scan through a proven broad ligament leiomyoma (L) and the displaced uterus (U) shows the infrequent problem of determining whether a pelvic mass arises from or merely abuts the uterus. In this case, CT cannot determine that the mass is actually between the adnexa and the uterus in the uterine ligament.

tures is important for differential diagnosis of gynecologic pelvic masses when women are referred for CT with a large abdominopelvic mass and suspected ovarian carcinoma or with a pelvic mass and gynecologic and urinary tract symptoms. Also, knowledge of CT findings in leiomyomas is important when they are an incidental finding in the pelvis.

REFERENCES

1. Casillas J, Joseph RC, Guerra JJ. CT appearance of uterine leiomyomas. Radiographics 1990;10:999.

2. Walsh JW. Computed tomography of gynecologic neoplasms. Radiol Clin North Am 1992;30:817.
3. Tada S, Tsukioka M, Ishii C, et al. Computed tomographic features of uterine myoma. J Comput Assist Tomogr 1981;5:866.
4. Sawyer RW, Walsh JW. CT in gynecologic pelvic diseases. Semin Ultrasound CT MR 1988;9:122.
5. Walsh JW. Imaging of uterine masses and tumors. In: Putman CE, Ravin CE, eds. Textbook of diagnostic imaging, ed 2. Philadelphia. WB Saunders, 1994:2057.
6. Foshager MC, Walsh JW. CT anatomy of the female pelvis: a second look. Radiographics 1994;14:51.
7. Togashi K, Nishimura K, Nakano Y, et al. Cystic pedunculated leiomyomas of the uterus with unusual CT manifestations. J Comput Assist Tomogr 1986;10:642.
8. Dodd GD, Budzik RF. Lipomatous uterine tumors: diagnosis by ultrasound CT and MR. J Comput Assist Tomogr 1990;14:629.

Clinical Gynecologic Imaging, edited
by Arthur C. Fleischer, Marcia C. Javitt,
R. Brooke Jeffrey, Jr., and Howard W. Jones III,
Lippincott-Raven Publishers, Philadelphia © 1997.

CHAPTER 6

Cervical Cancer

Overview

David L. Tait, MD

EPIDEMIOLOGY

Carcinoma of the uterine cervix will account for 15,800 new cases of cancer in 1995, making it the seventh most common malignancy in women after breast, lung, colorectal, endometrial, and ovarian cancer and lymphoma in the United States. Among gynecologic cancers, cervical cancer ranks third as a cause of death, with 4800 deaths estimated annually.[1] Cervical cancer is prevalent worldwide and a leading cause of death in several Latin American countries as well as Romania, Poland, and Singapore. Populations with lower frequency of cervical cancer include Jewish women and nuns.

The average age at diagnosis of cervical cancer is 52 years with a bimodal distribution of cases with peaks at 35 to 39 years and 60 to 64 years. Cervical cancer occurs more frequently in women from lower socioeconomic groups. Other risk factors include early age of first intercourse, a high number of sexual partners, multiparity, a history of cervical dysplasia, and a history of sexually transmitted diseases. The concept of a sexually transmitted risk factor was demonstrated in a study from India that showed a higher incidence of cervical cancer in monogamous women whose husbands had multiple lifetime sexual partners.[2] Sexual inactivity and nulliparity lower the risk of developing cervical cancer.

Over the past several years, many agents have been described as potential etiologic agents in cervical cancer, including herpesvirus type 2 and *Trichomonas.* Currently, there is a strong body of evidence suggesting human papillomavirus as the cause of cervical cancer. Human papillomavirus has many serotypes causing several different diseases. Human papillomavirus types 1, 2, 6, and 11 are responsible for common warts, plantar warts, and genital warts. Types 16, 18, 31, and 39 are oncogenic viruses and have been found in up to 90% of cervical cancers.[3] The E6 and E7 viral proteins interact with host recessive oncogenes *p53* and retinoblastoma, respectively, to cause a loss of growth regulation within the host cell.[4] The role of human papillomavirus in cervical cancer is not completely understood.

CLINICAL EVALUATION

The two most common symptoms of cervical cancer are vaginal bleeding and vaginal discharge. As many as 90% of patients experience some type of vaginal bleeding, which includes postmenopausal bleeding, postcoital bleeding, menorrhagia, or intermenstrual bleeding. Although postmenopausal bleeding is emphasized as the hallmark symptom in carcinoma of the endometrium, some series have demonstrated it to be the most common symptom in cervical cancer.[5] A serosanguineous yellow vaginal discharge can be a more subtle symptom of cervical cancer. This may be attributed to vaginal infection or cervicitis and the diagnosis of cancer overlooked. Other more nonspecific symptoms are urinary frequency or dysuria, pelvic pain, constipation, and rectal bleeding. Constitutional symptoms such as nausea, vomiting, and weight loss may be more indicative of advanced disease producing urinary or intestinal obstruction.

Frequently, patients with cervical cancer have a normal physical examination outside the pelvis. Specific findings suggestive of metastatic disease include supraclavicular and cervical adenopathy, leg edema, and hepatomegaly. The most significant physical findings are found on pelvic examination. Speculum examination of the cervix may reveal a normal cervix if the cancer is occult. Most commonly a necrotic, ulcerated, or bleeding mass is visualized on the cervix. The rectovaginal examination provides the most information about local tumor spread. Detailed palpation of the parametria, uterosacral ligaments, and distal rectal mucosa allows assessment for local spread of disease.

Screening for cervical cancer by cytologic examination or Papanicolaou smear has decreased the prevalence of invasive carcinoma.[6] A Papanicolaou smear may provide the first indication of a cervical abnormality. This may lead to a colposcopic examination and cervical biopsies or a cervical conization, yielding the diagnosis of a microinvasive or occult carcinoma. In the cervix containing a grossly visible abnormality, biopsy with Kevorkian or Tischler forceps is warranted. After histologic confirmation of invasive cancer, laboratory studies including a complete blood cell count, Sequential Multiple Analyzer-12, and urinalysis are obtained. Radiographs in the workup include a chest radiograph and intravenous pyelogram.

STAGING

The International Federation of Gynecology and Obstetrics (FIGO) staging system for carcinoma of the cervix is based on clinical evaluation. This includes physical examination, radiographic studies of the chest and kidney, and biopsies. Studies not used for clinical staging include CT (except for information about ureteral anatomy that may be substituted for intravenous pyelography), MRI, lymphangiograms, arteriograms, and laparotomy or laparoscopy findings. The key component to clinical staging is the bimanual

pelvic and rectal examination performed under general anesthesia. With patient relaxation achieved under anesthesia, precise evaluation of cancer spread into the parametria and uterosacral ligaments can be accomplished. If there is suspicion of tumor invasion into the bladder or rectum, cystoscopy and sigmoidoscopy with biopsies can also be performed at the same time.

The official staging system for cervical carcinoma is shown in Table 6-1. It can be summarized as follows: in stage I the tumor is confined to the cervix; in stage II the tumor is confined to the vagina or parametrium, but not to the pelvic sidewall; in stage III the tumor has extended to

TABLE 6-1. *FIGO* staging for carcinoma of the cervix uteri (1995)*

Stage	Description
0	Carcinoma in situ, intraepithelial carcinoma
I	The carcinoma is strictly confined to the cervix.
IA	Invasive cancer identified only microscopically. All gross lesions even with superficial invasion are stage IB cancers. Invasion is limited to measured stromal invasion with maximum depth of 5 mm and no wider than 7 mm.†
IA1	Measured invasion of stroma no greater than 3 mm in depth and no wider than 7 mm
IA2	Measured invasion of stroma greater than 3 mm and no greater than 5 mm in depth, and no wider than 7 mm
IB	Clinical lesions confined to the cervix or preclinical lesions greater than stage IA
IB1	Clinical lesions no greater than 4 cm
IB2	Clinical lesions greater than 4 cm
II	The carcinoma extends beyond the cervix but has not extended to the pelvic wall. The carcinoma involves the vagina but not as far as the lower third.
IIA	No obvious parametrial involvement
IIB	Obvious parametrial involvement
III	The carcinoma has extended to the pelvic wall. On rectal examination, there is no cancer-free space between the tumor and the pelvic wall. The tumor involves the lower third of the vagina. All cases with a hydronephrosis or nonfunctioning kidney are included unless they are known to be due to other causes.
IIIA	No extension to the pelvic wall
IIIB	Extension to the pelvic wall and/or hydronephrosis or nonfunctioning kidney
IV	The carcinoma has extended beyond the true pelvis or has clinically involved the mucosa of the bladder or rectum. A bullous edema as such does not permit a case to be allotted to stage IV
IVA	Spread of the growth to adjacent organs
IVB	Spread to distant organs

* FIGO, International Federation of Gynecology and Obstetrics.

† The depth of invasion should not be more than 5 mm taken from the base of the epithelium, either surface or glandular; from which it originates. Vascular space involvement, either venous or lymphatic, should not alter the staging.

the pelvic sidewall or hydronephrosis is present; and in stage IV the tumor has locally invaded the bladder or rectum or there is distant metastasis.

TREATMENT

Stage IA

Microinvasive carcinoma of the cervix (stage IA) can be subdivided into two groups, stage IA1 and stage IA2, which reflect depth of invasion and volume of tumor. Ideally, "microinvasion" should represent the group of patients with virtually no risk for lymph node involvement, dissemination, or recurrence. The FIGO system has defined stage IA1 as less than or equal to 3 mm depth of invasion with a maximum width of 7 mm. These patients can be successfully treated with a simple hysterectomy either vaginally or abdominally. Young patients who desire future fertility can be offered conservative therapy with a cervical cone biopsy. Recurrence rates of 1% or less have been reported with this form of management.[7] However, these patients require close follow-up with examination and Papanicolaou smear performed every 3 months.

Stage IA2, defined as 3 to 5 mm of invasion by FIGO, has a 4.8% incidence of lymph node spread.[8] This produces a significant risk of failure when treated by hysterectomy alone. A modified radical (type II) hysterectomy with the addition of a pelvic lymphadenectomy is the preferred treatment of choice. Additionally, stage IA2 as well as stage IA1 could be treated with radiation therapy (see later).

Stages IB and IIA

Stages IB and IIA can be treated with either radical surgery or radiation therapy. The choice of treatment modality depends on the preference of the gynecologic oncologist or radiation oncologist, the medical condition of the patient, and the characteristics of the lesion. The treating physician has the luxury of choice between the equally efficacious therapies.

Surgery for stage IB and IIA cervical cancer consists of radical hysterectomy and pelvic lymphadenectomy. Tissues removed include the uterus, cervix, upper 3 to 5 cm of vagina, parametria and cardinal ligaments, and the pelvic lymph nodes to include the obturator, external iliac, and internal iliac chains. This approach has particular advantage in the younger patient as ovarian preservation is possible and sexual dysfunction is less likely than with radiation therapy.[9] Complications are related to the risk of surgery and anesthesia, such as hemorrhage, infection, thromboembolic events, or atelectasis. Most importantly, radical hysterectomy carries a significant risk of urinary tract injury. The risk of ureteral injury or ureterovaginal or vesicovaginal fistula is 1% to 2%.[10] In addition, detrusor dysfunction from denerva-

tion of the detrusor muscle can produce persistent voiding difficulty.

Radiation therapy is the most commonly used treatment of cervical cancer worldwide and is applicable to all stages. Treatment of stage IB and IIA cervical cancer uses a combination of external and intercavitary therapy. The total dose of radiation required to treat cervical cancer is 7500 to 8500 cGy delivered to point A. Point A is defined as a reference point 2 cm lateral to the axis of the endocervical canal and 2 cm superior to the lateral vaginal fornix. First, the patient will receive 4500 to 5000 cGy as external beam therapy to the pelvis in divided doses over approximately 5 weeks. This is followed by one or two intracavitary system or brachytherapy applications. Immediate complications include diarrhea, abdominal cramping, dysuria, skin reactions, or bone marrow suppression with anemia and leukocyte suppression. Complications often occurring years after therapy are bowel and urinary fistulas, radiation proctitis or cystitis, and fibrosis of the vagina.

Survival rates for stage IB carcinoma range between 85% and 95% with no difference in efficacy of surgery and radiation present.[10,11] Stage IIA offers less overall survival, averaging 75%.[12]

Stage IIB–IV

Patients with stage IIB, III, and IVA cervical cancer are treated with radiation. These patients often have large pelvic tumors that produce a high rate of treatment failure within the pelvis. In addition, the increasing incidence of pelvic and paraaortic lymph node metastasis that accompanies advanced stage disease results in frequent systemic recurrence. The survival rates are 65% for stage IIB, 35% for stage IIIB, and 20% for stage IVA.

Patients with stage IVB cervical cancer have systemic disease at diagnosis and overall have a very poor prognosis. Treatment consists of combination radiation and chemotherapy. Five-year survival rates are 10% or less.

RECURRENCE

Recurrent cervical cancer can be divided into two categories: local or central recurrence and distant recurrence. Identifying a patient with a recurrence that is located centrally within her pelvis is important because 25% to 50% of these patients can be cured by pelvic exenteration.[13] This operation consists of removal of the uterus, cervix, vagina, bladder, and rectum. Reconstruction of the bladder and vagina is possible.

Metastatic disease is treated with palliative chemotherapy. Cisplatin is the most active single agent, with response rates of 20%.[14] The Gynecologic Oncology Group is evaluating multidrug combinations including cisplatin, ifosfamide, and bleomycin.

REFERENCES

1. Cancer statistics 1995. CA 1995;45·12.
2. Agarwal SS, Sehgal A, Sardana S, et al. Role of male factor behavior in cervical carcinogenesis among women with one lifetime sexual partner. Cancer 1993;72:1666.
3. Lorincz AT, Reid R, Jenson AB, et al. Human papillomavirus infection of the cervix: relative risk associations of 15 common anogenital types. Obstet Gynecol 1992;3:328.
4. Scheffner M, Munger K, Byrne JL, Hawley PM. The state of the *p53* and retinoblastoma genes in human cervical carcinoma cell lines. Proc Natl Acad Sci 1991;88:5523.
5. Pardanani NS, Tischler LP, Brown WH. Carcinoma of the cervix: evaluation of treatment in a community hospital. NY Stage J Med 1975;75:1018.
6. Guznick DS. Efficacy of screening for cervical cancer: a review. Am J Public Health 1978;68:125.
7. Burghardt E, Girardi F, Lahousen M, et al. Microinvasive carcinoma of the uterine cervix (International Federation of Gynecology and Obstetrics Stage IA). Cancer 1991;67:1037.
8. Simon NL, Gore H, Shingleton HM, et al. Study of superficially invasive carcinoma of the cervix. Obstet Gynecol 1986;68:19.
9. Abitol NM, Davenport JH. Sexual dysfunction after therapy for cervical carcinoma. Am J Obstet Gynecol 1974;119:181.
10. Artman LE, Hoskins WE, Bibro MC, et al. Radical hysterectomy and pelvic lymphadenectomy for stage IB carcinoma of the cervix: twenty-one years experience. Gynecol Oncol 1987;28:8.
11. Symmonds RE. Morbidity and complications of radical hysterectomy with pelvic lymph node dissection. Am J Obstet Gynecol 1986;94:663.
12. Perez CA, Camel HM, Walz BJ, et al. Radiation therapy alone in the treatment of carcinoma of the uterine cervix: a 20 year experience. Gynecol Oncol 1986;23:127.
13. Lawhead RA, Jr, Clark DG, Smith DH, et al. Pelvic exenteration for recurrent or persistent gynecologic malignancies: a 10-year review of the Memorial Sloan-Kettering Cancer Center experience (1972–1981). Gynecol Oncol 1989;33:279.
14. Jobson V, Homesley H, Muss H, et al. Chemotherapy of advanced squamous carcinoma of the cervix: a phase I-II study of high-dose cisplatin and cyclophosphamide. Am J Clin Oncol 1984;7:341.

Magnetic Resonance Imaging in Cervical Cancer

Kaori Togashi, MD

THE ROLE OF MRI

Clinical International Federation of Gynecology and Obstetrics (FIGO) staging criteria is the main determinant in guiding treatment decisions in patients with cervical cancer. However, clinical FIGO staging does have inherent inaccuracies. Discrepancies between clinical and surgical staging are found in more than 30% of patients,[1] and, furthermore, clinical staging does not address other prognostic factors, such as tumor size or lymphadenopathy. Thus the role of noninvasive tumor evaluation by imaging is important. MRI is the most reliable imaging modality in evaluating cervical cancer and offers direct tumor visualization, accurate assessment of the depth of stromal invasion, and reliable staging accuracy. MRI is indicated in patients with large tumors. Endocervical lesions and predominantly infiltrative tumors should also be evaluated by MRI. At present, MRI is not incorporated in the FIGO staging system; however, recent works have shown that the use of MRI decreases the number of diagnostic tests and invasive procedures.[2]

TECHNIQUE

T2-weighted images are mandatory to image the uterus, the tumor, and surrounding structures.[3,4] Sagittal images allow clear appreciation of the relationship of tumor to the cervix, corpus, and vagina. Axial images have an important role in assessing parametrial tumor extension. Off-axis scans may be of value in assessment of the parametrium.[5]

Use of pelvic phased-array coil offers fascinating images of the uterus.[6] However, the use of the pelvic phased-array coil does not significantly improve the overall staging accuracy compared with use of the body coil, although it does improve the detection of stromal invasion and the accuracy of tumor sizing.[7] Use of endorectal surface coil[8] or endovaginal coil[9] also offers fascinating results; however, further investigation is required to determine the appropriate importance compared with use of standard MRI.

The role of contrast medium enhancement is limited.[10,11] The use of contrast media causes consistent overestimation of tumor size, depth of stromal invasion, and tumor extension.[10,11] Gadolinium-enhanced imaging is primarily used for advanced disease with suspected bladder and rectum invasion. Dynamic study may help identify preinvasive diseases[12] or may improve the accuracy in staging.

TUMOR DEPICTION

MRI is able to identify invasive carcinoma as a relatively hyperintense mass, thus helping to identify clinically problematic lesions and to evaluate the depth of stromal invasion and an exact tumor size.[3,4,13] In addition, Papanicolaou smears are usually highly sensitive as screening methods, but there are several pitfalls and then MRI may help identify malignancy.

On T2-weighted images, 95% of invasive disease is identified as a relatively hyperintense mass that is sharply marginated or ill defined (Fig. 6-1).[3,13] Preinvasive disease, which constitutes more than 70% of cervical cancer, cannot be identified. Cervical cancer usually shows homogeneous hyperintensity, but adenocarcinoma of mucin-producing type is embedded with multiple tiny cysts (Fig. 6-2).[14] The hyperintense area well corresponds to the tumor extent, and the peripheral low intensity stripe well corresponds to the uninvolved stroma, being in accord (within 5 mm) with measurements determined by pathologic examination.[4,13,15,16] The accuracy in evaluating the depth of stromal invasion is almost 80%.[17,18]

MRI contributes to the identification of clinically problematic lesions, such as masses totally within the canal, tumors with an unexpected cephalad limit, or deep stromal invasions developing beneath relatively normal epithelium. The demonstration of these lesions may help obviate diagnostic conization. At the same time, MRI is an accurate method of defining tumor size. Tumor size is important to predict the prognosis of the patients; however, clinical examination often overestimates it in exophytic lesions and underestimates it in endophytic-infiltrative lesions. Recently, it has been suggested that a large tumor may be better treated with preoperative chemotherapy. Accurate assessment of tumor size by MRI is becoming much more important.[19,20]

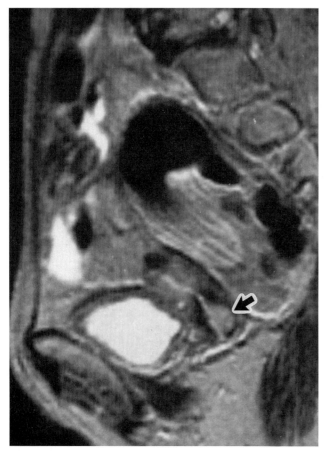

FIG. 6-1. Cervical cancer. Sagittal T2-weighted image. Small endocervical tumor is clearly identifiable as a hyperintense mass *(arrow),* although clinical examination failed to identify the lesion. MRI offers direct tumor visualization and accurate assessment of the tumor size and the depth of stromal invasion. Endocervical lesions and predominantly infiltrative tumors should be evaluated by MRI. (From Togashi K, Konishi J. Magnetic resonance imaging in the evaluation of gynecological malignancy. Magn Reson Q 1990;6:250.)

Pitfalls

Other cervical lesions that may exhibit hyperintense signal include cervical myomas, nabothian cysts, postbiopsy changes, or, rarely, cervicitis seen in patients with uterine prolapse. Papanicolaou smears are usually highly sensitive, but we must be careful about the presence of carcinoma in a patient with negative Papanicolaou smears and biopsy specimens. Adenocarcinoma arising from deep gland simulates hyperintense myoma, and adenoma malignum (minimally deviated adenocarcinoma) mimics a cluster of nabothian cysts.[14,21] These conditions are famous for their delayed diagnosis in spite of early clinical manifestation, such as heavy watery discharge, but they are identifiable on MRI. Another pitfall is malignant lymphoma. Lymphoma can be mistaken for poorly differentiated adenocarcinoma on histologic samples. If the lesion shows extensive involvement of the uterus in spite of relatively preserved endometrium and

epithelium, specific stain may be necessary under certain clinical conditions.[22]

STAGING

Staging is mandatory in selecting the way of treatment. The overall accuracy of MRI in staging cervical cancer is 76% to 83%.[4,13,17,18] Comparative studies have reported the overall staging accuracy is 70% for clinical staging, 63% for CT, and 83% for MRI or 69% for CT and 77% for MRI.[17,18] At present, MRI is the most reliable method of staging and has advantages over CT, especially in the assessment of parametrial status. Comparative studies reported that the accuracy for parametrial evaluation was 78% for clinical evaluation, 70% for CT, and 92% for MRI.[17,18]

Anatomic Review

In assessing parametrial status, it is important to review the anatomic aspect. The cervix and vaginal fornix is not directly surrounded by fat but is surrounded by the parametrium, that is, loose connective tissue mixed with abundant vessels. Thus, it is difficult to distinguish the cervix from

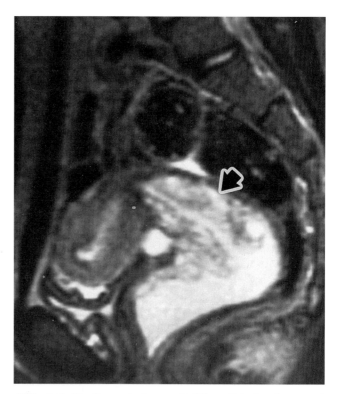

FIG. 6-2. Mucin-producing well-differentiated adenocarcinoma. Sagittal T2-weighted image. The lesion *(arrow)* is embedded with multiple tiny cysts. Papanicolaou smears are usually highly sensitive, but carcinoma does present with negative Papanicolaou smears and biopsy specimens, such as adenocarcinoma arising from deep glandular tissue or adenoma malignum. Although they are clinically problematic, these lesions can be identifiable on MRI.

the parametrium on T1-weighted images and T2-weighted images are mandatory to evaluate parametrium.[23] The other important thing is that the cervix consists of the supravaginal cervix and vaginal cervix. The supravaginal cervix is directly adjacent to the parametrium. In this condition, tumor protrusion from the disrupted stroma represents parametrial invasion. In contrast, vaginal cervix is separated from the cervix by the vaginal fornix. In this condition, tumor protrusion from the stroma does not mean parametrial invasion. Parametrial invasion should be suspected only when the vaginal fornix is disrupted.[23]

Parametrial Assessment: IB Versus IIB

On axial T2-weighted images, normal cervical stroma appears as a ring of distinct hypointensity.[3] Preservation of this hypointense stromal ring is a reliable sign of intact parametrium (IB) (Fig. 6-3A). This finding has a very high specificity, almost 100%, and is of great value in the exclusion of parametrial invasion.[4,13,15–18] Segmental disruption of the hypointense stroma indicates full-thickness stromal invasion.[4,13,15–18] If the lesions are sharply marginated, remaining within the configuration of the ring, they are still confined to the cervix (IB) (see Fig. 6-3B). In contrast, if the supravaginal tumor protrudes through the defect, there is parametrial involvement (IIB) (see Fig. 6-3C).

With disrupted or completely lost hypointense stroma, parametrial assessment is frequently difficult, resulting in low accuracy (60%).[13] Other difficulties are found in tumors within the vaginal cervix. In this condition, parametrial invasion should be suspected only when the thin vaginal fornix is disrupted (Fig. 6-4).

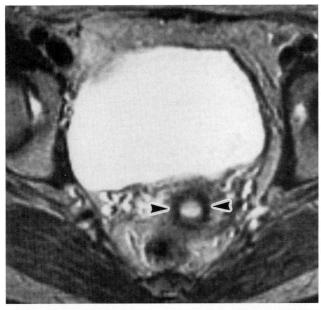

A

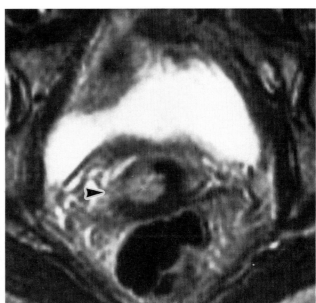

B

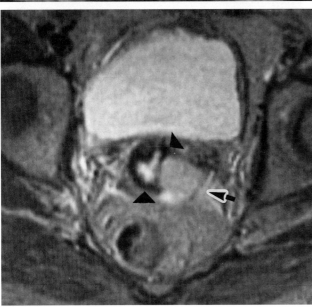

C

FIG. 6-3. Parametrial evaluation. T2-weighted axial images. **(A)** Ib, **(B)** Ib, **(C)** IIb. MRI is the most reliable imaging modality of staging, especially in the assessment of parametrial status. **(A)** Preservation of the hypointense stromal ring (arrowheads) is a reliable sign of intact parametrium. **(B)** Segmental disruption indicates full-thickness stromal invasion. If the lesion (arrow) still remain the contour of the ring (arrowheads), the parametrium is intact. **(C)** If the supravaginal tumor (arrow) protrudes through the defect (arrowheads), there is parametrial involvement. (From Togashi K. MRI of the female pelvis. Tokyo, Igaku-Shoin, 1993.)

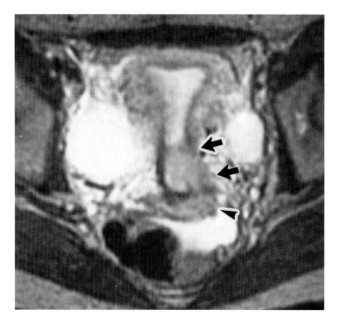

FIG. 6-4. Parametrial evaluation. T2-weighted axial image. Cervical cancer, stage IIB. The tumor disrupts both the supravaginal cervical stroma *(arrows)* and the vaginal fornix *(arrowhead)* and irregularly protrudes into the left parametrium. Parametrial invasion should be suspected based on the disrupted stromal ring in the supravaginal tumor and on the disrupted vaginal fornix in the tumor within the vaginal cervix.

Pelvic Wall Invasion: IIIB

The criteria for pelvic wall invasion are difficult to determine because of rare surgically proved cases. If the lesion extends to any of the pelvic musculature or the iliac vessels, it is obvious that the lesion involves the pelvic wall (IIIB) (Fig. 6-5).[4,13] However, even in the presence of abundant fat planes between the tumor and muscles, fine strands between them or complete loss of parametrial signal associated with the disrupted stroma may also indicate pelvic wall invasion.[23]

Vaginal Invasion: IIA and IIIA

The sensitivity of MRI in the detection of vaginal invasion is excellent, with an accuracy of 93%.[4] Segmental disruption of the low intensity signal of the vagina or demonstration of a thick hyperintense vagina indicates vaginal invasion (IIA) (Fig. 6-6).[4,13] Involvement in the lower third of vagina indicates the disease is stage IIIA. However, we must be careful in assessing a thin, stretched vaginal fornix, because it may not be identified even if it is intact.

Bladder Invasion and Rectal Invasion: IVB

MRI seems to be reliable and very sensitive in evaluating bladder invasion.[3,23] A relatively large number of cases of bladder invasion may be missed if reliance is placed on the clinical examination alone. On MRI, the segmental disruption of the low intensity wall is a reliable indicator that the lesion involves the muscle layer (Fig. 6-7).[4,13] Bullous edema may also be identified as a hyperintense band along the disrupted muscle wall. Possible weakness of MRI is an evaluation of vesicoureteral junction, because the ureter is not identifiable on MRI.

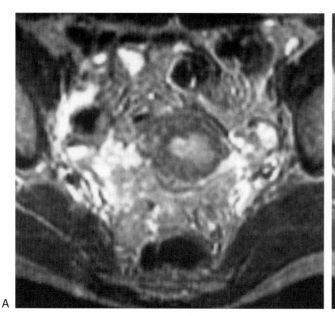

A

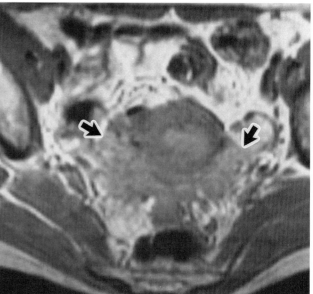

B

FIG. 6-5. Pelvic wall involvement. The lesion obviously involved the ureter on DIP and CT (not shown) and was assigned to stage IIIB. **(A)** T2-weighted image. **(B)** Proton-density—weighted image. The lesion directly extends to the vessels *(arrows)* and also exhibits fine strands radiating to the muscles. These findings are more easily assessed on **B** than on **A**.

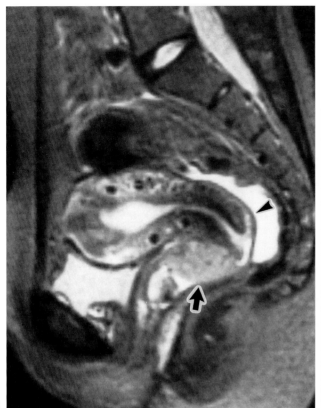
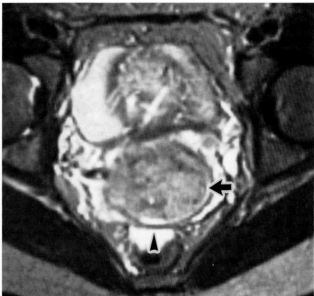

A

B

FIG. 6-6. Vaginal invasion. T2-weighted sagittal **(A)** and axial **(B)** image. Vaginal invasion is indicated as segmental disruption of the hypointense wall *(arrow)*. Arrowhead indicates intact posterior vaginal fornix. (From Togashi K. MRI of the female pelvis. Tokyo, Igaku-Shoin, 1993.)

Whereas the bladder wall has a tight ligamentous attachment to the cervix, the rectum is separated from the posterior vaginal fornix by cul-de-sac; thus to see a direct rectal invasion is a rare occurrence. Rectal invasion is identified by the segmental thickening or loss of hypointense signal of the anterior rectal wall adjacent to the tumor.[4,13] Prominent strands between the tumor and the rectum may be another sign of invasion.

LYMPH NODE EVALUATION

Lymph node evaluation should be based on the size and location of the nodes. Thus MRI has the same accuracy for this evaluation as CT.[24–26] Signal intensity of the lymph nodes is not helpful to distinguish benign from malignant nodes. Although the signal of fast flowing blood was first described to be easily distinguished from that of lymph nodes, stagnant pelvic flow shows variable signal intensities.

The size criteria for positive lymph nodes is under debate; as a result, the reported accuracy varies.[27,28] The common reported accuracy ranges between 70% and 80%. Kim and colleagues[27] have proposed a minimal axial diameter of more than 1 cm as a sign of lymph nodes metastasis.[27] With this criteria, they reported 93% accuracy on MRI.[27] They

also reported the ratio of mean maximal axial diameter to minimal axial diameter was 1.09 for true-positive nodes and 1.76 for false-positive nodes.[27] Considering the shape of lymph nodes, their proposal seems to be reasonable. The site of lymph nodes is also important. It means regional nodes should be the first site for metastasis. Pelvic nodes should be involved in carcinoma of the cervix, in contrast to paraaortic nodes in endometrial carcinoma or carcinoma of the ovary.

RESIDUAL TUMOR OR RECURRENCE VERSUS FIBROSIS

Residual Tumor After Irradiation or Chemotherapy

A Papanicolaou smear is usually highly accurate, but it is less reliable shortly after irradiation.[29] MRI is promising.[30–32] In one report a 97% negative predictive value with apparently normal cervix was shown (Fig. 6-8).[31] A distinct hyperintense mass has an 86% positive predictive value.[31] However, diffuse hyperintense signal of the cervix or hyperintense mass within the canal is indeterminate. In addition, we must be careful about the presence of a delayed responder. A delayed responder may have viable tumor on both MRI and histologic samples even 6 months after the

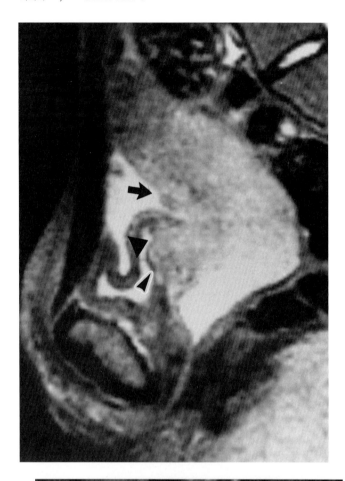

FIG. 6-7. Bladder invasion. T2-weighted sagittal image. Huge tumor *(arrow)* is adjacent to the bladder wall. Segmental disruption of the hypointense bladder wall *(arrowheads)* indicates involvement of the muscle layer of the bladder.

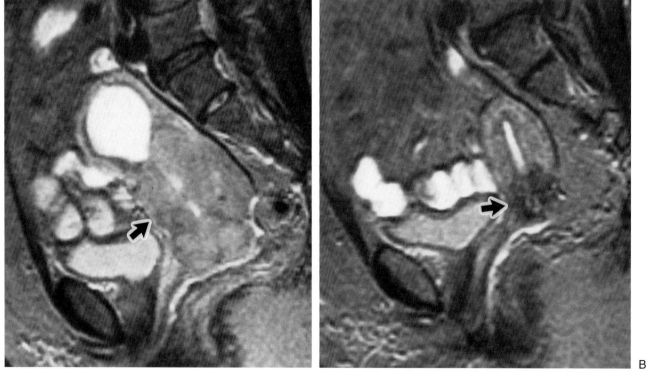

FIG. 6-8. Evaluation of residual tumor, true negative case T2-weighted sagittal image. **(A)** Huge cervical tumor *(arrows)* and hematometra are observed at the initial examination. **(B)** After twice intraarterial infusion chemotherapy, the cervix is apparently normal with distinct hypointense stroma *(arrow)*. Tumor-free cervix was confirmed by surgery.

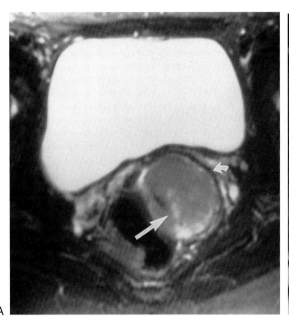
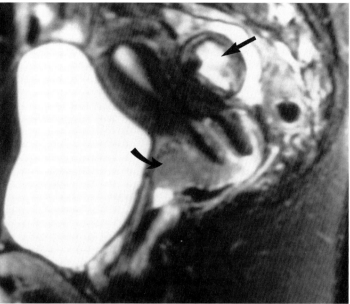

A   B

FIG. 6-9. Cervical cancer, stage IB *(curved arrow in A, between arrows in B)* shown in axial **(A)** and sagittal **(B)** scan planes. A degenerating fibroid *(straight white arrow)* is seen in **B**. Images were obtained with phased-array coil. (Courtesy of R. Brooke Jeffery, MD.)

irradiation but will still improve and have a good prognosis.[30] Most important is the course of the lesion under observation.

Recurrence Versus Fibrosis

The distinction between fibrosis and recurrent tumor has been very difficult and problematic. Even with MRI it is difficult to distinguish tumor from early fibrosis within a year (Fig. 6-9).[33] However, after 1 year, MRI contributes to distinguishing recurrence from late fibrosis.[33] Late fibrosis shows distinct hypointensity on T2-weighted images; in contrast, recurrent tumor exhibits hyperintensity. MRI is especially excellent in evaluating the vaginal stump, which is the common site of the recurrence. The vaginal stump may have a variable shape but should have hypointensity even after irradiation and surgery.[34]

REFERENCES

1. Van Nagell Jr, Roddick JW Jr, Lowin DM. The staging of cervical cancer; inevitable discrepancies between clinical staging and pathologic findings. Am J Obstet Gynecol 1971;10:973.
2. Hricak H, Powell CB, Sterm J. Cost-effectiveness of MR imaging for cancer of the cervix in patients evaluated for radical hysterectomy. Radiology 1994;193(p):278.
3. Togashi K. Nishimura K, Itoh K, et al. Uterine cervical cancer: assessment with high-field MR imaging. Radiology 1986;160:431.
4. Hricak H, Lacey CG, Sandles LG, et al. Invasive cervical carcinoma: comparison of MR imaging and surgical findings. Radiology 1988; 166:623.
5. Baumgartner BR, Bernardino ME. MR imaging of the cervix: off-axis scan to improve visualization of zonal anatomy. AJR 1989;153:1001.
6. Smith RC, Reinhold C, Lange RC, et al. Fast spin-echo MR imaging of the female pelvis: I. Use of a whole-volume coil. Radiology 1992; 184:665.
7. Yu KK, Hricak H, Subak LL, et al. Preoperative staging of cervical carcinoma with MR imaging: comparison of body versus phased array coil. Radiology 1995;197(p):321.
8. Milestone BN, Schnall MD, Lenkinski RE, et al. Cervical carcinoma: MR imaging with an endorectal surface coil. Radiology 1991;180:91.
9. deSouza NM, Hawley IC, Schwieso JE, et al. The uterine cervix on in vitro and in vivo MR images: a study of zonal anatomy and vascularity using an enveloping cervical coil. AJR 1994;163:607.
10. Hricak H, Hamm B, Semelka RC, et al. Use of GD-DTPA in the MR evaluation of carcinoma of the uterus. Radiology 1991;181:95.
11. Sironi S, De Cobelli F, Scarfone G, et al. Carcinoma of the cervix: value of plain and gadolinium-enhanced MR imaging in assessing degree of invasiveness. Radiology 1993;188:797.
12. Yamashita Y, et al. Carcinoma of the cervix: dynamic MR imaging. Radiology 1992;182:643.
13. Togashi K, Nishimura K, Sagoh T, et al. Carcinoma of the cervix: staging with MR imaging. Radiology 1989;171:245.
14. Togashi K. Differential diagnosis of gynecological disease by MRI. Tokyo, Igaku-Shoin, in press.
15. Lien HH, Blomlie V, Kjorstad K, et al. Clinical stage I carcinoma of the cervix: value of MR imaging in determining degree of invasiveness. AJR 1991;156:1191.
16. Sironi S, Belloni C, Taccgni GL, et al. Carcinoma of the cervix: value of MR imaging in detecting parametrial involvement. AJR 1991;156: 753.
17. Kim SH, Choi BI, Lee HP, et al. Uterine cervical carcinoma: comparison of CT and MR findings. Radiology 1990;175:45.
18. Kim SH, Choi BI, Han JK, et al. Preoperative staging of uterine cervical carcinoma: comparison of CT and MRI in 99 patients. J Comput Assist Tomogr 1993;17:633.
19. Sironi S, Belloni C, Taccagni G, et al. Invasive cervical carcinoma: MR imaging after preoperative chemotherapy. Radiology 1991;180: 719.
20. Kim KH, Lee BH, Do YS, et al. Stage IIb cervical carcinoma: MR evaluation of effect of intraarterial chemotherapy. Radiology 1994;192: 61.
21. Yamashita Y, Yakahashi M, Katabuchi H, et al. Adenoma malignum: MR appearances mimicking nabothian cysts. AJR 1994;162:649.

22. Kawakami K, Togashi K. Malignant lymphoma of the uterus. J Comput Assist Tomogr 1995;19:238.

23. Togashi K. MRI of the female pelvis. Tokyo, Igaku-Shoin, 1993.

24. Lee JKT, Heiken JP, Ling D, et al. Magnetic resonance imaging of abdominal and pelvic lymphadenopathy. Radiology 1984;153:181.

25. Dooms GC, Hricak H, Crooks LE, Higgins CB, et al. Magnetic resonance imaging of the lymph nodes: comparison with CT. Radiology 1984;153:719.

26. Hawnaur JM. Review: staging of cervical and endometrial carcinoma. Clin Radiol 1993;47:7.

27. Kim SH, Kim SC, Choi BI, Han MC. Uterine cervical carcinoma: evaluation of pelvic lymph node metastasis with MR imaging. Radiology 1994;190:807.

28. Matsukuma K, Tsukamoto N, Matsuyama T, et al. Preoperative CT study of lymph nodes in cervical cancer: its correlation with histological findings. Gynecol Oncol 1989;33:158.

29. Shield PW, Wright RG, Free K, Daunter B. The accuracy of cervico-vaginal cytology in the detection of recurrent cervical carcinoma following radiotherapy. Gynecol Oncol 1991;41:223.

30. Flueckiger F, Ebner F, Poschauko H, et al. Cervical cancer: serial MR imaging before and after primary radiation therapy: a 2-year follow up study. Radiology 1992;184:89.

31. Hricak H, Swift PS, Campos Z, et al. Irradiation of the cervix uteri: value of unenhanced and contrast enhanced MR imaging. Radiology 1993;189:381.

32. Weber TM, Sostman HD, Spritzer CE, et al. Cervical carcinoma: determination of recurrent tumor extent versus radiation changes with MR imaging. Radiology 1995;194:135.

33. Ebner F, Kressel HY, Mintz MC, et al. Tumor recurrence versus fibrosis in the female pelvis: differentiation with MR imaging at 1.5 T. Radiology 1988;166:333.

34. Brown JJ, Gutierrez ED, Lee JKT. MR appearance of the normal and abnormal vagina after hysterectomy. AJR 1992;158:95.

Computed Tomography of Cervical Cancer

R. Brooke Jeffrey, Jr., MD

INITIAL TUMOR STAGING

Magnetic resonance imaging, using either a pelvic array or endorectal coil, is the imaging method of choice to initially stage patients with clinically suspected invasive carcinoma of the cervix. CT is generally a second-line imaging option in patients who are not suitable candidates for MRI (eg, those with a cardiac pacemaker or claustrophobia). A comparative study of CT and MRI by Subak and associates[1] demonstrated that, when compared with radical hysterectomy specimens, MRI was superior to CT in demonstrating tumor size, stromal invasion, and overall staging. Both CT and MRI were comparable in assessing lymphadenopathy. Similar results were obtained by Kim and colleagues,[2] who documented that MRI was superior to CT in overall lesion detection and evaluation of parametrial invasion. In general, CT is most accurate in staging advanced disease (stage III or IV).

Most prior reports evaluating the accuracy of CT for cervical carcinoma, however, were performed using earlier generation CT scanners and not newer helical or spiral CT.[3-6] It is quite possible that with thin-section (3–5 mm) spiral CT technique and optimal contrast medium enhancement of parametrial vessels, the sensitivity of spiral CT would be substantially greater than with conventional CT performed at 10-mm slice collimation. With current spiral CT technique it is important to initiate scanning at the symphysis pubis and then scan craniad to the level of the iliac crest during the vascular phase of the contrast injection. This is to identify the parametrial vascular plexus during peak contrast medium enhancement. Delayed scans, also with thin sections, may be of value in more precisely delineating stromal invasion of the cervix.

The goal of preoperative imaging with either CT or MRI is to determine which patients are potential candidates for radical hysterectomy. If there is clear-cut evidence of tumor extension beyond the cervix with parametrial invasion (stage IIB), radical hysterectomy is contraindicated. Patients are then treated with external beam radiation rather than surgery. Thus, the identification of parametrial invasion is critically importance for accurate clinical staging and patient management. Carcinoma of the cervix is typically hypoattenuating on contrast medium–enhanced CT because it is considerably

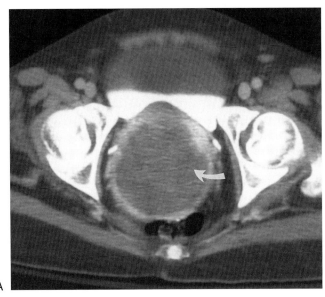
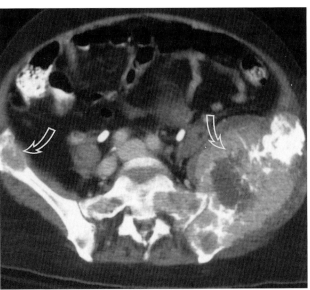

A   B

FIG. 6-10. Necrotic cervical carcinoma with bony metastasis. Note large, low-attenuating cervical mass in **A** *(arrow)*. The low attenuation is due to extensive necrosis. There are bilateral lytic metastases to the iliac crests in **B** *(arrows)*.

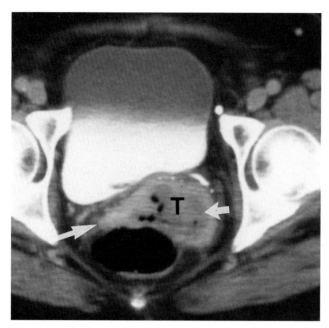

FIG. 6-11. Carcinoma of the cervix with left parametrial invasion. Note the triangular configuration of the normal right parametrium *(long white arrow)*. A low-density tumor extends into the left parametrium *(short white arrow)*. Gas is noted within the cervical tumor (T) from a recent biopsy.

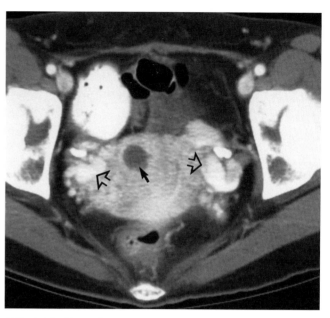

FIG. 6-12. Normal enhancing parametrial vessels. A nabothian cyst is noted in the cervix *(black arrow)*. Normal enhancing parametrial vessels are evident on this spiral CT *(open arrows)*. Without excellent contrast medium enhancement these vessels could be easily misconstrued as a soft tissue mass representing parametrial tumor invasion.

less vascular than the adjacent cervical stroma (Fig. 6-10).[7] It may also be hypodense due to ulceration or necrosis. Parametrial invasion on CT can be diagnosed when there is soft tissue nodularity or infiltration along the lateral cervical margin or if tumor is identified encasing the pelvic ureter.[7] Unlike MRI, CT cannot clearly delineate the fibrous stroma of

the cervix (Fig. 6-11), and, thus, infiltration of the paracervical fat must be relied on to diagnose parametrial tumor extension with CT (Fig. 6-12). It is important not to mistake the normal cardinal ligament or normal parametrial vessels for parametrial tumor extension. The cardinal ligaments may be slightly asymmetric in their appearance, although they tend

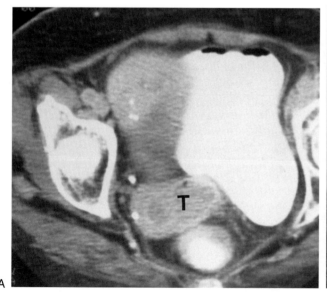

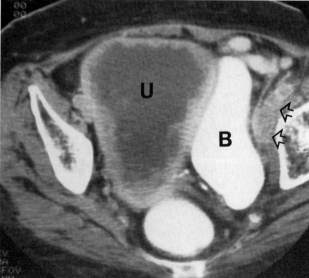

A   B

FIG. 6-13. Metastatic carcinoma of the cervix. In **(A)** note the hypoattenuating tumor (T) within the cervix. In **(B)** there are low-density secretions within the obstructed uterus (U). Note the displacement of the urine-filled bladder to the left (B). Metastatic lymphadenopathy is evident to the external iliac nodes *(open arrows)*.

on CT to have a predominantly triangular configuration with distal tapering.

The accuracy of CT for diagnosing parametrial invasion based on older generation scanners is only 30% to 58%.[4,5,8,9] In part, this may have been due to the difficulty in differentiating normal vessels or ligaments from parametrial tumor invasion. Parametritis secondary to recent dilatation and curettage or cervical conization may at times cause slight soft tissue infiltration around the lateral margin of the cervix. Therefore, for parametrial invasion to be confidently diagnosed there must be clear-cut evidence of a soft tissue mass with infiltration, rather than ill-defined edema in the paracervical tissues.

Carcinoma of the cervix may obstruct the uterus, leading to distention endometrial cavity with blood and secretions. The obstructed uterus has a characteristic CT appearance because the endometrial cavity contains low attenuating complex fluid (Fig. 6-13). Cervical carcinoma invading the pelvic sidewall indicates stage IIIB disease. This is evident on CT as a heterogeneous mass extending to either obturator internus or piriformis muscles (Fig. 6-14). Identification of hydronephrosis due to obstruction of the pelvic ureter also indicates stage IIIB disease.

Stage IV carcinoma of the cervix may be diagnosed when there is CT evidence for either bladder or rectal invasion (Fig. 6-15). Paraaortic or inguinal lymphadenopathy also indicates stage IV disease (Fig. 6-16). The CT criteria for bladder or rectal invasion include loss of adjacent fat planes and nodular thickening of either the bladder or rectal wall.[10,11] In general, paraaortic lymph nodes larger than 1 cm in short

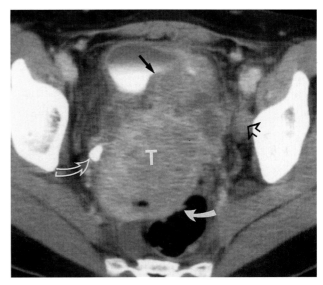

FIG. 6-15. Stage IV carcinoma of the cervix with invasion of the bladder and rectum. Note the large tumor mass (T) from carcinoma of the cervix. There is nodular invasion of the posterior wall of the bladder *(black arrow)* and of the rectum *(curved white arrow)*. Note the normal enhancing white ureter *(open curved white arrow)* and the lack of visualization of the left ureter due to tumor encasement. Metastasis to obturator lymph node is evident *(open black arrow)*.

axis size are suggestive of metastatic involvement. This is particularly true of lymph nodes that are low in attenuation owing to the decreased vascularity of squamous cell carcinoma of the cervix.

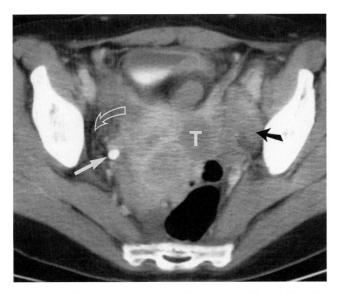

FIG. 6-14. Stage III carcinoma of the cervix with pelvic sidewall extension. Note heterogeneous tumor (T) extending to the left pelvic sidewall *(black arrow)*. There is lack of visualization of the left ureter due to obstruction by the mass. Note the normal enhancing right ureter *(white arrow)* and adjacent normal fat planes of the right hemipelvis *(open curved arrow)*.

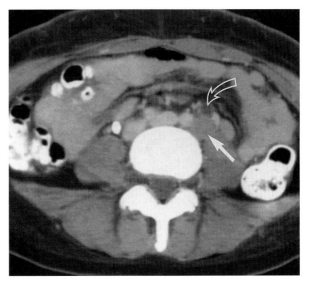

FIG. 6-16. Paraaortic nodal metastasis from carcinoma of the cervix. Note the characteristic low-attenuating left paraaortic nodal metastasis *(straight arrow)* and the obstructed left ureter *(curved open arrow)* from stage IV carcinoma of the cervix.

One potential new role of CT in the evaluation and staging of patients with cervical carcinoma is assessment of prognosis by accurately determining tumor depth (ie, maximum anteroposterior dimensions). Shepherd and colleagues[12] retrospectively reviewed the CT scans of 56 patients with carcinoma of the cervix. Patients with a tumor depth greater than 4 cm were noted to have significantly increased risk for metastases to lymph nodes and had an overall poor prognosis. Therefore, assessment of maximal tumor depth by CT may provide important prognostic information that cannot be obtained by simple International Federation of Gynecology and Obstetrics (FIGO) staging alone.

RECURRENT CERVICAL CARCINOMA

CT may be of considerable clinical value in diagnosing recurrent cervical carcinoma (Fig. 6-17 and 6-18).[13–15] CT is significantly more accurate in assessing recurrent cervical carcinoma than in the initial tumor staging.[14,15] Serial CT may be used to guide response to radiation therapy or chemotherapy and to detect metastatic disease involving the lymph nodes, liver, or lungs. If at all possible, a pelvic CT scan obtained 6 weeks after completion of radiation therapy is extremely useful as a baseline for subsequent follow-up CT. Fibrotic pelvic soft tissue masses may result from radiation therapy alone and not tumor recurrence. Radiation therapy may cause thickening of the uterosacral ligaments, as well as discrete presacral or pelvic sidewall masses due to fibrosis. In selected patients, CT-guided biopsy may be used to help differentiate radiation fibrosis from tumor recurrence. However, false-negative results may occur owing to sampling error, because tumor cells are intermixed within a large amount of collagenous tissue. MRI, or potentially positron emission tomographic scanning, may be of value in assess-

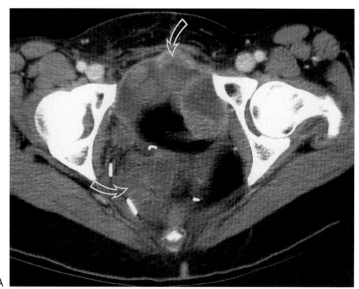

A

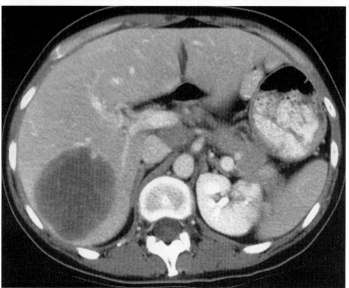

B

FIG. 6-17. Recurrent cervical carcinoma after radical hysterectomy. Note extensive pelvic tumor occurrence in **A** *(arrows)*. Metastasis to the liver is also noted in **B.**

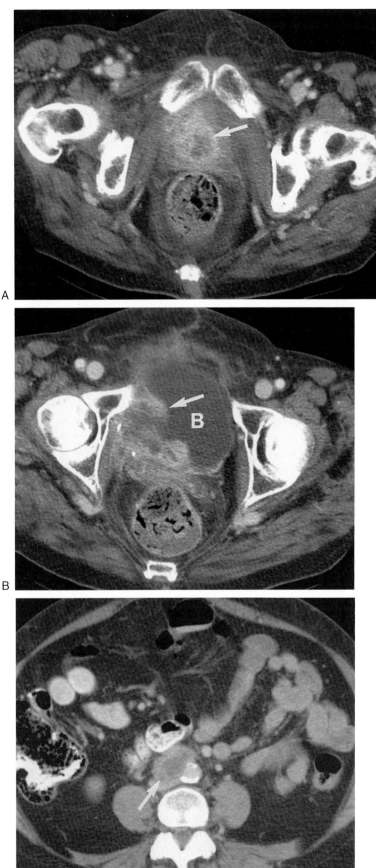

FIG. 6-18. Recurrent cervical carcinoma after radiation therapy. Patient presented with vaginal bleeding. In **(A)**, note enhancing heterogeneous mass within the vagina *(arrow)*. In **(B)**, note large recurrent right pelvic sidewall mass *(arrow)* invading the bladder (B). In **(C)**, low-density retroperitoneal lymph node metastases are evident *(arrow)*.

ing these patients as well. Serial follow-up scans demonstrating an enlarging mass are clear evidence for tumor recurrence.

REFERENCES

1. Subak LL, Hricak H, Powell CB, et al. Cervical carcinoma: computed tomography and magnetic resonance imaging for preoperative staging. Obstet Gynecol 1995;86:43.
2. Kim SH, Choi BI, Han JK, et al. Preoperative staging of uterine cervical carcinoma: comparison of CT and MRI in 99 patients. J Comput Assist Tomogr 1993;17:633.
3. Kim SH, Choi BI, Lee HP, et al. Uterine cervical carcinoma: comparison of CT and MR findings. Radiology 1990;175:45.
4. Kilcheski TS, Arger PH, Mulhern CJ, et al. Role of computed tomography in the presurgical evaluation of carcinoma of the cervix. J Comput Assist Tomogr 1981;5:378.
5. Walsh JW, Goplerud DR. Prospective comparison between clinical and CT staging in primary cervical carcinoma. AJR 1981;137:997.
6. Walton LA, McCartney WH, Vesterinen E. The use of computerized tomography to obviate celiotomy in recurrent carcinoma of the cervix. Gynecol Oncol 1981;12:166.
7. Walsh JW. Computed tomography of gynecologic neoplasms. Radiol Clin North Am 1992;30:817.
8. Grumbine FC, Rosenshein NB, Zerhouni EA, Siegelman SS. Abdominopelvic computed tomography in the preoperative evaluation of early cervical cancer. Gynecol Oncol 1981;12:286.
9. Villasanta U, Whitley NO, Haney PJ, Brenner D. Computed tomography in invasive carcinoma of the cervix: an appraisal. Obstet Gynecol 1983;62:218.
10. Walsh JW, Jones CMI. Diagnostic imaging techniques in gynecologic oncology. In: Hoskins WJ, Perez CA, Young RC, eds. Gynecologic oncology principles and practice. Philadelphia, JB Lippincott, 1992.
11. Walsh JW, Vick CW. Staging of female genital tract cancer. In: Walsh JW, ed. Computed tomography of the pelvis. New York, Churchill Livingstone, 1985:163.
12. Shepherd SF, Collins CD, Fryatt IJ, et al. Computerized axial tomographic scan measurements as prognostic indicators in patients with cervical carcinoma. Br J Radiol 1995;68:600.
13. Bandy LC, Clarke PD, Silverman PM, Creasman WT. Computed tomography in evaluation of extrapelvic lymphadenopathy in carcinoma of the cervix. Obstet Gynecol 1985;65:73.
14. Franchi M, La FA, Babilonti L, et al. Clinical value of computerized tomography (CT) in assessment of recurrent uterine cancers. Gynecol Oncol 1989;35:31.
15. Walsh JW, Amendola MA, Hall DJ, et al. Recurrent carcinoma of the cervix: CT diagnosis. AJR 1981;136:117.

Clinical Gynecologic Imaging, edited
by Arthur C. Fleischer, Marcia C. Javitt,
R. Brooke Jeffrey, Jr., and Howard W. Jones III,
Lippincott-Raven Publishers, Philadelphia © 1997.

CHAPTER 7

Pelvic Inflammatory Disease

Pelvic Inflammatory Disease: Overview

Ted L. Anderson, MD, PhD

Pelvic inflammatory disease (PID) is a microbial process involving the female reproductive tract that continues to have a profound impact on medical, social, and fiscal aspects of society. Our understanding of the pathogenesis and management of this complex process is constantly evolving. Indeed, its scope has been expanded by the Centers for Disease Control and Prevention (CDC) to incorporate any combination of upper genital tract infections, including endometritis, salpingitis, oophoritis, tuboovarian abscess, and pelvic peritonitis.[1]

Considered to represent an ascending polymicrobial infection, PID is most frequently associated with sexually transmitted microorganisms, particularly *Neisseria gonorrhoeae* and *Chlamydia trachomatis,* which account for approximately two thirds of the cases. However, it is now widely recognized that aerobic and anaerobic bacteria comprising the normal vaginal flora may be solely responsible for as many as one third of cases. Further, up to half of women with

PID of sexually transmitted etiology will have concomitant involvement by vaginal flora.[2] Other organisms occasionally associated with PID include a myriad of anaerobes and respiratory microorganisms from the endometrium or cul-de-sac, including *Haemophilus influenzae,* group B *Streptococcus, Escherichia coli,* and *Bacteroides* species. The extent of mycoplasmic involvement in PID remains unclear.[3]

EPIDEMIOLOGY

In 1988 it was estimated that 10% of reproductive-aged American women had been treated for PID.[4] A more recent CDC study examining hospital admissions from 1988 to 1990 for women between the ages of 15 and 44 found that PID accounted for almost 20% of all gynecologic diagnoses, representing an average annual rate of 49.3 per 10,000 hospital discharges.[5] Notably, this probably reflects only a fraction of total PID cases per year; inpatient treatment has con-

TABLE 7-1. *Risk factors for pelvic inflammatory disease*

Presence of *Neisseria gonorrhoeae, Chlamydia trachomatis,*
  or bacterial vaginosis
Low socioeconomic status
Adolescence (age <19)
Multiple sexual partners
Previous episodes of pelvic inflammatory disease
Intrauterine contraceptive device
Intercourse during last menstrual period
Absence of contraception use (especially barrier)
Recent pelvic surgery
Douching

tinued to decline since the mid 1980s whereas the number of women consulting physicians as outpatients has increased.[6] With over 1 million American women affected per year, it is evident that the incidence of PID continues to rise at an alarming rate.

In addition to the public health implications, the growing fiscal impact of PID is staggering. It has been estimated that greater than 100,000 surgical procedures are performed each year as an direct or indirect consequence of PID. Costs related to the treatment of PID and its associated sequelae, including ectopic pregnancy and infertility, were estimated at $5 billion in 1992 and are projected to be as high as $10 billion by the year 2000.[7,8]

Common risk factors for development of PID have been identified and are listed in Table 7-1. However, risk assessment is predicated on an understanding of the variables of host susceptibility, including both propensity for acquisition of infection and facilitation of pathogen spread. For example, not only are adolescents frequently associated with higher risk behavior, but this population of patients has a larger zone of cervical ectopy and greater permeability of cervical mucus. Lower socioeconomic status has been associated with an increased prevalence of sexually transmitted disease and these patients are less likely to seek adequate or timely medical health care. In addition to increased exposure through retained high-risk behaviors, patients with a history of PID have damaged fallopian tubes that are more susceptible to infection. There are both behaviorial and biologic components that must be considered when assessing the possibility of a PID diagnosis.

DIAGNOSIS

The diagnosis of PID continues to be enigmatic for clinicians because of the inherent diversity in its presentation; associated complaints described by patients are plethoric. The diagnostic goal is to establish guidelines with sufficient sensitivity to avoid missing mild cases, but with sufficient specificity to avoid unwarranted antibiotic therapy.[7] This has led to the development of established diagnostic criteria,[1] the recent revision of which is presented in Table 7-2.

Although common symptoms of PID include fever, lower abdominal pain (often dull and constant), and vaginal discharge, this is not invariant. Indeed, some patients may describe only nonspecific pelvic discomfort, dysmenorrhea, or dyspareunia, more typically associated with endometriosis. Alternatively, there may be menorrhagia or vaginal discharge in the absence of concurrent abdominal pain.[9] As such, a diagnosis of PID should be entertained in any patient with genitourinary symptoms. Other important entities to consider in the differential diagnosis include appendicitis, ectopic pregnancy, ovarian cyst or torsion, gastroenteritis, diverticulitis, dysfunctional uterine bleeding, cystitis, or pyelonephritis.[2,10–12] Therein lies the import of a careful sexual history to reveal one or more associated risk factors as described earlier.

Any combination of genital tract symptoms in the "at risk" patient may indicate PID, but none is specific enough to warrant definitive diagnosis solely on historical grounds. The pelvic examination, including evaluation of vaginal and endocervical secretions is a key component of the diagnosis. Adnexal tenderness, which may be unilateral, is almost invariably noted, although a distinct mass or adnexal fullness may not be appreciated. Tenderness elicited on moving the cervix from side to side ("chandelier sign") is a sign of peritoneal irritation. Leukorrhea has been touted as a finding of critical importance in differentiating PID from pain of other etiologies.[7] Defined as a polymorphonuclear leukocyte to epithelial cell ratio of greater than 1:1 observed on a wet mount of vaginal secretions, leukorrhea has been described to be present in over 95% of patients with laparoscopically confirmed PID.[13] Similarly, a green or yellow discharge from an erythematous, edematous, and friable cervix (mucopurulent endocervicitis) in the presence of pelvic organ tenderness is always indicative of PID. Conversely, the absence of mucopurulent endocervicitis should raise suspicion for a noninfectious etiology of pain.

TABLE 7-2. *Diagnostic criteria for pelvic inflammatory disease*

ALL OF THE FOLLOWING:
Lower abdominal pain with tenderness on examination
Adnexal tenderness (may be unilateral)
Cervical motion tenderness

PLUS ONE OR MORE OF THE FOLLOWING:
"ROUTINE CRITERIA"
Temperature >38.3°C (100.9°F)
Leukocytosis (WBC > 10,500/mm^3)
Elevated C-reactive protein
Elevated erythrocyte sedimentation rate
Laboratory evidence of gonococcal or chlamydial infection
  (eg, cervicitis, antigen test, Gram stain)
"ELABORATE CRITERIA"
Endometrial biopsy with evidence of endometritis
Tuboovarian abscess documented by diagnostic imaging
Laparoscopic abnormalities consistent with pelvic infection

LABORATORY TESTING

Other than bacteriologic or immunologic testing, there are no laboratory tests that are pathognomonic for PID. Furthermore, while Gram stain, bacterial culture, or antigen identification testing is helpful, the results of these tests are often not available at the time of initial diagnosis. All patients should have a pregnancy test and complete blood cell count with differential.

INVASIVE TESTING

Histologic confirmation of acute or chronic endometritis by endometrial biopsy provides diagnostic certainty for PID.[14] Although obtained with relative ease and minimal discomfort to the patient, the results are seldom available before 24 hours. As such, endometrial biopsy has limited usefulness in this setting other than diagnostic confirmation.

Laparoscopy has long been hailed as the "gold standard" for PID diagnosis in that it allows visualization of pelvic organs and permits direct culture of involved sites. Diagnostic criteria include pronounced hyperemia and edema of the tubal wall along with exudate on the serosal surface or at the fimbriated ends. However, in the absence of blocked tubes, the presence of exudate is most specific and guards against diagnostic bias[15]; a histologically positive endometrial biopsy is a useful adjunct in this setting. Routine laparoscopy is rarely performed owing to the expense and operative risk. However, in cases of diagnostic uncertainty, especially when there is high suspicion of need for urgent intervention (eg, appendicitis, ovarian torsion, or ectopic pregnancy), laparoscopy may play an integral role in diagnosis and therapeutic intervention. As many as one third of patients with a clinical diagnosis of PID do not have laparoscopic evidence of true salpingitis. Although it is possible that some of these patients with an apparently normal pelvic anatomy may have mucosal inflammation not evident by examination of the tubal serosa, the most common findings include ectopic pregnancy, ovarian cysts, appendicitis, or endometriosis.[16]

ROLE OF SONOGRAPHY

Sonography continues to be an invaluable tool in the assessment of acute pelvic pain. When compared with laparoscopy, it offers the significant advantages of real-time imaging with immediate interpretation in a low-cost noninvasive modality. Sonography provides additional diagnostic benefit in the obese patient, in whom the physical examination findings may be less conclusive, and in whom there is greater potential morbidity associated with laparoscopic evaluation.

Sonographic evaluation of the abdomen and pelvis has long provided obvious benefits in the differential diagnosis of appendicitis, ectopic pregnancy, ovarian cysts, and inflammatory adnexal complexes resulting from advanced stages of PID. More recently, the improved resolution

achieved by placing high-frequency transvaginal transducers in close proximity to pelvic soft tissues, especially when combined with Doppler analysis technology, has permitted elucidation of adnexal pathology at earlier stages in the progression of PID. As fluid accumulates within the tube, especially if adhesions have resulted in distal occlusion, the tapered fusiform shape and lack of peristalsis allow it to be distinguished from fluid-filled loops of small bowel.[17] Although sonographic findings may be minimal in women with mild salpingitis, greater than 90% sensitivity has been reported in identifying tubal and periovarian inflammation, as confirmed by laparoscopic findings.[18]

In addition to readily available and cost-efficient diagnostic capabilities, sonography also provides a mechanism for therapeutic intervention, such as guided drainage of tuboovarian abscess,[19] and for following patients to assess the effectiveness of treatment.

TREATMENT

Predicated on the consensus that PID is a polymicrobial process, it is generally accepted that antibiotic therapy should provide broad-spectrum coverage. The current CDC recommendations, including both inpatient and outpatient multiagent regimens,[1] are presented in Table 7-3. Differences in these regimens reflect costs, spectrum of coverage, and route of administration. In prescribing a treatment regimen, additional considerations must include the issues of patient education, compliance, treatment of partners, and follow-up care.

An increasing number of patients with PID are being

TABLE 7-3. *Treatment guidelines for pelvic inflammatory disease*

OUTPATIENT REGIMEN A
Cefoxitin, 2 g IM, and probenecid, 1 g, orally, or ceftriaxone, 250 mg IM, or equivalent cephalosporin
Doxycycline, 100 mg orally bid × 14 days

OUTPATIENT REGIMEN B
Ofloxacin, 400 mg orally bid × 14 days
Clindamycin, 450 mg orally qid × 14 days, or metronidazole, 500 mg orally bid × 14 days

INPATIENT REGIMEN A
Cefoxitin, 2 g IV qid, or cefotetan, 2 g IV bid, or equivalent cephalosporin
Doxycycline, 100 mg IV or orally bid

INPATIENT REGIMEN B
Clindamycin, 900 mg IV tid
Gentamicin loading dose (2 mg/kg) IV or IM, then maintenance (1.5 mg/kg) tid

An inpatient regimen is continued for at least 48 hours after the patient clinically improves, after which doxycycline, 100 mg orally bid, or clindamycin, 450 mg orally qid is continued to total 14 days of therapy (may be completed on an outpatient basis).

TABLE 7-4. *Criteria for hospitalization*

Severe illness (temperature >101°F, WBC >15,000/mm³, upper peritoneal signs, shock)
Uncertain diagnosis (need to exclude ectopic pregnancy or appendicitis)
Inability to tolerate or unlikely to comply with outpatient therapy
Suspected anaerobic infection (intrauterine device or recent uterine instrumentation)
Suspected pelvic or tuboovarian abscess
Failure to respond to 48 hours of outpatient treatment
Infection with human immunodeficiency virus
Pregnancy

treated on an outpatient basis. There are no data to suggest that hospitalized patients have better outcomes than those managed as outpatients. As such, the decision of whether a patient requires inpatient therapy is based largely on severity of illness, need for intravenous therapy, and predicted effectiveness of outpatient therapy or follow-up (eg, medical or social factors affecting compliance). Criteria for hospitalization have been established by the CDC[1] and are outlined in Table 7-4.

With an increasing understanding of the pathogenesis and natural history of PID, along with more sensitive tools for accurate early diagnosis, including sonography, diagnostic laparoscopy is required in fewer patients. However, surgical intervention is still of benefit to assess severity of disease or for therapeutic intervention. Indeed, approximately one third of patients hospitalized with acute PID, and the majority of patients hospitalized with chronic PID, still require surgical intervention to drain abscesses, resect or repair pelvic organs, or remove intrauterine devices that have become embedded or extrauterine.[12,20]

SEQUELAE

The most common adverse sequelae of PID are infertility (predominantly tubal factor), ectopic pregnancy, and chronic pelvic pain. All of these are related to tubal damage and adhesion formation as a consequence of PID.

Although the endpoint is virtually identical, the mechanism by which different organisms cause tubal damage varies. Gonococcal infections elicit a complement-mediated inflammatory response with migration of polymorphonuclear leukocytes and transudation of plasma into tissues. The reparative process of removing debris and infiltration of fibroblasts results in scarring and adhesiogenesis.[21] Conversely, chlamydial infections evoke cell-mediated immune responses whereby a chronic hypersensitivity reaction to chlamydial antigens is believed to result in tissue destruction.[22]

The incidence of infertility after PID has been demonstrated to be related to both severity and frequency of disease, with approximately a 10-fold increase after a single episode and almost a doubling of incidence with each subse-

quent episode.[23] In addition to mechanical factors, chronic antigen exposure in women with asymptomatic chlamydial infections ("silent salpingitis") may be conducive to development of an autoimmune response. Possible cross-reactivity of antibodies generated in this manner with human sperm antigens, even after the infection is treated, may also contribute to infertility.[24] Similar to the increased incidence of infertility, those patients who do get pregnant are at increased risk for ectopic pregnancy; varied reports have provided estimates between 4- to 10-fold increased risk.[23,25]

Multiple studies have documented an association between PID and subsequent chronic pelvic pain, with some estimates as high as 24% incidence.[23,26] Additional related morbidity includes menstrual disturbances and dyspareunia.[27]

FITZ-HUGH–CURTIS SYNDROME

Fitz-Hugh–Curtis syndrome results from extension of the inflammatory process out of the pelvis to the subdiaphragmatic space, either by transperitoneal or lymphatic dissemination.[28] Occurring in 5% to 10% of PID cases, perihepatitis or focal peritonitis is caused by a purulent exudate adherent to the liver capsule. Of note, the inflammatory process appears to be limited to the hepatic capsule with sparing of parenchymal tissue; liver enzymes are typically not elevated.

Patients with this syndrome may present in the acute phase with pleuritic pain and right upper quadrant tenderness with possible radiation to the shoulder or back. Indeed, Fitz-Hugh–Curtis syndrome is frequently mistaken initially for pneumonia, pancreatitis, or cholecystitis; pelvic manifestations usually direct the correct diagnosis. Development of "violin string" adhesions between the visceral peritoneum of the anterior liver surface and the parietal peritoneum of the anterior abdominal wall occurs with progression to the chronic phase. This is frequently diagnosed retrospectively as an incidental laparoscopic finding. Treatment during the acute phase is identical to that of salpingitis. When the chronic phase is diagnosed laparoscopically, lysis of asymptomatic adhesions is not typically indicated.

CONCLUSION

Pelvic inflammatory disease continues to present both public health and economic burdens. In addition to immediate treatment concerns, long-term sequelae constitute a growing concern and consume an expanding share of health care expenditures. Although accurate identification of PID with confidence continues to escape clinicians, sonography is playing an ever-increasing role in early diagnosis of PID and in distinguishing among the diagnostic possibilities in acute pelvic pain. This is of particular importance in the cost-containment arena of managed care. Clearly, early diagnosis, effective treatment, and prevention of recurrence play key roles in decreasing associated morbidity.

REFERENCES

1. Centers for Disease Control and Prevention. 1993 Sexually transmitted diseases treatment guidelines. MMWR 1993;42:1.
2. Sweet RL. Pelvic inflammatory disease. In: Sweet RL, Gibbs RS, eds. Infectious diseases of the female genital tract. Baltimore, Williams & Wilkins, 1990:241.
3. Soper DE, Brockwell NJ, Dalton HP, Johnson D. Observations concerning the microbial etiology of acute salpingitis. Am J Obstet Gynecol 1994;170:1008.
4. Aral SO, Mosher WD, Cates W. Self-reported pelvic inflammatory disease in the United States, 1988. JAMA 1991;266:2570.
5. Velebil P, Wingo PA, Xia Z, et al. Rate of hospitalization for gynecologic disorders among reproductive-age women in the United States. Obstet Gynecol 1995;86:765.
6. Rolfs RT, Galaid EI, Zaidi AA. Pelvic inflammatory disease: trends in hospitalizations and office visits 1979–1988. Am J Obstet Gynecol 1992;166:983.
7. Soper DE. Pelvic inflammatory disease. Infect Dis Clin North Am 1994;8:821.
8. Washington AE, Katz P. Cost of and payment source for pelvic inflammatory disease: trends and projections, 1983 through 2000. JAMA 1991;226:2565.
9. Wolner-Hanssen PW, Kiviat NB, Holmes KK. Atypical pelvic inflammatory disease: subacute, chronic, or subclinical upper genital tract infection in women. In: Holmes KK, Mardh P-A, Sparling PF, et al, eds. Sexually transmitted diseases, 2nd ed. New York, McGraw-Hill, 1990;615.
10. Adelman A. Abdominal pain in the primary care setting. J Fam Pract 1987;25:27.
11. Bongard F, Landers DV, Lewis F. Differential diagnosis of appendicitis and pelvic inflammatory disease. Am J Surg 1985;150:90.
12. McCormack WM. Pelvic inflammatory disease. N Engl J Med 1994;330:115.
13. Westrom L. Diagnosis and treatment of salpingitis. J Reprod Med 1983;28:703.
14. Kiviat NB, Wolner-Hanssen P, Eschenbach DA, et al. Endometrial histopathology in patients with culture-proved upper genital tract infection and laparoscopically diagnosed acute salpingitis. Am J Surg Pathol 1990;14:167.
15. Soper DE. Diagnosis and laparoscopic grading of acute salpingitis. Am J Obstet Gynecol 1991;164:1370.
16. Cates W, Rolfs RT, Aral SO. Sexually transmitted diseases, pelvic inflammatory disease, and infertility: an epidemiologic update. Epidemiol Rev 1990;12:199.
17. Fleischer AC, Entman SE. Sonographic evaluation of pelvic masses with transabdominal and transvaginal scanning. In: Fleischer AC, Romero R, Manning FA, et al, eds. The principles and practice of ultrasonography in obstetrics and gynecology, ed 4. Norwalk, CT, Appleton & Lange, 1991:537.
18. Patten RM, Vincent LM, Wolner-Hanssen P, et al. Pelvic inflammatory disease: endovaginal sonography with laparoscopic correlation. J Ultrasound Med 1990;9:681.
19. Nosher JL, Winchman HK, Needell GS. Transvaginal pelvic abscess drainage with US guidance. Radiology 1987;165:872.
20. Hillis SD. PID prevention: clinical and societal stakes. Hosp Pract 1994;29:129.
21. Rice PA, Schachter J. Pathogenesis of pelvic inflammatory disease: what are the questions? JAMA 1991;266:2587.
22. Witkin SS, Leger WJ. New directions in the diagnosis and treatment of pelvic inflammatory disease. J Antimicrob Chemother 1993;31:197.
23. Westrom L, Joesoef R, Reynolds B, et al. Pelvic inflammatory disease and fertility: a cohort study of 1,844 women with laparoscopically verified disease and 657 control women with normal laparoscopic results. Sex Transm Dis 1992;19:185.
24. Kurpisz M, Clark GF, Mahony MC, et al. Mouse monoclonal antibodies against human sperm: evidence for immunodominant glycosylated antigenic sties. Clin Exp Immunol 1989;78:250.
25. Westrom L. Pelvic inflammatory disease: bacteriology and sequelae. Contraception 1987;36:111.
26. Safrin S, Schachter J, Dahrouge D, et al. Long-term sequelae of acute pelvic inflammatory disease: a retrospective cohort study. Am J Obstet Gynecol 1992;166:1300.
27. Adlet MW, Belsey EH, O'Conner BH. Morbidity associated with pelvic inflammatory disease. Br J Vener Dis 1982;58:151.
28. Lopez-Zeno JA, Keith LG, Berger GS. The Fitz-Hugh–Curtis syndrome revisited: changing perspectives after half a century. J Reprod Med 1985;30:567.

Transvaginal Sonography in Pelvic Inflammatory Disease

Marcela Böhm-Vélez, MD

Pelvic inflammatory disease (PID) is a broad term for infection of the upper genital tract involving the endometrium, fallopian tubes, ovaries, and adjacent pelvic, perihepatic, and peritoneal spaces. The infection is usually due to an organism that ascends from the lower genital tract through the endometrium and fallopian tubes into the pelvic peritoneum predominantly in sexually active premenopausal women. Less common, pathogens can reach the fallopian tubes by hematogenous spread (eg, tuberculosis) and contiguous spread from adjacent pelvic infection (eg, appendicitis).[1]

In the past decades, the incidence and prevalence of PID in women has increased.[1] Morbidity and economic costs associated with acute PID appear to be substantial; therefore, early accurate diagnosis and treatment is important to prevent sequelae including ectopic pregnancy, tubal disease, and infertility.[2–5]

RISK FACTORS

Multiple predisposing factors have been identified for the development of PID. Young age is a risk factor for PID, with PID common among sexually active adolescents. For teenagers, there is an estimated risk of 1 in 8 compared with 1 in 80 for women aged 24 years or older.[3] One explanation may be that adolescent girls have "cervical ectopy" or columnar epithelium in the endocervical canal extending into the vagina. This columnar epithelium is susceptible to virulent pathogens. With age, the columnar epithelium recedes and is replaced with squamous epithelium, which is more resistant to infection. In addition, in adolescents, menstrual cycles may be anovulatory to begin with, and the low viscosity of the cervical mucus in these cycles facilitates the proximal transport of pathogens.[3] PID is rare in sexually inactive women and probably results from spread of infection from appendix, rectosigmoid, or other extragenital sites.

Contraceptives play a role in PID. Condoms, diaphragms, or spermicides may protect women from acquiring infection by preventing vaginal bacteria from ascending into the uterine cavity. On the other hand, the intrauterine contraceptive device (IUD) can increase the risk by one and one-half to four times, depending on the type of IUD employed.[6] Most cases associated with PID are seen within the first 4 months after insertion of the IUD. The tail of the IUD provides a path for travel of bacteria through the cervix to the endometrium and then, by means of the lymphatics and veins, into a fallopian tube, usually causing a unilateral infection. Prior use of IUDs may result in infertility, explained by subclinical episodes of salpingitis that cause tubal occlusion.[7]

Multiple sexual partners increase the risk of developing PID by five times.[8] An important continuous source of infection is the untreated man with silent urethral infection. Forty percent of men with urethral *Neisseria gonorrhoeae* infections are asymptomatic.[9] History of previous PID increases the possibility of subsequent infection in 20% to 25% of the cases. The damaged tubal epithelium, by previous episodes of PID, is susceptible to bacterial colonization and recurrent infection.[8]

PATHOGENESIS

The major etiologic agents associated with acute PID are *Neisseria gonorrhoeae* and *Chlamydia trachomatis.*[9] The gonococci attach to the nonciliated mucosal epithelial cells and release endotoxin, causing the loss of cilia. Gonococcal infection may be limited to mucosal surface of the tube, while *C. trachomatis* and anaerobic bacteria cause infection below the basement membrane. When subepithelial connective tissues, muscularis, and serosal surfaces become involved in the inflammatory process, permanent tubal damage may occur. During the early stage of infection the tubal lumen remains open and infected material is frequently spilled through the fimbriated end, producing a peritonitis.

Specimens for culture can be collected from cervical smears, endometrial biopsy, peritoneal fluid, or fluid from fallopian tubes through transvaginal or laparoscopic procedures.[10] Most reliable are specimens recovered directly from the infected fallopian tube. Positive tubal gonococcal cultures are usually obtained only during early stages, because as the disease progresses the microorganism becomes intracellular or inhibited by leukocytes.

CLINICAL PRESENTATION

The clinical manifestations of PID are varied and nonspecific. The combination of various classic signs and symptoms are seen in only 20% of patients. The most common symptom is pelvic pain, which is usually bilateral, continuous, and aggravated by motion, making the bimanual examination difficult and nondiagnostic. The development of pain in the first 7 days of menses for the majority of the patients with *N. gonorrhoeae* infection suggests that the infection spreads from the cervix to tubes during menses. The cervical mucus that mechanically protects bacterial penetration is lost during menses, allowing entry of bacteria into the endometrium. Fever and chills are present only in 40% of patient with severe PID.

Four to 20% of patients develop the Fitz-Hugh–Curtis syndrome, also known as perihepatitis, which is an inflammatory reaction of the liver capsule and peritoneum of the adjacent abdominal wall. Clinically, patients present with right upper quadrant pain similar to that seen in patients with acute cholecystitis.[11,12]

The number of diagnostic tests used in PID suggest the difficulty in diagnosis and nonspecificity in the findings.

IMAGING

The imaging modalities that are available include sonography (transabdominal and transvaginal), CT, and MRI. Sonography should be the initial study because it is highly accurate in the diagnosis of PID and is also effective for management and treatment. Spirtos and co-workers[13] found that transabdominal sonographic findings were consistent with PID in 94% of patients with severe PID, in 80% of patients with moderate PID, and in 65% of patients with mild PID. Swayne and associates[14] correlated transabdominal sonographic features with pathologic findings in patients with PID but were unable to differentiate between the various entities of the PID spectrum such as pyosalpinx, hydrosalpinx, chronic salpingitis, tuboovarian complex, and tuboovarian abscess. Even though the transabdominal technique gives more global extent of the process and is able to identify masses high in the pelvis, the high-frequency intravaginal probe closer to the pelvic structures provides a higher resolution and can better characterize and determine the origin of the mass. Bulas and colleagues[15] compared transabdominal sonography with transvaginal sonography in 84 patients with the clinical diagnosis of PID and found transvaginal sonography to provide additional information in 71% of the patients. The improved resolution provided by the intravaginal probe allows differentiation of ovarian from tubal pathologic processes and of the various stages of PID without laparoscopy.[16] The ability to identify the severity of the disease contributes to deciding on the best management of the patient.[15]

SONOGRAPHIC FINDINGS

A normal pelvic sonogram in the right clinical setting does not exclude inflammatory disease. Mild tubal erythema

present in early cases of PID may not be visualized with ultrasound.[14] However, the majority of the patients with PID have various sonographic abnormalities that have been described.

Free Fluid

A small amount of anechoic free fluid in the cul-de-sac can be seen in early stages of PID and is indistinguishable from normal, physiologic fluid in mid cycle after follicular rupture.[17] Free pelvic fluid has been detected by transvaginal sonography in 77% with and 21% without endometritis.[18] In PID, the free fluid may represent a response to the inflammatory process or spillage of fluid from the tubes into the peritoneal cavity. However, as the disease progresses or the tuboovarian abscess ruptures, greater amounts of fluid may accumulate and have increase echogenicity, representing either inflammatory exudate, pus, or blood. An increase in echogenicity in the fluid may signal severity of the inflammatory disease. Kohkichi and colleagues[19] found that 47.2% of the patients with PID had echogenic free fluid in the cul-de-sac. However, in young females, echogenic free fluid in the adnexa or cul-de-sac can also be seen in the presence of ectopic pregnancy, ovarian torsion, or nongynecologic abscess.[20]

Uterus

Bowie and colleagues[21] described the transabdominal sonographic findings of ill-defined uterine borders in patients with PID and called it the "indefinite uterus." This sign occurs in both acute and chronic PID.[14]

Blurring of the margins of the uterus, adnexa, and other pelvic structures can be seen in the presence of both inflammatory and noninflammatory disease such as endometriosis, ovarian tumor, and fibroids. Periuterine inflammatory changes have been identified in only 25% of patients with PID using the transvaginal technique.[16] Fixation of the pelvic organs by adhesions in PID can be seen by the lack of motion of the pelvic structures when the transvaginal transducer is gently pushed and pulled. This feature is called the absence of "the sliding organ sign" and was described by Timor-Tritsch.[22] Uterine enlargement described with transabdominal sonography is only seen with transvaginal sonography in 25% of patients who were laparoscopically or by biopsy confirmed to have PID.[16] This is probably because the size of the uterus can be difficult to evaluate with the narrow field of view of the intravaginal probe.

Endometritis, present in nearly all patients with salpingitis, can be clinically silent and sonographically inapparent. It may be depicted sonographically by increased endometrial echogenicity and increased thickness of more than 14 mm.[23] The endometrial thickness is a nonspecific finding that requires clinical correlation. Acoustic enhancement posterior to the endometrial echoes is frequently seen. Areas of de-

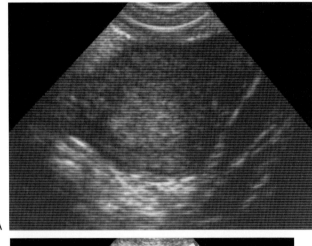

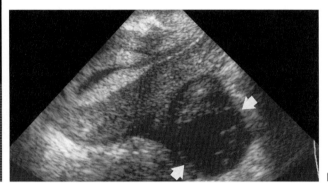

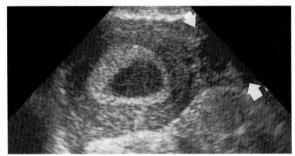

FIG. 7-1. Endometritis can present as a thickened echogenic endometrium (**A,** coronal transvaginal view) or a complex endometrial fluid collection that can mimic a pseudogestational sac of an ectopic pregnancy. Arrows outline left adnexal abscess. (**B**) Sagittal view. (**C**) Coronal view.

creased echogenicity within the echogenic endometrium may represent blood, pus, or secretions. Variable amounts of fluid can be seen within the endometrium, broadening the differential diagnosis (Fig 7-1).[24] The endometrial fluid collections may mimic pseudogestational sacs seen in ectopic pregnancy, and, in these cases, a pregnancy assay is necessary for interpretation.[25] Transvaginal sonography has been shown to depict the endometrium better than the transabdominal technique.[26] The enhanced resolution obtained with the intravaginal probe may detect endometritis earlier than with transabdominal sonography.[27]

Fallopian Tubes

The fallopian tubes are normally narrow, measuring no more than 4 mm in diameter and not usually seen with ultrasound unless their lumen contains fluid or tubes are surrounded by fluid.[22] Transvaginal sonography can help predict tubal inflammation with a sensitivity of approximately 90%.[16,18]

In acute inflammation, the tubes dilate, elongate, and become tortuous, which is the most frequent sonographic finding of PID (Fig. 7-2). Visualization of a hydrosalpinx does not indicate the acuteness of the process because tubal distention can be seen as a sequela of previous infection or surgery. The dilated fallopian tubes may contain internal echoes representing pus (pyosalpinx) or blood (hematosalpinx) (Fig. 7-3).[28,29] Tessler and colleagues[30] described four transvaginal sonographic features of salpingitis. The most common was the fluid-filled tubular structure. The other

findings included well-defined echogenic walls, folded configuration, and linear echoes protruding into the lumen. Increased interface within the endosalpinx secondary to purulent exudate suggest acuteness of process and is referred

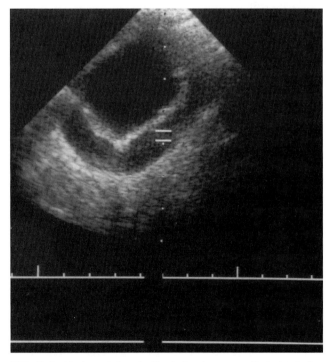

FIG. 7-2. Hydrosalpinx. In the left adnexa, a dilated tubular structure with no flow is seen on Doppler imaging.

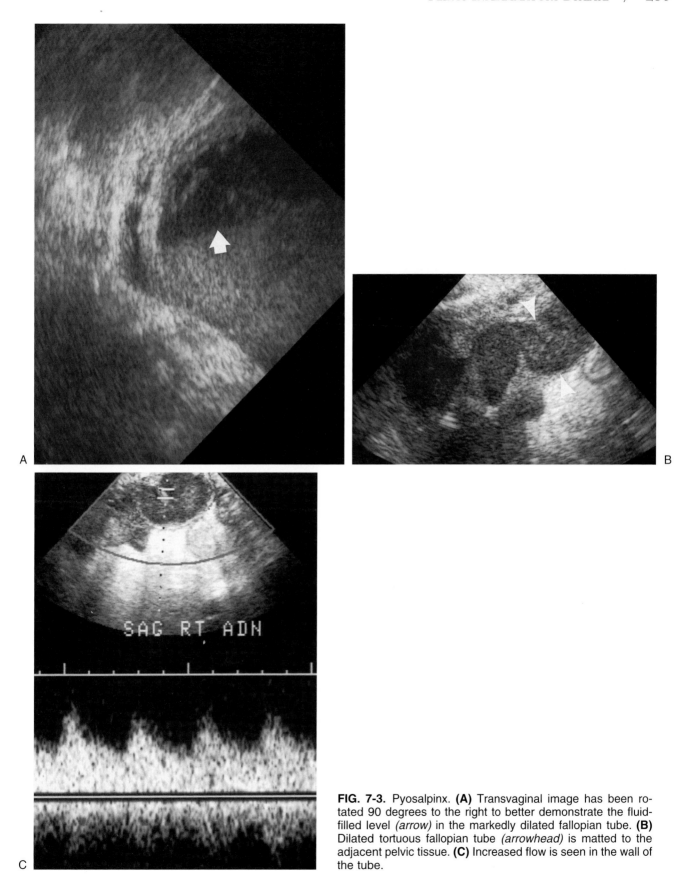

FIG. 7-3. Pyosalpinx. **(A)** Transvaginal image has been rotated 90 degrees to the right to better demonstrate the fluid-filled level *(arrow)* in the markedly dilated fallopian tube. **(B)** Dilated tortuous fallopian tube *(arrowhead)* is matted to the adjacent pelvic tissue. **(C)** Increased flow is seen in the wall of the tube.

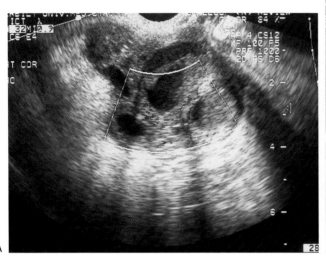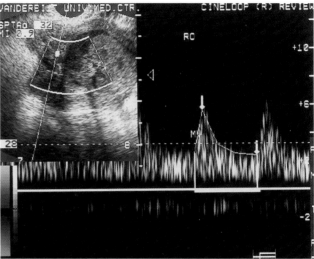

A   B

FIG. 7-4. Tuboovarian complex. **(A)** Large complex mass containing tubular structures representing matted fallopian tubes. Increased flow is seen around the inflamed fallopian tubes. **(B)** Doppler waveform in the periphery of the mass shows low impedance flow. (Courtesy of Arthur C. Fleischer, MD.)

to as the "string sign." This finding has been described in 50% of the patients with PID.[31] Tubal wall thickening may also be seen in other entities, such as chronic interstitial salpingitis, endometriosis, torsed fallopian tube, and fallopian tube carcinoma.[32]

Dilated tubular structures seen in the pelvis can also represent dilated pelvic veins or fluid-filled loops of bowel. Blood within the vessels may be identified by real-time sonography or duplex Doppler, color flow Doppler, or power Doppler imaging. Visualization of peristalsis within a viscus may help to distinguish bowel from dilated fallopian tube or vascular structures.

Dilated fallopian tubes may appear as complex, septated cystic masses (Fig. 7-4).[33,34] When large, dilated, convoluted fallopian tubes are not distinguished with ultrasound from the contiguous ovary, the diagnosis of tuboovarian complex is suspected. Even though the ovary is relatively resistant to infection, continuous spillage of purulent exudate from the tube into the periovarian space can cause involvement of the ovary.

Ovary

In the early stages of PID the only sonographic abnormality of the ovary may be an enlargement and loss of the typical corticomedullary differentiation.[31] Ovaries with increased stroma containing several follicles having a polycystic appearance are seen with transvaginal sonography in 47% of patients with PID (Fig. 7-5).[18] The configuration of the ovaries may be due to edematous changes in the stroma not allowing the follicles to rupture normally.

When a tuboovarian abscess occurs, it can be easily identified sonographically. Tuboovarian abscesses may be completely cystic, complex, or solid (Fig. 7-6). Transvaginal sonography can better depict septations, debris levels, and

irregularities in the walls of these masses. Visualization of gas within a mass may suggest an abscess. A follow-up study after a symptomatic patient has been treated with antibiotics can be useful in narrowing the diagnostic possibilities. If a complex adnexal mass decreases in size, an abscess can be inferred.

Nonspecific adnexal masses are identified sonographically in 38.9% of patients with PID and usually represent tuboovarian abscesses; less common they are pelvic adhesions.[31,35] Pelvic adhesions secondary to PID, endometriosis, or surgical changes may also present as complex masses. The masses probably represent fixation of the ovaries to the adjacent omentum and loops of bowel.

Tuboovarian abscess in postmenopausal women is rare and associated with increased mortality and morbidity. It may be related to recurrent PID. *Escherichia coli* is a more common etiologic agent. Vaginal bleeding is usually the pre-

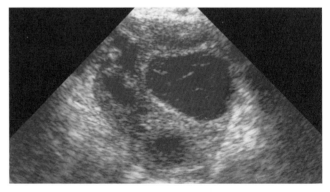

FIG. 7-5. Polycystic-appearing ovary. Ovary with increased stroma containing multiple follicles has been described in patients with inflammatory disease to the ovary.

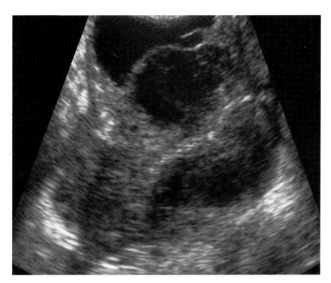

FIG. 7-6. Tuboovarian abscess. A large complex mass with thick septations and echogenic debris was evident in a patient with fever and chills.

senting sign, and occasionally fever and sepsis are associated. Diagnosis is made with exploratory laparotomy.[36,37]

MANAGEMENT

Tuboovarian abscesses that are refractory to medical therapy can be drained using ultrasound guidance (Fig. 7-7). Transvaginal sonographic guided technique avoids the risk of general anesthesia, surgical morbidity, and abdominal wall complications. The advantages of the transvaginal approach include that the loops of bowel, bladder, and uterus, in addition to the neurovascular structures encountered through the transgluteal approach, can be avoided.[38] Feld and co-workers[39] aspirated 41 pelvic collections by transvaginal sonography, causing either complete cure or tempo-

rizing the abscess in 78% of the patients. The two recurrences were in patients who had inflammatory bowel disease. Transabdominal sonography can also be used to guide the transvaginal drainage of pelvic abscesses in certain cases.[40]

When transvaginal sonography is limited, such as collections extending to the presacral space or into the ischiorectal fossa, the transrectal approach may be the best route. Kuligowska and colleagues[41] described a one-step method for treating pelvic abscesses by transrectal sonographically guided needle aspiration-lavage. Their technique does not require catheter placement or prolonged drainage. Complete aspiration for microbiologic cultures without catheter drainage may be the reasonable treatment in patients with no purulent aspirate.

In certain instances the transabdominal approach may be helpful. These include when the fluid collection is high in the pelvis and not accessible to the transvaginal probe or when the inflamed vaginal or rectal wall is very tender and there is a resistance to the needle.

DIFFERENTIAL DIAGNOSIS

The differential diagnosis for a nonspecific adnexal mass in a premenopausal female should include an ectopic pregnancy, hemorrhagic cyst, endometrioma, and neoplasm (benign or malignant). An ectopic pregnancy can present sonographically as a small fluid collection surrounded by an echogenic rim or a complex mass, usually extraovarian. However, usually a pregnancy assay is necessary for the diagnosis.[42,43] Identification of a yolk sac or embryo within the mass increases the sensitivity for diagnosing an ectopic pregnancy. Sonographically, a hemorrhagic cyst is seen as an intraovarian mass containing fine septations and internal echoes. A rim of ovarian tissue can usually be identified. An endometrioma or a chocolate cyst usually has homogeneous low-level internal echoes. However, the echogenicity of this

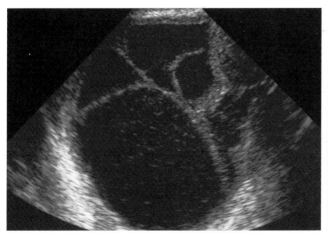
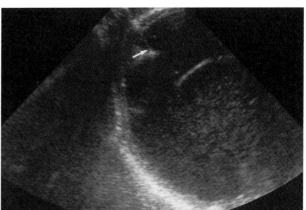

A   B

FIG. 7-7. Management of a large pelvic abscess. **(A)** Large pelvic abscess contains septation and echogenic debris. Transvaginal guided aspiration was performed. **(B)** An 18-gauge needle *(arrow)* is seen within the abscess.

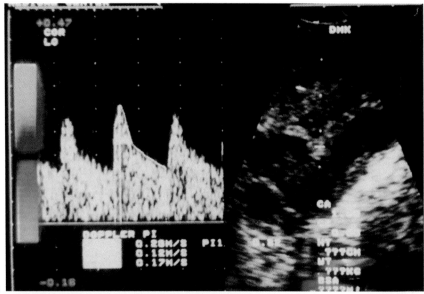

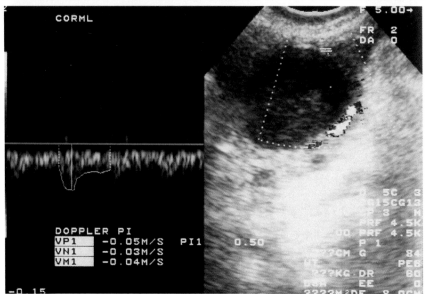

FIG. 7-8. Low resistant waveforms. **(A)** Tuboovarian abscess shows increased flow in the wall of the fallopian tube. **(B)** Similar waveform can be seen in the wall of an appendiceal abscess. (Courtesy of Arthur C. Fleischer, MD.)

ectopic endometrial tissue that undergoes cyclic changes depends on the age of hemorrhage. The actual implants in endometriosis are not detected sonographically because of their size of less than 5 mm. The patient usually presents with symptoms similar to PID. The pain may be caused by bleeding into these masses, and fever may be due to superimposed infection. Rupture of an endometrioma can result in fibrosis and adhesions, indistinguishable sonographically from the complex masses associated with PID. Ovarian neoplasms are intraovarian masses that may be cystic, complex, or solid. The cystadenomas are predominantly cystic whereas cystadenocarcinomas are cystic masses usually with thick and multiple septations that occasionally contain solid components.

Color flow, duplex, and power Doppler imaging may offer an alternative method in evaluating these nonspecific adnexal masses. Increased blood flow to an inflammatory mass causes a low pulsatility index (PI) of the uterine artery in

patients with severe acute PID (Fig. 7-8). Tinkelman and colleagues[44] found that PI in the uterine artery in patients with severe PID was between 1.5 and 2, which was lower than in the control group. In patients with PID, the PI did not change between different stages of the menstrual cycle, as was seen in the control group. As the infection subsided, the PI values approached normal level. Only in chronic infection did the PI value remain low in spite of normal C-reactive protein. A low resistance waveform can be identified in the margins of a tuboovarian complex and probably is due to vasodilatation and angioneogenesis that occurs in the first week of the inflammatory process.[45] Angioneogenesis is a process in which the macrophages secrete angioneogenesis factor and new capillary beds are formed. The increased blood flow in the capillaries is demonstrated with Doppler by a low PI and resistive index (RI) value. As the infectious process heals, scar forms and there is an increase resistance to flow with higher PI and RI values. With the

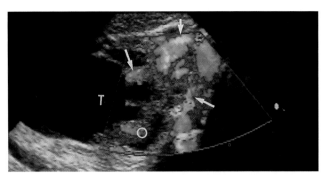

FIG. 7-9. Hydrosalpinx. Power Doppler reveals small vessels *(arrows)* within the ovary (O). Fimbriated portion of dilated fallopian tube (T) is seen.

addition of power Doppler technique to the transvaginal probes, identification of smaller vessels is possible (Fig. 7-9).

Duplex Doppler color flow or power Doppler imaging can help in narrowing the differential diagnosis. In the differential diagnosis for a menstruating female with a negative pregnancy test and presentation of acute pain is ovarian torsion. Ovarian torsion occurs from extensive mobility of adnexal supporting ligaments and is frequently associated with a mass. Sonographically, an enlarged hypoechoic ovary measuring from 23 to 44 cm^3 with loss of its corticomedullary differentiation or a complex or solid mass is visualized. The absence of flow confirms the diagnosis.[46] However, owing to the dual arterial supply to the ovary, the presence of flow does not exclude ovarian torsion.[47]

In a postpartum patient with fever and chills, in addition to abscess, the differential diagnosis includes ovarian vein thrombophlebitis. Doppler, color flow, and power Doppler imaging can also be helpful in diagnosing postpartum ovarian vein thrombophlebitis. This syndrome involves the pelvic, ovarian, iliac, and femoral veins and the inferior vena cava and occurs in 0.05% to 0.18% of all pregnancies.[48] The patient presents 1 to 5 days after delivery with pelvic pain and fever that persists up to 72 hours on antibiotic therapy. Clinically, there is a palpable mass usually on the right side. Complications include pulmonary emboli, which are seen in 21% of the cases. The treatment consists of both antibiotics and heparin. The diagnosis is confirmed when the fever decreases within 48 to 72 hours after initiating heparin. On sonography, an 8- to 10-cm nonspecific adnexal mass usually on the right, in addition to thrombus in the ovarian vein, inferior vena cava, or iliac or femoral veins can be identified (Fig. 7-10). MRI and CT may be helpful in the diagnosis of this entity.[49]

CONCLUSION

Sonography should be the first imaging modality when evaluating PID. The sonographic findings are usually nonspecific and must be correlated with the clinical history and laboratory findings. Transvaginal sonography has been shown to differentiate the various stages of PID and contributes to the selection of optimal management and treatment.

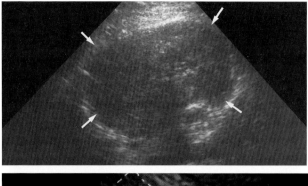

A

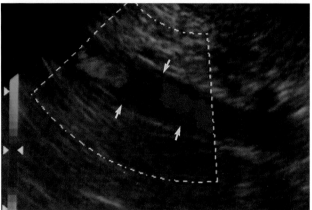

B

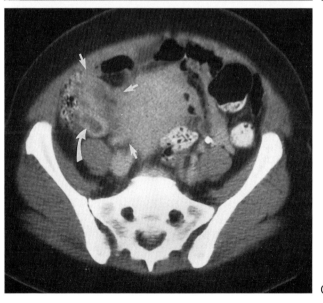

C

FIG. 7-10. Postpartum ovarian vein thrombophlebitis. Visualization of a right hypoechoic adnexal mass *(arrows)* **(A)** and thrombosis *(arrows)* in the iliac vein with color flow Doppler imaging **(B)** confirms the diagnosis. **(C)** CT scan reveals an ill-defined soft tissue density *(arrows)* with a thrombosed pelvic vein *(curved arrow)*.

REFERENCES

1. Freij BJ. Acute pelvic inflammatory disease. Semin Adolescent Med 1986;2:143.
2. Paavonen J. Pelvic inflammatory disease. Semin Dermatol 1990;9:126.
3. Westrom L. Incidence, prevalence, and trends of acute pelvic inflam-

matory disease and its consequences in industrialized countries. Am J Obstet Gynecol 1980;138:880.

4. Curran JW. Economic consequences of pelvic inflammatory disease in the United States. Am J Obstet Gynecol 1980;138:845.

5. Washington AE, Arno PS, Brooks MA. The economic cost of pelvic inflammatory disease. JAMA 1986;225:1735.

6. Lee NC, Rubin GL, Ory HW, et al. Type of intrauterine device and the risk of pelvic inflammatory disease. Obstet Gynecol 1983;62:1.

7. Williams CE, Lamb GHR, Lewis-Jones HG. Pelvic actinomycosis: beware the intrauterine contraceptive device. Br J Radiol 1990;63:134.

8. Eschenbach DA. Acute pelvic inflammatory disease. Urol Clin North Am 1984;11:65.

9. Eschenbach DA, Buchanan TM, Pollack HM, et al. Polymicrobial etiology of acute pelvic inflammatory disease. N Engl J Med 1975;293:166.

10. Sweet RL, Schacter J, James J, et al. Microbiology and pathogenesis and acute salpingitis as determined by laparoscopy: what is the appropriate site to sample? Am J Obstet Gynecol 1980;138:985.

11. Banerjee B, Rennison A, Boyes BE. Case reports: sonographic features in a case of Fitz-Hugh–Curtis syndrome masquerading as malignancy. Br J Radiol 1992;65:342.

12. Schoenfeld A, Fisch B, Cohen M, et al. Ultrasound findings in perihepatitis associated with pelvic inflammatory disease. J Clin Ultrasound 1992;20:339.

13. Spirtos NJ, Bernstine RL, Crawford WL, Fayle J. Sonography in acute pelvic inflammatory disease. J Reprod Med 1982;27:312.

14. Swayne LC, Love MB, Karasick SR. Pelvic inflammatory disease: sonographic-pathologic correlation. Radiology 1984;151:751.

15. Bulas DI, Ahlstrom PA, Sivit CJ, et al. Pelvic inflammatory disease in the adolescent: comparison of transabdominal and transvaginal sonographic evaluation. Radiology 1992;183:435.

16. Patten RM, Vincent LM, Wolner-Hanssen P, Thorpe E. Pelvic inflammatory disease and endovaginal sonography with laparoscopy correlation. J Ultrasound Med 1990;9:681.

17. Golden N, Cohen H, Gennari G, Neuhoff S. The use of pelvic ultrasonography in the evaluation of adolescents with pelvic inflammatory disease. Am J Dis Child 1987;141:1235.

18. Cacciatore B, Leminen A, Ingman-Friberg S, et al. Transvaginal sonographic findings in ambulatory patients with suspected pelvic inflammatory disease. Obstet Gynecol 1992;80:912.

19. Kohkichi H, Toshiyuki H, Showa A, et al. Ultrasonographic evaluation of pelvic inflammatory disease. Acta Obstet Gynaecol Jpn 1989;41:895.

20. Berland LL, Lawson TL, Foley WD, Albarelli JN. Ultrasound evaluation of pelvic infections. Radiol Clin North Am 1982;20:367.

21. Bowie JD. Ultrasound of gynecological pelvic masses: the indefinite uterus and other patterns associated with diagnostic error. J Clin Ultrasound 1977;5:323.

22. Timor-Tritsch IE, Rottem S, Thaler J. Review of transvaginal ultrasonography: a description with clinical application. Ultrasound Q 1988;6:1.

23. Fleischer AC, Mendelson EB, Böhm-Vélez M, Entmann SS. Transvaginal and transabdominal sonography of the endometrium. Semin Ultrasound CT MR 1988;9:81.

24. Laing FC, Filly RA, Marks WM, Brown TW. Ultrasonic demonstration of endometrial fluid collections unassociated with pregnancy. Radiology 1980:471.

25. Nyberg DA, Laing FC, Filly RA, et al. Ultrasonographic differentiation of the gestational sac of early intrauterine pregnancy from the pseudogestational sac of ectopic pregnancy. Radiology 1983;146:755.

26. Mendelson EB, Böhm-Vélez M, Joseph N, et al. Endometrial abnormalities: evaluation with transvaginal sonography. AJR 1988;150:139.

27. Mendelson EB, Böhm-Vélez M, Joseph N, et al. Gynecologic imaging, comparison of transabdominal and transvaginal sonography. Radiology 1988;166:321.

28. Subramanyam BR, Raghavendra BN, Balthazar EJ, et al. Hematosalpinx in tubal pregnancy: endovaginal vs. transabdominal sonography. AJR 1990;155:307.

29. Mikkelsen AL, Felding C. Laparoscopy and ultrasound examination in women with acute pelvic pain. Gynecol Obstet Invest 1990;30:163.

30. Tessler FN, Perella RR, Fleischer AC, Grant EG. Endovaginal sonographic diagnosis of dilated fallopian tubes. AJR 1989;153:523.

31. Hata K, Hata T, Aoki S, et al. Ultrasonographic evaluation of pelvic inflammatory disease. Acta Obst Gynaecol Jpn 1989;41:895.

32. Sherer DM, Liberto L. Abramovicz JS, et al. Endovaginal sonographic features associated with isolated torsion of the fallopian tube. J Ultrasound Med 1991;10:107.

33. Reuter K, Cohen S, Daly D. Ultrasonic presentation of giant hydrosalpinges in asymptomatic patients. J Clin Ultrasound 1987;15:45.

34. Uhrich PC, Sanders RC. Ultrasonic characteristics of pelvic inflammatory masses. J Clin Ultrasound 1976;4:199.

35. Dewbury KC, Joseph AE. The role of ultrasound scanning. Scand J Gastroenterol Suppl 1994;203:5.

36. Kremer S, Kutcher R, Rosenblatt R, et al. Postmenopausal tubo-ovarian abscess: sonographic considerations and clinical significance. J Ultrasound Med 1992;11:613.

37. Fisher M, Drugan A, Gaven J, et al. Case report: postmenopausal tubo-ovarian abscess. Acta Obstet Gynecol Scand 1986;65:661.

38. Aboulghar MA, Mansour RT, Serour GI. Ultrasonographically guided transvaginal aspiration of tuboovarian abscesses and pyosalpinges: an optional treatment for acute pelvic inflammatory disease. Am J Obstet Gynecol 1995;172:1501.

39. Feld R, Eschelman DJ, Sagerman JE, et al. Treatment of pelvic abscesses and other fluid collections: efficacy of transvaginal sonographically guided aspiration and drainage. AJR 1994;163:1141.

40. Nosher TL, Winchman HK, Needell GS. Transvaginal pelvic abscess drainage with US guidance. Radiology 1987;165:872.

41. Kuligowska E, Keller E, Ferrucci JT. Treatment of pelvic abscesses: value of one-step sonographically guided transrectal needle aspiration and lavage. AJR 1995;164:201.

42. Böhm-Vélez M, Mendelson EB, Freimanis MG. Transvaginal sonography in evaluating ectopic pregnancy. Semin Ultrasound CT MR 1990;11:44.

43. Frates MC, Laing FC. Sonographic evaluation of ectopic pregnancy: an update. AJR 1995;165:251.

44. Tinkanen H, Kujansuu E. Doppler ultrasound studies in pelvic inflammatory disease. Gynecol Obstet Invest 1992;34:240.

45. Tinkanen H, Kujansuu E. Doppler ultrasound findings in tubo-ovarian infectious complex. J Clin Ultrasound 1993;21:175.

46. Rosado WM Jr, Trambert MA, Gosink BB, et al. Adnexal torsion: diagnosis by using Doppler sonography. AJR 1992;159:1251.

47. Fleischer AC, Stein SM, Cullinan JA, Warner MA. Color Doppler sonography of adnexal torsion. J Ultrasound Med 1995;14:523.

48. Grant TH, Schoettle BW, Buchsbaum MS. Postpartum ovarian vein thrombosis: diagnosis by clot protrusion into the inferior vena cava at sonography. AJR 1993;160:551.

49. Baran GW, Frisch KM. Duplex Doppler evaluation of puerperal ovarian vein thrombosis. AJR 1987;149:321.

Clinical Gynecologic Imaging, edited
by Arthur C. Fleischer, Marcia C. Javitt,
R. Brooke Jeffrey, Jr., and Howard W. Jones III,
Lippincott-Raven Publishers, Philadelphia © 1997.

CHAPTER 8

Pelvic Pain

Pelvic Pain: Overview

Howard W. Jones III, MD

One of the most vexing problems for both the patient and clinician is discerning the cause of pelvic pain. The symptoms are largely subjective, the physical findings often equivocal, and results of laboratory tests and imaging studies frequently within normal limits. Nevertheless, the symptom of pelvic pain is common and a carefully considered approach to diagnosis will provide the best chance to identify and remedy the patient's complaints with the most economic use of testing.

In this subchapter dysmenorrhea, which is pain associated with the ovulatory menstrual cycle, is not formally considered. This type of pelvic pain is due to prostaglandin release and is noted most often in teenagers and young women. It often resolves with the first pregnancy.

When considering the diagnosis of pelvic pain, it is usually helpful to both localize the pelvic organ involved and also attempt to identify the etiology of the pain. For example, ectopic pregnancy may involve the fallopian tube and be a pregnancy-related event. Acute pelvic inflammatory disease also involves the fallopian tube, but the cause is infectious. Symptoms of pelvic pain and fever can also be seen in acute

appendicitis, which is also an infection but involves the appendix. By careful evaluation of the history and physical findings and appropriate use of imaging and laboratory studies, it is usually possible to make a diagnosis and develop a treatment plan.

ACUTE PELVIC PAIN

History

Because the causes and management of acute pelvic pain differ significantly from those of chronic pain, they are considered separately here. Acute pelvic pain is often abrupt in onset, and its duration is usually measured in hours or days. In addition to the onset of the pain, its severity, character, and location need to be established. As with most pelvic conditions, a menstrual history is absolutely crucial. A ruptured ectopic pregnancy can be fatal, and therefore pregnancy-associated diagnoses must be considered. The date of the last menstrual period, type of contraception, regularity

245

TABLE 8-1. *Causes of acute pelvic pain*

GYNECOLOGIC
Endometriosis
Infection
  Pelvic inflammatory disease
  Tuboovarian abscess
Ovarian
  Adnexal torsion
  Corpus luteum cyst
  Endometrioma
  Follicular cyst
  Neoplasm
  Ovulation
  Ruptured cyst
Uterine
  Fibroids: degeneration, torsion
  Dysmenorrhea

PREGNANCY-RELATED
Abortion: septic, spontaneous
Ectopic pregnancy
Intrauterine pregnancy

GASTROINTESTINAL
Appendicitis
Constipation
Diverticulitis
Gastroenteritis
Inflammatory bowel disease

UROLOGIC
Acute cystitis
Ureteral calculi

of menses, any other vaginal bleeding, and sexual activity should all be a part of the history. In young unmarried women, an accurate history of sexual activity and possible pregnancy may be difficult to obtain and require sensitivity and a nonjudgmental approach by the physician. Fever is another symptom that may be helpful in identifying an infectious process.

A past history of similar episodes and any past surgical history may also be important. Finally, any gastrointestinal or urinary tract symptoms should be specifically asked about, such as whether the patient has experienced a change in bowel or bladder habits.

The differential diagnosis of acute pelvic pain is listed in Table 8-1. From the history it should be possible to have a good idea about the cause of the pain (eg, inflammatory, pregnancy-related, endometriosis).

Physical Examination

Vital signs may be a clue to infection when a fever is present, or acute anemia may be noted if the patient has tachycardia. The abdominal examination may provide an indication of the acuity of the situation. Many patients have tenderness to deep palpation in one or both lower quadrants, but rebound tenderness is an important finding of significant peritoneal inflammation. Normal bowel sounds are somewhat reassuring, whereas hypoactive bowel sounds may be a response to inflammation and hyperactive sounds usually suggest an obstruction. Superpubic tenderness can be found in patients with acute cystitis or endometritis. Costovertebral tenderness is uncommon in women complaining of pelvic pain but is easy to check and completes the urinary tract examination.

The pelvic examination is a key part in the evaluation of acute pelvic pain. The speculum examination allows the clinician the opportunity to check for uterine bleeding or vaginal or cervical discharge. On bimanual examination, pelvic tenderness can be carefully evaluated and the size and character of the uterus and ovaries can be palpated. In cases of severe pain and tenderness, the patient's discomfort will preclude a good examination, which makes imaging studies such as sonography particularly useful. Cervical motion tenderness is characteristic of acute pelvic inflammation seen with pelvic inflammatory disease. Except for the rare case associated with an intrauterine device, pelvic inflammatory disease is almost always associated with bilateral adnexal tenderness. Unilateral tenderness is common with ovarian cysts, adnexal torsion, ectopic pregnancy, or appendicitis. The size, consistency, and mobility of the uterus and ovaries should also be noted. Nodularity in the uterosacral ligaments is characteristic of endometriosis but is a relatively uncommon finding.

Laboratory Workup

The single most important laboratory test in a patient with pelvic pain is a pregnancy test. Although history of last menstrual period, contraception, and sexual activity will usually rule out the possibility of pregnancy, this is such an important diagnosis that almost every women in the reproductive age group who presents with acute pelvic pain should have a rapid pregnancy test. The current immunologic tests are positive at greater than 5.0 mIU of β-human chorionic gonadotropin (β-hCG), which means that by the time of the first missed period the tests are often positive.

A routine complete blood cell count is also a valuable test because an elevated white blood cell count is indicative of infection and a low hematocrit or hemoglobin is seen with acute (or chronic) blood loss. The erythrocyte sedimentation rate is a very nonspecific indication of infection and not often used.

Imaging studies, especially sonography, are very useful in the evaluation of acute pelvic pain and are discussed in another section of this chapter.

Management

There are really three possible management options for patients with acute pelvic pain: surgery, medical therapy, and observation. Careful follow-up with mild analgesics is appropriate for functional corpus cysts such as follicular or corpus luteum cyst, ovulation pain, and dysmenorrhea.

Pelvic inflammatory disease, diverticular abscess, and cystitis all require antibiotics,[1] although, as with endometriosis, if there is a mass—endometrioma or abscess—surgical excision or drainage is usually required.

Both endometriosis and ectopic pregnancy can be managed with either medical therapy or surgery. Oral contraceptives, danazol, and gonadotropin-releasing hormone analogues have been very successful for the treatment of endometriosis, although long-term management is not usually possible.[2] Surgical treatment of endometriosis associated with infertility or with endometriomas is recommended. The extent of the endometriosis and tubal obstruction may be evaluated preoperatively with pelvic sonography or hysterosalpinogography or both. In many instances, laparoscopy may be used instead of traditional open pelvic surgery. These minimally invasive techniques result in fewer postoperative adhesions and a more rapid recovery.

Ectopic pregnancy may be treated with methotrexate if the diagnosis can be made early.[3] Although some larger lesions can be successfully managed by chemotherapy, if the tubal ectopic pregnancy is greater than or equal to 3 cm in diameter and the β-hCG level is less than 5000 mIU/mL, a success rate of 80% or greater can be expected using either intramuscular methotrexate at 1 mg/kg or transvaginal sonographic-guided aspiration of the gestational sac followed by methotrexate instillation. Laparoscopic salpingostomy or salpingectomy may be used for larger ectopic pregnancies, and exploratory laparotomy may still be necessary if the ectopic pregnancy has ruptured with significant hemoperitoneum.

Pelvic masses, neoplastic ovarian cysts, and uterine fibroids all should be managed surgically, but again the laparoscopic approach is widely used so the size and character of the mass, as well as the presence of intraperitoneal fluid or blood, will help the surgeon decide on the best approach.

CHRONIC PELVIC PAIN

Pelvic pain that has been present for 6 months or longer is defined as chronic and is much more difficult to diagnose and treat (Table 8-2). In some cases, uterine fibroids or endometriosis can be identified, but in many cases the diagnosis is unclear and almost always there is a significant psychological component to the pain. This does not mean that the pain is imaginary but rather that the chronic symptom of pelvic pain has resulted in certain lifestyle and emotional changes that will not and cannot be instantly cured by an operation or new medication. Many of these problems are related to sexual intercourse or the inability to hold a job because of the pain. Steege and Stout[4] have proposed the term *chronic pelvic pain syndrome,* which they define as pelvic pain for more than 6 months with at least three of the following four criteria: (1) inadequate relief of symptoms by prior therapies,

TABLE 8-2. *Causes of chronic pelvic pain*

GYNECOLOGIC
Adhesions
Chronic pelvic inflammatory disease
Endometriosis
Ovarian remnant
Pelvic floor myalgia
Pelvic congestion
Pelvic relaxation
Retained ovary syndrome
Uterine fibroids

ABDOMINAL WALL FACTORS
Myofascial pain
Trigger points

GASTROINTESTINAL
Constipation
Diverticulitis
Inflammatory bowel disease
Irritable bowel syndrome

UROLOGIC
Interstitial cystitis
Urethral syndrome

PSYCHOLOGICAL

(2) impaired physical functionality, (3) altered family role, and (4) at least one vegetative sign of depression.

In many cases it is not possible to "cure" pelvic pain as one might cure appendicitis or a twisted ovarian cyst. It may need to be "treated" or "managed" much the way one would manage a patient with migraine headaches. Because of the multifaceted nature of chronic pelvic pain, such patients may be best evaluated and managed by a team approach involving a clinical psychologist.[5] The general clinician needs to be able to initiate the workup and eliminate specific conditions such as uterine fibroids, large adnexal masses, and chronic pelvic inflammatory disease for which appropriate therapy can be recommended.

History

In addition to a careful history concerning the character of the pain as discussed previously in the section on acute pelvic pain, it is most important to take a detailed history of the types of treatment the patient has already received. Typically, such women have seen a number of physicians and have had several surgical procedures. In some cases the patient will arrive with an armload of records and radiographs. In any case it may be useful to document the surgical findings with operative notes and pathology reports. It is also important to speak with the previous treating physicians because the written notes may not convey the complete picture and the patient's description of the procedures, therapy, and results may differ from observations and records made at the time.

How does the pain affect the patient's life? Is it present all the time? What causes the pain? Does anything relieve the pain? Is the patient able to work? Can she do normal household tasks? How has the pain affected her relationship with her spouse? Her family? Does the pain make intercourse impossible? Symptoms of depression such as sleeplessness, inability to concentrate, and feelings of inadequacy should also be sought. Has she been treated with antidepressants? What type of pain medication has she used? This is an indicator of the severity of the pain and may be a clue to drug abuse.

In many cases a history of sexual or physical abuse may be elicited in women who develop chronic pelvic pain.[6] Because of the sensitive nature of such history, it is useful to establish a certain rapport with the patient before embarking on this area of questioning.

Physical Examination

As with acute pelvic pain patients, the pelvic examination is the most important part of the examination. However, a complete physical examination is indicated because these patients often have a variety of symptoms in addition to pelvic pain. Previous abdominal incisions should be carefully examined and palpated to search for hernias or trigger points that initiate the pain.

Laboratory Workup

Even with longstanding pelvic pain, it is important to be sure a life-threatening condition does not exist. Malignant ovarian tumors, uterine sarcomas, and colon cancer can produce chronic pelvic symptoms so these diagnoses need to be ruled out, along with diverticular and chronic tuboovarian abscess. History and physical examination, as well as a careful review of the patient's previous workup, will allow the clinician to select the appropriate laboratory work. In addition to a complete blood cell count, tumor markers such as CA 125 and carcinoembryonic antigen may be helpful. Sonography, CT, and MRI, as well as barium examination or intravenous pyelography, may be indicated, but the usefulness of repeated studies in patients who have had a previous normal study at another facility within the past year or so should be questioned.

Management

In most cases it is the desire of the physician to cure the patient—to surgically correct a problem or prescribe a medication that alleviates the women's symptoms. But in some cases of chronic pelvic pain this is not possible.[7] In some cases a small pelvic mass can be identified on imaging studies and the diagnosis of endometriosis[8] or ovarian remnant[9] made, and surgical removal recommended. Enlarged pelvic or uterine veins are associated with the diagnosis of pelvic congestion syndrome--a controversial diagnosis that some authors believe is a cause of pelvic pain.[10] Hysterectomy is generally recommended as the treatment of choice, but Sichlau and coworkers[11] have described transcatheter embolectomy in three women with good results.

The role of pelvic adhesions in chronic pelvic pain is also controversial. Undoubtedly, some women with adhesions have pain, but they often have a long history of pelvic infection and several operations so it is important to carefully evaluate these women before making a diagnosis of adhesions. It is also important to be sure the patient and her family understand the possibility that surgery will not cure her symptoms and the risk of complications, including a worsening of the symptoms. In experienced hands, laparoscopy may be used to evaluate the presence of adhesions and to perform adhesiolysis.[12]

If an enlarged uterine fibroid or a chronic inflammatory condition can be identified and surgically removed or treated with antibiotics, a true cure can be achieved; but all too often the cause of the pain remains unclear, and treatment is far less likely to be successful if the diagnosis is unknown or incorrect. In many cases prolonged management of this chronic pain is required. The secondary gain of this pelvic pain must be considered, and antidepressants may prove useful.[13] Classic psychotherapy is rarely helpful, but clinical psychologists or psychiatrists may be involved in the patient's care. A team approach, including psychologists, physical therapists, anesthesiologists, and gynecologists has been recommended by some authors.

REFERENCES

1. Lipscomb GH, Ling FW. Relationship of pelvic infection and chronic pelvic pain. Obstet Gynecol Clin North Am 1993;20:699.
2. Lu PY, Ory SJ. Endometriosis: current management. Mayo Clin Proc 1995;70:453.
3. Fernandez H, Baton C, Benifla J-L, et al. Methotrexate treatment of ectopic pregnancy: 100 cases treated by primary transvaginal injection under sonographic control. Fertil Steril 1993;59:773.
4. Steege JF, Stout AL. Resolution of chronic pelvic pain following laparoscopic adhesiolysis. Am J Obstet Gynecol 1991;165:278.
5. Milburn A, Reiter RC, Rhomberg AT. Multidisciplinary approach to chronic pelvic pain. Obstet Gynecol Clin North Am 1993;20:643.
6. Walling MK, Reiter RC, O'Hara MW, et al. Abuse history and chronic pain in women: I. Prevalences of sexual abuse and physical abuse. Obstet Gynecol 1994;84:193.
7. McDonald JS. Management of chronic pelvic pain. Obstet Gynecol Clin North Am 1993;20:817.
8. Sutton CJB, Ewen SP, Whitelaw N, Haines P. Prospective, randomized, double-blind, controlled trial of laser laparoscopy in the treatment of pelvic pain associated with minimal, mild, and moderate endometriosis. Fertil Steril 1994;62:696.
9. Siddall-Allum J, Rae T, Rogers V, et al. Chronic pelvic pain caused by residual ovaries and ovarian remnants. Br J Obstet Gynaecol 1994;101:979.
10. Gupta A, McCarthy S. Pelvic varices as a cause for pelvic pain: MRI appearance. Magn Reson Imaging 1994;12:679.
11. Sichlau MJ, Yao JST, Vogelzang RL. Transcatheter embolotherapy for the treatment of pelvic congestion syndrome. Obstet Gynecol 1994;83:892.
12. Steege JF. Repeated clinic laparoscopy for the treatment of pelvic adhesions: A pilot study. Obstet Gynecol 1994;83:276–279.
13. Waller KG, Shaw RW. Endometriosis, pelvic pain, and psychological functioning. Fertil Steril 1995;63:796.

Conventional and Color Doppler Transvaginal Sonography in Pelvic Pain

Arthur C. Fleischer, MD

In this subchapter the discussion is focused on the use of diagnostic imaging in the evaluation of women with pelvic pain. There are many causes of pelvic pain. Some can be detected and evaluated by sonography, MRI, and other imaging procedures, but in some patients the cause of the pain remains uncertain. The real-time capability of transvaginal sonography affords depiction of causes that may be functional, such as hemorrhagic ovarian cysts. Interestingly enough, only 63% of women undergoing laparoscopy for pelvic pain with normal pelvic examinations had abnormal findings.[1] Conversely, 18% of women with pain and abnormal pelvic examinations had no abnormalities at laparoscopy. Thus, there is not always a correlation between the presence of pelvic pain and the abnormality of the pelvic organs. Ovarian abnormalities accounted for approximately 10% in this series of women with pelvic pain who underwent laparoscopy; 27% had pelvic adhesions, 22% had pelvic inflammatory disease, and 3% had unsuspected endometrioma.

The disorders that are emphasized here include

- Adnexal torsion
- Endometriosis/adenomyosis
- Ureteral calculi
- Appendicitis and other bowel related disorders such as ischemic bowel disease
- Pelvic congestion syndrome

Disorders such as ectopic pregnancy and endometriosis are covered elsewhere in this volume.

ADNEXAL TORSION

Color Doppler sonography has an important role in the evaluation of women presenting with lower abdominal and pelvic pain. In particular, the possibility of adnexal torsion can be assessed using this modality.

In this subchapter the evaluation of patients with sus-

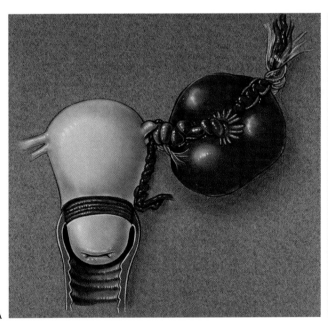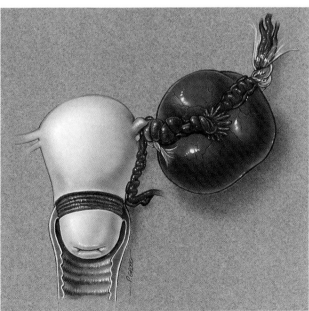

A   B

FIG. 8-1. Diagrams showing adnexal (ovarian) torsion in early **(A)** and late **(B)** phase. In the acute phase (first hour) there is engorgement of the ovary and tube that is followed by gangrenous changes later.

pected adnexal torsion with color Doppler sonography is discussed. The importance of recognition of certain flow patterns is emphasized as they relate to ovarian viability.

Clinical Features

The female patient may have a variety of disorders that result in lower abdominal and pelvic pain.[2,3] Transvaginal and transabdominal sonography play a pivotal role in distinguishing adnexal causes from nongynecologic causes, such as appendicitis or distal ureteral obstruction due to a renal calculus (Figs. 8-1 through 8-5).[4] Patients with adnexal torsion may present several times to the emergency department.[5] Their symptoms may be attributed to appendicitis, urinary tract infection, inflammatory bowel disease, endometriosis, or functional ovulatory pain. It is not uncommon for patients who have the final diagnosis of adnexal torsion

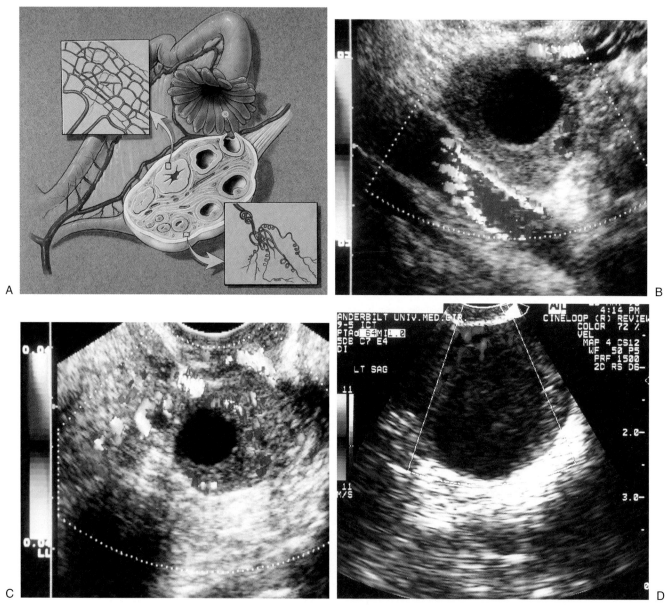

FIG. 8-2. Normal adnexal blood flow. **(A)** Diagram of arterial flow to ovary. The ovary is supplied by the main ovarian artery, which branches from the aorta and the adnexal branch of the uterine artery. There are arterial anastomoses with the tubal blood supply as well. Intraovarian arterial flow depends on the proximity to a developing follicle or corpus luteum. Near a corpus luteum, the flow has low resistance and high diastolic flow, whereas in areas away from developing follicles the intraovarian arterioles are spiral and have a high resistance. Venous flow roughly parallels arterial flow. **(B)** Transvaginal color Doppler sonogram showing intraovarian blood flow derived from both the adnexal branch of the uterine artery and the main ovarian artery. The internal iliac vein is seen immediately adjacent to the ovary. **(C)** Same as **B** in a coronal plane. **(D)** Intraovarian blood flow surrounding a hemorrhagic corpus luteum.

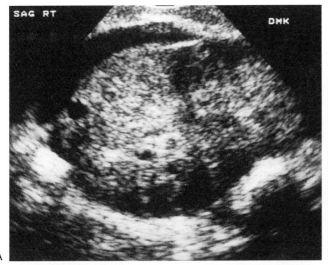
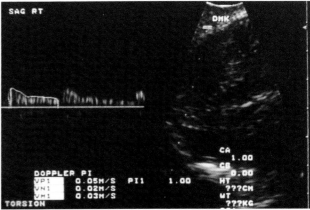

A

B

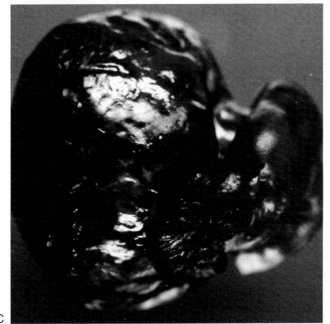

C

FIG. 8-3. Enlarged ovary in an 18-year old young woman presenting with a 3-day history of acute pelvic pain. A similar episode was experienced 1 and 2 months before this admission. **(A)** Transvaginal sonogram showing enlarged right ovary containing several immature follicles in the periphery. **(B)** Triplex transvaginal color Doppler sonogram showing slow arterial flow in the region of the adnexal branch of the uterine artery. **(C)** Resected specimen showing gangrenous ovary.

to be treated mistakenly for urinary tract infection or other disorders. The pain associated with adnexal torsion is usually intense and localized to either adnexal region. It may be intermittent; this can be attributed to intermittent episodes of incomplete torsion. Expeditious and confident identification of adnexal torsion by color Doppler imaging may result in salvage of the ovaries and fallopian tubes.

The pathophysiology of torsion is variable depending on the cause. In some cases there is massive edema of the ovary probably related to vasodilatation with leakage of blood into the endometrium combined with hindered venous outflow.[6] In others, thrombus within the ovarian vein may contribute to venous engorgement of the ovary, further precipitating torsion. I have documented the presence of thrombi within the smaller intraovarian veins in some cases of torsion (Fig. 8-6). In other cases, torsion is associated with a mass or hemorrhage within the ovary (Figs. 8-7 and 8-8). Some clini-

cians attribute torsion to relatively lax ligamentous support of the ovary, particularly in children. Tubal torsion should be suspected in women who have undergone tubal ligation (Figs. 8-9 and 8-10). The ligated tubal segment may become filled with fluid and be predisposed to torsion. Ovulation stimulation may be associated with enlarged ovaries that contain numerous follicles. These ovaries tend to torse, and quick recognition of torsion may lead to conservative surgery.[7] Adnexal torsion may also be encountered in pregnant patients, possibly related to the results of corpus luteum cysts that persist during pregnancy (see Fig. 8-10).

Sonographic Findings

It has been my observation that torsion associated with venous obstruction results in an enlarged but morphologi-

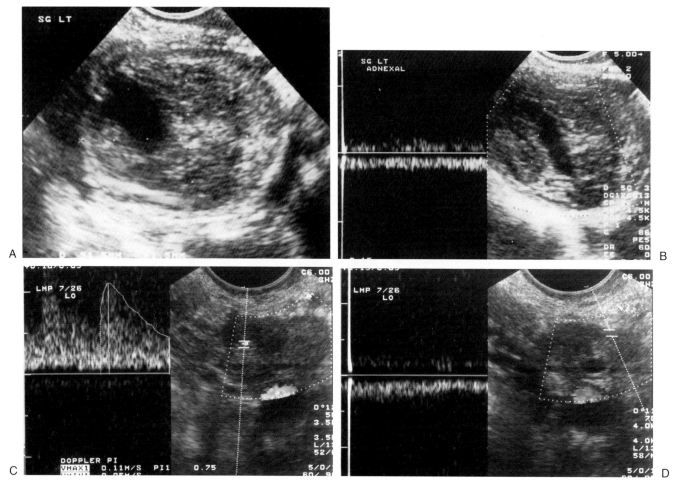

FIG. 8-4. Enlarged ovary found to be viable at surgery in a 28-year-old woman presenting with 2 weeks of intermittent left lower quadrant pain. **(A)** Transvaginal sonogram demonstrating 5 × 6-cm ovary with hypoechoic area. **(B)** Triplex transvaginal color Doppler sonogram demonstrating arterial and venous flow. At surgery, this ovary appeared viable, was untwisted, and became perfused, as determined by visual inspection. Same patient's left ovary 1 year later showing normal intraovarian arterial **(C)** and venous flow **(D)**.

cally recognizable ovary.[5] The sonographic findings most likely correlate with the presence or absence of intraovarian hemorrhage and chronicity and completeness of the torsion. It is possible that because the ovary has a dual arterial blood supply, torsion in one arterial system may be compensated by increased flow from blood in the other arterial system. Chronic torsion may be associated with the establishment of collateral arterial and venous flow. As in testicular torsion, repeated episodes might even be associated with a reactive hyperemia.

The blood supply to the ovary is derived from the adnexal branch of the uterine artery as well as from the main ovarian artery, which is a direct branch from the aorta. This vascular arrangement is illustrated in Figure 8-1, and the sonographic findings are shown in the accompanying color Doppler sonograms. The arterial blood supply to the ovary is derived from these two large branches, with numerous arterioles extending to the capsule of the ovary and small penetrating arterioles within the ovary itself. In an area that lacks follicular devel-

opment these intraovarian arteries are coiled, whereas in areas of corpora lutea formation, a low impedance vascular arcade can be recognized on transvaginal color Doppler sonography.

The ovarian blood supply may vary from usually five to six branches that penetrate the capsule to two large branches with multiple twigs. The arterial flow may be derived predominantly from either the adnexal branch of the uterine artery or the main ovarian artery.[8]

The Doppler waveforms derived from intraovarian vessels depend on their proximity to functional follicles or corpora lutea. Venous blood supply within and support surrounding the ovary can also be routinely detected on color Doppler imaging. If torsion is suspected on one side, it is important for the sonographer to document the presence of flow within the ovary on the unaffected side. It is also important to recognize that the proper gain, pulse repetition frequency, and black/white and color Doppler read/write priority settings are used because the lack of flow can be produced if the

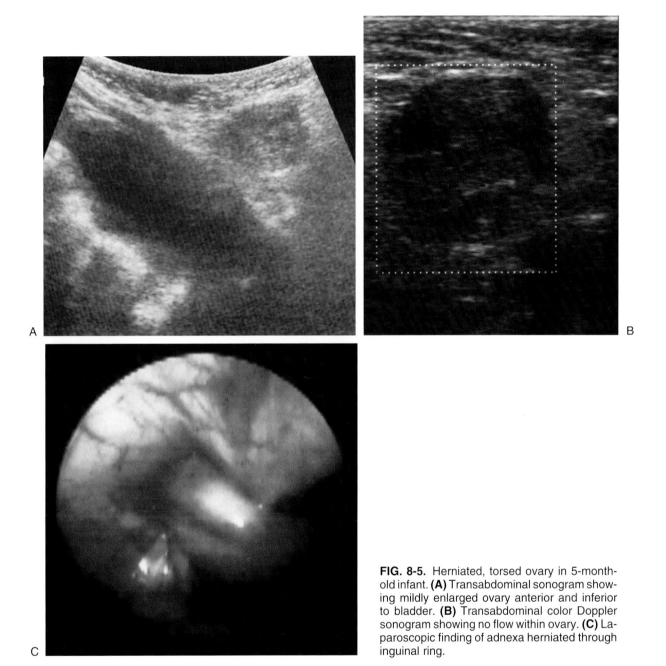

FIG. 8-5. Herniated, torsed ovary in 5-month-old infant. **(A)** Transabdominal sonogram showing mildly enlarged ovary anterior and inferior to bladder. **(B)** Transabdominal color Doppler sonogram showing no flow within ovary. **(C)** Laparoscopic finding of adnexa herniated through inguinal ring.

color priority is not set high enough relative to the gray scale imaging setting.

Rarely, torsion is encountered in normal-sized ovaries.[9] Ovarian and adnexal torsion often produces ovarian enlargement. This may be either diffuse enlargement or focal enlargement related to areas of hemorrhage or an intraovarian mass.[10,11] When central edema is present, the ovaries may be enlarged with central increased echogenicity. Multiple immature follicles may be present along the periphery of the ovary, the result of central ovarian edema. Hemorrhage within the ovary usually produces hypoechoic areas that are either homogeneous or contain delicate linear and punctate echogenicities arising from fibrin strands.

Isolated tubal torsion usually produces enlargement of the tube, as identified by its fusiform shape and hypoechoic center.[12] Thickening of the tubal wall may be recognized in some cases of adnexal torsion (see Figs. 8-8 and 8-9). Absent or reversed diastolic flow is usually associated with gangrenous changes in the wall.

Color Doppler Sonographic Findings

The diagnosis of adnexal torsion by color Doppler sonography is not as simple as documenting the presence or absence of flow.[13,14] Rather, the color Doppler sonographic

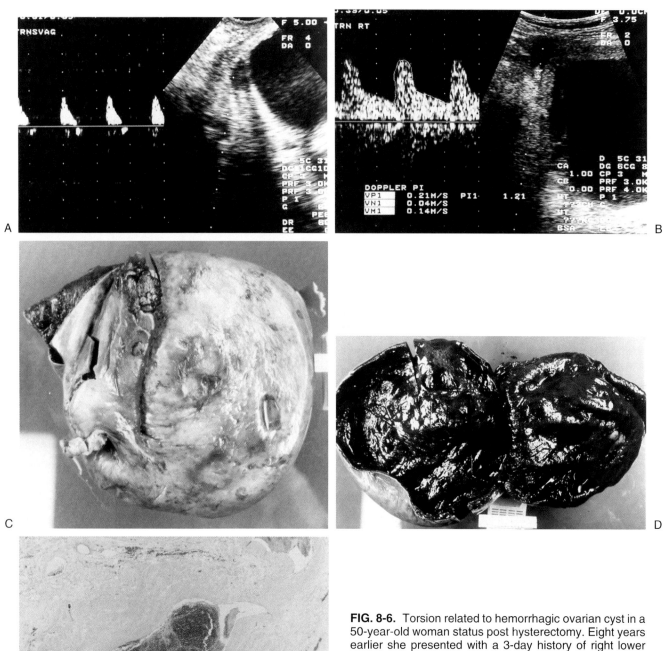

FIG. 8-6. Torsion related to hemorrhagic ovarian cyst in a 50-year-old woman status post hysterectomy. Eight years earlier she presented with a 3-day history of right lower quadrant and flank pain. **(A)** Transvaginal color Doppler sonogram showing absent diastolic flow in adnexal branch of uterine artery. The ovary contains a hemorrhagic mass. **(B)** Same as **A** showing an area of intermediate impedance flow adjacent to hemorrhagic mass. **(C)** Excised specimen showing torsed vascular pedicle but perfused tube. **(D)** Opened specimen showing areas of hemorrhage. **(E)** Low-power photomicrograph showing thrombus within an intraovarian vein.

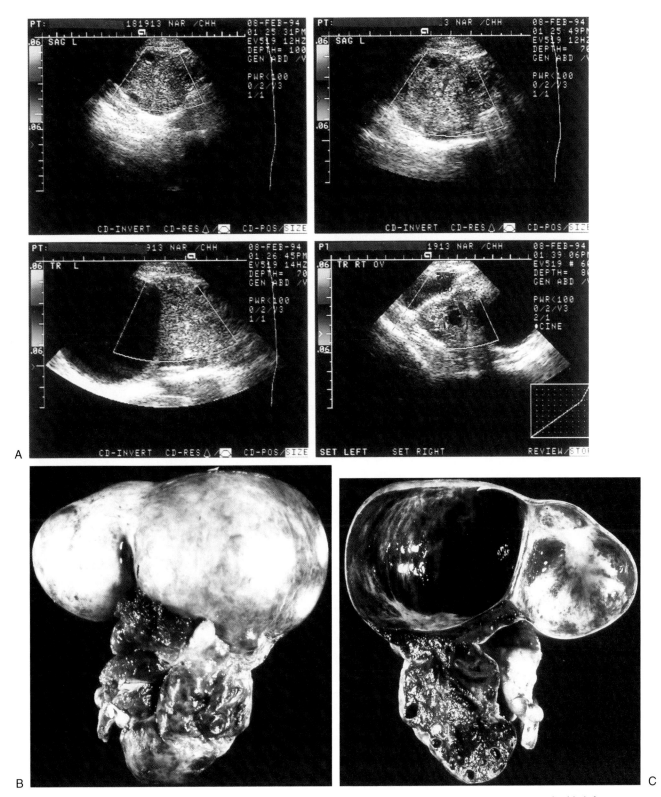

FIG. 8-7. Torsion associated with an ovarian tumor in a 34-year-old woman who presented with left lower quadrant pain for several days. She had a similar episode 5 months earlier. **(A)** Composite transvaginal color Doppler sonogram showing enlarged left ovary demonstrating intraovarian flow adjacent to cystic mass. The right ovary *(bottom right)* also had intraovarian flow surrounding a corpus luteum. **(B)** Excised specimen showing gangrenous ovary and mass projecting from left ovary. **(C)** Opened specimen showing hemorrhagic ovarian mass and normal ovary containing several corpora lutea, immature follicles, and one corpus luteum. **(A** through **C,** courtesy of Mary Warner, MD.)

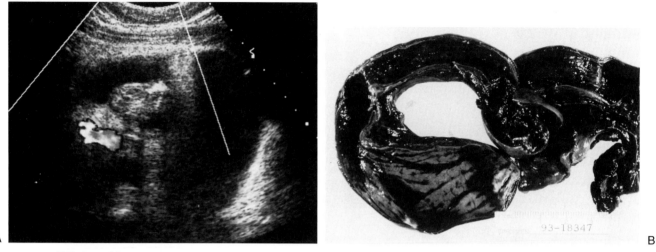

FIG. 8-8. Bilateral tubal torsion in a 35-year-old woman status post bilateral tubal ligation. **(A)** Fusiform mass without flow in patient status post tubal ligation. **(B)** Excised specimen showing hydrosalpinx and hemorrhagic wall of tube.

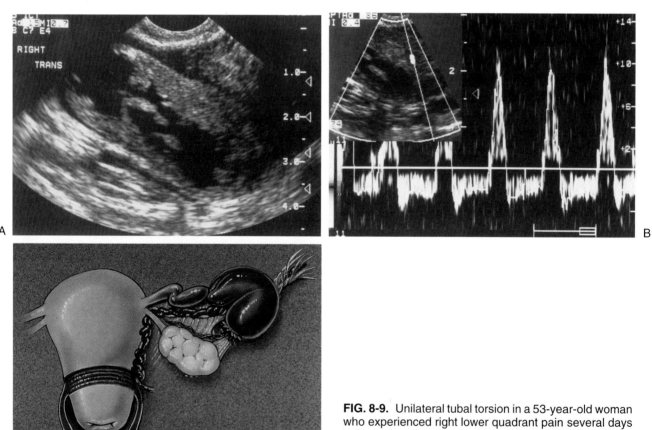

FIG. 8-9. Unilateral tubal torsion in a 53-year-old woman who experienced right lower quadrant pain several days before admission. She had undergone bilateral tubal ligation 8 years ago. **(A)** Transvaginal sonogram showing fusiform mass with thickened wall. **(B)** Reversed diastolic flow thin wall of tube. **(C)** Diagram of unilateral tubal torsion. (**C** drawn by Paul Gross, MS.)

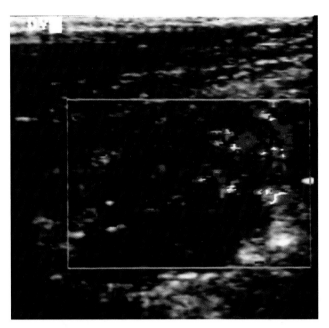

FIG. 8-10. Torsion during pregnancy. Enlarged ovary in a patient with severe left-sided pain during the mid trimester. Color Doppler sonogram showing flow to the hilar region of the ovary. At surgery this was considered a viable ovary because it "pinked up" after untwisting. (Courtesy of Mary Warner, MD.)

findings are related to the chronicity and completeness of torsion as well as its cause. In chronic torsion, there may be arterial collaterization of flow; but in acute torsion, the first and only finding may be lack of venous flow within the ovary. Experimental data suggest that chronic torsion may be associated with nonpulsatile arterial waveforms that mimic venous waveforms.[15]

My colleagues and I have reviewed 14 cases of documented torsion and have found that the presence of central venous flow is usually associated with a viable adnexa.[5] With torsion, arterial flow may be seen in the capsular branches but is usually absent in the intraovarian branches (see Figs. 8-3 and 8-10). One color Doppler sonographic finding that may help distinguish viable from nonviable ovaries is the presence of central venous flow in potentially viable torsed ovaries.[5] Color Doppler sonography may help monitor the presence of flow in ovaries that have been surgically determined.

In torsion related to areas of hemorrhage or a mass, absent flow is usually present in the area of the mass whereas flow may be present within the ovary itself (see Fig. 8-7). In particular, focal areas of corpora lutea formation may still demonstrate significant flow whereas areas around the mass are avascular (see Fig. 8-7). Tubal torsion may be recognized by a fusiform structure created by the hydrosalpinx.[8,16] Flow within the thickened wall may be seen, but absent or reversed diastolic flow on waveform analysis is sometimes demonstrated (see Fig. 8-8).

Discussion

There have only been a few reports of color Doppler sonographic findings in documented adnexal torsion.[2,13,14] Fortunately, this is a relatively rare condition even though as sonologists and sonographers we are requested frequently to exclude this possibility, not uncommonly in the middle of the night.

The flow pattern distribution depicted by color Doppler sonography has diagnostic significance rather than waveform analysis for assessing the presence or absence of flow within the ovary. Torsed ovaries in young girls may demonstrate flow. In our report of 14 cases, flow was found in approximately 40%.[17] Similarly, in a report of four cases of proven torsion, flow was documented in one that was successfully treated by untwisting the pedicle.[18] There still exists the caveat that detorsing of a vessel containing a clot may further precipitate pulmonary embolization.[19]

The improved delineation of flow by power color Doppler sonography may improve the detection of focal areas of absent flow associated with adnexal torsion. Early and prompt diagnosis of adnexal torsion may contribute to conservative surgery, which may spare the ovary from removal.

PELVIC CONGESTION SYNDROME

Pelvic congestion syndrome can be associated with chronic pelvic pain. On transvaginal color Doppler sonography, it is manifested by dilated arcuate, ovarian, and uterine veins that contain slow "to and fro" flow in dilated venous structures (Figs. 8-11 through 8-15). There is significant controversy as to the clinical importance of these findings because some patients with these findings will not experience significant pelvic pain (see Fig. 8-14).

To comprehend the relationship between impaired venous return from the pelvis and this syndrome, it is important to appreciate certain anatomic features that may predispose to this condition. The right ovarian vein drains directly into the inferior vena cava, whereas the left empties into the left renal vein. The ovarian vein usually contains several valves that can become incompetent. Dilatation of the vein occurs during pregnancy owing to increased flow, and the diameter of the ovarian vein is usually less than 5 mm. Ovarian vein thrombosis may result in reduced venous return, further predisposing the patient to edema of the ovarian stroma.

Venous drainage from the adnexal structures also includes the uterine plexus, which drains the parametrium, and the ovarian veins, which drain the ovarian blood flow into the internal iliac vein.[20] The uterine and vaginal plexus drains by means of the uterine veins, usually three on each side, which form at the level of the cervix and run to the lateral pelvic wall and into the internal iliac vein. The fundal part of the uterine plexus drains partially into the uterine veins and partially into the ovarian venous plexus.

It has been our experience that ovarian and uterine veins

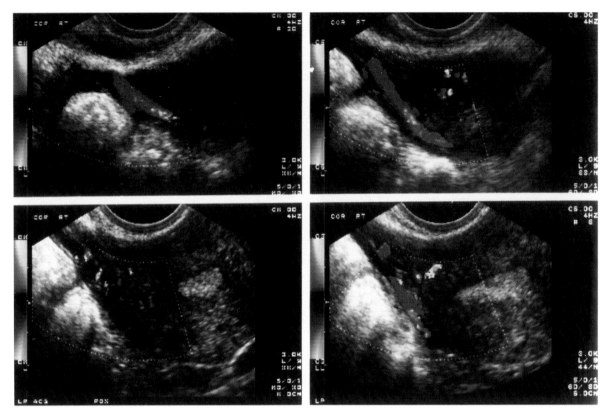

FIG. 8-11. Composite transvaginal color Doppler sonogram showing uterine vein extending into myometrium as arcuate vein and arcuate arteries in between the outer and middle layers of myometrium.

may be somewhat more dilated in multiparous than in nulliparous women, particularly in those with a retroflexed uterus. It may be postulated that this position of the uterus may contribute to a diminution in venous return. It can further be hypothesized that decreased venous return from the ovary may contribute to ovarian edema and, therefore, eventually make the ovary more susceptible to ovarian torsion.

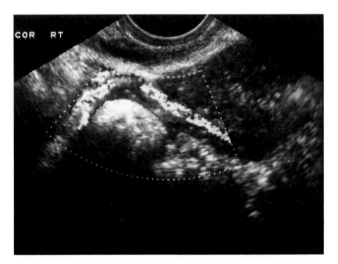

FIG. 8-12. Close-up transvaginal color Doppler sonogram showing uterine vein extending into arcuate vein.

Transvaginal color Doppler sonography demonstrates distended venous structures in the adnexa (Figs. 8-16 and 8-17; see also Figs. 8-13 through 8-15). The diameter of these venous structures is usually greater than 3 to 4 mm, and the flow within them is slow (less than 3 cm/s) and sometimes lacks respiratory variation or periodicity.

The correlation of these sonographic findings to the clinical syndrome associated with pelvic congestion has been described.[21] This syndrome is characterized by pain produced with adnexal palpation, dysmenorrhea, dysfunctional bleeding, or painful intercourse. Before transvaginal color Doppler sonography, the diagnosis was made on phlebography by direct injection into the uterus.

Treatment is directed toward alleviation of the anatomic situation associated with pelvic congestion, namely, surgical correction of uterine retroflexion. Some have treated this condition with embolization of the ovarian veins or medically with nonsteroidal analgesics. Antithrombotic drugs have also been used to variable success. The reader is referred to several articles that describe the syndrome and its treatment in greater detail for further information.[22,23]

MISCELLANEOUS CAUSES OF PELVIC PAIN

Transvaginal sonography and transvaginal color Doppler sonography can be used to diagnose several causes of pelvic

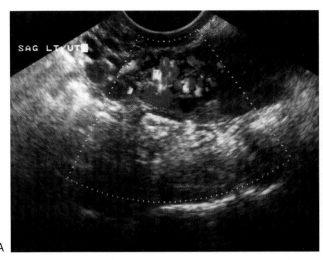
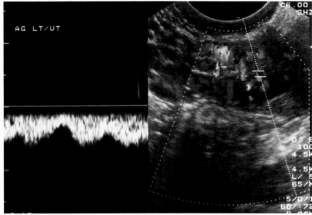

FIG. 8-13. Transvaginal color Doppler sonography of distended pelvic (parauterine) veins. **(A)** Dilated uterine veins in the left adnexal area. **(B)** Pulsatile venous waveform.

pain that are relatively rare, such as distal ureteral calculi, appendicitis and other bowel disorders, and adenomyosis (Fig. 8-18).

The distal ureter can be evaluated with transvaginal sonography.[24] Calculi within a distended ureter near the uretrovesical junction can be determined by observing for the urine jet arising from the ureteral orifice (see Fig. 8-18).

Appendicitis can be recognized by either transabdominal or transvaginal sonography by an abnormally thickened (over 3 mm single wall thickness) bowel loop in the right lower quadrant (Fig. 8-19). Although usually best depicted by the transabdominal approach, the proximity of bowel within the cul-de-sac to the transvaginal sonography probe may allow diagnosis by this approach.[25,26]

Ischemic bowel appears as an abnormally thickened aper-

istaltic loop. Color Doppler imaging may show absent flow to the bowel wall.[27]

Adhesions secondary to previous surgery may be seen if fluid is on either side of them. Otherwise, adhesive disease may be implied if the uterus and ovaries do not move independently when the probe is introduced (''sliding organ sign''). This topic is described in greater detail in Chapter 7.

CONCLUSION

Transvaginal color Doppler sonography has an important role in the evaluation of women with pelvic pain, primarily in establishing or excluding adnexal torsion, which requires immediate surgical intervention.

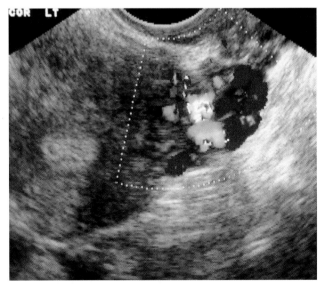

FIG. 8-14. Transvaginal color Doppler sonogram showing distended uterine veins in an asymptomatic patient.

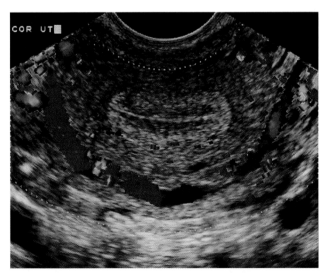

FIG. 8-15. Transvaginal color Doppler sonogram showing distended arcuate veins coursing between outer and middle layers of myometrium.

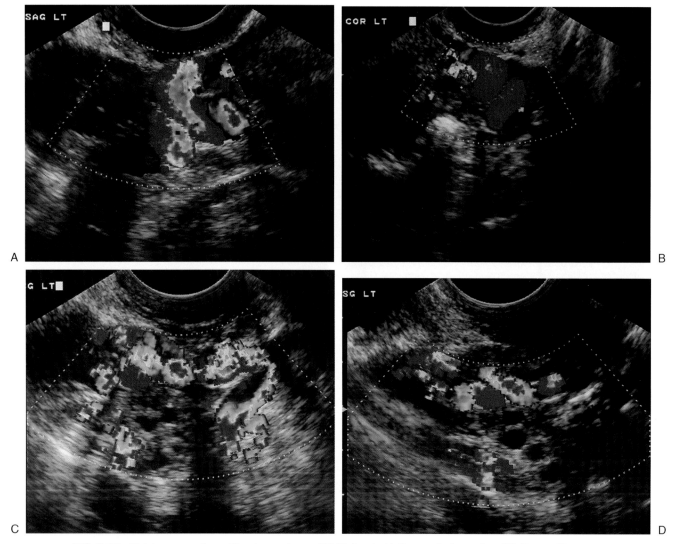

A

B

C

D

FIG. 8-16. Pelvic congestion without symptoms. **(A)** Distended left parauterine veins. **(B)** Coronal image of **A. (C)** Distended paraovarian vessels of a different patient from that shown in **A** and **B. (D)** Coronal image of **C.**

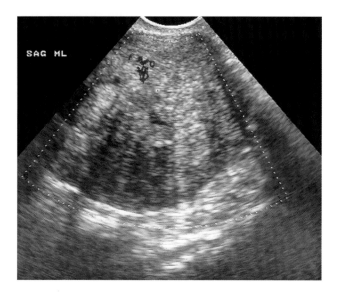

FIG. 8-17. Amplitude color Doppler sonogram of adenomyosis. No significant increased flow was seen within the abnormal myometrium.

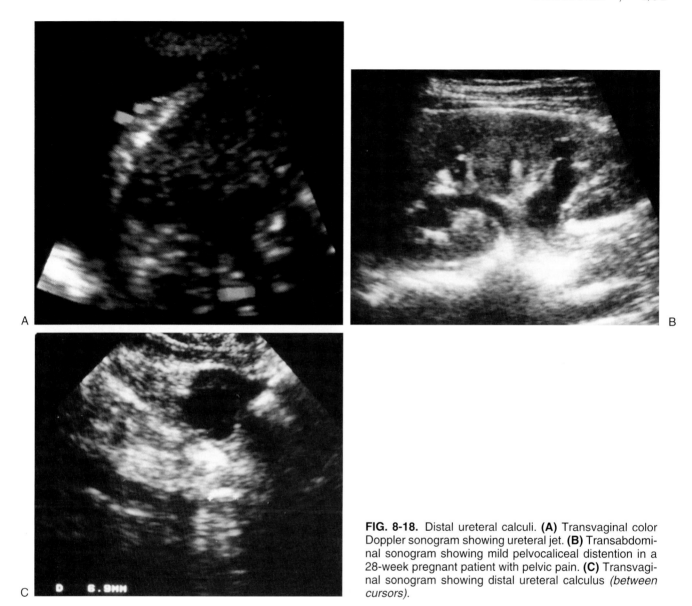

FIG. 8-18. Distal ureteral calculi. **(A)** Transvaginal color Doppler sonogram showing ureteral jet. **(B)** Transabdominal sonogram showing mild pelvocaliceal distention in a 28-week pregnant patient with pelvic pain. **(C)** Transvaginal sonogram showing distal ureteral calculus *(between cursors)*.

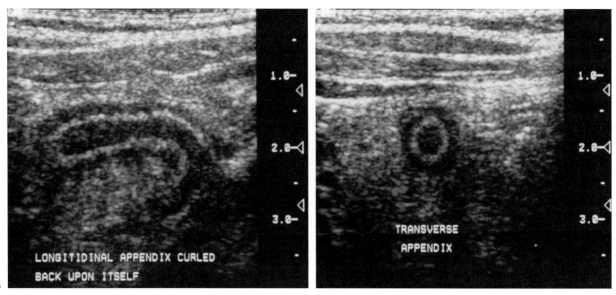

FIG. 8-19. Transabdominal sonogram of appendicitis. **(A)** A fusiform mass is depicted at McBurney's point, which represented an abnormal appendix. **(B)** Same as **A,** seen on short axis. (Courtesy of ATL, Inc)

REFERENCES

1. Cunanan RG, Courey NG, Lippes J: Laparoscopic findings in patients with pelvic pain. Am J Obstet Gynecol 1983;146:589.
2. Quillin SP, Siegel MJ. Transabdominal color Doppler ultrasonography of the painful adolescent ovary. J Ultrasound Med 1994;13:549.
3. Bider D, Mashiach S, Dulitzky M, et al. Clinical, surgical and pathologic findings of adnexal torsion in pregnant and nonpregnant women. Surg Gynecol Obstet 1991;173:363.
4. Laing FC, Benson CB, Disalvo DN, et al. Distal ureteral calculi: detection with vaginal US. Radiology 1994;192:545.
5. Fleischer A, Stein S, Cullinan J, Warren M: Color Doppler sonography of adnexal torsion J Ultrasound Med 1995;14:523.
6. Lee AR, Kim KH, Lee BH, et al. Massive edema of the ovary: imaging findings. AJR 1993;161:343.
7. Mashiach S, Bider D, Moran O, et al. Adnexal torsion of hyperstimulated ovaries in pregnancies after gonadotropin therapy. Fertil Steril 1990;53:76.
8. Elchalal U, Caspi B, Schachter M, et al. Isolated tubal torsion: clinical and ultrasonographic correlation. J Ultrasound Med 1993;2:115.
9. Worthington-Kirsch RL, Raptopoulos V, Cohen IT: Sequential bilateral torsion of normal ovaries in a child. J Ultrasound Med 1986;5:663.
10. Graif M, Itzchak Y. Sonographic evaluation of ovarian torsion in childhood and adolescence. AJR 1988;150:647.
11. Warner MA, Fleischer AC, Edell SL, et al. Uterine adnexal torsion: sonographic findings. Radiology 1985;154:773.
12. Baumgartel P, Fleischer A, Cullinan J. Color Doppler sonography of isolated tubal torsion. *Ultra Ob Gyn* 7:367–370, 1996.
13. Rosado WM, Trambert MA, Gosink BB, et al. Adnexal torsion: diagnosis by using Doppler sonography. AJR 1992;159:1251.
14. Van Voorhis BJ, Schwaiger J, Syrop CH, et al. Early diagnosis of ovarian torsion by color Doppler ultrasonography. Fertil Steril 1992; 58:215.
15. Bude RO, Kennelly MJ, Adler RS, Rubin JM. Preliminary investigations: nonpulsatile arterial waveforms: observations during graded testicular torsion in rats. Acad Radiol 1995;2:879.
16. Sherer DM, Liberto L, Abramowics JS, et al. Endovaginal sonographic features associated with isolated torsion of the fallopian tube. J Ultrasound Med 1991;10:107.
17. Stark JE, Siegel MJ. Ovarian torsion in prepubertal and pubertal girls: sonographic findings. AJR 1994;163:1479.
18. Willms AB, Schlund JF, Meyer WR. Endovaginal Doppler ultrasound in ovarian torsion: a case series. Ultrasound Obstet Gynecol 1995;5: 129.
19. Gordon JD, Hopkins KL, Jeffrey RB, Giudice LC. Adnexal torsion: color Doppler diagnosis and laparoscopic treatment. Fertil Steril 1994; 61:383.
20. Kennedy A, Hemingway A. Radiology of ovarian varices. Br J Hosp Med 1990;44:38.
21. Bonilla-Musoles F, Ballester M. Transvaginal color Doppler in the diagnosis of pelvic congestion syndrome. In Kurjak A, ed. Transvaginal color Doppler, ed 2. London, Parthenon Press, 1993;207.
22. Beard RW, Reginald PW, Wadsworth J. Clinical features of women with chronic lower abdominal pain and pelvic congestion. Br J Obstet Gynaecol 1988;95:153.
23. Hobbs JT. The pelvic congestion syndrome. Br J Hosp Med 1990;43: 200.
24. Laing FC, Benson CB, DiSalvo D, et al. Distal ureteral calculi: detection with vaginal US. Radiology 1994;192:545.
25. Puylaert JBCM. Acute appendicitis: US evaluation using graded compression. Radiology 1986;158:355.
26. Puylaert J. TVS for Dx of appendicitis. Letter to Editor. AJR 1994; 163:746.
27. Jeffery R, Sommer F, Debotcu J. Color Doppler sonography of focal gastrointestinal lesions: initial clinical experience. J Ultrasound Med 1994;13:473.

Magnetic Resonance Imaging of Acute and Chronic Pelvic Pain Disorders

Eric K. Outwater, MD

The clinical presentation of various causes of pelvic pain has been discussed in earlier chapters. It is diagnostically helpful to classify pelvic pain as acute or chronic at presentation because these presentations have separate differential diagnoses and, therefore, different imaging strategies for their evaluation. The differential diagnosis of pelvic pain is long and encompasses gynecologic, urologic, gastrointestinal, musculoskeletal, neurologic, and, frequently, idiopathic causes. MRI offers advantages over sonography in that many of these systems are evaluated in a complete examination of the pelvis, whereas sonography examines chiefly the uterus and adnexae.

ACUTE PELVIC PAIN

In patients presenting with acute pelvic pain, numerous diagnostic possibilities are evident. These include both gynecologic (eg, hemorrhagic ovarian cyst, a ruptured ectopic pregnancy, spontaneous abortion, and ovarian torsion) and nongynecologic (eg, appendicitis, inflammatory bowel disease). In this discussion of the MRI features of disorders associated with acute pelvic pain, the focus is on the gynecologic causes.

Ovarian Cysts

Patients with functional ovarian cysts can frequently present with acute pelvic pain. Functional ovarian cysts can develop hemorrhage within the cyst into the peritoneal cavity or can serve as predisposing factors to ovarian torsion. Bleeding within corpus luteum cysts occurs as a normal physiologic process, sometimes associated with mild degrees of pain. More severe presentations may be due to larger volumes of hemorrhage in these corpus luteum cysts. Corpus luteum cysts can display a wide variety of appearances on sonography.[1,2] With MRI, typical hemorrhagic corpus luteum cysts show intermediate high signal intensity on T1-weighted sequences and intermediate high signal intensity on T2-weighted sequences. The walls of corpus luteum cysts are generally distinctly evident, measure between 1 and 3 mm in thickness, and show intense enhancement after the administration of gadolinium (DTPA) (Fig. 8-20). It is not always possible to distinguish hemorrhagic corpus luteum cysts from endometriomas by MRI,[3] but in general most endometriomas present a distinct appearance from hemorrhagic corpus luteum cysts (Fig. 8-21). Corpus luteum cysts generally do not show the profound degrees of T2 shortening (low signal intensity on the T2-weighted sequences), which are typical for endometriomas. In addition, endometriomas generally show high signal intensity on T1-weighted images homogeneously throughout the cyst contents, with an intensity similar to that of fat (see Fig. 8-21). Acute or subacute hemorrhage generally gives distinctly different mixed signal intensity on T1-weighted sequences or a ring of high signal intensity in the periphery. Any mass that is evident as high signal intensity on T1-weighted images should be differentiated from a lipid-containing mass (eg, dermoid cyst) by chemical shift imaging (Fig. 8-22).[4–7]

Ectopic Pregnancy

The MRI findings in an ectopic pregnancy have not been well described. A hemorrhagic adnexal mass is generally present.[8] In the setting of a positive β-human chorionic gonadotropin test and without a normal intrauterine gestational sac, the following possibilities are likely: (1) early pregnancy; (2) an ectopic pregnancy with or without tubal rupture; (3) gestational trophoblastic disease with theca-lutein cysts or adnexal metastases; and (4) spontaneous abortion in progress or retained products of conception. In general, these entities are difficult to distinguish by sonography and may also be difficult to distinguish by MRI. All may be associated with some degree of endometrial abnormality.[8] Gestational trophoblastic disease has a distinct appearance with multiple signal voids around an endometrial or myometrial mass, owing to numerous enlarging vessels.[8–12] Adnexal metastases appear similar.[8] In general, however, patients with suspected ectopic pregnancy require transvaginal sonography to identify the intrauterine gestational sac or, in the event of actual ectopic pregnancy, to identify the tubal ring of the ectopic pregnancy. Transvaginal sonography in this case is diagnostic in the majority of cases.[13] If MRI is performed, signs of acute or subacute hematoma are usually evident (Fig. 8-23).[14,15]

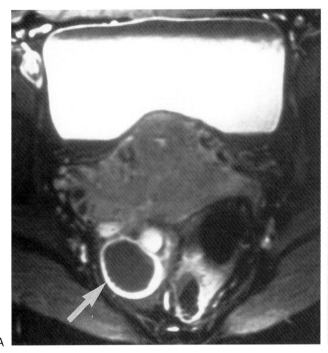
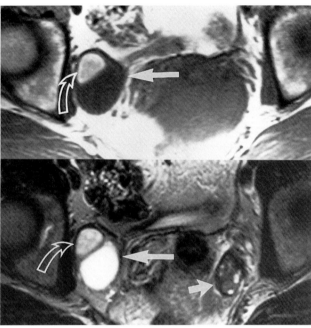

A   B

FIG. 8-20. Corpus luteum cysts. (A) Gadolinium-enhanced T1-weighted fat-saturated image shows characteristic intense wall enhancement of surgically proven corpus luteum cyst *(arrow)*. (B) T1-weighted spin-echo *(top)* and T2-weighted fast spin-echo *(bottom)* images show a corpus luteum cyst anteriorly *(curved arrows)* adjacent to a follicular cyst *(long straight arrows)*. Note the slightly lower signal intensity in the center of the luteal cyst, a finding characteristic of subacute hematoma and atypical for endometriomas. Both cysts proven at surgery. (Fig. 8-20 (A) reprinted with permission from: Outwater EK. MR imaging of the pelvis. In: Haaga J, Lanzieri C, Sartoris D, Zerhouni E, eds. Computed tomography and magnetic resonance imaging of the whole body. vol 2. St. Louis, CV Mosby Co., 1994:1393.)

Pelvic Inflammatory Disease

The diagnosis of pelvic inflammatory disease can be made by the clinical combination of fever and a tender pelvic mass in a nonpregnant sexually active female that resolves with conservative therapy and antibiotics. Transvaginal sonography may show tubal dilatation and a mass. Tubal enlargement on MRI can also easily be shown by the tortuous folding of a fluid-filled structure.

Multiplanar T2-weighted images are the key in diagnosing hydrosalpinges. What appears to be a multiloculated adnexal mass may be clearly identified as a dilated folded tube on images acquired in a second plane. Fast spin-echo T2-weighted images in three planes are helpful when hydrosalpinx is a diagnostic consideration. The contents of dilated tubes are variable on MRI with hemorrhagic components manifested by short T1 of the tubular lumen.[16] The normal fallopian tube has an interdigitating enfolded mucosa that fills the tubular lumen. When this tube is dilated, these mucosal enfoldings become attenuated but can still be identified in many cases of mild to moderate tubal dilatation as longitudinal thin ridges along the course of the dilated tube. The signal intensity of the tuboovarian abscess fluid itself may be variable. This may appear as simple fluid with only mild T2 shortening, or it may be hemorrhagic with T1 shortening.[17] The outer margin of the tuboovarian abscess will be infiltrative owing to surround edema. The appearance may not be separable from endometriosis in all cases. The walls of tuboovarian abscesses enhance as do the walls of endometriosis.[18]

Ovarian Torsion

Ovarian torsion can be identified on MRI. Previous studies using older body coil techniques have identified some patients with ovarian torsion. Congested vessels, low signal intensity serpiginous structures along the expected course of the fallopian tube, evidence of hemorrhage, and an underlying mass have been described.[19] Deviation of the uterus toward the side of the torsion is an additional feature.[19] In the cases of torsion with infarction, a high signal intensity rim on the T1-weighted sequences in absence of gadolinium enhancement has been described.[20] High-resolution techniques obtained with multicoil techniques reveal some additional features of the ovarian torsion. Namely, the torsion knot within the fallopian tube itself can be identified. This appears as a very low signal intensity spiculated focus on fallopian tube on T2-weighted sequences (Fig. 8-24). Enlargement of the tube from edema can, in addition, be evident. In adults, torsion is due to the presence of an underlying ovarian mass, very commonly a dermoid cyst or ovarian fibroma. When the underlying ovary

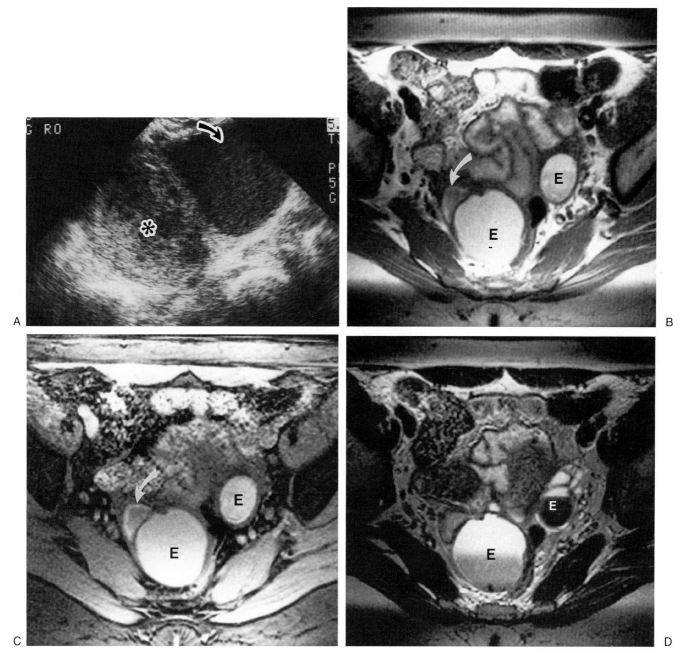

FIG. 8-21. Characteristic MRI findings in endometriomas. **(A)** Sagittal transvaginal sonogram shows heterogeneous cystic mass anteriorly *(asterisk)* and homogeneous cystic mass posteriorly. The posterior mass is characteristic of an endometrioma *(curved arrow)*. T1-weighted spin-echo image **(B)** and fat-saturated T1-weighted gradient-echo image **(C)** show masses of high signal intensity in both ovaries (E). Note the somewhat thick rims to these masses. The signal intensity approaches that of fat. The fat-saturated image in **C** demonstrates that the contents of these masses do not contain lipid and that, therefore, these are hemorrhagic masses. **(D)** T2-weighted fast spin-echo image shows characteristic findings of shading with components to the endometriomas (E) of low signal intensity. Note that the resolving corpus luteum cyst shows lower signal intensity on the T1-weighted image in **A** than the endometriomas.

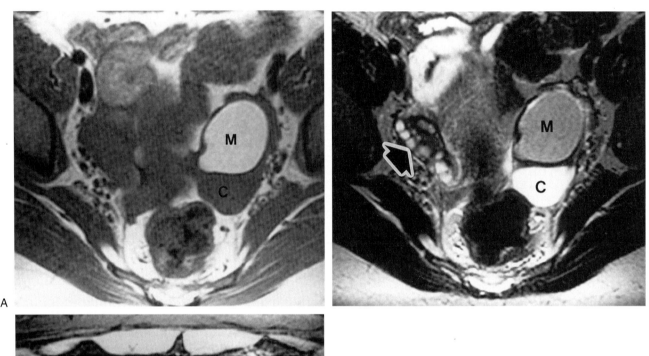

A

B

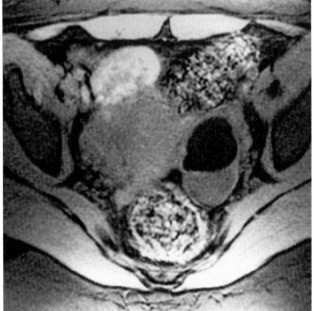

C

FIG. 8-22. Chemical-shift imaging of adnexal mass shown by high signal intensity. T1-weighted spin-echo image **(A)** and T2-weighted fast spin-echo image **(B)** show two cystic masses in the left ovary. The anterior mass (M) shows high signal intensity on the T2-weighted image, and the T2-weighted image shows lower signal intensity than that expected for a simple cyst, one of which lies posteriorly in the ovary (C). The anterior mass (M) is compatible with an endometrioma or ovarian dermoid. **(C)** Fat-saturated image shows lost signal within the anterior cyst, indicating the presence of lipid in this dermoid cyst. Note the normal right ovary.

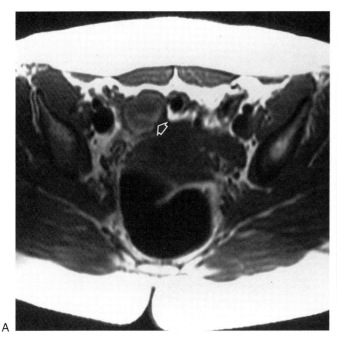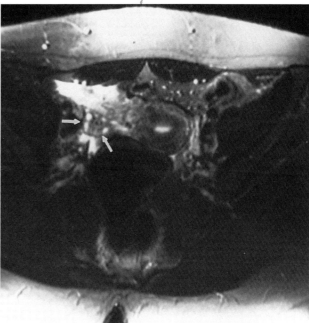

A   B

FIG. 8-23. Tubal pregnancy. **(A)** Axial spin-echo image shows a heterogeneous mass in the right adnexa with peripheral high signal intensity *(arrow)*. **(B)** Axial fast spin-echo image at the superior aspect of the mass shows an ovary with preserved morphology and several small follicular cysts *(arrows)*, thus establishing an extraovarian origin to the hemorrhagic mass.

can be identified, edema and hemorrhage within the ovary can be appreciated by MRI. However, the critical diagnostic features in the case of ovarian torsion rely on the identification of the torsion knot; these features are specific.

CHRONIC PELVIC PAIN

Chronic pelvic pain in women of childbearing age is a frequent clinical problem for gynecologists, and the elucidation of its underlying cause is often elusive.[21] Common conditions that may result in chronic pelvic pain include pelvic inflammatory disease, vaginal or vulvar infections, leiomyomas and adenomyosis, and endometriosis. A complete differential diagnosis for chronic pelvic pain, however, is extremely long; and numerous causes must be considered in the patients who have an unrevealing initial workup.[21]

Although the potential for MRI in patients with chronic pelvic pain has not been elucidated, there are a number of common disorders that MRI can depict. These include endometriosis, leiomyomas, and adenomyosis. However, in most patients who are referred for further evaluation of chronic pelvic pain these causes have already been excluded by sonography and laparoscopy.

Endometriosis

Endometriosis is a common condition and a frequent cause of chronic pelvic pain. It is often asymptomatic, however, and

the severity of abnormalities bears an inconstant relationship to clinical symptoms.[22] MRI features of endometriosis have been previously described.[23–28] Basically, endometriomas can be distinguished from the vast majority of adnexal masses, both benign and malignant.[26] Ovarian cysts with very high signal intensity on T1-weighted images, with similar signal intensity to that of fat, and which show lower than expected signal intensity on T2-weighted sequences are strongly suggestive of endometriomas (see Fig. 8-21).[26] Multiple hyperintense cysts are also suggestive of endometriomas. Cysts that display high signal intensity on T1- and T2-weighted sequences or only intermediate signal intensity on T1-weighted images are less suggestive of endometriomas.[26] A more helpful feature in the diagnosis of patients with endometriosis is the presence of small implants of endometriosis.[23–25] These appear as nodules, particularly in the cul-de-sac, which have low signal intensity on T2-weighted sequences and enhance with gadolinium-DTPA (see Fig. 8-25).[24] Frequently, small areas of hemorrhage within them are seen on the T1-weighted sequences. These are more easily seen on T1-weighted, fat-suppressed images (Fig. 8-26).[23,25] Additional imaging features of endometriomas include a low signal intensity rim due to hemosiderin and a somewhat thick, shaggy wall due to the fibrotic attachments to the adjacent fat and organs. This low signal intensity on the T2-weighted images has been termed *shading.* This may appear as a gradient of high to low signal intensity within the cyst owing to the viscous concentrated blood products present within these "chocolate" cysts (see Fig. 8-21). The presence of endome-

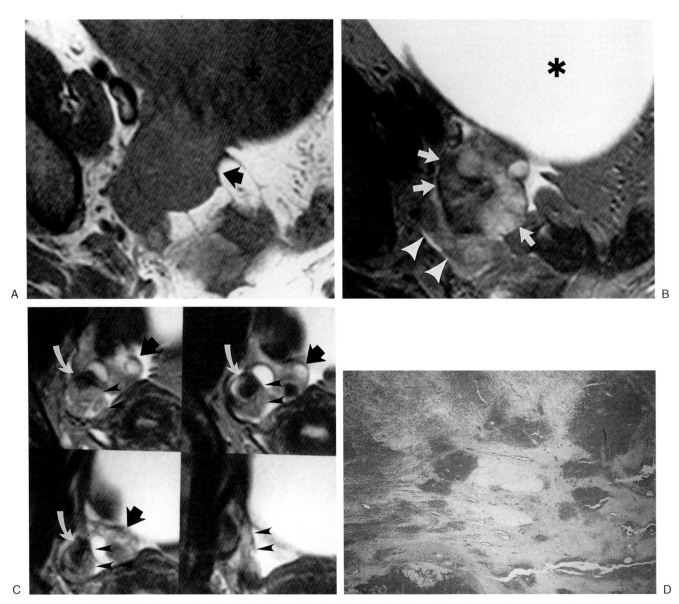

FIG. 8-24. Ovarian torsion due to simple cyst. **(A)** Axial spin-echo T1-weighted image shows an enlarged right adnexa *(arrow)* containing a low signal intensity cyst anteriorly *(asterisk)*. **(B)** Axial T2-weighted fast-spin echo image demonstrates the enlarged edematous ovary *(arrows)* and a coiled edematous tube posteriorly *(arrowheads)*. **(C)** Coronal T2-weighted fast spin-echo images shows the right adnexa from posteriorly upper left to anterior lower right. The enlarged fallopian tube *(arrowheads)* extends posteriorly from the uterine cornua inferolaterally to the ovary *(black arrow)*. Note the low signal intensity torsion knot *(curved arrow)*. **(D)** Histology shows extensive hemorrhage and edema in the ovarian stroma. (Reprinted with permission from: Outwater EK, Schiebler ML. Magnetic resonance imaging of the ovary. MRI Clin N Am 1994;2:245.)

trial implants and fibrotic implants outside the ovaries is a more specific feature of endometriosis because some endometriomas may present a nonspecific appearance on MRI that is difficult to separate from many other hemorrhagic masses.[3]

Pelvic Adhesive Disease

Pelvic adhesive disease is believed to be an important cause of chronic pelvic pain.[21] Endometriosis, prior surgery, or pelvic inflammatory disease can result in extensive adhesions. MRI can identify some adhesions if they distort normal anatomy or are particularly dense. These appear as ill-defined areas of peritoneal enhancement after administration of gadolinium-DTPA. Interfaces between the uterus and cul-de-sac may become obscured by perceptible amounts of low signal intensity fibrotic areas on T2-weighted scans. In patients with endometriosis, these adhesions may be particularly dense and nodular, with foci of hemorrhage representing islands of endometriosis within the adhesions. Most

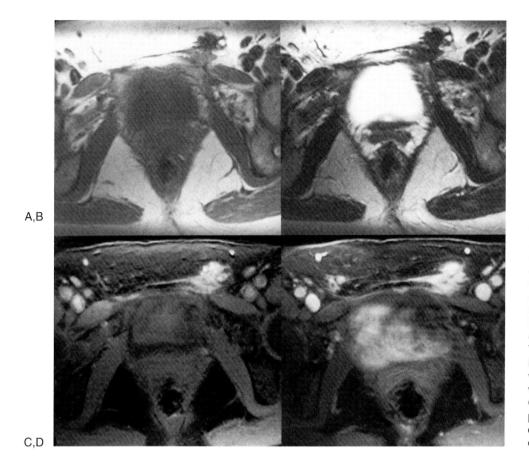

A,B

C,D

FIG. 8-25. Fibrotic masses of endometriosis. T1-weighted spin-echo image **(A)**, T2-weighted fast spin-echo image **(B)**, and fat-saturated gradient-echo images before **(C)** and after **(D)** the administration of gadolinium dimeglumine demonstrate a mass in the left inguinal canal surrounding the round ligament. The mass has areas of high signal intensity on the T1-weighted images and very low signal intensity on the T2-weighted images compatible with hemorrhage and fibrosis. Gadolinium enhancement is present. These findings are typical of fibrotic implants from endometriosis.[24]

adhesive disease, however, that is obvious on laparoscopy is not detectable by MRI or sonography.

Adenomyosis

Similar to endometriosis, adenomyosis is a common condition affecting premenopausal women and one that often has an uncertain relationship to the production of clinical symptom etiology. Adenomyosis occurs in 15% to 20% of hysterectomy specimens.[29,30] It is generally acknowledged that moderate adenomyosis may give rise to menorrhagia or cyclic pelvic pain.[30] Because, unlike leiomyomas, adenomyosis forms a very indistinct boundary between the smooth muscle hypertrophy around the island of ectopic endometrial epithelium and stroma, it is not possible to easily resect adenomyosis short of a hysterectomy.

The MRI findings of adenomyosis are generally only appreciated on T2-weighted images.[31,32] Sagittal T2-weighted images usually display the uterine anatomy to the best advantage (Fig. 8-26). The subendometrial myometrium is termed the *junctional zone* and normally shows very low signal intensity on T2-weighted images. This low signal intensity

results from the compact nature of the smooth muscle in this location,[33–35] similar to the packed smooth muscle in the vaginal wall, rectal wall, and bladder wall. Therefore, the signal intensity on T2-weighted images of these structures is similar. In contrast, the outer myometrium has a looser arrangement of myometrial smooth muscle fibers and numerous interspersed vessels, leading to an overall higher signal intensity.[33–35]

Adenomyosis appears as ill-defined low-signal areas within the myometrium.[31,32,36] This may produce a focal or diffuse thickening of the junctional zone (Fig. 8-27), or low-signal intensity masses may be seen outside the junctional zone.[31,36] A junctional zone measuring greater than 12 mm is indicative of adenomyosis.[37] This low signal is due to the proliferation of smooth muscle that occurs around the islands of ectopic endometrium.[30] The islands of ectopic endometrium appear as high-signal intensity foci on T2-weighted images. These small islands of adenomyosis usually enhance after the administration of gadolinium-DTPA. MRI is more accurate than transvaginal sonography for the diagnosis of adenomyosis.[37,38] It can easily distinguish between leiomyomas, which are well defined and frequently have high signal intensity rims, and adenomyosis, which is ill defined.[31,32]

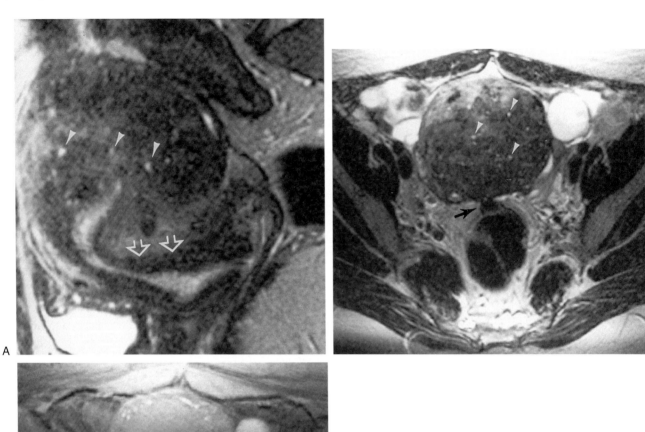

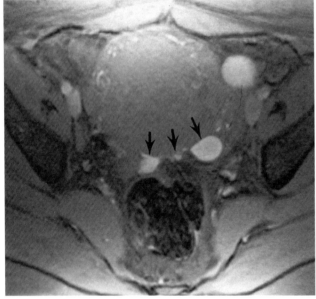

FIG. 8-26. Endometriosis and adenomyosis. Sagittal T2-weighted fast spin-echo image **(A)** and axial T2-weighted fast spin-echo image **(B)** show marked thickening of the myometrium with low signal intensity tissue resembling that of junctional zone. Normal junctional zone in the lower uterine segment is denoted by white arrows. Note the punctate high signal intensity foci within the myometrium representing the glandular epithelium of the adenomyosis *(arrowheads).* The axial T2-weighted fast spin-echo image **(B)** and the axial gradient-echo T1-weighted fat-saturated image **(C)** at slightly different levels show the hemorrhagic and fibrotic deposits of endometriosis *(black arrows)* in the left ovary and cul-de-sac in this patient with proven coexistent endometriosis and adenomyosis.

Pelvic Congestion Syndrome

Pelvic congestion syndrome is a controversial entity that again has a very unclear and uncertain relationship between any radiographic findings and the patient's clinical symptoms.[21,39,40] Dilated paraovarian gonadal veins have been described as a feature of this syndrome; however, it is clear that many patients who have no pain or other symptoms have prominent parauterine and gonadal veins. Large parauterine veins and gonadal veins can be identified postpartum or in multiparous women by MRI, and caution in ascribing significance to these findings is advised.

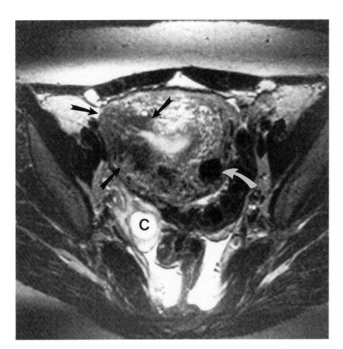

FIG. 8-27. Focal adenomyosis. Axial T2-weighted fast spin-echo image shows focal low signal intensity around the right cornua of the uterus *(black arrows)*. This gives the impression of a focal thickening of the junctional zone. Note the infiltrative nature of the abnormality compared with the well-defined margins of the leiomyoma *(curved white arrow)*. A corpus luteum cyst (C) in the right ovary is seen.

REFERENCES

1. Baltarowich KH, Kurtz AB, Pasto ME, et al. The spectrum of sonographic findings in hemorrhagic ovarian cysts. AJR 1987;148:901.
2. Okai T. Transvaginal sonographic appearance of hemorrhagic functional ovarian cysts and their spontaneous regression. Int J Gynecol Obstet 1994;44:47.
3. Outwater EK, Schiebler ML, Owen RS, Schnall MD. MRI characterization of hemorrhagic adnexal masses: a blinded reader study. Radiology 1993;186:489.
4. Guinet C, Buy JN, Ghossain MA, et al. Fat suppression techniques in MR imaging of mature ovarian teratomas: comparison with CT. Eur J Radiol 1993;17:117.
5. Stevens SK, Hricak H, Campos Z. Teratomas versus cystic hemorrhagic adnexal lesions: differentiation with proton-selective fat-saturation MR imaging. Radiology 1993;186:481.
6. Kier R, Smith RC, McCarthy SM. Value of lipid- and water-suppression MR images in distinguishing between blood and lipid within ovarian masses. AJR 1992;158:321.
7. Szumowski J, Plewes DB. Separation of lipid and water MR imaging signals by Chopper averaging in the time domain. Radiology 1987; 165:247.
8. Barton J, McCarthy S, Kohorn E, et al. Pelvic MR imaging findings in gestational trophoblastic disease, incomplete abortion, and ectopic pregnancy: are they specific? Radiology 1993;186:163.
9. Hricak H, Demas BE, Braga CA, et al. Gestational trophoblastic neoplasm of the uterus: MR assessment. Radiology 1986;161:11.
10. Ha HK, Jung JK, Jee MK, et al. Gestational trophoblastic tumors of the uterus: MR imaging—pathologic correlation. Gynecol Oncol 1995; 57:340.
11. Mirich DR, Hall JT, Kraft WL, et al. Metastatic adnexal trophoblastic neoplasm: contribution of MR imaging. J Comput Assist Tomogr 1988; 12:1061.
12. Szolar DH. MRI appearance of gestational choriocarcinoma within the myometrium. Eur J Radiol 1994;18:61.
13. Frates MC, Laing FC. Sonographic evaluation of ectopic pregnancy: an update. AJR 1995;165:251.
14. Kuhl CK, Heuck A, Kreft BP, et al. Combined intrauterine and ovarian pregnancy mimicking ovarian malignant tumor: imaging findings. AJR 1995;165:369.
15. Ha HK, Jung JK, Kang SJ, et al. MR imaging in the diagnosis of rare forms of ectopic pregnancy. AJR 1993;160:1229.
16. Outwater EK, , Mitchell DG. MR imaging of hydrosalpinx and hematosalpinx. J Magn Reson Imaging 1994;4(P):51.
17. Mitchell DG. Magnetic resonance imaging of the adnexa. Semin Ultrasound CT MR 1988;9:143.
18. Hricak H, Carrington B. MRI of the pelvis: a text atlas. Norwalk, CT, Appleton & Lange, 1991.
19. Kimura I, Togashi K, Kawakami S, et al. Ovarian torsion: CT and MR imaging appearances. Radiology 1994;190:337.
20. Kawakami K, Murata K, Kawaguchi N, et al. Hemorrhagic infarction of the diseased ovary: a common MR finding in two cases. Magn Reson Imag 1993;11:595.
21. Rapkin AJ, Reading AE. Chronic pelvic pain. Curr Probl Obstet Gynecol Fertil 1991;14:105.
22. Fukaya T, Hoshiai H, Yajima A. Is pelvic endometriosis always associated with chronic pain? A retrospective study of 618 cases diagnosed by laparoscopy. Am J Obstet Gynecol 1993;169:719.
23. Ascher SM, Agrawal R, Bis KG, et al. Endometriosis: appearance and detection with conventional and contrast-enhanced fat-suppressed spin-echo techniques. J Magn Reson Imaging 1995;5:251.
24. Siegelman ES, Outwater EK, Wang T, Mitchell DG. Solid enhancing masses in endometriosis: MR imaging observations. AJR 1994;163: 357.
25. Sugimura K, Okizuka H, Imaoka I, et al. Pelvic endometriosis: detection and diagnosis with chemical shift MR imaging. Radiology 1993; 188:435.
26. Togashi K, Nishimura K, Kimura I, et al. Endometrial cysts: diagnosis with MR imaging. Radiology 1991;180:73.
27. Arrivé L, Hricak H, Martin MC. Pelvic endometriosis: MR imaging. Radiology 1989;171:687.
28. Zawin M, McCarthy S, Scoutt L, Comite F. Endometriosis: appearance and detection at MR imaging. Radiology 1989;171:693.
29. Zaloudek C, Norris JH. Mesenchymal tumors of the uterus. In: Kurman RJ, ed. Blaustein's pathology of the female genital tract. New York, Springer-Verlag, 1994:518.
30. Azziz R. Adenomyosis: current perspectives. Obstet Gynecol Clin North Am 1989;16:221.
31. Togashi K, Nishimura K, Itoh K, et al. Adenomyosis: diagnosis with MR imaging. 1988;166:111.
32. Togashi K, Ozasa H, Konishi I, et al. Enlarged uterus: differentiation between adenomyosis and leiomyoma with MR imaging. Radiology 1989;174:531.
33. Brown HK, Stoll BS, Nicosia SV, et al. Uterine junctional zone: correlation between histologic findings and MR imaging. Radiology 1991; 179:409.
34. McCarthy S, Scott G, Majumdar S, et al. Uterine junctional zone: MR study of water content and relaxation properties. Radiology 1989;171: 241.
35. Scoutt LM, Flynn SD, Luthringer DJ, et al. Junctional zone of the uterus: correlation of MR imaging and histologic examination of hysterectomy specimens. Radiology 1991;179:403.
36. Mark AS, Hricak H, Heinrichs LW, et al. Adenomyosis and leiomyoma: differential diagnosis with MR imaging. Radiology 1987;163:527.
37. Reinhold C, McCarthy S, Bret M, et al. Uterine adenomyosis: a prospective comparative analysis with endovaginal US and MR imaging. Radiology 1993;189(P):300.
38. Ascher SM, Arnold LL, Patt RH, et al. Adenomyosis: prospective comparison of MR imaging and transvaginal sonography. Radiology 1994; 190:803.
39. Giacchetto C, Catizone F, Cotroneo GB, et al. Radiologic anatomy of the genital venous system in female patients with varicocele. Surg Gynecol Obstet 1989;169:403.
40. Beard RW, Highman JH, Pearce S, Reginald PW. Diagnosis of pelvic varicosities in women with chronic pelvic pain. Lancet 1984;2:946.

Clinical Gynecologic Imaging, edited
by Arthur C. Fleischer, Marcia C. Javitt,
R. Brooke Jeffrey, Jr., and Howard W. Jones III,
Lippincott-Raven Publishers, Philadelphia © 1997.

CHAPTER 9

Fertility Disorders

Fertility Disorders: Clinical Aspects as They Relate to Imaging

Michael P. Diamond, MD

The role of imaging studies in the evaluation of infertility falls into two major subcategories. The first is the identification and documentation of the integrity of the reproductive tract as a conduit for the passage of gametes and embryos. The second is for the identification of pathologic processes within the abdominal cavity itself that may be a cause of or a contributing factor to infertility. An important corollary to the second category is the identification of a pathologic process coexistent with infertility but not necessarily cause and effect.

ROLE OF IMAGING STUDIES

The value of imaging studies as diagnostic procedures resides in their ability to guide clinical therapy, to predict clinical outcome, to provide guidance in the selection of which of many possible alternatives to pursue, and to allow for appropriate preparation for performance of therapeutic interventions. Additionally, if it is possible to identify that the likelihood of success is discouragingly small, these couples can consider alternatives such as adoption or in vitro fertilization and embryo transfer (as an alternative to surgery) or may consider abandoning their attempts at conception. Accurate identification of the pathologic process present is immensely important to plan the appropriate surgical interventions. Assessment can reveal information that will help make the decision as to whether the surgical approach should be at laparotomy or laparoscopy, and which instruments should be available at the time of each of these procedures. Additionally, the concordant need of hysteroscopy, falloposcopy, fluoroscopy, and other procedures is based on accurate determination of the clinical situation.

The ideal imaging study would contain many characteristics, including the following:

1. The technique should have high accuracy in identifying the presence or absence of abnormalities and their identification.
2. High resolution capabilities are needed so that small masses or other types of abnormalities such as vails of adhesions could be accurately diagnosed and their location specifically identified.
3. The procedure should be noninvasive.
4. The procedure should require minimum amounts of time to perform.
5. The equipment should have low complexity so that it would be available for use by practitioners without access to tertiary care service and could be widely disseminated.
6. The technique should be physician independent so that individuals other than the leading world authorities are able to make highly accurate diagnosis.
7. The technique should be able to be priced so that it could be widely used and available to all who might benefit from its performance.
8. The technique should have no potential of doing harm to the tissues that are imaged. This is of particular importance in obstetrics where there is concern for the developing fetus. Other potential sources of concern in this regard are whether the imaging modality may cause risks of cancer or whether exposure of oocytes to this technique would cause any teratogenic effects.

Many of the imaging techniques available today, including sonography, MRI, and CT, offer several of these characteristics, but none as yet is able to meet all these criteria with the degree of achievement that would be desirable.

Among couples who present with infertility, tuboperitoneal disease is thought to be a contributing factor in up to 40%, with still additional couples having uterine abnormalities that further contribute to difficulty in conceiving. Thus, a standard portion of the infertility evaluation is evaluation of the uterine cavity and fallopian tubes. Classically, this procedure has been performed by hysterosalpingography and provides the opportunity to evaluate the uterine cavity to assess its contour, size, and the presence or absence of intrauterine filling defects. These defects may take the form of myomas, polyps, adhesions, septums, or foreign bodies. An alternative to the performance of a hysterosalpingogram is hysteroscopy, either in the office or the operating room suite, or the performance of what we have come to call sonohysterography.

Sonohysterography involves the instillation of saline into the uterine cavity through a narrow catheter such as a pediatric feeding tube. The saline instillation allows distention of the uterine cavity, which is performed concurrently with transvaginal sonographic imaging of the uterus. This technique also allows identification of the size, shape, and contour of the uterine cavity as well as the identification of the filling defects. It also has potential advantages of avoiding the use of ionizing radiation. Sonohysterograms also allow identification of uterine abnormalities, such as fibroids, which are present but not extending into the uterine cavity that are not usually identifiable by hysterosalpingography, as well as determination of the thickness of the endometrium both before and during fluid instillation. These determinations may be of value in determining growth or development of the endometrium as a predictor of embryo implantation or the diagnosis of endometrial hyperplasia and cancer.

A second type of information able to be obtained from hysterosalpingograms is the status of the fallopian tubes. In particular, issues to be assessed are whether the tubes are patent or whether there is a block, and if so whether the block is at the uterine cornua (proximal), midtubal, or distal. Additionally, if the tube does have a distal blockage, characteristics of the appearance of the resulting hydrosalpinx can be a predictive value in subsequent success of operative corrections. Better success after neosalpingostomies is achievable in tubes that still have rugal patterns manifest and are not excessively large. Hysterosalpingograms are also able to give some idea about the presence of intraabdominal adhesions, although this is often suggested rather than definitive. As dye fills a patent fallopian tube, it should spread fairly freely throughout the lower abdominal cavity, particularly if a patient is asked to move from side to side to help disseminate the dye. If, however, the dye remains loculated in areas surrounding the distal ends of the tubes, this is a strong suggestion that adhesions are present. Unfortunately, dissemination of dye often occurs in individuals with extensive adhesions in situations where the adhesions are in areas such that loculation does not occur.

Sonohysterosalpingograms are able to provide some information about tubal patency by identifying a collection of fluid inside the abdominal cavity. However, at this time, it is more difficult to assess each tube individually. Perhaps with the development of new distending contrast media the use of sonohysterosalpingography for the determination of tubal patency will be better able to be evaluated.

Another imaging alternative for evaluation of the fallopian tube is falloposcopy. This can be done at the time of either laparoscopy or laparotomy by placing a narrow scope through the fimbria of the fallopian tube. An alternative is to advance a falloposcope or catheter into the fallopian tube at the time of either hysteroscopy, fluoroscopy, or sonographic-guided procedures. This would allow evaluation of the fallopian tubes and help make better identification of a tubal pathologic process including areas of scarring or strictures. Additionally, in patients with hydrosalpinx, this procedure offers the additional advantage of being able to look at the tubal mucosa and using this information as a prediction of pregnancy outcome. Patients who have "bald" tubes have a low likelihood of conceiving, while those in whom mucosal folds are present inside the cells and that appear to be normal would be more likely to be successful in conception.

Imaging of intraabdominal structures is also becoming an increasingly important aspect of obstetric and gynecologic care. The widespread use of sonography for assessment of the developing fetus goes far beyond the scope of this chapter; to mention a few uses, these include identification of multiple gestations, dating of pregnancy, establishment of intrauterine growth retardation, evaluation for congenital malformations, diagnosis of antepartum bleeding, and assessment of fetal well being. In gynecology, diagnostic imaging studies are used for evaluation of pelvic masses, evaluation of pelvic pain, diagnosis of ectopic pregnancies, and identification of abnormalities, such as endometriosis and bowel obstruction.

A wide variety of techniques are used for diagnostic imaging of intraabdominal processes. These include the use of radiographs (for diagnosis of bowel obstruction and identification of calcifications), radiographs with contrast material (such as intravenous pyelography to identify size and location of kidneys and ureter), as well as sonography, CT, and MRI. Because of the current differential price between sonography and either CT or MRI, sonography is often the first approach. Additionally, availability of sonographic equipment is much more widespread, with ability to perform sonographic procedures much more readily available.

Probably the classic example of the use of sonography in gynecologic practice as a diagnostic aid is the identification and localization of a pregnancy. Whereas establishing that a pregnancy has occurred is usually performed by pregnancy testing, localization and assessment of viability is often much more difficult, often requiring additional modalities.

Nomograms have been established that identify timing at which landmarks should be identified by sonography. (The absolute numbers often vary because of different standards used in performing human chorionic gonadotropin assays.) It is now often possible to identify each uterine sac by 5 to 6 weeks' gestation with identification of fetal heart motion 1 to 2 weeks later. Sonography is often very useful for these purposes. Timing at which these landmarks are able to be identified can be made earlier by performing transvaginal sonography as opposed to transabdominal scanning. Transvaginal scanning also offers a second advantage in addition to earlier identification of intrauterine pregnancies. The second advantage is a better ability to identify masses in the adnexa that would be consistent with ectopic pregnancies. The use of color Doppler flow imaging has further explained the usefulness of sonography in the evaluation of the developing gestation. These new techniques can be further used to assess viability of an intrauterine pregnancy by the degree of flow going to an intrauterine gestation. Additionally, the adnexal mass, which may have represented either an ectopic pregnancy or a corpus luteum cyst, can now often be differentiated by the use of these additional technologies. Unfortunately, however, use of these new modalities requires more expensive machines and more extensive training, making them less readily available to the general practitioner.

Other intraabdominal processes for which diagnostic imaging is helpful include evaluation of tuboovarian abscesses, ovarian masses, tubal enlargement, uterine fibroids, endometriosis (particularly endometriomas), ovarian torsion, appendicitis, and diverticulitis. Additionally, neoplasms of the reproductive tract, urinary tract, and intestinal tract are able to be evaluated and often diagnosed with a high degree of certainty with imaging technologies. Thus, these techniques are helpful in patients in whom adequate pelvic examinations cannot be performed either due to patient obesity, patient discomfort, or inability of the patient to allow performance of an adequate examination. Additionally, in patients in whom an adequate examination is able to be performed, image modalities can be used to confirm the findings of physical examination or to allow evaluation of areas of examination not believed to have been adequately evaluated by examination alone.

Sonography is helpful with the initial evaluation of adnexal masses. Often, masses can be localized as to ovarian origin or origin from another site and precise sizes can be established. Furthermore, characteristics of the mass can be ascertained, including whether they are solid or cystic, whether there are internal septations, the thickness of septations, and the presence of fluid levels in the tissue within these masses. Thus, it has been helpful in raising or lowering suspicion of a malignant neoplasm and in guiding subsequent therapy. Evaluation of these adnexal masses can further be improved by the use of color Doppler flow imaging.

Although CT and MRI have also been helpful in the evaluation of the pelvis, their price often relinquishes them to secondary purposes in the pelvis. These modalities are useful for evaluation of larger masses extending into the abdominal cavity and also for evaluation of retroperitoneal structures including lymph nodes. MRI has also been found helpful in the differentiation of ovarian masses, particularly endometriomas because of the characteristic appearance of the blood in the endometrioma. (The differential diagnosis would include a corpus luteum cyst.) MRI has also been of benefit in the evaluation of complex adnexal pelvic masses and in differentiating myomas from ovarian processes. It has also been used for the differentiation of benign myomas from malignant leiomyosarcomas and in evaluation of malformations of the reproductive tract.

CONCLUSION

A great deal of information can be obtained by diagnostic imaging studies. Whereas previously they have been used solely to guide subsequent clinical therapy, their use has often been criticized as to whether the findings actually helped change clinical interventions. It is hoped that in the future use of these modalities will not only be able to help guide clinical interventions but also be able to identify situations in which interventions can be avoided and the abnormalities monitored by successive scans, thereby eliminating the expense and morbidity of an interventional procedure.

Transvaginal Sonography in Gynecologic Fertility Disorders

Arthur C. Fleischer, MD, Jaime M. Vasquez, MD, and
Donna M. Kepple, RDMS

Transvaginal sonography has a vital role in the management of infertility disorders related to a variety of gynecologic disorders.[1,2] Specifically, this imaging technique has its greatest clinical applications in follicular monitoring and guided follicular aspiration. Other procedures that may benefit from sonographic guidance include embryo transfer and transcervical cannulization of the fallopian tube for gamete intrafallopian tube transfer (GIFT) procedures. Other applications of sonography in infertility include evaluation of the endometrium in patients with possible luteal phase inadequacy, assessment of tubal patency, and detection and follow-up of disorders that may be related to infertility, such as endometriosis. Transvaginal sonography also has a vital role in the monitoring of pregnant women, making sure there is no likelihood of an ectopic pregnancy and detecting and monitoring complicated intrauterine pregnancies. It also has a role in evaluating women with suspected uterine malformations. In this subchapter the most frequently used applications are discussed with particular emphasis on the role of transvaginal transducer/probes.

CLINICAL ASPECTS AS RELATED TO SONOGRAPHY

Infertility, as defined by the inability to conceive after 1 year of unprotected intercourse, affects 10% to 15% of couples in the United States. Whereas 80% of couples who are between 18 and 28 years of age will conceive during a 1-year period, and another 10% the following year, 10% of couples in the United States (approximately 2.4 million couples) have a fertility disorder. In approximately two thirds of the cases, the cause for infertility can be related to the female partner, and in one third the cause can be related to the male partner. The most common gynecologic disorders related to infertility include occlusive tubal disease or endometriosis (30% to 50%), ovulation disorders (40%), cervical factors (10%), and luteal phase abnormalities (5%).[3] For between 5% and 10% of cases, the cause of infertility is unexplained.[3,4]

Over the past 10 to 15 years, there have been significant advances in the medical treatment of gynecologic infertility, as well as more refined techniques for the surgical management of these disorders. Together, these techniques are now referred to as assisted reproductive technology. More recently, the use of transvaginal sonography has afforded the development of several minimally invasive procedures such as transvaginal aspiration of follicles and cannulation of the fallopian tube for GIFT procedures. Tubal patency can also be assessed with contrast medium–enhanced transvaginal sonography.

The most common medical treatment for gynecologic infertility involves induction of ovulation with either human menopausal gonadotropin (hMG) or clomiphene citrate. These medications are given after pituitary block with gonadotropin-releasing hormone analogues such as leuprolide (Lupron). For patients receiving these medications, transvaginal sonography has an important role in documenting normal or abnormal follicular development (Fig. 9-1).[5] Although transvaginal sonography is preferred for follicular monitoring, transabdominal scanning is sometimes helpful in the patient with ovaries that have been sutured to the peritoneum, bladder, or uterus. Performance of follicular monitoring by the transvaginal technique also allows the operator to become familiar with the lie of the ovaries and the location of the dominant follicles before their transvaginal aspiration. Occasionally, transvaginal sonography can be used in combination with other tests such as luteinizing hormone (LH) assay and cervical mucus scoring to better define the time of ovulation.[6] Transvaginal sonography can depict textural changes in the endometrium characteristic of mid cycle. The relative phase of endometrial development (proliferative, mid-cycle, or secretory) can be determined by assessment of endometrial thickness and texture (Fig. 9-2). Color Doppler sonography affords detection of flow changes in ovarian blood flow associated with ovulation. As shown in several studies, formation of a corpus luteum is associated with a decreased impedance of arterial flow within the ovary. Velocities also show differences depending on whether ovulation has occurred (Fig. 9-3). Sonographic determination of the time of ovulation may also be helpful for patients

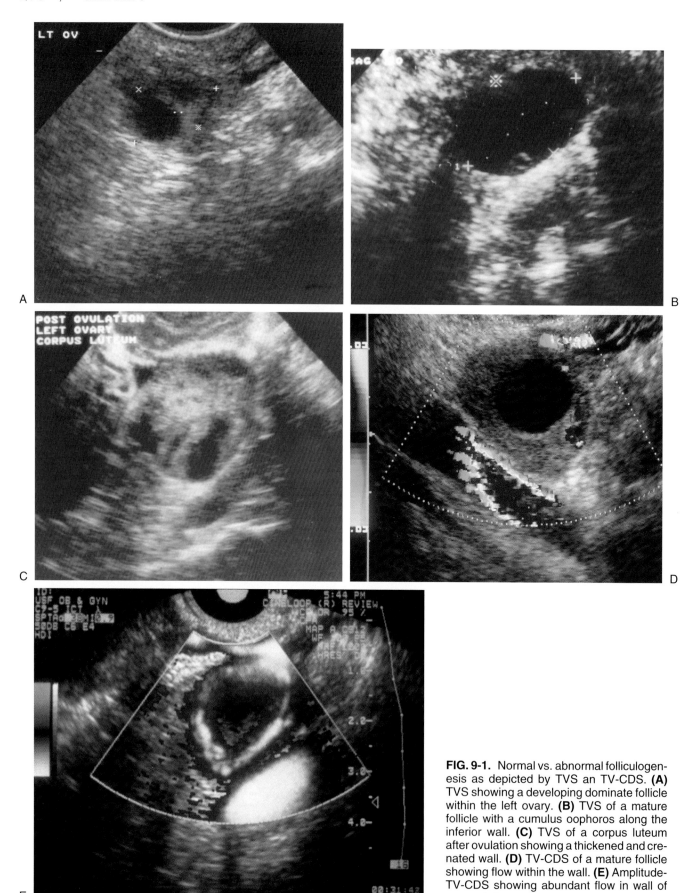

FIG. 9-1. Normal vs. abnormal folliculogenesis as depicted by TVS an TV-CDS. **(A)** TVS showing a developing dominate follicle within the left ovary. **(B)** TVS of a mature follicle with a cumulus oophoros along the inferior wall. **(C)** TVS of a corpus luteum after ovulation showing a thickened and crenated wall. **(D)** TV-CDS of a mature follicle showing flow within the wall. **(E)** Amplitude-TV-CDS showing abundant flow in wall of corpus luteum.

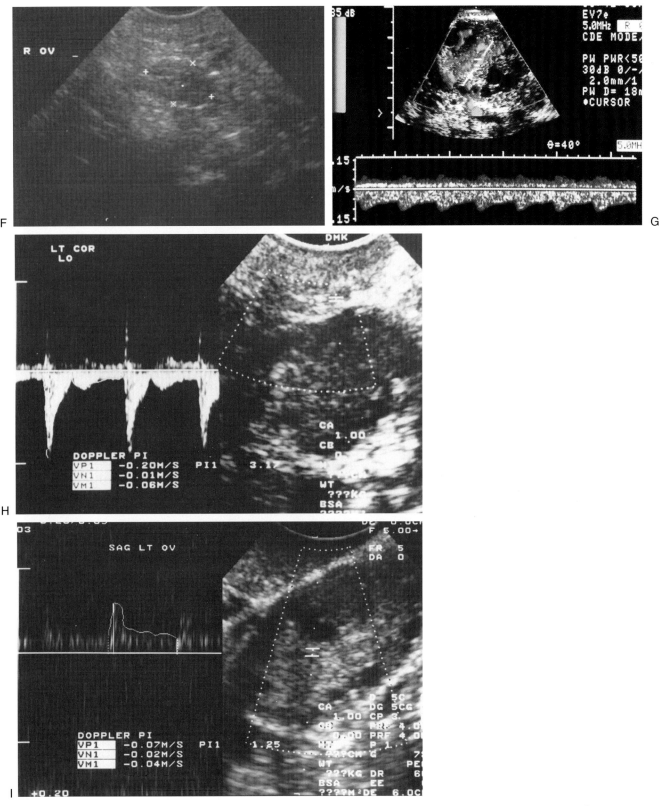

FIG. 9-1. *Continued.* **(F)** TVS showing no follicular development within the right ovary *(between cursors)* after ovulation induction. **(G)** Amplitude TV-CDS showing cluster of immature follicles and low impedance arterial flow in an intraovarian arteriole. TV-CDS of a polycystic ovary showing different waveforms in hilum **(H)** and stroma **(I)** of the ovary. Persistent high impedance intraovarian flow can be seen in faulty folliculogenesis after ovulation induction. **(E,** courtesy of Anna Parsons, MD.)

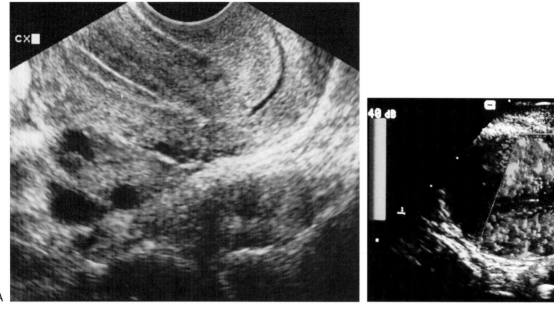

FIG. 9-2. Endometrial development as depicted by TVS. **(A)** Multilayered mid-cycle endometrium. The endometrial interfaces include the outer echogenic basalis, the relatively hypoechoic functionalis, and the echogenic median echo arising from refluxed mucus. The cervical mucus is hyperechoic. The ovary is depicted adjacent to the uterine corpus and contains several immature follicles. **(B)** TV-CDS (C,D,E) showing flow within the myometrium and same flow within the basal layer of endometrium. **(B,** courtesy of Acuson, Inc.)

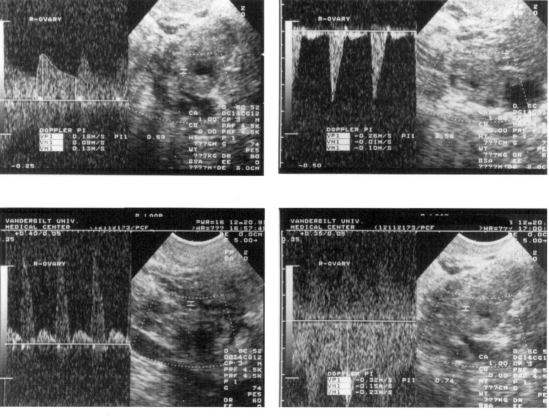

FIG. 9-3. Differences in impedance within the same ovary. Composite TV-CDS shows various flows in different area within same ovary. High impedance waveforms are seen in the region of the adnexal branch of the uterine artery, whereas low impedance flow is present and near the corpus luteum.

undergoing timed insemination (ie, artificial insemination by husband, artificial insemination by donor).

In vitro fertilization and embryo transfer (IVF-ET) is now offered in several centers primarily for patients who have absent or significantly diseased tubes. It also has been used for some other infertility disorders related to cervical factors, oligospermia, and immune factors. For this procedure, transvaginal sonography not only has an important role in follicular monitoring but also plays a vital role in guiding follicular aspiration.[2]

The actual success rate (as defined by the percentage of "take-home babies" divided by the number of stimulated cycles) for IVF-ET is between 12% and 18%.[7] In some subpopulations this rate is higher, approximating the natural rate at which fertilized ova progress to delivering of a live neonate (approximately 30%).[8] The primary factors that influence the success or failure of IVF-ET include the number of mature oocytes retrieved and the number and quality of fertilized ova transferred.[9] Other factors that may influence the success or failure of this procedure include the endometrial "receptivity" to the implanting conceptus and, possibly, the method used for follicular aspiration.

A new procedure has been developed that involves transfer of sperm and ova directly into the tube (gamete intrafallopian tube transfer [GIFT] or zygote intrafallopian transfer [ZIFT]) for some couples with unexplained infertility. This procedure involves follicular aspiration and mixing of ovum and sperm, with replacement of the mixture or fertilized zygote back into the fallopian tubes. Embryo replacement is done either by laparoscopic cannulation of the fallopian tube or, more recently, by sonographically guided catheterization of the fallopian tube through the endocervical and endometrial lumina.[10]

Besides these specific treatments for infertility, sonography is occasionally used to document the progression or regression of endometriosis or to confirm the presence of polycystic ovaries and other adnexal masses such as tuboovarian abscesses that may be associated with gynecologic infertility.[11] Although most endometriomas are small (approximately 5 mm) and are located on the serosal surfaces of bowel or other intraabdominal organs or ligaments, they may not be detectable on sonography. Larger ones (over 2 cm) that are located separate from bowel and contain hypoechoic hemorrhage can be delineated and followed during and after treatment.[12] The enlarged and rounded ovaries that contain immature subcapsular follicles of women with polycystic ovaries can be diagnosed, even though in up to 30% of women with this disorder the ovaries may not be abnormally enlarged.[11,13]

Thus, most common indications for sonography in infertility include the following:

• Serial monitoring of follicular development
• Guided follicular aspiration
• Assessment of endometrial development
• Assessment of tubal patency

Transvaginal sonography is occasionally used for guiding embryo replacement, transluminal GIFT procedures, and evaluation of the endometrial cysts or submucosal fibroids.[14,15] Whether the technique that is used for follicular aspiration actually influences the success or failure of IVF-ET requires more extensive worldwide experience.[16] However, it is clear that sonographically guided procedures have several advantages over laparoscopic aspiration (eg, decreased anesthesia exposure, operative manipulation, and operative risk), that now make it the procedure of choice for most patients undergoing in vitro fertilization.

Color Doppler sonography affords physiologic assessment of the ovaries and endometrium. Lack of the typical low impedance, high diastolic flow within a corpus luteum coupled with poor uterine or endometrial perfusion may suggest luteal phase inadequacy.[17] Color Doppler sonography may also be helpful in the assessment of tubal patency, because it is quite sensitive to the flow created when contrast medium is injected within the uterine lumen.[18]

INSTRUMENTATION

Transvaginal sonography has become the method of choice for evaluation of the uterus and ovaries. The transvaginal transducer/probe allows more detailed depiction of the uterus and ovary than transabdominal scans for several reasons. First, the uterus and adnexal structures are closer to the transducer, allowing higher-frequency transducers to be used (between 6 and 10 MHz). Second, because the beam does not have to transverse the abdominal wall there is less beam scattering. In contrast to transabdominal scanning, however, transvaginal scanning displays images in nonconventional imaging planes. In addition, the regions of interest are limited to 6 to 10 cm and do not afford as global delineation of the pelvic structures as transabdominal scanning. In transvaginal sonography, surrounding bowel loops are usually not interposed between the probe and the adnexa. If they are, gentle manual abdominal palpation or manipulation of the probe, or both, can be used to displace intervening bowel.

Needle guides have been developed that can be attached to transvaginal probes and greatly facilitate guided follicular aspiration. After the probe is draped with a condom, these needle guides can be placed directly on the transducer/probe, allowing for direct and continuous visualization of the aspirating needle as it is advanced into the ovary. The "line of sight" generated on the monitor closely approximates the needle path that will be traversed.

There are several types of transvaginal transducer/probes available. These include curved linear-array, phased-array, and mechanical-sector devices. The field of view of most of these probes is 100 degrees. The curved linear-array affords a large sector field of view as the curved linear-array probes. Phased-array probes may have resolution problems in the lateral aspects of the image owing to side lobe artifacts. Color Doppler capabilities have been added to transvaginal scanners. The addition of color Doppler sonography does not significantly increase the intensities used for imaging because the color Doppler imaging affords specific selection of the vessels and areas to be interrogated by pulsed Doppler techniques. Flow can be assessed by waveform analysis, which reveals relative impedance to flow, and by overall assessment of the color shown in area of uterus, which is related to the relative vessel density of a particular area.

FOLLICULAR MONITORING

Sonography has a vital role in depicting follicular development in patients treated for infertility who receive ovulation-induction medications.[19] Although the maturity of the oocyte can only be indirectly inferred by the size of the follicle, the sonographic information can be coupled with estradiol values to provide an accurate assessment of the presence or absence and number of mature follicles.[20-22] The anatomic information obtained with sonography concerning the size and development of maturing follicles and corpus luteum can be used to distinguish physiologic from insufficient or abnormal cycles.[23] For example, the maximal follicle size in insufficient cycles has been reported to be significantly smaller than in normal ones, and the absence of a corpus luteum has been found more often in insufficient cycles.[23] In addition, the undesirable development of multiple immature follicles rather than development of a single dominant follicle can be recognized in patients with polycystic ovaries.[23]

Although its actual contribution to infertility is controversial, some infertility specialists describe an abnormality in ovulation termed *luteinized unruptured follicle syndrome* as a cause of unexplained infertility.[24] In this disorder there is failure of ovulation of the oocyte, which remains trapped within the follicle. The presence of this abnormality can only be confirmed by observation at laparoscopy of the absence of a stigma (healed rent in the ovarian capsule where ovulation occurred) on the ovarian capsule. Because this may no longer be present at 2 hours post ovulation, the presence of this syndrome is difficult to confirm. With sonography, one can observe failure of the follicle to deflate and the absence of intraperitoneal fluid associated with ovulation. This syndrome may be more common in women with endometriosis and may not be present on consecutive cycles.[8,25]

Abnormalities in folliculogenesis can be further assessed with transvaginal color Doppler sonography. This technique depicts physiologic changes in flow impedance and velocity associated with follicular enlargement and corpus luteum formation. A significant drop in impedance occurs with development of the vascular "arcade" that occurs in the follicular wall within a corpus luteum. In addition, a slow increase in velocity and blood flow within the intraovarian arterioles occurs during folliculogenesis (see Fig. 9-3). This steady increase is interrupted in patients with luteinized unruptured follicles.

Spontaneous Cycles

At the time of birth, the female neonate has approximately 2 million primary oocytes within each ovary. When menarche begins approximately 200,000 remain per ovary. During the childbearing years, approximately 200 oocytes will be ovulated. This indicates that approximately 99.9% of primary oocytes become atretic or do not develop at all.

Maturation of the oocyte and follicle is responsive primarily to changes in follicle-stimulating hormone (FSH), LH, and circulating levels of estrogen (E_2). With the elaboration and release of FSH in the late secretory phase, there is development of one and sometimes two follicles in a subsequent cycle. It is not uncommon to observe two follicles developing to approximately 10 mm, with one becoming dominant and growing and the other regressing. Luteinizing hormone reinitiates meiosis of the oocyte, and ovulation typically occurs within 36 hours of its "surge" in circulating levels. Estradiol is synthesized by the granulosa cells and provides important feedback to the pituitary in the production of FSH and LH. With development of a corpus luteum an increase in vascularity within the wall is observed on transvaginal color Doppler sonography. If this process does not occur, luteal inadequacy is likely.

Beginning with menarche, during spontaneous cycles, there is usually development of one or sometimes two dominant follicles. Sonography can depict the developing follicles, beginning at the time they measure between 3 and 5 mm. In the spontaneous cycle, there is usually one or at the most two follicles that develop to approximately 10 mm. As the follicle matures, more fluid is elaborated into its center and the number of granulosa cells lining the inside wall of the follicle increases. The oocyte, which is less than 0.1 mm, is surrounded by a cluster of granulosa cells. This complex is termed the *cumulus oophorus*. It measures approximately 1 mm and can be depicted occasionally inside mature follicles (see Fig. 9-1). As the follicle reaches maturity, its inner dimensions range from 17 to 25 mm.[26] However, within the same individual, the size of a mature follicle is relatively constant cycle to cycle. Intrafollicular echoes may be observed with mature follicles, probably rising from clusters of granulosa cells that shear off the wall near the time of ovulation. After ovulation, the follicular wall becomes irregular as the follicle becomes "deflated." The fresh corpus luteum usually appears as an echogenic structure approximately 15 mm in size.

On transvaginal color Doppler sonography, folliculogenesis can be assessed by changes in impedance and velocity in intraovarian arterioles. With formation of a corpus luteum, impedance drops a reflection of the vascular arcade that develops within the wall of the corpus lutea. Velocities increase up to 40 cm/s as the corpus luteum becomes functional. Changes in velocity of impedance do not occur in cycles that are not associated with the development of dominant follicles.[27,28]

In addition to delineation of changes in follicle size, morphology, and blood flow, sonography can depict the presence of intraperitoneal fluid and endometrial changes (see Figs. 9-1 and 9-2). It is not uncommon to have 1 to 3 mL in the cul-de-sac before ovulation. When ovulation occurs, there is typically between 4 and 5 mL within the cul-de-sac. When the patient is scanned with a fully distended bladder, the fluid may be located outside the cul-de-sac, surrounding bowel loops in the lower abdomen and upper pelvis.

Induced Cycles

In patients whose infertility can be attributed to an ovulation abnormality, ovulation induction is indicated. Ovulation induction is also used in IVF-ET to increase the number of oocytes aspirated. This increase in turn increases the number of fertilized concepti that may be transferred, thereby increasing the chance of pregnancy.

As previously mentioned, the two medications that are most commonly used for ovulation induction include clomiphene citrate and hMG. Although both medications result in the development of multiple follicles, they act by different mechanisms. Sonography has a vital role in monitoring follicular development in women receiving ovulation-induction medication.[25]

Patients undergoing ovulation induction are usually examined every other day beginning at day 10. Patients undergoing IVF-ET are examined by sonography starting earlier in their cycles and usually daily in an attempt to carefully monitor their follicular development.

Transvaginal sonography has an important role to detect cysts associated with leuprolide pretreatment that may impair the ability to induce ovulation with clomiphene citrate or hMG.

Clomiphene citrate is considered an estrogen antagonist and exerts its effect by binding estrogen receptor sites in the pituitary and hypothalamus. This, in turn, influences the pituitary to synthesize more FSH, thereby recruiting more follicles. Because the process of selection and dominance may be overridden, multiple, relatively synchronous follicles usually develop. Although the preovulatory E_2-LH feedback may be intact in clomiphene citrate–treated patients with an intact hypothalamus, some patients are given human chorionic gonadotropin (hCG) to induce final oocyte maturation.

Follicular development with clomiphene citrate can be quite different than that observed in spontaneous cycles (see Fig. 9-1). Specifically, each follicle seems to develop at an individual rate and at times may be accelerated or slowed down. Therefore, the largest follicle on a given date may not be the same one that is the largest 2 days later, and it may not even be the same one that is most mature. Furthermore, correlation of E_2 and follicle size is poor and the maximum preovulatory diameter can range from 19 to 24 mm.

As opposed to clomiphene citrate, treatment with hMG does not require an intact hypothalamus or pituitary. In hMG-treated patients, there seem to be two distinct patterns of follicular development.[29] In those amenorrheic women with no exogenous estrogen activity and dormant ovaries, the response to endogenous gonadotropin is to develop a small number of large follicles (see Fig. 9-1C). The growth rate and E_2 secretion are linear, correlate well, and are of equal predictive value. A high pregnancy rate is achieved in this group. In contrast, patients with estrogenic activity who harbor antral follicles at different stages of development react very differently. Stimulation of these patients requires less hMG and usually results in the rapid recruitment of many follicles with different growth rates with varying degrees of E_2 secretory capacity. Also, the rate at which E_2 increases is exponential, increasing the risk of hyperstimulation. Thus, there is a dissociation between follicle size and E_2 levels, suggesting the growth rate and functional maturity are asynchronous. This group of women particularly benefits from combined E_2 and sonographic follicular monitoring. Because hMG contains both FSH and LH and a spontaneous LH surge is less frequent when stimulating with hMG, hCG may be required to induce final follicular maturation. Sonographic delineation of follicle size is crucial because hCG is best administered once follicles reach 15 to 18 mm.

For in vitro fertilization, follicles are typically aspirated when they reach 15 to 18 mm in average dimension and when there is evidence by estradiol values of a mature follicle (approximately 400 pg/mL per mature follicle).[21] Another sonographic sign of a mature follicle is the presence of low-level, intrafollicular echoes. These echoes probably arise from sheets of granulosa cells that have separated from the follicular wall. In one study involving patients who underwent ovulation induction, a greater pregnancy rate was achieved in those patients whose follicles demonstrated such intrafollicular echoes.[2]

Sonography has an important role in decreasing the likelihood of ovarian hyperstimulation. Ovarian hyperstimulation disorder occurs in various degrees of severity in most patients who undergo ovulation induction, ranging from mild abdominal discomfort, probably due to the distention of the ovarian capsule, to severe circulatory compromise and electrolyte imbalance, probably secondary to ascites or pleural effusions that may develop. The more severe form, ovarian hyperstimulation syndrome, is usually associated with massive stromal edema of the ovary. The enlarged ovaries may be prone to torsion. The symptoms associated with ovarian hyperstimulation syndrome usually begin 5 to 8 days after hCG is given, but they can be most severe in patients who actually achieve pregnancy. Studies have shown that hyperstimulation is unlikely in women whose ovaries contain several large (over 15 mm) follicles and tends to occur when there are several small or intermediate-size follicles.[30]

Although sonographic findings of enlarged ovaries with multiple immature follicles may suggest the possibility of hyperstimulation, this syndrome can be more accurately predicted by extremely high levels of E_2 (over 3000 pg/mL).

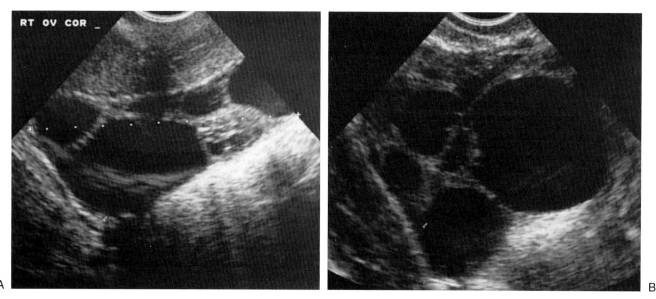

FIG. 9-4. Ovarian hyperstimulation as depicted by TVS. **(A)** Markedly enlarged right ovary containing multiple follicles of various sizes. **(B)** Markedly enlarged left ovary of same patient as in A, containing multiple follicles of various sizes.

Despite the superovulation required for in vitro fertilization, hyperstimulation is only rarely encountered. This is probably a reflection of close monitoring that these patients receive but also may be secondary to drainage and collapse of the aspirated follicles. On sonography, patients with ovarian hyperstimulation syndrome usually have enlarged ovaries (over 10 cm) that may contain several hypoechoic areas (Fig. 9-4). The hypoechoic areas may correspond to atretic follicles or to regions of hemorrhage within the ovary. Color Doppler sonography usually shows increased diastolic flow within the intraovarian arteries. In addition, venous flow may become nonphasic, a sign of reduced venous return. The

pregnancies that occur with ovarian hyperstimulation syndrome may be very early (less than 4 weeks), and no definitive sonographic findings may be found. Intraperitoneal fluid is commonly present. With supportive therapy, this syndrome usually regresses spontaneously.

After induced ovulation, the stimulated follicles usually undergo regression but may persist and enlarge over the remainder of the cycle. The presence of physiologic ovarian cysts (over 3 cm) may preclude ovulation induction during that cycle, because the previously induced follicles may not have totally regressed and the remaining ovarian tissue may not be as responsive to ovulation-induction medication.

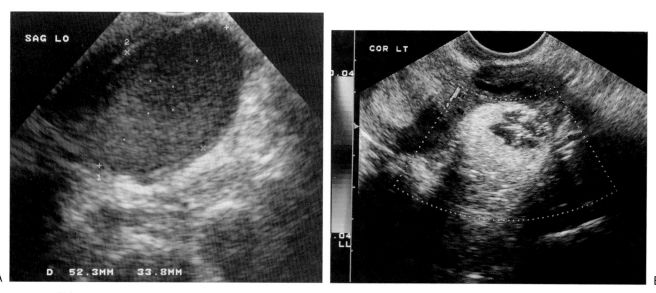

FIG. 9-5. Adnexal masses associated with infertility. **(A)** TVS of an endometrioma *(between cursors)* demonstrating ground glass texture. **(B)** TV-CDS of a dermoid cyst in an infertile patient showing little intratumoral flow.

Theoretically, the risk of torsion, rupture, or both may also be increased in these women.

Sonography can also detect other adnexal masses such as endometriomas, which may mimic physiologic cysts or follicles (Fig. 9-5). Endometriosis typically exhibits a ground-glass internal texture resulting from internal organized clot. Some demonstrate echogenic clots and echogenic borders secondary to the fibrosis that these masses incite.

Sonography is also helpful in decreasing the likelihood of multiple gestation that may occur with fertilization of multiple ova. However, it is difficult to predict which pregnancies will result in multiple births. Clearly, however, when there are more than four mature follicles, the chance for multiple gestation beyond twinning is more probable than if only two or three mature follicles are induced.

SONOGRAPHIC-GUIDED FOLLICULAR ASPIRATION

Transvaginal sonographic-guided follicular aspiration has now become the preferred procedure of choice for oocyte retrieval over the previously used laparoscopic technique. The major advantages to this technique include decreased exposure to general anesthesia, lower chance for operative complications, and feasibility of performing this procedure on an outpatient basis. The success rate as determined by the number of fertilizable oocytes retrieved and pregnancies produced is comparable to the laparoscopic technique.[31] The procedure is also advantageous in patients with pelvic adhesions because laparoscopic access to the ovary could be hampered in those cases.[32] Most importantly, acceptance of the procedure by patients is high and it can be performed as an outpatient procedure.[33,34]

There are several methods for follicular aspiration that involve sonographic guidance. These include transvaginal sonography for guidance of transvesicular aspiration and transabdominal sonographic guidance for transurethral aspiration. Although transvaginal sonography with transvaginal aspiration is most frequently used, the actual method that is used can be tailored to each patient according to the anatomic position of the ovary and other structures. For example, the transvaginal aspiration is the preferred route when the ovaries are in the cul-de-sac, whereas the transurethral approach may be used for aspiration of follicles in ovaries that are located near the dome of the bladder.

With all of these aspiration techniques, a long (30-cm) 18-gauge needle is used that is scored at the tip, which results in its enhanced sonographic visualization. The aspiration procedure is performed under local anesthesia and with supplemental intravenous or intramuscular medication. It is most often performed as an outpatient procedure.

For the transvaginal aspiration with transvaginal transducers, a needle guide is attached to the transducer/probe (Fig. 9-6). This allows the needle to traverse in the beam path of the transducer. The cursor is displayed on the scanning screen, which indicates the path of the needle. After a condom containing sterile gel is placed over the transducer and a sterile needle guide is attached, the operator manipulates the transducer to optimally delineate the ovary. The desired follicle is brought into the "line of sight" and the needle is introduced transvaginally. After the initial aspiration, the follicle is filled with buffered medium and flushed so that chances for retrieving a mature oocyte are maximized.

This aspiration technique has been associated with a low complication rate. One complication that has been described is inadvertent introduction of the needle into a vessel in the pelvis.[35] This problem can be avoided if the operator carefully examines any round structure in both long and short axis to distinguish a pulsatile vascular structure from a follicle.

Another technique that can be used for follicular aspiration that does not require a transvaginal probe involves transvaginal aspiration when the transducer is held on the abdominal wall.[36] This procedure is less accurate than the transvaginal route with a needle guide because it involves two operators and the beam may not be in the plane of the needle.

A modification of this procedure has been described using an approach through the catheterized urethra.[9] For this technique, a Foley catheter is placed within the urethra. The wall of the Foley catheter serves as a sheath for introduction of the needle into the bladder. This is particularly suited for ovaries that are located high along the dome of the bladder. This technique, however, involves passage of the needle through the bladder. This passage of a needle through the bladder and anterior peritoneum may be more painful than the transvaginal route. The transvesical approach with transabdominal monitoring is now considered less desirable than any of the previously mentioned techniques, owing primarily to the pain associated with needle passage through the bladder wall and peritoneum.

Whether the route of follicular aspiration actually affects the outcome of IVF-ET can be questioned.[37] Most studies, however, indicate a conception rate that is higher than or equal to that achieved using laparoscopic technique.[31]

Transvaginal sonographic-guided aspiration of recurrent endometriomas has been advocated by some as treatment for this disorder.[38] A larger needle (16 gauge) may be needed to aspirate some of the formed clot.

SONOGRAPHIC-GUIDED EMBRYO TRANSFER AND TUBAL CANNULATION

Sonography is also being used for transcervical cannulization of the uterine lumen.[39] This can be used for two procedures, including embryo replacement and cannulization of the fallopian tube required in GIFT procedures.

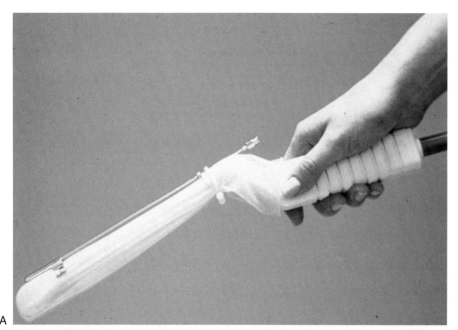

A

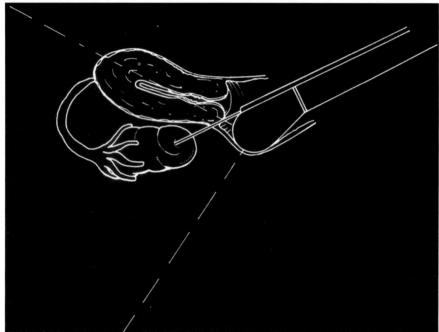

B

FIG. 9-6. TVS-guided follicular aspiration. **(A)** A needle guide is attached to the probe over a sterile sheath and provides a restricted path for the needle. **(B)** Diagram of guided follicular aspiration.

Sonographic guidance for embryo replacement has been described in one series.[14] This procedure involves transabdominal sonographic monitoring of the catheter in which the embryo is loaded. Optimally, the embryo should be instilled when the tip of the catheter extends to the top of the endometrial lumen. Embryo placement into the proper position may be identified by observing the echogenic air bubble, which is loaded before the embryo at the tip of the catheter. Although several institutions do not use sonographic monitoring for embryo replacement, it has been shown that this technique can facilitate more accurate placement of the transferred embryo.[14]

A technique for sonographic guidance of placement of a catheter into the fallopian tubes for GIFT procedure has been described.[10] For this procedure, a catheter is placed transcervically and manipulated into the area of the uterine cornu. The catheter is slowly introduced, under sonographic guidance, into the tubal ostia. Once the catheter is in the distal isthmic portion of the fallopian tube, the sperm and ova may be introduced through the cannula directly into the tube.

ENDOMETRIAL ASSESSMENT

Besides the factors involved in obtaining a fertilized ovum, the developmental state of the endometrium may also

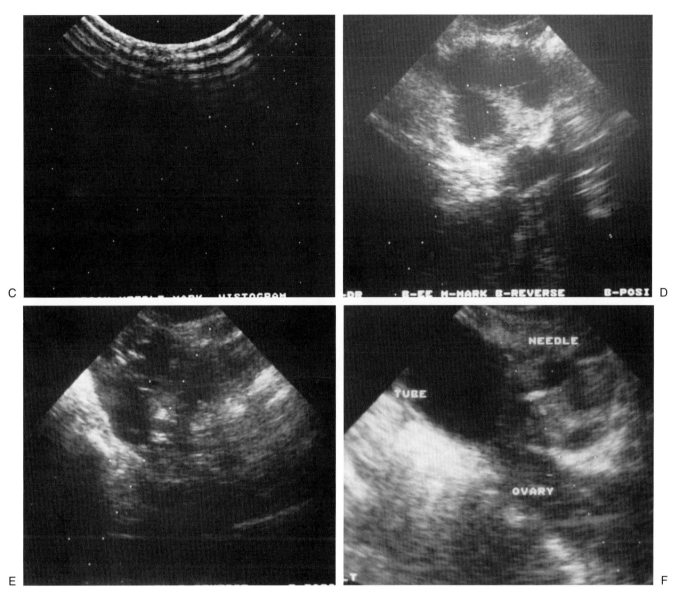

FIG. 9-6. *Continued.* **(C)** Picture of the monitor screen showing needle path. **(D** and **E)** TVS-guided follicular aspiration. Prior to aspiration, the desired follicle is lined up with the needle path **(D)**. After the needle is advanced into the follicle, the follicular contents are aspirated **(E)**. The needle tip is echogenic. **(F)** TVS-guided follicular aspiration in a patient with a hydrosalpinx adjacent to the right ovary.

be a factor that influences the probability that conception will occur (Fig. 9-7).[20] Because the endometrium can also be delineated on scans performed for follicular monitoring, several investigators have evaluated this mucous membrane in an attempt to study whether there is an optimal thickness or texture.[39–42] Clearly, there is an association of the texture of the endometrium as depicted sonographically and the circulating levels of estrogen and progesterone.[20] In spontaneous and induced cycles, the sonographic appearance of the endometrium varies according to its specific phases of development. In the menstrual phase, the endometrium appears as a thin, broken echogenic interface. In the proliferative phase, it thickens and becomes isoechoic, measuring 5

to 8 mm in anteroposterior width. Its relative hypoechogenicity is related to the relatively orderly organization of the glandular elements within the endometrium. As ovulation approaches, the endometrium becomes more echogenic, probably related to development of secretions within the endometrial glands and the numerous interfaces that arise from distended and tortuous glands. In the periovulatory period, there may be a hypoechoic area within the most central portion of the endometrium, probably within the compactum layer. This finding has been described as a means of confirming ovulation has occurred. However, with transvaginal sonography, we have observed this finding both before and immediately after ovulation. During the secretory phase, the

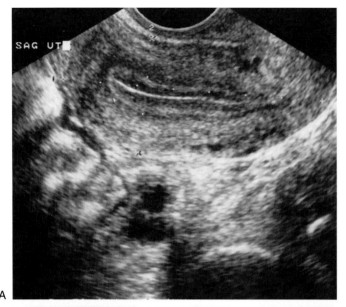

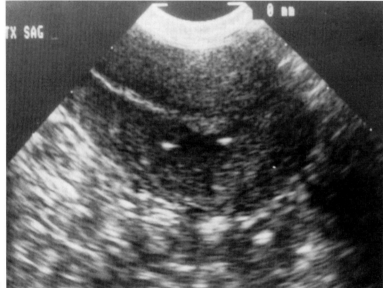

FIG. 9-7. Endometrium in conception vs non-conception cycles. **(A)** Conception. A multilayered endometrium in a patient who conceived after ovulation induction. **(B)** Non-conception. The endometrium is thin and does not exhibit a multilayered appearance. The echogenic foci probably represented scars within the inner myometrium from previous D&C. (**B,** courtesy of Deland Burks, MD.)

endometrium achieves its greatest thickness (between 6 and 12 mm) in echogenicity. Stromal edema also causes the endometrium to become more echogenic during the luteal phase. In addition to the echogenic endometrium, a hypoechoic band beneath the endometrium can be identified, probably arising from the inner layer of the myometrium.

The fact that medications used for ovulation induction may alter the development of the endometrium has been shown by both sonographic and histologic studies.[40] However, the relative importance of these changes to success or failure of achieving pregnancy is only speculative. One study, which evaluated the endometrial thickness in the secretory phase, has shown that conception was unlikely in endometria that measured less than 13 mm at 11 days post ovulation.[41,42] Other studies have indicated that the texture of the endometrium may be related to the success or failure of pregnancy. Specifically, the presence of a multilayered

endometrium within 1 to 2 days of embryo transfer was associated with a high postovulatory conception.[43,44]

Sonography may have a role in further evaluation of patients who have luteal phase inadequacy. It is conceivable that these patients could have underdeveloped endometria, which could be characterized sonographically as thinner and less echogenic than expected.

Color Doppler sonography has shown that uterine blood flow can also predict the probability of pregnancy.[45] In one study, pregnancies did not occur in women with high impedance (pulsatility index >3.0) uterine arterial flow.

TUBAL PATENCY ASSESSMENT

Transvaginal sonography has been used to detect intraperitoneal spillage of saline or contrast medium injected into the uterus and tubes. Some clinicians have used a specific contrast medium consisting of a suspension of galactose monosaccharide microparticles (Echovist) and color Doppler sonography as a means to assess tubal patency. The advantage of this technique includes preclusion of radiation and high tolerance of the patient. Patency can be inferred when there is spillage into the cul-de-sac, whereas tubal obstruction may result in filling of the uterine lumen without spillage.

In the past few years there has been great interest in the evaluation of tubal patency by sonographic methods. The first reported studies assessed tubal patency with transabdominal sonographic methods.[46,47] When they observed the collection of instilled fluid in the cul-de-sac, the authors indirectly concluded that one or both fallopian tubes were patent. On the basis of the comparison of sonosalpingographic and hysterosalpingographic findings they concluded

that in spite of advantages such as simplicity and cost-effectiveness, sonosalpingography should be indicated only in cases in which hysterosalpingography is contraindicated.

More recently, other investigators[48] have compared transvaginal sonosalpingography with chromotubation by laparoscopy in patients with unknown tubal function. In their study, transvaginal sonosalpingography and laparoscopy were completely consistent in 29 cases (76.3%) and partially consistent in 8 cases (21.05%). Transvaginal sonosalpingography accurately showed patency in 26 patients and bilateral nonpatency in three patients. Thus, they concluded that transvaginal sonosalpingography is a safe and accurate screening and diagnostic technique in the evaluation of tubal patency.

Deichert and colleagues[49] have used pulsed-wave Doppler imaging to improve the sensitivity to flow through the tube after injected fluid. They used transvaginal hysterosalpingo-

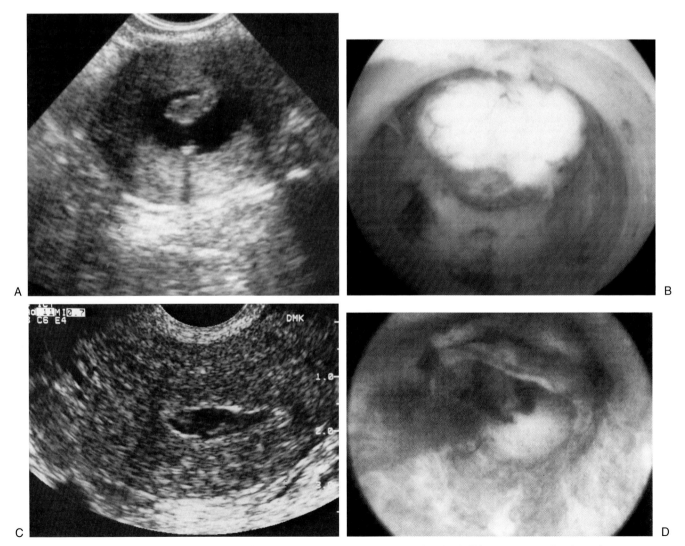

FIG. 9-8. Sonohysterography. **(A)** Endometrial polyp surrounded by fluid. **(B)** Hysteroscopic view of polyp shown in **A.** **(C)** Thick interface crossing endometrial lumen representing an adhesion. **(D)** Hysteroscopic view of adhesion.

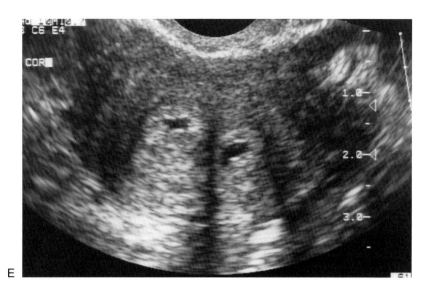

E

FIG. 9-8. *Continued.* **(E)** SHG showing two fluid-filled lumina separated by a myometrial septum. (**B** and **D,** courtesy of E. Eisenberg, MD.)

contrast sonography. They administered Echovist transcervically, then performed transvaginal hysterosalpingo-contrast sonography, and followed up with either chromolaparoscopy or hysterosalpingography. The diagnostic efficacy of gray scale and pulsed-wave Doppler imaging were then compared with each other and against one of the conventional control procedures. These investigators concluded that pulsed-wave Doppler imaging in transvaginal hysterosalpingo-contrast sonography is recommended as a supplement to gray scale imaging in cases of suspected tubal occlusion and if there is intratubal flow demonstrable only over a short distance.

Finally, Stern and colleagues[50] compared the results of color Doppler sonographic hysterosalpingography and radiographic hysterosalpingography with chromopertubation at the time of laparoscopy. Saline was administered transcervically during transvaginal color Doppler sonography in 238 women. Traditional radiographic hysterosalpingography was performed in 89 women, and laparoscopy and chromopertubation were performed in 121 women. Forty-nine women had all three procedures performed. Correlation between color Doppler sonographic hysterosalpingography and radiographic findings with chromotubation occurred in 81% versus 60% ($P < .001$) of all women studied. In the 49 women who had all three procedures, color Doppler sonographic hysterosalpingography results correlated with chromotubation more often than radiographic hysterosalpingography (82% versus 57%; $P < .05$).

In conclusion, color Doppler sonographic hysterosalpingography appears to be an efficacious method of establishing fallopian tube patency in patients with infertility. It can be performed in an outpatient setting and has high patient acceptance. Future infertility therapeutic approaches that may involve transvaginal sonography include early tubal screening in the diagnosis of infertility, visualization and documentation of transcervical tuboplasties, and gamete or embryo tubal transfers after transvaginal sonographic-guided ova retrievals.

The availability of positive (echogenic) contrast media for evaluation of the tubes has created much interest in sonographic techniques for assessment of tubal patency over standard radiographic ones. Albunex can be injected within the area of the tubal ostia for this purpose. Usually, the tubal lumen can be depicted by transvaginal sonography and the relationship of the fimbriated end of the tube to the ovary can be demonstrated. This topic is discussed in greater detail Chapter 10.

Sonographic Assessment of Intrauterine Lumen

Sonohysterography is being more extensively used for assessment of intraluminal disorders such as endometrial polyps, submucosal fibroids, intrauterine synechiae, and uterine malformation. The procedure uses a thin, flexible catheter that is placed through the cervix into the lumen with its tip near the fundus. Slow injection of 3 to 10 mL of sterile saline usually produces adequate distention of the lumen for the assessment of endometrial polyps, submucous fibroids, or synechiae (Fig. 9-8). This procedure should be performed in the secretory phase of the menstrual cycle when the endometrium is most echogenic. Endometrial polyps and submucosal fibroids appear as echogenic structures that project into the lumen, whereas synechiae are typically echogenic linear interfaces.[51]

Uterine Malformations

The transvaginal sonographic depiction of the endometrium, particularly in the secretory phase, can be helpful in the evaluation and detection of uterine malformations. Bicornuate uteri can be recognized by the two endometrial interfaces that are fused (Fig. 9-9). One can differentiate a septate from a bicornuate uterus by the configuration of the fundus

(*text continued on page 294*)

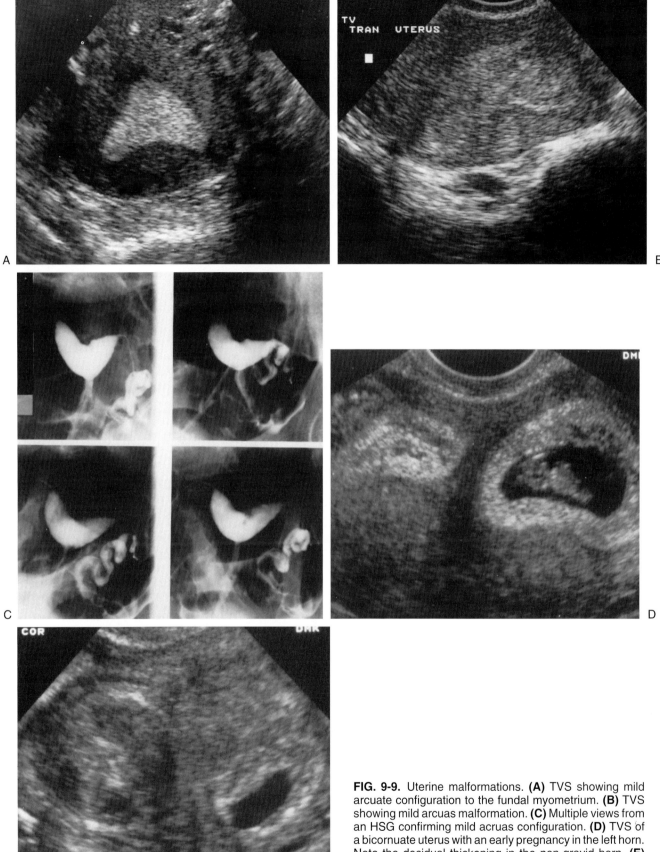

FIG. 9-9. Uterine malformations. **(A)** TVS showing mild arcuate configuration to the fundal myometrium. **(B)** TVS showing mild arcuas malformation. **(C)** Multiple views from an HSG confirming mild acruas configuration. **(D)** TVS of a bicornuate uterus with an early pregnancy in the left horn. Note the decidual thickening in the non-gravid horn. **(E)** TVS simulating the appearance of a bicornuate uterus with a pregnancy in one horn. This actually represented an intramural fibroid on the right adjacent to an early IUP.

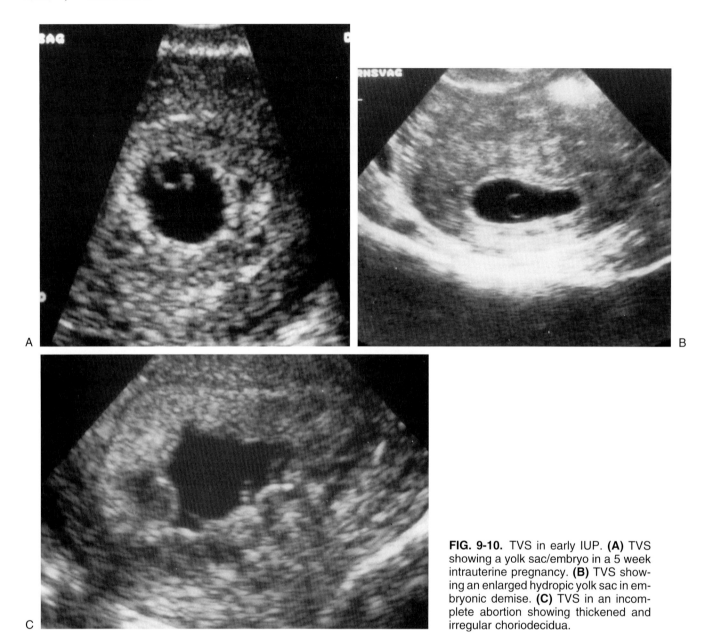

FIG. 9-10. TVS in early IUP. **(A)** TVS showing a yolk sac/embryo in a 5 week intrauterine pregnancy. **(B)** TVS showing an enlarged hydropic yolk sac in embryonic demise. **(C)** TVS in an incomplete abortion showing thickened and irregular choriodecidua.

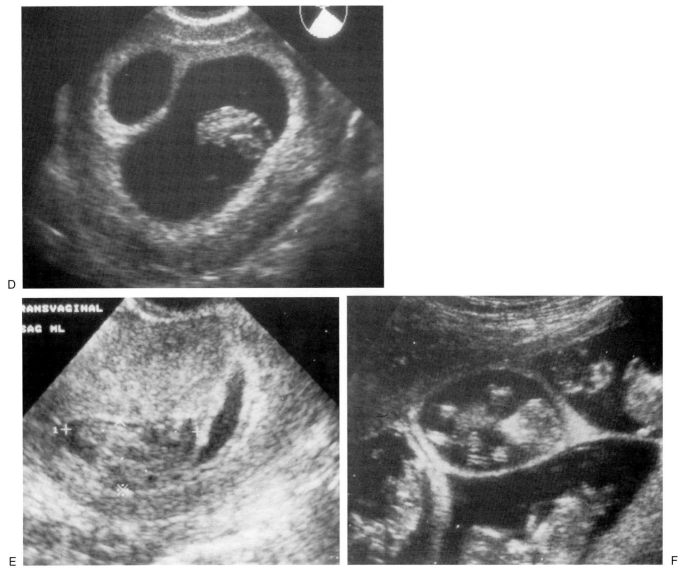

FIG. 9-10. *Continued.* **(D)** TVS showing a "blighted ovum" adjacent to a normal early pregnancy. **(E)** TVS showing retrochorionic hemorrhage. *(between cursors).* **(F)** TVS of a quadruplet 10-week pregnancy in a patient who had undergone an ovulation induction.

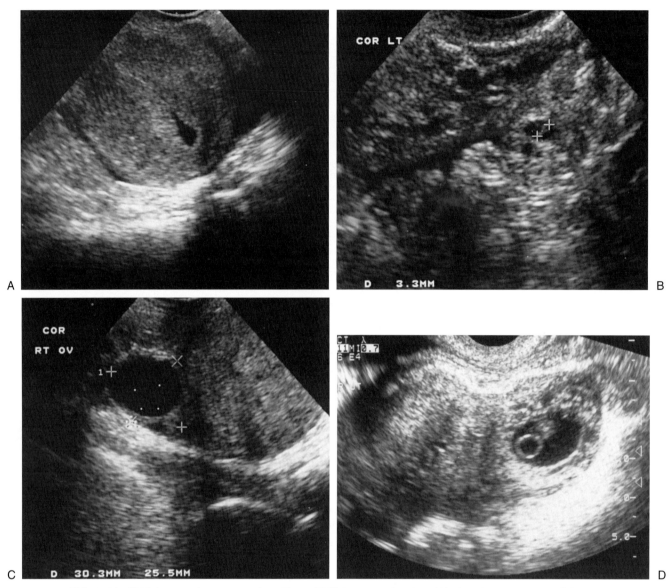

FIG. 9-11. TVS in ectopic pregnancies. Three TVS images showing **(A)** decidual thickening **(B)** an unruptured ectopic in the left adnexa and **(C)** a corpus luteum within the right ovary. **(D)** TVS showing unruptured ectopic pregnancy in the left adnexa.

because bicornuate uteri should have a cleft between the two horns whereas septated uteri do not.

Complicated Early Pregnancies

Transvaginal sonography has an important role in establishing early intrauterine pregnancies as early as 5 weeks post menstrual cycle. At this stage, a 5- to 10-mm hypoechoic area is present within the decidua (Fig. 9-10). As the gestational sac enlarges to over 10 mm, a yolk sac can be seen within the gestational sac. At 6 weeks the embryo/yolk sac can be seen. β-hCG determination is helpful in correlating the transvaginal sonographic findings. In general,

a gestational sac is seen when the β-hCG level is approximately 3000 mIU/mL.[52]

Ectopic pregnancies are common in women with infertility histories, probably owing to their association with scarred but patent tubes. On transvaginal sonography the unruptured ectopic typically appears as a ringlike structure separate from the ovary and uterus (Fig. 9-11).[53] On transvaginal color Doppler sonography flow within the decidua can be seen in some ectopic pregnancies.[54] The waveforms seen in ectopic pregnancies are highly variable, ranging from low impedance, high diastolic flow to absent or reversed diastolic flow. This range is probably a reflection of the various flow patterns seen in viable versus dying ectopic pregnancies (Fig. 9-12). The decidualized endometrium shows high imped-

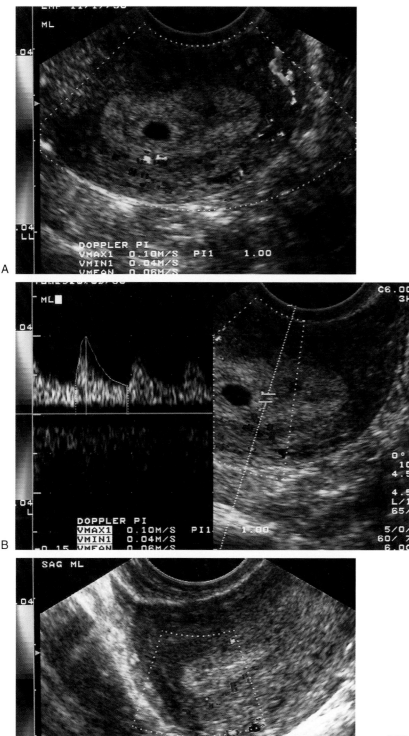

FIG. 9-12. TV-CDS in normal and abnormal early pregnancy. **(A)** TV-CDS in a 5 week IUP showing vascularity within decidua. **(B)** Same patient as in **A** showing intermediate impedance, low velocity flow within decidual arteriole. TV-CDS of an unruptured ectopic pregnancy showing poor myometrial flow **(C)**, high velocity flow in the wall of the ectopic.

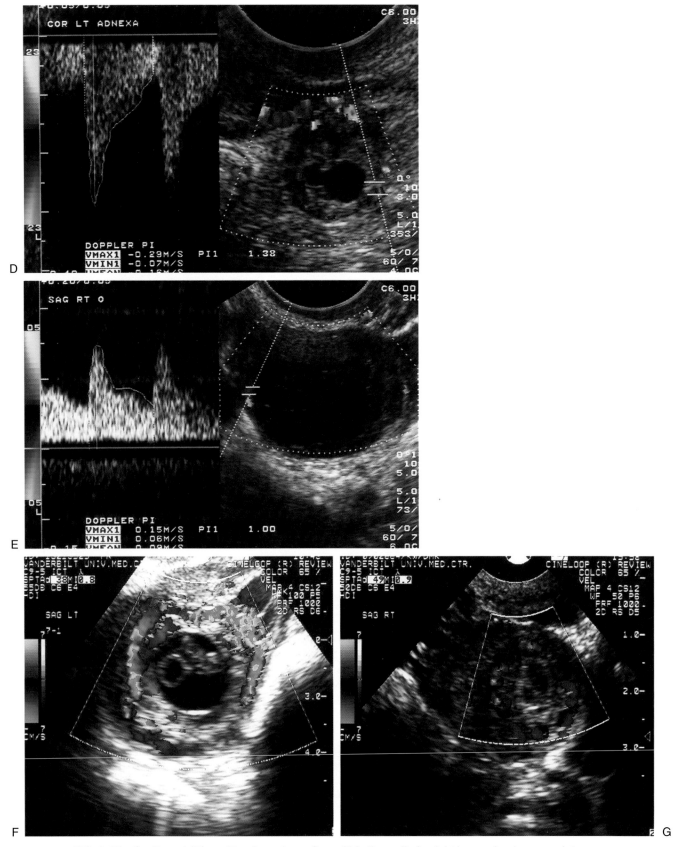

FIG. 9-12. *Continued.* **(D),** and low impedance flow within the wall of a right hemorrhagic corpus luteum **(E). (F)** TV-CDS showing vascularity surrounding an unruptured ectopic. **(G)** TV-CDS of a corpus luteum simulating the appearance of an unruptured ectopic.

ance flow because chorionic villi arterioles are not transformed by trophoblastic infiltration as in normal early intrauterine pregnancies. The corpus luteum may also exhibit a "ring of fire" flow pattern, but this can usually be documented to be within the confines of the ovary.

With the increased use of methotrexate treatment of ectopic pregnancies, transvaginal color Doppler sonography may have a role in decisions of who to treat and how much methotrexate to use.[55] Nonetheless, the goal of the sonologist is to identify ectopic pregnancies as early as possible to salvage the tube for future pregnancies and reduce complications of treatment.

Another common problem seen in women with infertility is nonviable intrauterine pregnancies, typically associated with a chromosomally abnormal fetus. In these pregnancies, the embryo/fetus may be absent (embryonic demise) or too small for the size of the gestational sac.[56] Other signs of nonviability include an amniotic cavity too large for the embryo or a hydropic yolk sac.[57,58] Retrochorionic hemorrhage may be present. If retrochorionic hemorrhage is extensive, the prognosis for pregnancy completion is guarded.

On the other hand, ovulation induction may be associated with multifetal pregnancy. In these cases it is important for the sonologist to ascertain the chorionicity of the placenta and relative size and viability of each of the fetuses to manage the patient optimally. In some, embryo reduction may be indicated. Transvaginal sonography serves as a guide for this procedure.

CONCLUSION

Sonography has a vital role in the management of certain gynecologic causes of infertility.[59] Its two major clinical applications involve follicular monitoring and guidance of follicular aspiration. The use of transvaginal transducer/probes has also enhanced their depiction sonographically and now allows a more in-depth knowledge of the processes leading to achievement of pregnancy in infertile or subfertile women.

REFERENCES

1. Quigley MM, In vitro fertilization 1986: new Procedures and new questions. Invest Radiol 1986;21:503.
2. Mendelson EB, Friedman H, Neiman HL, et al. The role of imaging in infertility management. AJR 1985;144:415.
3. Hann LE, Crivello M, McArdle C, et al. In vitro fertilization: sonographic perspective. Radiology 1987;163:665.
4. Hammond M, Talbert L. Infertility: a practical guide for the physician. Chapel Hill, NC, Health Sciences Consortium, 1981:2.
5. Fleischer AC, Pittaway DE, Wentz AC, et al. The uses of sonography for monitoring ovarian follicular development. In: Sanders RC, Hill M, eds. Ultrasound annual. New York, Raven Press. 1983.
6. Fleischer AC, Wentz A, Jones H, James AE. Sonography of the ovary. In: Callen P, ed. Ultrasonography in obstetrics and gynecology. Philadelphia, WB Saunders, 1983.
7. Raymond CA. In vitro fertilization enters stormy adolescence as experts debate the odds. JAMA 1988;259:464, 469.
8. Bigger J. In vitro fertilization and embryo transfer in human beings. N Engl J Med 1982;304:336.
9. Parson J, Booker M, Goswamy R, et al. Oocyte retrieval for in vitro fertilization by ultrasonically guided needle aspiration via the urethra. Lancet 1985;10:867.
10. Jansen RPS, Anderson JC. Catheterization of the fallopian tubes from the vagina. Lancet 1987;10:309.
11. Nicolini U, Ferrazzi E, Bellotti M, et al. The contribution of sonographic evaluation of ovarian size in patients with polycystic ovarian disease. J Ultrasound Med 1985;4:347.
12. Friedman H, Vogelzang RL, Mendelson EB, et al. Endometriosis detection by US with laparoscopic correlation. Radiology 1985;157:217.
13. Hann LE, Hall DA, McArdle CR, et al. Polycystic ovarian disease: sonographic spectrum. Radiology 1984;150:531.
14. Strickler RC, Christianson C, Crane JP, et al. Ultrasound guidance for human embryo transfer. Fertil Steril 1985;43:54.
15. Fleischer AC, Pittaway DE, Beard LA, et al. Sonographic depiction of endometrial changes occurring with ovulation induction. J Ultrasound Med 1984;3:341.
16. Marrs RP. Does the method of oocyte collection have a major influence on in vitro fertilization? Fertil Steril 1986;46:193.
17. Fleischer AC, Kepple DM, Vasques J. Conventional and color Doppler transvaginal sonography in gynecologic infertility. Radiol Clin North Am 1992;30:693.
18. Schlief R, Deichert U: Hysterosalpingo-contrast sonography of the uterus and fallopian tubes: results of a clinical trial of a new contrast medium in 120 patients. Radiology 1991;178:213.
19. Nyberg DA, Laing FC, Jeffrey RB. Sonographic detection of subtle pelvic fluid collections. AJR 1984;143:261.
20. Hackeloer BJ. The role of ultrasound in female infertility management. Ultrasound Med Biol 1984;10:35.
21. Marrs RP, Vargyas JM, March CM. Correlation of ultrasonic and endocrinologic measurements in human menopausal gonadotropin therapy. Am J Obstet Gynecol 1983;145:417.
22. McArdle CR, Seibel M, Weinstein F, et al. Induction of ovulation monitored by ultrasound. Radiology 1983;148:809.
23. Geisthovel F, Skubsch U, Zabel G, et al. Ultrasonographic and hormonal studies in physiologic and insufficient menstrual cycles. Fertil Steril 1983;39:277.
24. Liukkonen S, Koskimies AI, Tenhunen A, Ylostalo P. Diagnosis of luteinized unruptured follicle (LUF) syndrome by ultrasound. Abstract. Fertil Steril 1984;41:26.
25. Ritchie WGM. Sonographic evaluation of normal and induced ovulation. Radiology 1986;161:1.
26. Fleischer AC, Daniell JF, Rodier J, et al. Sonographic monitoring of ovarian follicular development. J Clin Ultrasound 1981;9:275.
27. Sladkevicius P, Valentin L, Marsal K. Blood flow velocity in the uterine and ovarian arteries during the normal menstrual cycle. Ultrasound Obstet Gynecol 1993;3:199.
28. Kupesic S, Kurjak A. Uterine and ovarian perfusion during the periovulatory period assessed by transvaginal color Doppler. Fertil Steril 1993; 60:439.
29. Tarlatizis BC, Laufer N, DeCherney AH. The use of ovarian ultrasonography in monitoring ovulation induction. J In Vitro Fertil Embryo Transfer 1984;1:226.
30. Blankstein J, Shalev J, Saadon T, et al. Ovarian hyperstimulation syndrome: prediction by number and size of preovulatory ovarian follicles. Fertil Steril 1987;47:597.
31. Feichtinger W, Kemeter P. Ultrasound-guided aspiration of human ovarian follicles for in vitro fertilization. In Sanders RC, Hill M, eds. Ultrasound annual. New York, Raven Press, 1986.
32. Taylor PJ, Wiseman D, Mahadevan M, Leader A. "Ultrasound rescue": a successful alternative form of oocyte recovery in patients with periovarian adhesions. Am J Obstet Gynecol 1986;154:240.
33. Hammarberg K, Enk L, Nilsson L, Wikland M. Oocyte retrieval under the guidance of a vaginal transducer: evaluation of patient acceptance. Hum Reprod 1987;2:487.
34. Schulman JD, Dorfmann AD, Jones SL, et al. Outpatient in vitro fertilization using transvaginal ultrasound-guided oocyte retrieval. Obstet Gynecol 1987;69:665.
35. Feichtinger W, Kemeter P. Transvaginal sector scan sonography for needle guided transvaginal follicle aspiration and other applications in gynecologic routine and research. Fertil Steril 1986;45:722.
36. Dellenbach P, Nisand I, Moreau L, et al. Transvaginal sonographically controlled follicle puncture for oocyte retrieval. Fertil Steril 1985;44:656.

37. Marrs RP. Does the method of oocyte collection have a major influence on in vitro fertilization? Fertil Steril 1986;46:193.

38. Aboulghar MA, Mansour RT, Serour GI, Rizk B. Ultrasonic transvaginal aspiration of endometriotic cysts: an optional line of treatment in selected cases of endometriosis. Hum Reprod 1991;6:1408.

39. Thickman D, Arger P, Tureck R, et al. Sonographic assessment of the endometrium in patients undergoing in vitro fertilization. J Ultrasound Med 1986;5:197.

40. Fleischer AC, Pittaway DE, Beard LA, et al. Sonographic depiction of endometrial changes occurring with ovulation induction. J Ultrasound Med 1984;3:341.

41. Rabinowitz R, Laufer N, Lewin A, et al. The value of ultrasonographic endometrial measurement in the prediction of pregnancy following in vitro fertilization. Fertil Steril 1986;45:824.

42. Glissant A, de Mouzon J, Frydman R. Ultrasound study of the endometrium during in vitro fertilization cycles. Fertil Steril 1985;44:786.

43. Fleischer AC, Herbert CM, Hill GA, et al. Transvaginal sonography of the endometrium during induced cycles. J Ultrasound Med 1991; 10:93.

44. Bourne T. In: Fleischer A, Emerson D, eds. Color Doppler sonograph in obstetrics gynecology. New York, Churchill Livingstone, 1993:45.

45. Steer CV, Campbell S, Tan SL, et al. Transvaginal color Doppler: a new technique for use after in vitro fertilization to identify optimum uterine conditions before embryo transfer. Fertil Steril 1992;57:372.

46. Richman TS, Biscomi GN, de Cherney A, et al. Fallopian tubal patency assessed by ultrasound following fluid injection. Radiology 1984;152: 507.

47. Randolph JR, Ying YK, Maier DB, et al. Comparison of real-time ultrasonography, hysterosalpingography, and laparoscopy/hysteroscopy in the evaluation of uterine abnormalities and tubal patency. Fertil Steril 1986;46:828.

48. Can Tufekci E, Girit S, Bayirli E, et al. Evaluation of tubal patency by transvaginal sonosalpingography. Fertil Steril 1992;57:336.

49. Deichert U, Schlief R, van de Sandt M, Daume E. Transvaginal hysterosalpingo-contrast sonography for the assessment of tubal patency with gray scale imaging and additional use of pulsed wave Doppler. Fertil Steril 1992;57:62.

50. Stern J, Peters AJ, Coulam CB. Color Doppler ultrasonography assessment of tubal patency: a comparison study with traditional techniques. Fertil Steril 1992;58:897.

51. Narayan R, Goswamy RK. Transvaginal sonography of the uterine cavity with hysteroscopic correlation in the investigation of infertility. Ultrasound Obstet Gynecol 1993;3:129.

52. Bree RL, Edwards E, Bohm-Velez M, et al. Transvaginal sonography in the evaluation of normal early pregnancy: correlation with hCG level. AJR 1989;153:75.

53. Fleischer AC. Ultrasound imaging: assessment of utero-ovarian blood flow with transvaginal color Doppler sonography: potential clinical applications in infertility. Fertil Steril 1991;55:684.

54. Emerson DS, Cartier MS, Altieri LA, et al. Diagnostic efficacy of endovaginal color Doppler flow imaging in an ectopic pregnancy screening program. Radiology 1992;183:413.

55. Atri M, Bret PM, Tulandi T. Spontaneous resolution of ectopic pregnancy: initial appearance and evolution at transvaginal US. Radiology 1993;186:83.

56. Bromley B, Harlow BL, Laboda LA, Benacerraf BR. Small sac size in the first trimester: a predictor of poor fetal outcome. Radiology 1991; 178:375.

57. Harrow MM. Enlarged amniotic cavity: a new sonographic sign of early embryonic death. AJR 1992;158:359.

58. Kurtz A, Needleman L, Pennel R. Can detection of the yolk sac in the first trimester of pregnancy be used to redirect the outcome of a pregnancy? A prospective sonographic study. AJR 1992;188:843.

59. Speroff L, Glass RH, Kase NG. Clinical gynecologic endocrinology infertility, ed 3. Baltimore, Williams & Wilkins, 1983.

Magnetic Resonance Imaging in the Diagnosis of Congenital Uterine Anomalies

Marcia C. Javitt, MD

Noninvasive evaluation of müllerian anomalies is often prompted by a workup of infertility or delayed menarche. The appropriate identification of müllerian anomalies is of paramount importance to provide an opportunity for proper treatment in cases which may have serious or adverse obstetric complications if untreated. Moreover, triaging patients to treatment by hysteroscopy with or without laparoscopic surgery versus laparotomy may be accomplished preoperatively.

Müllerian anomalies have a prevalence of about 3%.[1] One in four of these women will have infertility problems.[1,2] Commonly in these patients there may be a history of repetitive fetal losses due to the increased incidence of spontaneous abortions, premature labor, fetal malpresentation, dystocia, and disordered uterine contractility in active labor.[3-5] Whether the clinical presentation is due to pelvic pain secondary to an obstruction of the uterus or vagina, primary amenorrhea, infertility, or obstetric complications, the radiologic evaluation must define the outer contour of the uterus as well as the internal morphology of the uterine canal. This is especially important because the treatments of bicornuate and septate uteri differ drastically.

Müllerian anomalies are classified according to the system adopted by the American Fertility Society.[4] (Table 9-1) This system is organized based not only on the morphology of the uterus, but also on the clinical presentation, the likely implications for pregnancy, and the surgical treatment options available. The müllerian and mesonephric ducts are closely approximated such that the required ascent of the ureteric buds from the mesonephric ducts to contact the mesonephros may be disrupted in association with müllerian anomalies. Because of the resulting high incidence of associated urinary tract abnormalities including ectopia or agenesis of the kidney with müllerian anomalies, visualization of the kidneys is necessary.[5] Congenital absence of the uterus, cervix, and vagina, also known as Mayer-Rokitansky-Kuster-Hauser syndrome has been divided into two types. Type A has normal fallopian tubes and usually normal kidneys. Type B can be associated with abnormalities of the kidneys and ureters as well as the ovaries and fallopian tubes.[6,7] (Figures 9-13,9-14)

The etiology of müllerian anomalies is developmental.

Embryologically the uterus is formed by the fusion of the two paramesonephric ducts at about the tenth week of fetal life.[5] The fusion of the two müllerian ducts begins in the lower half of the uterus and extends cephalocaudally. The initial uterine cavity forms inferiorly with a septum of residual tissue superiorly. Normally the septum should gradually dissolve and disappears by the twentieth week of fetal life, leaving behind the fully formed uterine cavity. If this process fails or is disrupted, there can result a "double uterus" from failure of fusion, or a persistent septum.[5]

The vaginal canal is created between the urogenital sinus and the müllerian tubercle when a cell cord between the two dissolves starting at the hymen and progressing cephalad toward the cervix. If the regression of the cell cord fails, there can result a residual or persistent cell cord, hypoplasia

TABLE 9-1. *Classification of müllerian anomalies by the American Fertility Society*

Hypoplasia/Agenesis
  vaginal
  cervical
  fundal
  tubal
  combined
Unicornuate
  communicating
  noncommunicating
  absent cavity within one horn
  absent horn
Didelphys
Bicornuate
  complete
  partial
Septate
  complete
  partial
Arcuate
DES-/Drug-Related

From the American Fertility Society. The American Fertility Society classifications of adnexal adhesions, distal tubal occlusion, tubal occlusion secondary to tubal ligation, tubal pregnancies, mullerian anomalies, and intrauterine adhesions. Fertil Steril 1988;49:944.

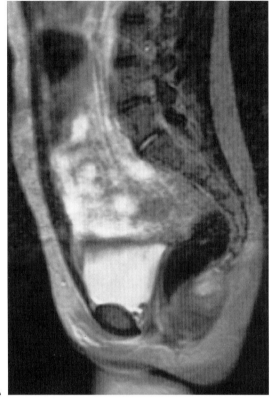
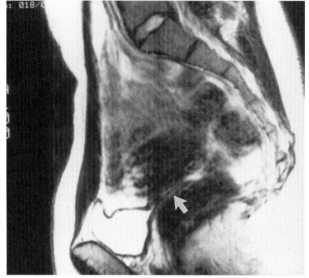

A   B

FIG. 9-13. Mayer-Rokitansky-Kuster-Hauser syndrome (Type A). **(A)** Sagittal T2-weighted scan shows absent uterus, cervix and vagina. **(B)** Sagittal T2-weighted scan in another patient shows absent vaginal canal, with a markedly hypoplastic uterus *(arrow)* containing a thin endometrial stripe. These two type A patients had no associated renal anomalies and normal ovaries.

or agenesis of the vaginal canal, or formation of a septum within the vagina.[5]

Although hysterosalpingography (HSG) provides an outline of the uterine cavity and fallopian tubes with contrast injection, there is no direct vision of the rest of the uterine wall, making classification of müllerian subtypes difficult. Only cavities which are patent or partially patent can be seen. In addition, HSG necessitates injection of contrast material as well as exposure to ionizing radiation. Though very useful for evaluation of tubal patency and uterine adhesions, HSG has not proved reliable for evaluating müllerian anomalies.[2]

Transvaginal US is probably the best initial imaging modality in the workup of suspected congenital uterine anomalies, because it is relatively noninvasive, lower in cost than MRI, and readily available. If the results of the US are inconclusive, then MRI is advisable, although its greater cost precludes its use as a primary screening modality. In one series comparing MRI, US and HSG, MRI was 100% accurate in diagnosing congenital uterine anomalies in 24 surgically proved cases, as compared with 92% for US, and less than 20% for HSG.[2]

The MRI examination of suspected müllerian anomalies

should include a T1-weighted image of the abdomen to assess the size shape and position of the kidneys, which can usually be accomplished rapidly by scanning in the coronal plane. In addition to the usual T2-weighted fast spin echo (FSE) sagittal scan, which shows the length and contour of the vaginal canal, uterine morphology, and zonal anatomy, an off-axis coronal scan plane is usually the best method to lay out the contour of the fundus, within which the distribution of the endometrial canal can be seen. This is prescribed from the sagittal images along the long axis of the uterus.

Axial images should be done with FSE T2-weighted technique. Sometimes short axis images prescribed from the sagittal scan are useful to show areas of communication or separation by septa or myometrium between the two sides of the uterus and to confirm the location and status of the ovaries. T1-weighted scans are always obtained usually in the sagittal, and sometimes in the axial planes or both, to show the relationship of an obstructed tract to the uterus and vagina. Hematometra and hematocolpos are usually bright in signal on both T1- and T2-weighted sequences because of the presence of subacute blood; however, their signal intensity will depend on the age and breakdown of the hemoglobin they contain.

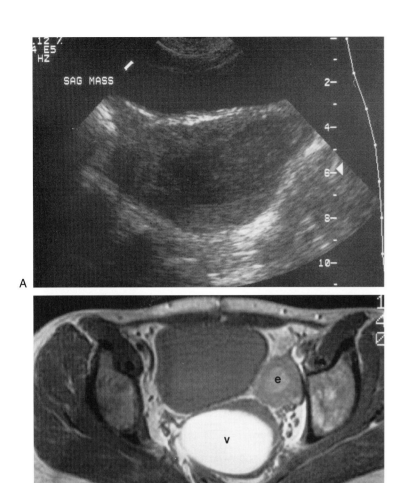

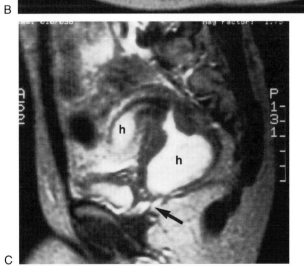

FIG. 9-14. Hematometrocolpos from vaginal dysgenesis **(A)** Sagittal US shows an ill-defined mass or complex collection in the mid-pelvis in this 14-year-old female who presented with amenorrhea. **(B)** Axial T1-weighted scan shows bright signal blood in the upper vaginal canal (v) and a distended endometrial canal (e). **(C)** Sagittal T2-weighted scan shows the distribution of the dilated bright signal blood filled hematometrocolpos (h) and the dysplastic portion of the vaginal canal with absent vaginal stripe *(arrow)*.

MÜLLERIAN AGENESIS

Müllerian hypoplasia or agenesis (class I anomaly) can be (a)vaginal, (b)cervical, (c)fundal, (d)tubal, or (e)combined. The incidence of vaginal agenesis is about 1:4000 live births.[8] The ovaries can be normal because they are derived separately from the mesodermal epithelium, the mesenchyme, and primordial germ cells.[8] Vaginal hypoplasia or agenesis can be treated with the Frank technique, with the use of dilators, or with the McIndoe procedure involving surgical reconstruction of a neovagina. If there is a normal functional uterus and cervix present, pregnancy is possible.[7] Otherwise, as is often the case, there may be a functioning or rudimentary uterus with a hypoplastic or absent cervix. (Figure 9-15,9-16) Hysterectomy may be recommended if there is severe menstrual pain, or additional surgery beyond the vaginal reconstruction may be attempted. Cervical reconstruction has a significant incidence of subsequent obstruc-

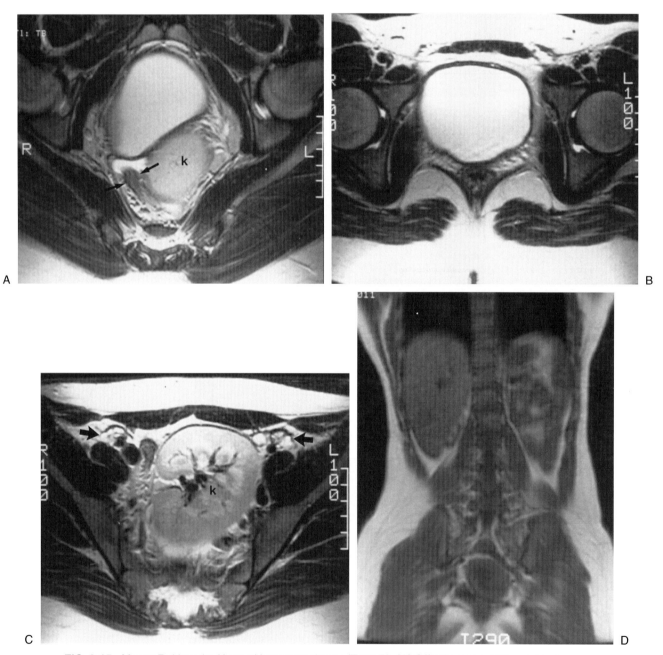

FIG. 9-15. Mayer-Rokitansky-Kuster-Hauser syndrome (Type B). **(A)** Off axis coronal T2 weighted scan. Note the rudimentary rightward deviated uterus (arrows) adjacent to a pelvic kidney (k). There is no endometrial stripe. **(B)** Axial T2-weighted scan shows absence of the upper half of the vaginal canal. **(C)** Axial T2-weighted scan. There is a large solitary pelvic kidney (k). The ovaries are normal *(arrows)*. *(D)* Coronal T1 weighted scan. There is no normotopic kidney in the retroperitoneum on either side. The type B is associated with renal, ovarian and fallopian tube anomalies.

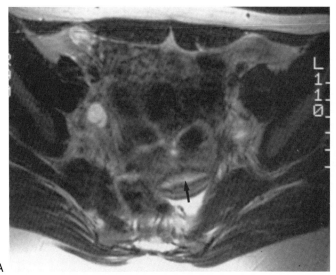

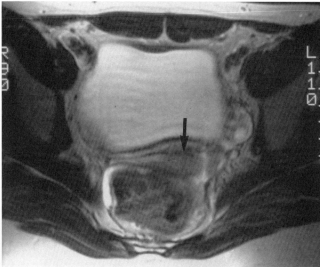

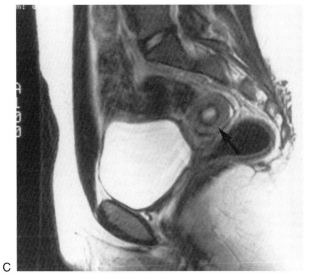

FIG. 9-16. Mayer-Rokitansky-Kuster-Hauser syndrome (Type A) with a hypoplastic uterus and hypoplastic cervix. **(A)** T2-weighted axial scan shows a small but definite uterus with an endometrial stripe *(arrow),* which is retroverted and deviated to the left. **(B)** T2-weighted axial scan shows a hypoplastic cervix (arrow) lacking normal zonal anatomy. **(C)** T2-weighted sagittal scan shows vaginal agenesis. Note the levoverted uterus (arrow).

tion.[9] If there is a uterus present, there is usually no associated wolffian duct anomaly. The incidence of absence of the kidney is approximately 15% if there is absence of the uterus and vagina, with an incidence of about 40% for all renal anomalies.[7] For the other class I müllerian anomalies, generally there are no well documented surgical treatment options. MRI shows the absent vaginal stripe and permits evaluation of the status of the uterine size and endometrial stripe.

UNICORNUATE UTERUS

The unicornuate uterus results from incomplete development of one of the two müllerian ducts. These class II anomalies can be:(a) with a communicating rudimentary horn,(b) with a noncommunicating rudimentary horn, (c) with a rudimentary horn but no endometrial cavity, or (d) no horn (Fig. 9-17).[4] The uterus is often deviated laterally and is lenticular in shape. If there is a rudimentary horn, there should be a

careful inspection to determine if there is an endometrial canal, whether it is lined with glandular tissue, and whether it communicates, all of which are best appreciated on FSE T2-weighted images. Due to the increased incidence of infertility, spontaneous abortions, premature labor, fetal growth retardation, ectopic pregnancies, pregnancies in the rudimentary horn, and endometriosis, the identification of an obstructed rudimentary horn (noncommunicating) may prompt surgical excision of that horn. There is a significant incidence of renal anomalies, about 25% in one series.[7,10] class II anomalies are usually not surgically treated.[5,7,9]

UTERUS DIDELPHYS

This class III anomaly is characterized by complete duplication of the uterine body and cervix which is due to a nonfusion of the müllerian ducts (Fig. 9-18). These patients are usually asymptomatic unless there is an associated vaginal septum causing hematocolpos. Complications of the uterus

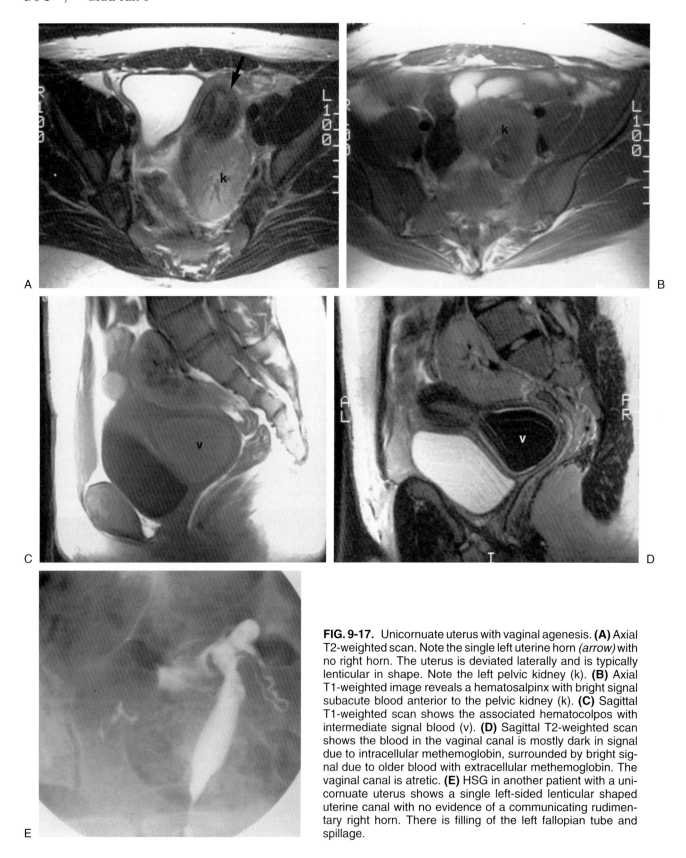

FIG. 9-17. Unicornuate uterus with vaginal agenesis. **(A)** Axial T2-weighted scan. Note the single left uterine horn *(arrow)* with no right horn. The uterus is deviated laterally and is typically lenticular in shape. Note the left pelvic kidney (k). **(B)** Axial T1-weighted image reveals a hematosalpinx with bright signal subacute blood anterior to the pelvic kidney (k). **(C)** Sagittal T1-weighted scan shows the associated hematocolpos with intermediate signal blood (v). **(D)** Sagittal T2-weighted scan shows the blood in the vaginal canal is mostly dark in signal due to intracellular methemoglobin, surrounded by bright signal due to older blood with extracellular methemoglobin. The vaginal canal is atretic. **(E)** HSG in another patient with a unicornuate uterus shows a single left-sided lenticular shaped uterine canal with no evidence of a communicating rudimentary right horn. There is filling of the left fallopian tube and spillage.

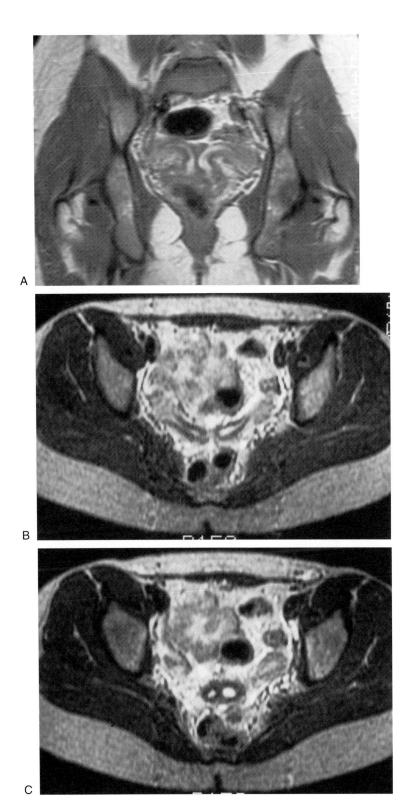

FIG. 9-18. Uterus didelphys. **(A)** Coronal proton density weighted scan. Note the two completely separate uterine canals, two cervices, and the vaginal septum. **(B, C, D)** Axial T2-weighted scans at the level of the uterine bodies, cervices, and vaginal canals respectively. Note the longitudinal vaginal septum *(arrow)*.

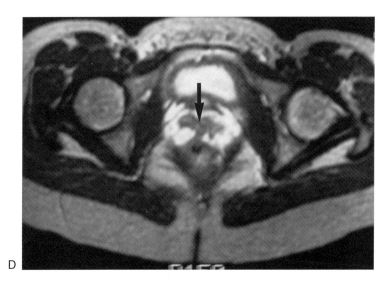

D

FIG. 9-18. *Continued.*

didelphys include preterm abortions, premature labor, fetal growth retardation, and malpresentation similar to the unicornuate uterus. The MRI appearance is that of two separate uterine bodies, two cervices, and, often, a vaginal septum. Unlike the longitudinal vaginal septum, if there is a transverse vaginal septum, there are usually symptoms of obstruction of the involved side. Vaginal septectomy may be performed. If a patient has a history of recurrent spontaneous abortion or premature labor attributable to the uterine anomaly, there can be an attempt at surgical union of the uterine bodies, but not the cervices because an incompetent cervix will usually result.[7] There is otherwise no surgical repair offered for the uterus didelphys.[9]

BICORNUATE UTERUS

The class IV anomaly results from lack of fusion of the uterine corpus, but there is a single cervix. The distinction of the bicornuate from the septate uterus is of paramount importance because the septate uterus is associated with greater incidence of fetal wastage and requires a different treatment than the bicornuate uterus (Fig. 9-19). The bicornuate uterus is treated by transabdominal surgical resection of the muscular division between the two sides of the uterus to fuse the two horns (Strassman metroplasty).[9] Preoperative evaluation of the anomaly is key. Although the signal intensity of the division between the two horns in the bicornuate uterus is usually that of myometrium and intermediate on T2-weighted scans, this is not reliable as a sole indicator of the bicornuate uterus, because the signal intensity has been variable and can be partially fibrous.[2,11,12,13]

The long axis view of the uterus (usually the off axis coronal) T2-weighted FSE scans are crucial to making the distinction. The fundal contour must be carefully inspected. There is a deep indentation in the bicornuate (and also didelphys) uteri, but the septate uterus is usually flat or with a tiny indentation (less than 1 cm). The bicornuate uterus has a wide intercornual distance.[14] The vertical septum between the two horns is usually intermediate signal intensity on T2-weighted images, but may also be hypointense if there is a fibrous portion, which is usually located inferiorly. The sensitivity and specificity of MRI for the diagnosis of bicornuate versus septate uteri has been reported as high as 100%.[2]

SEPTATE UTERUS

The class V septate uterus is the most common müllerian anomaly, and is due to partial or complete failure of resorption of the midline septum (Fig. 9-20—9-22). It is associated with a very high incidence of preterm labor and spontaneous abortions (90%) usually in the midtrimester. The exact cause has not been confirmed, but has been attributed to inadequate vascular supply within the septum to support implantation, or possibly to septal endometrial incompetence.[2,7] The treatment of the septate uterus is hysteroscopic metroplasty.[2,7,9] On MRI, the off-axis coronal T2-weighted FSE scans are critical and permit identification of a normal or near normal fundal contour and normal intercornual distance. If present, a small fundal notch should not exceed 1 cm. The fibrous septum is of low-signal intensity whether partial or complete, and may be constituted of muscle superiorly and of fibrous tissue inferiorly.

ARCUATE UTERUS

The arcuate uterus (class VI) is only slightly different morphologically from normal, with little or no increase in the incidence of spontaneous abortions as compared with the general population.[5] (Fig. 9-23) The MR imaging appearance is close to normal with only a slight prominence of the fundal myometrium with respect to the endometrial canal, and no outer contour abnormality.

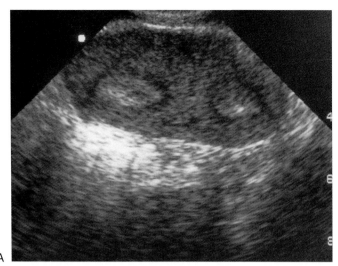

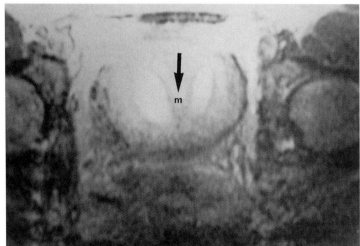

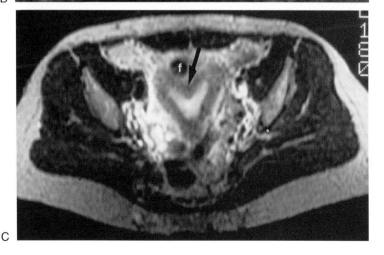

FIG. 9-19. Bicornuate uterus. **(A)** US shows two uterine horns separated by myometrium. **(B)** Axial T2-weighted image shows the two endometrial canals widely separated by a myometrial septum (m). **(C)** Another patient with a long axis view of a bicornuate uterus with a pedunculated fundal fibroid (f). Note the deep indentation in the fundus *(arrow)*, which is characteristic of the bicornuate uterus.

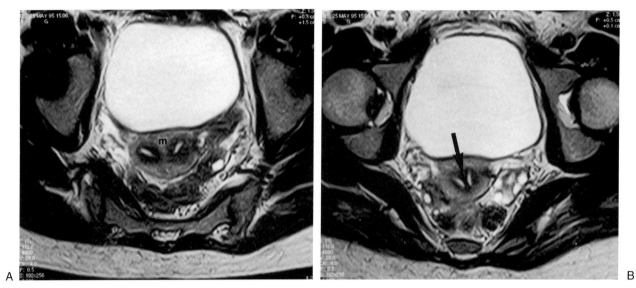

FIG. 9-20. Septate uterus. **(A)** T2-weighted off axis coronal scan. Note the near normal fundal contour. The septum is made of muscle tissue superiorly (m). **(B)** T2-weighted off axis coronal scan. The septum inferiorly is made of fibrous tissue *(arrow)*.

DIETHYLSTILBESTROL-EXPOSURE-RELATED ANOMALIES

Diethylstilbesterol (DES) was used until the 1970s in the treatment of abortions, preeclampsia, diabetes, and preterm labor and was administered to nearly 3 million women.[5] For female offspring exposed to DES in utero, an increased incidence of vaginal and cervical clear-cell adenocarcinoma have been documented.[5] (Fig. 9-24) Structural abnormalities have been observed in up to two thirds of women exposed to DES in utero making it the single most common cause of müllerian anomalies. These include hypoplastic uterine cavity, shortened upper uterine segment, T-shaped uterus, hypoplastic cervix, transverse septa, circumferential vaginal or cervical ridges, and cervical hood or collar. Vaginal adenosis, cervical ectropion, and hypoplastic cervix have been noted. In addition, abnormal fallopian tubes with shortening, narrowing and absent fimbria have been described.[5,15] There is an increased incidence of infertility, spontaneous abortions, ectopic pregnancies, and preterm labor in women with these structural abnormalities.[15—18]

The T-shaped uterus has special significance in that se-

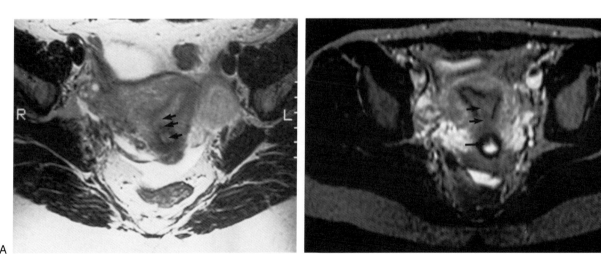

FIG. 9-21. Septate uterus. **(A)** T2-weighted off axis coronal scan. There is a low signal vertical fibrous septum running the length of the endometrial canal *(arrow)*. The fundal contour is smooth and near normal. The appearance of the fundal myometrium can be referred to as subseptate. **(B)** Another patient with the same configuration.

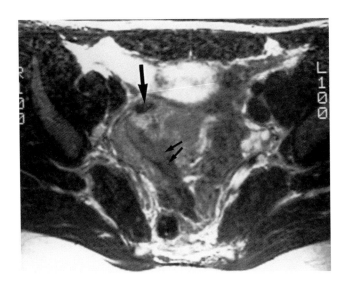

FIG. 9-22. Septate uterus with fundal fibroid. T2-weighted off axis coronal scan. Contrast the appearance of the fundal contour in this case of a septate uterus with a fundal fibroid with that in Figure 9-19**C.** The outer contour is smooth without an indentation, but there is a small convex contour abnormality from the fundal fibroid *(arrow).* The fibrous septum is thin but visible *(small arrows).* This patient underwent myomectomy with hysteroscopic metroplasty.

lected patients may benefit from surgical reconstruction. In this instance, the "T" is unroofed and redundant tissue is removed.[7,19]

MRI findings are best seen on off-axis coronal T2-weighted FSE scans and include abnormalities of uterine size and shape such as T-shaped uterus, constriction bands, and hypoplasia; however, HSG offers evaluation of tubal patency, which renders MRI an adjunctive examination.[20,21]

No effective treatment can be rendered for these class VII anomalies. Cervical cerclage can be offered if cervical incompetency complicates pregnancy.[5]

CONCLUSIONS

Because of its lower cost, wide availability, and noninvasiveness, US is probably the best primary modality to evaluate patients with suspected congenital uterine anomalies. If results of US with transvaginal scanning are inconclusive, MRI should be used as an adjunctive procedure and for problem solving. The use of HSG will likely not be supplanted in the near future in the evaluation of infertility in this setting because it is currently the only accepted and readily available method of evaluating tubal patency.

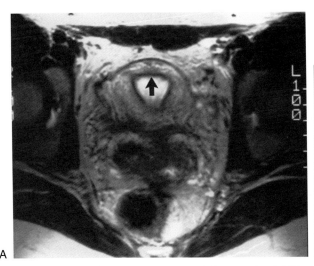
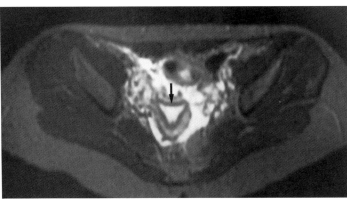

A

B

FIG. 9-23. Arcuate uterus. **(A)** Normal axial T2-weighted scan. The outer fundal contour is normal. The endometrial canal makes a smooth curvilinear convex margin *(arrow)* with the myometrium. **(B)** Arcuate uterus axial T2-weighted scan. The outer fundal contour is normal but the endometrial canal makes a concave inward curve *(arrow)* with respect to the myometrium.

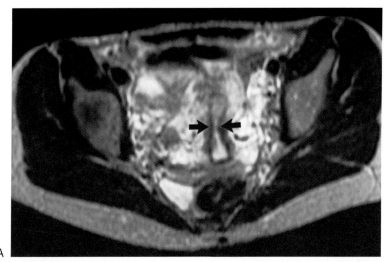

A

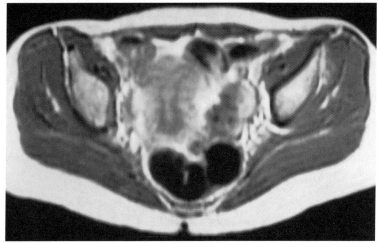

B

FIG. 9-24. Diethylstilbestrol (DES) Exposure-related anomalies. **(A)** Axial proton density-weighted image. The uterine body has a segmental constriction *(arrows)*. *(B)* Axial T2-weighted scan. Another patient with DES exposure. The uterus is T-shaped. Multifocal constrictions are seen in the endometrial canal.

REFERENCES

1. Golan A, Langer R, Bukovsky I, et al. Congenital anomalies of the müllerian system. Fertil Steril 1989;51:747.
2. Pellerito JS, McCarthy SM, Doyle MB, et al. Diagnosis of uterine anomalies: relative accuracy of MR imaging, endovaginal sonography, and hysterosalpingography. Radiology 1992;183:795.
3. Buttram VC. Müllerian anomalies: a proposed classification (analysis of 144 cases). Fertil Steril 1979;32:40.
4. The American Fertility Society. The American Fertility Society classifications of adnexal adhesions, distal tubal occlusion, tubal occlusion secondary to tubal ligation, tubal pregnancies, müllerian anomalies, and intrauterine adhesions. Fertil Steril 1988;49:944.
5. Cunningham FG, MacDonald PC, Gant NF, et al. Developmental Abnormalities of the Reproductive Tract, in Williams Obstetrics, 19th edition, p.721.Norwalk, Appleton and Lange, 1993.
6. Strubbe EH, Willemsen WN, Lemmens JA, et al. Mayer-Rokitansky-Kuster-Hauser syndrome: distinction between two forms based on excretory urographic, sonographic, and laparoscopic findings. Am J Roentgenol 1993;160:331.
7. Jones HW. Müllerian duct anomalies, in Wallach EE, and Zacur HA, (eds), Reproductive medicine and surgery, p.1093. St.Louis, Mosby-Year Book, Inc., 1995.
8. Moore KL. The Developing human: clinically oriented Embryology,p.278. Philadelphia, W.B. Saunders 1988.
9. Mattingly RF, Thompson JD. Surgery for anomalies of the müllerian ducts, in Mattingly RF, Thompson JD, (eds), Te Linde's operative Gynecology, 6th edition, p.345. Philadelphia, J.B. Lippincott, 1985.
10. Donderwinkle PFJ, Dorr JRJ, Willemsen WNP. The unicornuate uterus: clinical implications. Eur J Obstet Gynecol 1992;47:135.
11. Mintz MC, Grumbach K. Imaging of congenital uterine anomalies. Semin Ultrasound CT MR 1988;9:167.
12. Mintz MC, Thickman DI, Gussman D, et al. MR evaluation of uterine anomalies. AJR 1987;148:287.
13. Fedele L, Dorta M, Brioschi D, et al. Magnetic resonance evaluation of double uteri. Obstet Gynecol 1989;74:844.
14. Carrington BM, Hricak H, Nuruddin RN, et al. Müllerian duct anomalies: MR imaging evaluation. Radiology 1990;176:715.
15. Haney AP, Hammond CB, Soules MR, et al, Diethylstilbestrol-induced upper genital tract abnormalities. Fertil Steril 1979;31:142.
16. Kaufman RH, Binder GL, Gray PM, et al. Upper genital tract changes associated with exposure in utero to diethylstilbestrol. Am J Obstet Gynecol 1977;32:611.
17. Kaufman RH, Adam E, Binder GL et al. Upper genital tract changes and pregnancy outcome in offspring exposed in utero to diethylstilbestrol. Am J Obstet Gynecol 1980;137:299.
18. Kaufman RH, Noller K, Adam E, et al. Upper genital tract abnormalities and pregnancy outcome in DES-exposed progeny. Am J Obstet Gynecol 1984;148:973.
19. Khalifa E, Toner JP, Jones HW. The role of abdominal metroplasty in the era of operative hysteroscopy. Surg Gynecol Obstet 1993;76:208.
20. Kipersztok S, Javitt M, Hill MC, et al. Comparison of magnetic resonance imaging and transvaginal ultrasonography in the evaluation of DES-exposed women. J Reprod Med 1996;41:347.
21. van Gils APG, Tjon A, Tham RTO, et al. Abnormalities of the uterus and cervix after diethylstilbestrol exposure: correlation of findings on MR and hysterosalpingography. AJR 1989;153:1235.

Sonosalpingography

Arthur C. Fleischer, MD; Anna K. Parsons, MD; Jeanne A. Cullinan, MD

Sonosalpingography (SSG) refers to a technique that evaluates the fallopian tubes using sonography. It is usually performed using transvaginal sonography coupled with a sonographic contrast. The contrast media that have been used include saline, air, and positive contrast agents, such as Echovist (galactose) (Schering, Berlin, Germany) and microbubbles suspended in albumen (Albunex, Mallinckrodt, St. Louis, MO).

The accuracy and ease of use of SSG make it a desirable and useful technique that can be used in the place of hysterosalpingography (HSG), which requires fluoroscopic monitoring. SSG is still associated with minimal pain or discomfort and does not reveal the anatomic detailed afforded by HSG. However, it has become a widely used technique because it can be performed with standard sonographic equipment and in a gynecologist's office without the need for sedation or preprocedural medications.

TECHNIQUE

SSG is performed with a high-frequency transvaginal sonography probe that is covered with a condom before placement into the vagina. The study is best recorded on videotape with a few representative still images recorded on paper or film.

SSG is best used after the uterine lumen is distended and examined with saline, a procedure called ''sonohysterography.''[1] Once in place, the catheter balloon needs to be inflated to prevent reflux of contrast out the endocervical canal. The HUS catheter that has a balloon is preferred. Initially, 3 to 5 cc of saline are preloaded within the catheter to prevent air from entering the cavity before saline introduction. Once the lumen is distended, the endometrial surfaces should be carefully examined for polyps or synechiae.

SSG is best performed during the follicular phase, when the endometrium is thinnest and chances of inadvertent dislodgement of an unsuspected gestational sac are low. Some have reported less pain when SSG is performed in the follicular phase.[2] Although most patients do not require anxiolytics or antibiotics, these premedications may be used in selected patients.

Once the endometrial lumen is examined, additional saline may be injected and followed for periovarian and/or cul-de-sac spill. Typically, the saline will contain air bubbles which ''sparkle'' around the ovary when released into the cul-de-sac. In most normal cases, the entire tube is seen as a rather serpiginous echogenic structure when contrast is used (Figs. 9-25, 9-26, 9-27).

If there is a question of spill, the intraluminal saline should be aspirated and a positive contrast injected. With contrast, the tubal ostium and tube should be readily apparent. Patients with tubal spasm may require reinjection and restudy after 5 to 10 minutes (Fig. 9-28).

Albunex contains microbubbles that are suspended within albumen. It should be warmed and used within minutes after aspirating from the vial. There are no known contraindications to its use except for allergy to blood products.

INDICATIONS AND CLINICAL APPLICATIONS

The accuracy of SSG is similar to HSG but slightly less (10%) than chromoperturbation when dye is injected directly into the tube and observed with laparoscopy. The main indication for SSG is evaluation of tubal patency, although additional applications may arise from more extensive use.

Tubal obstruction is typically the sequelae of pelvic inflammatory disease but may also result from adhesions that cross the tube and obstruct it from external compression. Previous salpingostomy associated with removal of ectopic pregnancy may also contribute to tubal obstruction. Hydrosalpinges can be confirmed using a sonographic contrast by demonstrating their continuity with the tubal lumen (see Fig. 9-28). It is conceivable that tubal cancers could be diagnosed using SSG as solid masses contiguous with the tubal lumen.

DIAGNOSTIC ACCURACY

Various reports have described the use of saline alone, saline and air, saline followed by color Doppler sonography,

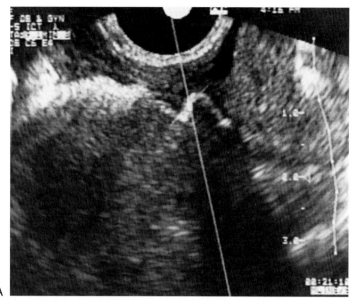

A

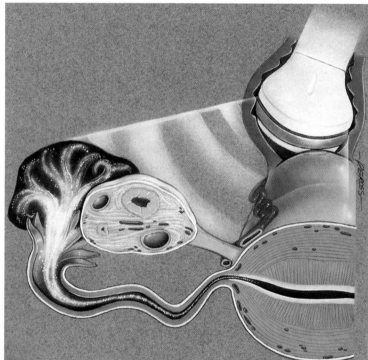

B

FIG. 9-25. Normal sonosalpingography. **(A)** Albunex-enhanced visualization of entire right tube. Doppler cursor is placed on isthmic portion. **(B)** Diagram of normal right tube as depicted with transvaginal sonography, using contrast. (Drawing by Paul Gross, M.S.).

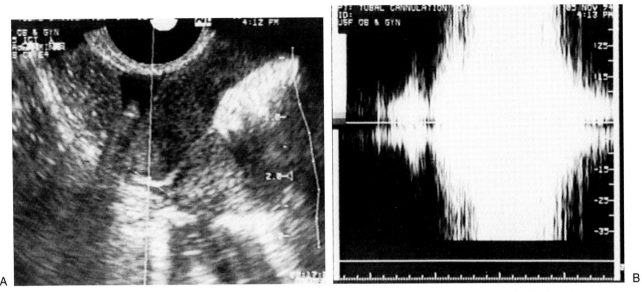

FIG. 9-26. Right tubal patency. **(A, B)** Initial tubal spasm followed by filling as documented with Doppler tracing **(B).**

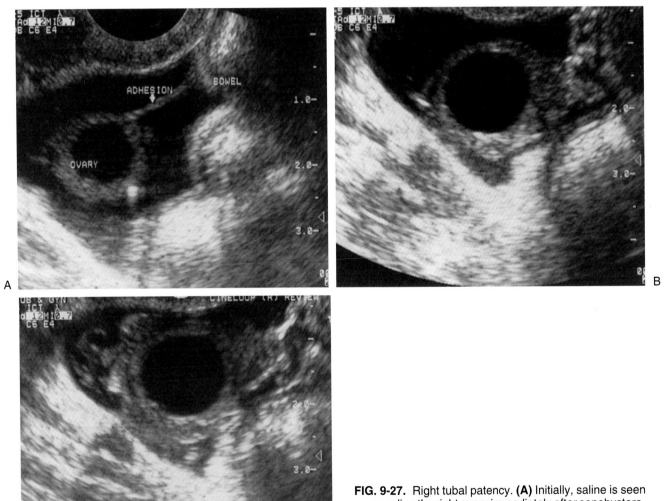

FIG. 9-27. Right tubal patency. **(A)** Initially, saline is seen surrounding the right ovary immediately after sonohysterogram. An adhesion is seen between a bowel loop and the ovary, which contains an immature follicle. **(B)** After injection of Albunex, there is echogenic contrast partially surrounding the ovary. **(C)** Fifty-six seconds later than **B,** contrast is seen surrounding the ovary.

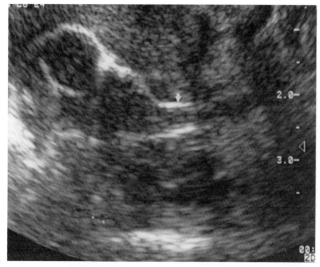

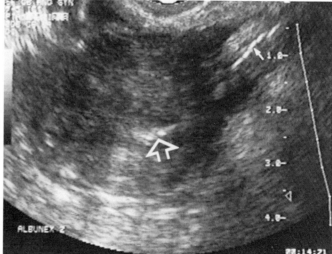

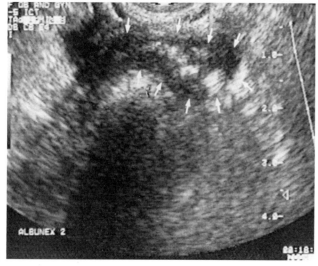

FIG. 9-28. Abnormal sonosalpingography findings. **(A)** Tubal spasm at cornua *(arrow).* This tube did not demonstrate spill, even after 5 minutes. **(B,C)** Contrast-filled hydrosalpinx *(arrows).* The thick-walled, abnormally distended left tube is depicted against the echogenic, contrast-filled lumen.

and contrast SSG for the evaluation of tubal patency.[3] The largest series of over 600 patients reported an 89.2% concordance of SSG with HSG and 90.2% for chromoperturbation.[2] Others have reported 81% and over 90% correlation between saline-CDS SSG and HSG.[4,5] The lowest accuracy (76%) has been observed using saline only.[6] The use of air and saline is reported to result in 80% sensitivity and 85% specificity for tubal obstruction.[7]

SUMMARY

SSG is a well-tolerated and inexpensive means to evaluate tubal patency. Because it can be performed in gynecologists' offices, it will probably supplant HSG as the initial test for tubal evaluation, with HSG reserved for difficult or inconclusive cases.

REFERENCES

1. Cullinan JA, Fleischer AC, Kepple DM, Arnold AL. Sonohysterography: a technique for endometrial evaluation. RadioGraphics 1995;15: 501.
2. Campbell S,. Bourne TH, Tan SL, Collins WP. Hysterosalpingo contrast sonography (HyCoSy) and its future role within the investigation of infertility in Europe. Ultrasound Obstet Gynecol 1994;4:245.
3. Schlief R, Deichert U. Hysterosalpingo contrast sonography of the uterus and fallopian tubes: results of a clinical trial of a new contrast medium in 120 patients. Radiology 1991;178:213.
4. Stern J, Peters AJ, Coulam CB. Color Doppler ultrasonography assessment of tubal patency: a comparison study with traditional techniques. Fertil Steril 1992;58:897.
5. Allahbadia GN. Fallopian tubes and ultrasonography: the Sion experience. Fertil Steril 1992;58:901.
6. Tüfekci EC, Girit S, Bayirli E, Durmuşoğlu F, Yalti S. Evaluation of tubal patency by transvaginal sonosalpingography. Fertil Steril 1992; 57:336.
7. Volpi E, Zuccaro G, Patriarca A, Rustichelli S, Sismondi P. Transvaginal sonographic tubal patency testing using air and saline solution as contrast media in a routine infertility clinic setting. Ultrasound Obstet Gynecol 1996;7:43.

Clinical Gynecologic Imaging, edited
by Arthur C. Fleischer, Marcia C. Javitt,
R. Brooke Jeffrey, Jr., and Howard W. Jones III,
Lippincott-Raven Publishers, Philadelphia © 1997.

CHAPTER 10

Special Imaging Procedures in Gynecology

Sonohysterography and Sonohysterosalpingography

Arthur C. Fleischer, MD, Jeanne A. Cullinan, MD, and
Anna K. Parsons, MD

Certain procedures in gynecologic imaging can be designated as "special" because they require specialized techniques or equipment. The most commonly performed special procedure is hysterosalpingography, which requires a fluoroscopic suite, specially designed catheters, and radiographic contrast media. The recently developed technique of saline infusion within the endometrial lumen under sonographic guidance, termed *sonohysterography,* is becoming more frequently used, particularly in the gynecologist's office or sonographic suites. It provides a means to detect polypoid endometrial lesions, submucosal fibroids, adhesions, and uterine malformations that affect the lumen. Sonohysterosalpingography combines the evaluation of the endometrial

lumen with saline with the contrast medium–enhanced evaluation of tubal patency. It is becoming more extensively used as a means to assess tubal patency because it has the advantage of lack of exposure to ionizing radiation and can be performed in the gynecologist's office or sonographic suite.

Sonohysterography has an important role in evaluation of the patient with unexplained postmenopausal bleeding and in those patients in whom the transvaginal sonogram shows endometrial thickening. Polyps usually result from endometrial overgrowth usually stimulated by excess circulating estrogen or hormone replacement. They are typically associated with intermenstrual bleeding or infertility or both.

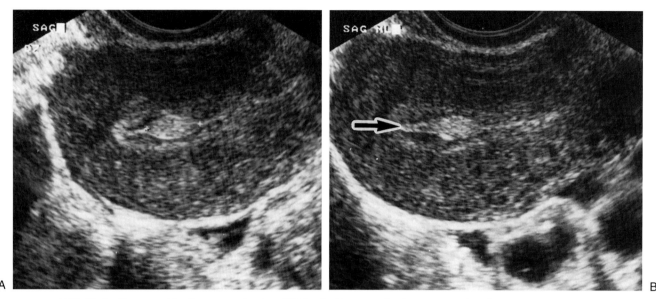

A
B

FIG. 10-1. Sonographically apparent polyp. **(A)** Sagittal transvaginal sonogram showing polyp *(between cursors)* separating endometrial surfaces. **(B)** Same patient as in **A.** The cleavage produced by the polyp separating the two endometrial layers is seen *(arrow).*

Carcinomas may also arise within polyps (Figs. 10-1 and 10-2).[1] Sonohysterography affords clear detection of the polyp and its pedicle.

Intraluminal fluid collections are frequently seen on transvaginal sonography. Although they may be associated with endometrial cancer in some patients, they are more frequently associated with benign conditions such as cervical stenosis.[2] This "natural sonohysterography" can be used to advantage to outline endometrial surfaces.

In this subchapter an overview to the clinical utility and

limitations of each of these procedures is provided and the circumstances in which they should be ordered are discussed.

SONOHYSTEROGRAPHY

With the more extensive use of transvaginal sonography, the possibility of improved delineation of the endometrial lumen with intraluminal fluid instillation became possi-

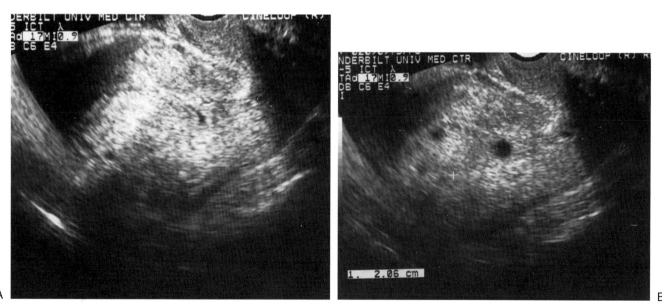

A
B

FIG. 10-2. Sonographically nearly inapparent polyp. **(A)** Transvaginal sonogram showing a large polyp occupying a markedly enlarged endometrial lumen. Only a sliver of fluid is seen surrounding this polyp, which on histologic examination showed clear cell carcinoma. **(B)** Short-axis view showing near conspicuity of polyp.

ble.[3-6] The technique uses sterile saline as a negative (hypoechoic) contrast medium to outline the endometrial lumen under continuous transvaginal sonographic visualization.[7]

Sonohysterography is primarily used for evaluation of endometrial polyps, for assessing the presence and extent of submucosal fibroids, and for detecting uterine synechiae and, in selected cases, uterine malformations that involve the endometrial lumen. The reader is referred to several excellent descriptions of the spectrum of sonographic findings with this technique.[7,8].

Sonohysterography involves placement of an insemination catheter or pediatric Foley or pediatric feeding tube into the uterine lumen through the endocervical canal. Once the cervix is cleansed with a cleansing solution and stabilized with a speculum, 3 to 10 mL of sterile saline is injected under sonographic visualization. The endometrium is imaged in both long and short axes (Figs. 10-3 and 10-4).

The procedure is best performed in the follicular phase. This avoids confusing images arising from sloughed endometrium or clot that may be encountered in the late secretory portion of the cycle and also decreases the possibility of dislodging an unsuspected early pregnancy. Because endometrial polyps are echogenic, the relatively hypoechoic proliferative phase endometrium is best shown against the relatively hypoechoic proliferative phase endometrium (Figs. 10-5 and 10-6). Conversely, submucosal fibroids may best be imaged in the secretory phase because they are typically hypoechoic and their relation to the displaced endometrium may be best delineated during this phase of the cycle (Fig. 10-7).

Contraindications to sonohysterography include hematometra or extensive pelvic inflammatory disease or an atrophic or stenotic vagina from aging or previous radiation therapy in which placement of a speculum might produce significant discomfort.

The standard procedure for transvaginal sonography is followed, including covering the probe with a condom and placement of the transvaginal probe within the vaginal fornix and mid vagina to optimally delineate the endometrial interfaces in both long and short axes. The procedure should be recorded on hard copy film or paper and videotaped for later review.

Typically, the patient does not experience significant discomfort if the catheter is properly placed in the fundus and only small amounts of fluid are allowed to be both within the lumen and reflux out of the cervix. Prophylactic antibiotics are usually not needed, but nonsteroidal antiinflammatory agents may be helpful in patients experiencing pelvic pain.

Typical Sonographic Findings

The normal endometrium is usually delineated in its entirety after the introduction of intraluminal fluid. On short axis, the normal areas of endometrial invagination in both tubal ostia can be seen. In general, the endometrium measures up to 4 mm in thickness per single layer and should have a relatively regular and homogeneous texture.

Endometrial polyps are typically echogenic and project into the endometrial lumen (see Figs. 10-5 and 10-6). Larger polyps may contain cystic spaces representing obstructed glands within the polyp. In the nondistended endometrium they typically displace the median echo, which may represent refluxed cervical mucus (see Fig. 10-1). As they enlarge, they can distend the cavity and may be apparent without iatrogenic distention of the endometrial lumen. Some are outlined by trapped intraluminal fluid.

Submucosal fibroids are typically hypoechoic and displace the endometrium (see Fig. 10-7). Their extent into the myometrial layers is important to determine in that superficial submucosal fibroids may be able to have the stalk

(text continued on page 326)

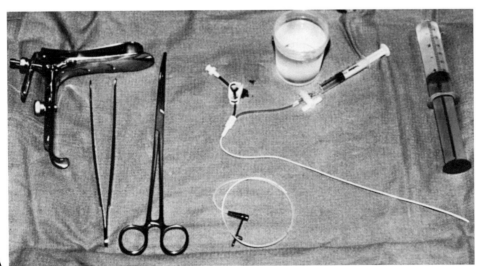

FIG. 10-3. Setup for sonohysterography and normal examples. **(A)** Setup used for sonohysterography consisting of long straight forceps, open lipped speculum, catheter, saline, long cotton-tipped applicator, and cleansing solution.

A

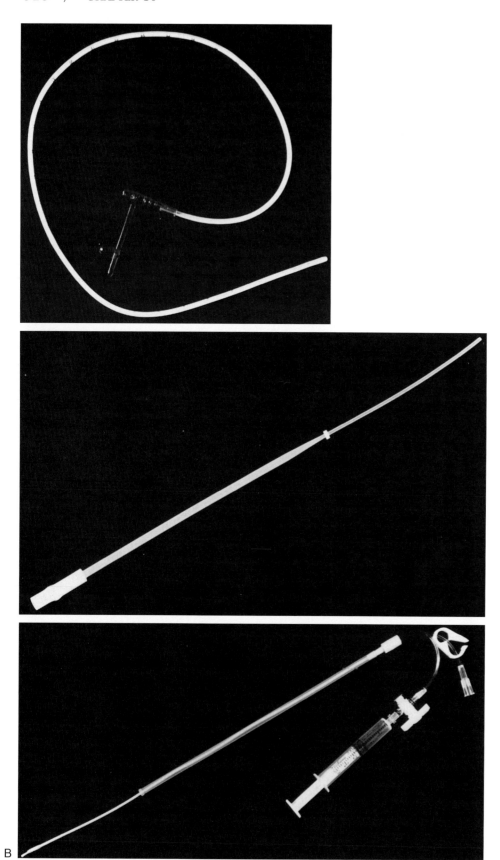

FIG. 10-3. *Continued.* **(B)** Catheters used for sonohysterography: *Top:* Pediatric feeding tube. *Middle:* Insemination catheter. *Bottom:* hysterosalpingography catheter.

B

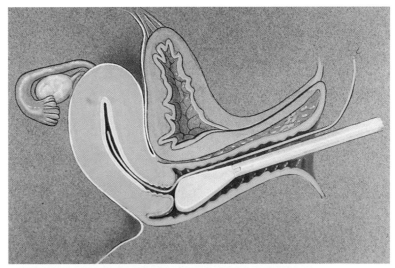

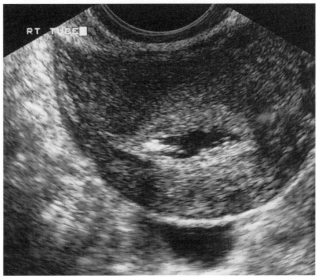

C

FIG. 10-3. *Continued.* **(C)** *(Top)* Diagram showing bendable pediatric catheter. The tip should be advanced into the fundus to obtain maximal dilatation. *(Bottom)* Semicoronal transvaginal sonogram during initial fluid instillation showing secretory phase endometrium. The catheter produces a linear interface.

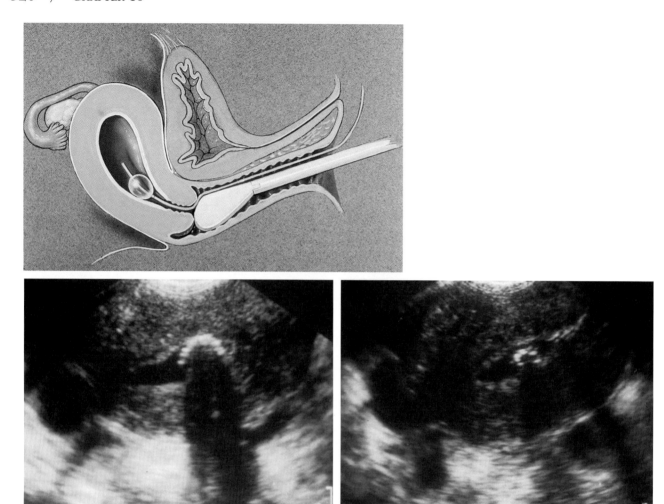

FIG. 10-3. *Continued.* **(D)** *(Left)* Diagram of sonohysterography using pediatric Foley catheter with inflatable balloon. *(Right)* Transvaginal sonogram showing same balloon when inflated *(Left)* and deflated *(Right)*.

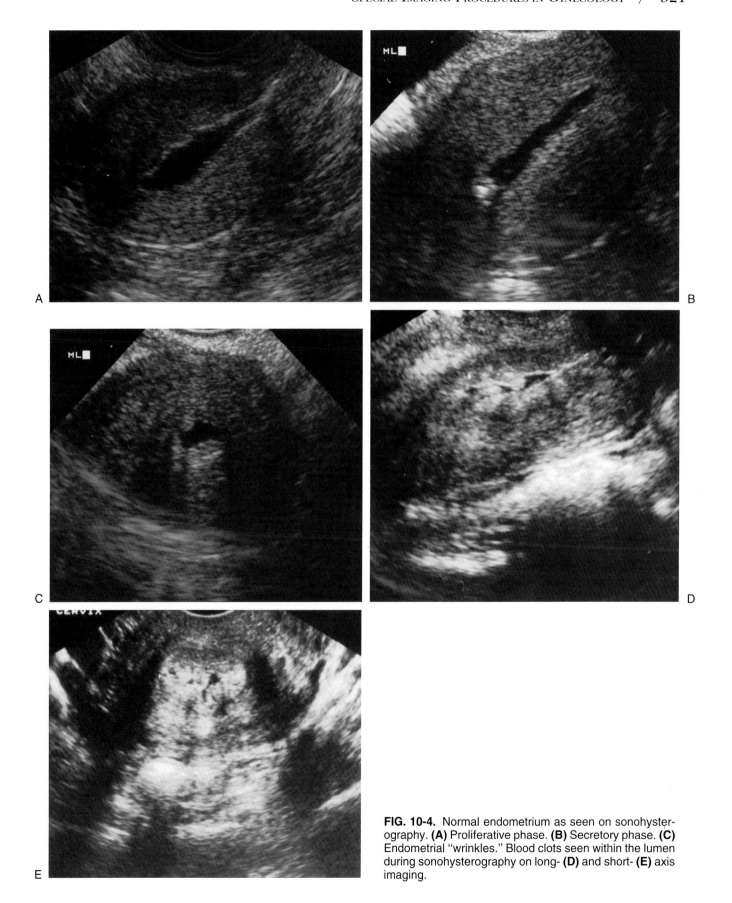

FIG. 10-4. Normal endometrium as seen on sonohysterography. **(A)** Proliferative phase. **(B)** Secretory phase. **(C)** Endometrial "wrinkles." Blood clots seen within the lumen during sonohysterography on long- **(D)** and short- **(E)** axis imaging.

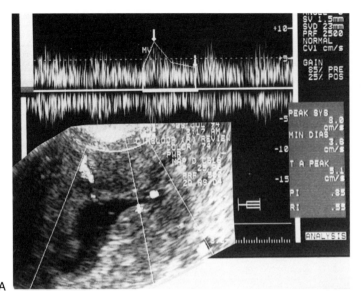

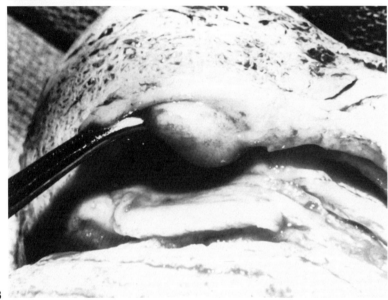

FIG. 10-5. Polyp imaged with color Doppler sonography shows vascularity. **(A)** Combined transvaginal sonogram and Doppler spectrum from vessel within polyp showing low impedance flow. **(B)** Sectioned uterus showing polyp.

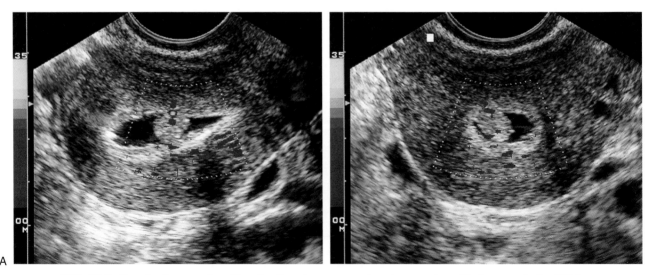

FIG. 10-6. Sonohysterography with color Doppler sonography shows polyp with its vascularity. **(A)** In the sagittal plane the power Doppler scan shows vascularity within the pedicle of the polyp. **(B)** The same as in **A** in the coronal plane.

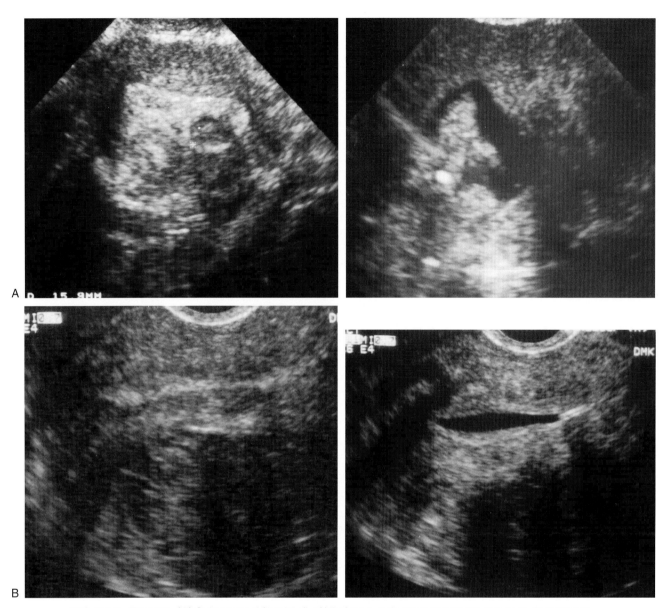

FIG. 10-7. Fibroids. **(A)** Submucosal fibroid. *(Left)* Before sonohysterography the hypoechoic submucosal fibroid is seen to displace overlying echogenic endometrium. *(Right)* After saline instillation the overlying endometrium and submucosal leiomyoma are seen. **(B)** Intramural fibroid. *(Left)* Before sonohysterography an intramural leiomyoma is seen extending into the outer layer of the myometrium. *(Right)* After saline instillation, the relationship of the normal endometrium to the intramural leiomyoma is clearly demonstrated.

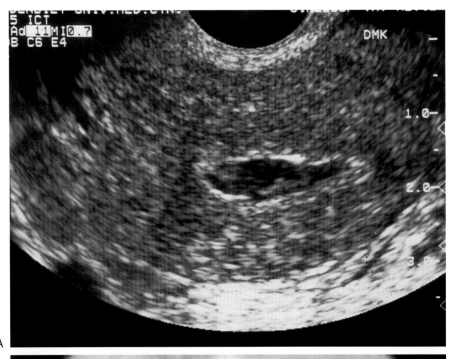

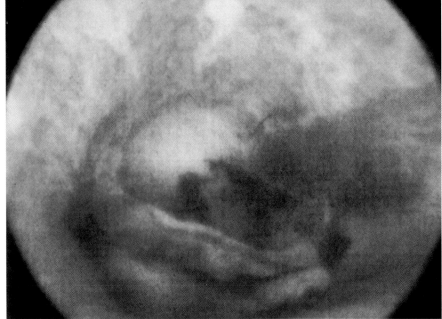

FIG. 10-8. Adhesions. **(A)** Sonohysterography showing linear adhesions crossing lumen. **(B)** Hysteroscopy shows the adhesion. **(B,** courtesy of E. Eisenberg, MD.)

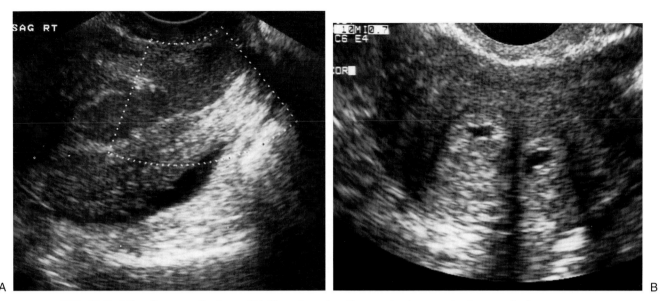

FIG. 10-9. Miscellaneous findings. **(A)** Hematometra. Presonohysterography transvaginal sonogram showed hematometria, a contraindication to sonohysterography. **(B)** Septate uterus. Sonohysterography showed two lumina separated by a thick septum. There was no fundal cleft.

removed by wire loop or alligator forceps whereas those that extend into the outer layers of myometrium will not be amenable to wire loop resection.

Synechiae typically occur as the sequelae of intrauterine instrumentation. They may be either echogenic or hypoechoic, depending on their fibrous content (Fig. 10-8). The hypoechoic synechiae are best delineated in the background of echogenic secretory phase endometrium.[9]

Certain uterine malformations that affect the lumen such as bicornuate or septated uteri may be evaluated using sonohysterography. The presence or absence of a fundal cleft is important in distinguishing bicornuate uteri from septated uteri (Fig. 10-9).

Color Doppler sonography may be helpful to identify the vascular pedicle of a polyp as well as the vascular rim of certain leiomyomas (see Fig. 10-6). Sonohysterography is helpful in determining whether a polyp has a wide or narrow pedicle because polyps or a thin pedicle are more easily removed than ones with a thick pedicle.

Sonohysterography is also particularly helpful in determining whether certain intraluminal cystic areas are within a polyp or the myometrium. Punctate cystic spaces are frequently seen within polyps as a result of glandular obstruction. They may also be seen within the myometrium in women who are on tamoxifen, possibly a result of reactivation of dormant adenomyosis.[10]

SONOHYSTEROSALPINGOGRAPHY

The use of contrast medium–enhanced evaluation of tubal patency has become more widespread with the availability of sonographic contrast agents, which are specifically designed for this purpose (Figs. 10-10 and 10-11). Injection of saline with evaluation by duplex Doppler or color Doppler sonography can be used but is not as definitive as establishment of tubal patency with a contrast medium.[11–16]

The best procedure for assessment of tubal patency involves initial evaluation of the endometrial lumen with sonohysterography followed by evaluation of the tube with sonohysterosalpingography. This sequence of studies allows for accumulation of fluid surrounding the ovary into the pelvic peritoneal cavity, which helps identify the fimbriated end of the tube for confirming contrast medium passage (Fig. 10-12). To achieve adequate tubal opacification, the balloon needs to be distended so as to obstruct retrograde passage of contrast medium out the endocervical canal.

High degrees (over 90%) of accuracy have been reported

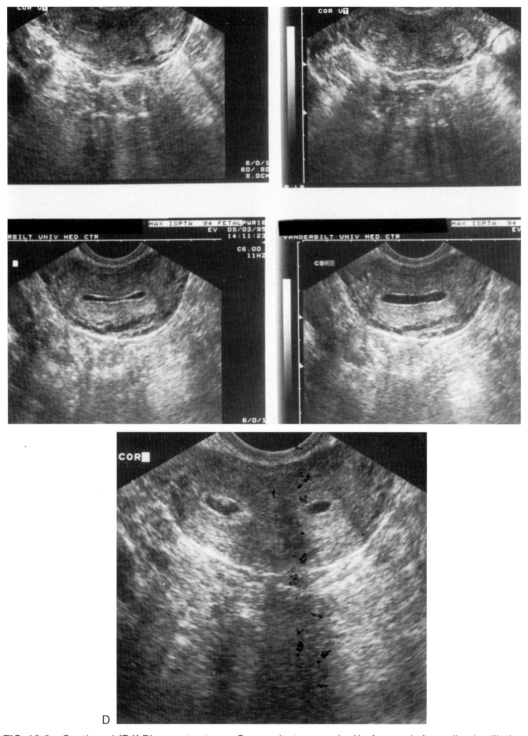

D

FIG. 10-9. *Continued.* **(D1)** Bicornuate uterus. Composite transvaginal before and after saline instillation. Two endometrial lumina are seen before *(top)* and after *(bottom)* saline instillation. **(D2)** The thin endometria are seen best on this coronal transvaginal sonogram taken through the fundus. A small fundal cleft is seen.

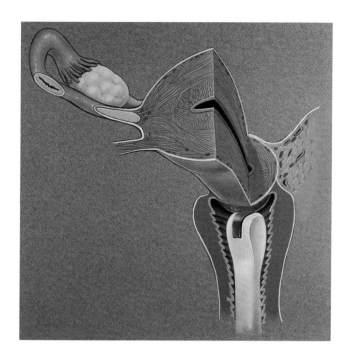

FIG. 10-10. Diagram showing transvaginal sonographic field of view for delineation of normal right tube. (Drawn by Paul Gross, MS.)

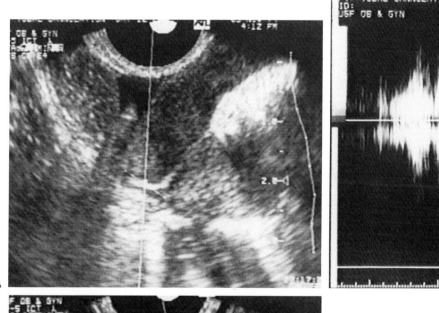

A

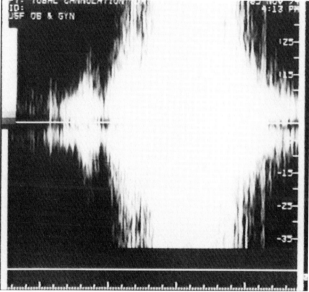

B

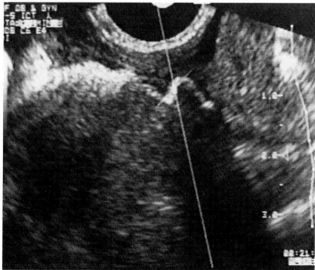

C

FIG. 10-11. Patent tubes shown by sonohysterosalpingography. **(A)** Initially after injection showing flow through right tubal ostia. **(B)** Doppler signal from sample volume showing flow. **(C)** Flow in right mid-ampullary tube showing intraperitoneal spillage.

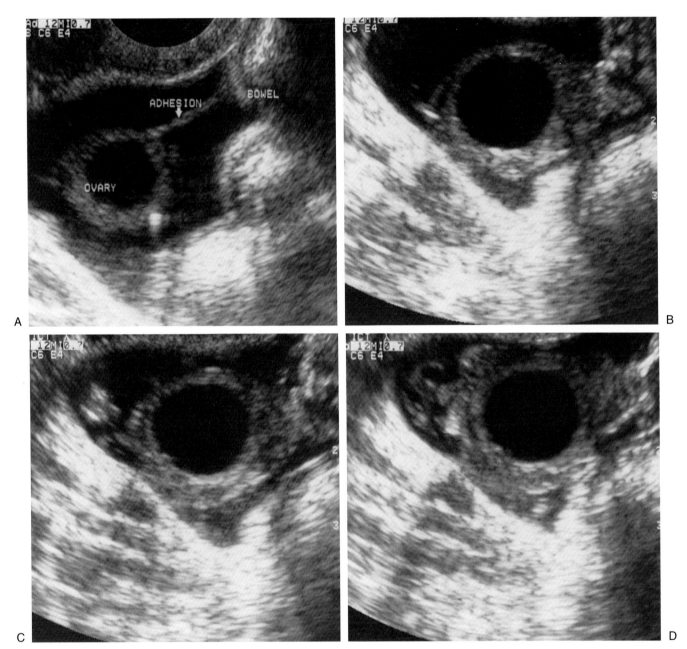

FIG. 10-12. Patent tube shown on sequential transvaginal sonographic images from a sonohysterosal-pingogram. **(A)** Initial scan showing ovary containing a mature follicle attached to bowel by an adhesion. Fluid is surrounding the ovary after sonohysterography in both long- **(B)** and short- **(C)** axis images. **(D)** Forty-six seconds later there is demonstration of flow out of the fimbriated end of the tube.

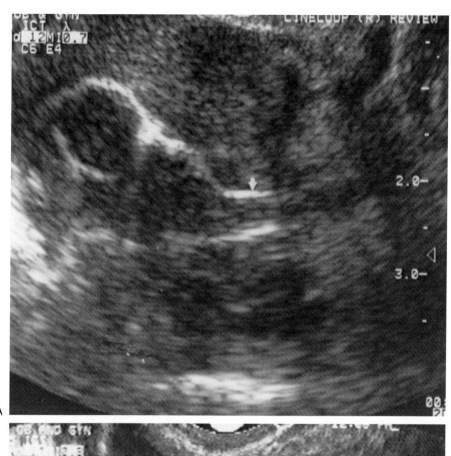

A

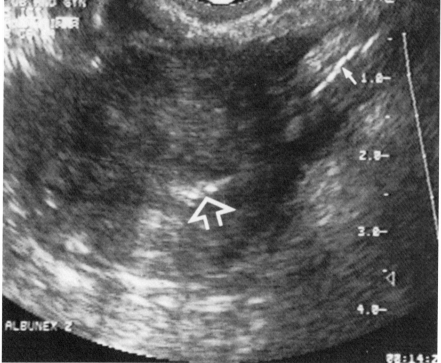

B

FIG. 10-13. Tubal spasm as demonstrated on sonohysterosalpingography. **(A)** Initially there was no filling of the tube past the left tubal ostia *(arrow)*. **(B)** Seven seconds later filling of the ampullary portion of the tube is evident *(arrow)*.

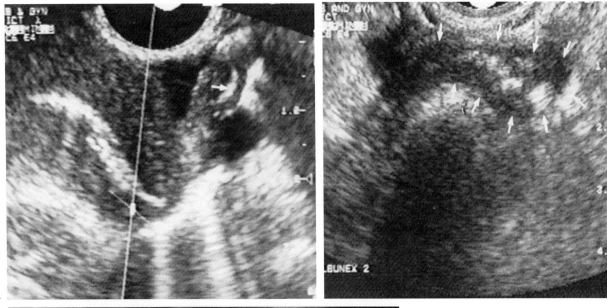

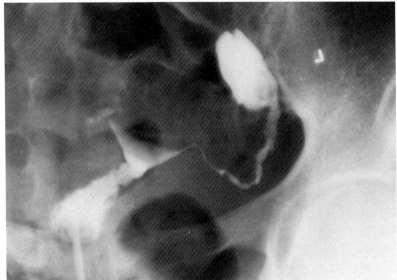

FIG. 10-14. Obstructed tube as shown by sonohysterosalpingography. **(A)** Initial scan showing contrast medium within lumen of ampullary portion of left tube. **(B)** Almost 5 minutes later there was no intraperitoneal spillage. Contrast medium is trapped within lumen *(arrows)* of thickened tube. **(C)** Hysterosalpingogram of same patient showed obstructed, distended tube.

for hystero-contrast sonography in a multicenter study.[11] These investigators used Echovist, a positive contrast media that consists of galactose-coated particles that are echogenic. Others have used Albunex, a contrast medium derived from microparticles suspended in human albumen.

With either sonographic contrast agent, tubal patency can be assessed. Tubal spasm and its accompanying discomfort is sometimes observed during the initial instillation but is usually transient. Although tubal spasm occurs in some patients, continuous sonographic evaluation after 10 to 15 minutes usually definitively establishes the presence or absence of tubal obstruction (Figs. 10-13 and 10-14).

It is anticipated that there will be more widespread use of sonohysterosalpingography with hysterosalpingography as a backup test for certain indications.

REFERENCES

1. Salm R. The incidence and significance of early carcinomas in endometrial polyps. J Pathol 1972; 108:47.
2. Pardo J, Kaplan B, Nitke S, et al. Postmenopausal intrauterine fluid collection: correlation between ultrasound and hysteroscopy. Ultrasound Obstet Gynecol 1994;4:224.
3. Syrop CH, Sahakian V. Transvaginal sonographic detection of endometrial polyps with fluid contrast augmentation. Obstet Gynecol 1992;79:1041.
4. Parsons AK, Lense JJ. Sonohysterography for endometrial abnormalities: preliminary results. J Clin Ultrasound 1993;21:87.
5. Goldstein SR. Use of ultrasonography for triage of perimenopausal patients with unexplained uterine bleeding. Am J Obstet Gynecol 1994; 170:565.
6. Dubinsky T, Parvey H, Gormaz G, Maklad N. Transvaginal hysterosonography in the evaluation of small endometrial masses. J Ultrasound Med 1995;14:1.
7. Cullinan J, Fleischer A, Kepple D, Arnold A. Sonohysterography: a technique for endometrial evaluation. Radiographics 1995;15:501.

8. Parsons A, Cullinan JA, Goldstein S, Fleischer AC. Sonohysterography, sonosalpingography and sonohysterosalpingography. In: Fleischer A, Romero R, Manning R (eds). Sonography in obstetrics and gynecology. Stamford, CT, Appleton & Lange, 1995.

9. Narayan R, Goswamy RK. Transvaginal sonography of the uterine cavity with hysteroscopic correlation in the investigation of infertility. Ultrasound Obstet Gynecol 1993;3:129.

10. Goldstein SR: Unusual ultrasonographic appearance of the uterus in patients receiving tamoxifen. Am J Obstet Gynecol 1994;170:447.

11. Campbell A, Bourne TH, Tan SL, Collins WP. Hysterosalpingo contrast sonography (HyCoSy) and its future role within the investigation of infertility in Europe. Ultrasound Obstet Gynecol 1994;4:245.

12. Schlief R, Deichert U. Hysterosalpingo-contrast sonography of the uterus and fallopian tubes: results of a clinical trial of a new contrast medium in 120 patients. Radiology 1991;178:213.

13. Allahbadia GN. Fallopian tubes and ultrasonography: the Sion experience. Fertil Steril 1992;58:901.

14. Deichert U, Schlief R, van de Sandt M, Daume E. Transvaginal hysterosalpingo-contrast sonography for the assessment of tubal patency with gray scale imaging and additional use of pulsed wave Doppler. Fertil Steril 1992;57:62.

15. Tüfekci EC, Girit S, Bayirli E, et al. Evaluation of tubal patency by transvaginal sonosalpingography. Fertil Steril 1992;57:336.

16. Stern J, Peters AJ, Coulam CB. Color Doppler ultrasonography assessment of tubal patency: a comparison study with traditional techniques. Fertil Steril 1992;58:897.

Hysterosalpingography

Amy S. Thurmond, MD

The first hysterosalpingogram was probably performed in 1910, only 15 years after the discovery of radiographs. It was one of the first specialized radiographic tests ever performed, using the placement of Bismuth paste in the cervical canal. A large body of information, therefore, has accumulated regarding the strengths and limitations of this test. At the same time, because it is old fashioned and lacks the glamour of MRI and some of the more technical examinations, it may have been neglected by radiologists and gynecologists in some institutions. The development of Fallopian tube catheterization in the 1980s and of sonohysterosalpingography (SHSG) in the 1990s has caused a resurgence in interest in the technique of hysterosalpingography (HSG) and the anatomy of the uterine cavity and Fallopian tubes.

Some authors have recommended that hysteroscopy and laparoscopy be used instead of hysterosalpingography, because hysterosalpingography may fail to diagnose pelvic adhesions in up to 30% of patients with this condition. HSG remains a mainstay in the initial evaluation of the infertile couple, however,[1] because of its availability as an outpatient procedure, absence of anesthesia requirements, speed of procedure, minimal morbidity, and relatively low cost. Good technique and careful interpretation of the findings will maximize the benefits of HSG. If there is suspicion of peritubal adhesions by history, and the hysterosalpingogram looks normal, laparoscopy may be considered.

HSG should not be performed when there is active vaginal bleeding. This is to prevent the flushing of clots into the peritoneal cavity. HSG should also not be performed if there is active pelvic infection, because it could exacerbate the infection. The procedure should not be performed within 6 weeks of pregnancy, uterine surgery, tubal surgery, or uterine curettage because the defects in the endometrial or tubal lining predispose to venous intravasation of contrast material. Clearly, HSG should not be performed if there is a possibility of a normal intrauterine pregnancy. To avoid irradiating an early pregnancy, the ''10-day rule'' can be used; that is, the procedure should not be performed if the interval of time from the start of the last menses is greater than 10 to 12 days. Because menses start usually 14 days after ovulation, if the patient has cycles that are longer than 28 days, then the 10-day rule can be stretched to 13 to 15 days. If the patient has irregular cycles or absent menses, some physicians recommend a pregnancy test before performing the examination. Previous reaction to iodinated contrast agent may be a contraindication to HSG if the risks outweigh the benefits.

The patient is placed supine with her knees flexed and heels apart. Stirrups on the table to support the feet can be used but are not necessary, because this positioning is required only until the HSG device is placed, at which point the patient can be placed comfortably flat on the table for imaging. The cervix is exposed with a speculum. Visualization of the cervix may be helped by elevating the patient's pelvis, particularly in thin women. The cervix and vagina are copiously swabbed with a cleansing solution such as Betadine and the HSG cannula is placed. A variety of cannulas can be used for HSG.[2–4] Once correct placement of the cannula is confirmed, the speculum should be removed. Leaving the speculum in is uncomfortable for the patient and a metal speculum obscures findings. Using fluoroscopic guidance, contrast agent at room temperature is slowly injected, usually 5 to 10 cc over 1 minute, and radiographs are obtained. Injection of contrast agent is halted when adequate free spill into the peritoneal cavity is documented, when myometrial or venous intravasation occurs, or when the patient complains of increased cramping, which usually occurs when the tubes are blocked.

The side effects and complications of HSG are for the most part the same as SHSG. Mild discomfort or pain is commonly experienced by women undergoing HSG.[5] Routine analgesia is not necessary, although oral Ibuprofen is a reasonable preprocedure medication. Reassurance and rapid and skillful completion of the examination are the best approach. Mild vaginal bleeding is common after HSG. Severe bleeding requiring curettage is unusual and is presumably related to underlying pathology such as endometrial polyps. Other side effects such as vasovagal reactions and hyperventilation may occur, and their incidence may be reduced if the examiner is experienced and calming.

Pelvic infection is a serious complication of HSG, causing tubal damage, and in the days before antibiotics, even death. In a private-practice setting, the overall incidence of post-HSG pelvic infection was 1.4%, occurring predominantly in women with dilated tubes.[6] Subsequently, when women with known dilated tubes were given prophylactic doxycycline, no postprocedure infections occurred.[6] For this reason, if dilated tubes are noted at the time of HSG, particularly if there is a dilated tube with free spill, doxycycline (200 mg orally) should be administered before the patient leaves the department and a prescription for 5 days' doxycycline, 100 mg orally, twice daily should be given to the patient. If the tubes are normal, there is no evidence to suggest prophylactic antibiotics are necessary. All women, however, should be warned about the symptoms of pelvic infection.

An allergic or idiosyncratic reaction related to the contrast medium can occur after HSG, although the incidence is unknown and is presumably quite low. A delayed reaction consisting of urticaria and severe hypotension 1 hour after a normal HSG without intravasation was reported. The delayed reaction was presumably related to peritoneal absorption.[7] To our knowledge, no deaths from idiosyncratic reactions to contrast media have been reported after HSG. The incidence of such reactions is sufficiently low that routine use of on-ionic contrast agents for HSG is not warranted. This may, however, be a reasonable option in the presence of history of previous reaction to iodinated contrast media.

Radiation exposure is a side effect not shared by SHSG. It is a concern, because the women being examined are of reproductive age. The incidence of irradiating an early pregnancy is quite low when HSG is routinely performed in the follicular phase of the cycle, as previously described. Although cases are few, there is nothing to suggest that inadvertent performance of an HSG in early pregnancy is harmful to the fetus.[8] Radiation exposure to the ovaries is minimal and can be reduced by using good fluoroscopic technique and obtaining only the number of radiographs necessary to make an accurate diagnosis.

Whether HSG helps women achieve pregnancy has been debated for many years. Multiple retrospective or nonrandomized studies showed an increased pregnancy rate following HSG, particularly when oil-based media were used.[5] Recently, a randomized, prospective study showed a significantly increased pregnancy rate after the use of oil medium when compared with 3 water-soluble media, including a nonionic agent.[9] Even though all of these studies are subject to criticism, there probably is an unexplained therapeutic benefit of HSG, particularly in patients with a normal uterus and Fallopian tubes, in whom the cause of infertility is unexplained.

TYPICAL FINDINGS

The fallopian tubes have a unique status in the body. Via the uterus, cervix, and vagina they connect the peritoneal cavity to the external world. Their function and anatomy is complex, and includes conduction of sperm from the uterine end towards the ampulla, conduction of ova in the other direction from the fimbriated end to the ampulla, and support as well as conduction of the early embryo from the ampulla into the uterus for implantation. The normal fallopian tube ranges in length from 7 cm to 16 cm, with an average length of 12 cm (Figure 10-15). The tube is divided into four regions: (1) the intramural or interstitial portion, which occurs in the wall of the uterine fundus and is 1 cm to 2 cm long; (2) the isthmic portion, which is about 2 cm to 3 cm long; (3) the ampullary portion, which is 5 cm to 8 cm long; and

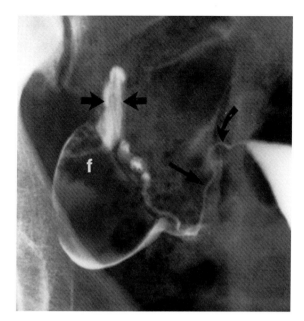

FIG. 10-15. Conventional contrast hysterosalpinography demonstrates the normal interstitial *(curved arrow)* and isthmic portions of the fallopian tube *(long arrow)*, as well as the ampulla with its rugal folds *(short arrows)*, and the outline of the velvety fimbria **(f)** draped over the ovary outlined by the spill of contrast media.

(4) the infundibulum, which is the trumpet-shaped distal end of the tube terminating in the fimbria (Figure 10-15). Patency of the fallopian tubes is established when contrast medium flows through them and freely around the ovary and loops of bowel at the time of salpingography, using either fluoroscopic or sonographic guidance.

Diverticulae in the isthmic segment of the tube are caused by salpingitis isthmica nodosa (SIN) (Figure 10-16). These

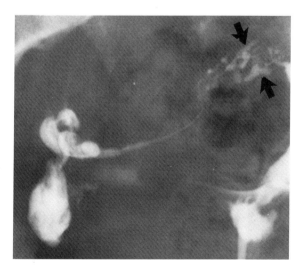

FIG. 10-16. The left fallopian tube demonstrates filling of small isthmic diverticulae (arrows). Overall caliber of the tube is normal and therefore this severe disease would likely be missed by sonography.

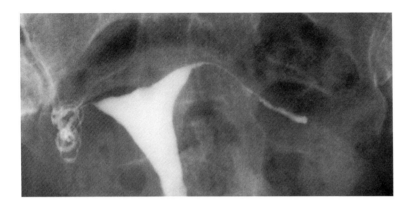

FIG. 10-17. The left fallopian tube is occluded in the distal isthmic portion. This also would be difficult to discern with sonography.

would be difficult to appreciate by sonography. SIN was described more than 100 years ago as irregular benign extensions of the tubal epithelium into the myosalpinx, associated with reactive myohypertrophy and sometimes inflammation. There is an association between SIN and pelvic inflammatory disease; however it is not clear whether SIN is caused by pelvic inflammation, or is congenital and predisposes to inflammation.

Obstruction of the tubes can occur anywhere along their length. Obstruction in the midisthmic portion would be difficult to discern with sonography, because of the small caliber of the tube and the absence of dilation when there is obstruction at this level (Figure 10-17).

Polyps are small, smooth filling defects, which can be single or multiple, and do not distort the overall size and shape of the uterine cavity (Figure 10-18). Leiomyomas are usually single, larger lobulated masses, which only partially project into the cavity, and often enlarge and distort the cavity (Figure 10-19). Adenomyosis also presents as a mass or uterine enlargement, although the margins of the mass are ill-defined and the multiple abnormal glandular structures within the mass may be filled with contrast agent (Figure 10-20). Synechiae are scars that result from uterine trauma such as complications of pregnancy, curettage, uterine surgery, or uterine infection. Synechiae are generally linear and irregular (Figure 10-21) and extend from one wall to the opposite wall allowing contrast agent to flow around them only in one dimension. For this reason, they are more easily

defined than the masses described above, which in general, allow contrast agent to flow around them in two dimensions. Synechiae may also manifest as absence of filling of the entire uterus or part of it, and can be confused with a müllerian defect (Figure 10-22).

Müllerian anomalies probably occur in 1% of women and are associated with renal anomalies in one quarter.[1] The anomalies have been classified into seven groups, based on their prognosis for future fertility and their surgical treatment.[10] Anomalies occur that do not fit neatly into any of these categories, however. When in doubt, it is best to completely describe the anatomy without attaching a label to it. Class I (segmental müllerian agenesis) is manifested by variable absence of the uterus or cervix. It presents as absence of menstrual bleeding at puberty and may be associated with pelvic pain because of retrograde menses. It may or may not be surgically correctable, depending on the findings. Class II (unicornuate uterus) is caused by absence of development of one of the müllerian ducts (Figure 10-23), and is almost always accompanied by absence of the kidney on the same side. There is an association with fertility and pregnancy difficulties and there is essentially no treatment. Class III (uterus didelphys) results in two separate uterine horns, cervices, and vaginas. In general it is not associated with fertility or pregnancy problems and therefore it is usually not treated. Class IV (bicarnuate uterus) is characterized by two separate uterine horns, usually one cervix, and one

(text continued on page 337)

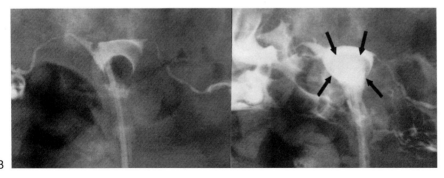

A,B

FIG. 10-18. Uterine polyp. **(A)** Polyp is obscured by the balloon used for injection. **(B)** Repeat injection is performed with the balloon inflated and reveals the polyp *(arrows)*.

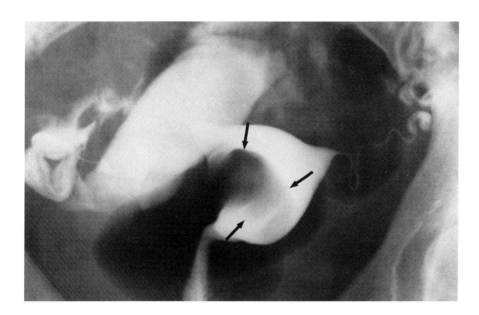

FIG. 10-19. A single lobulated filling defect that distorts the cavity is a myoma *(arrows)*.

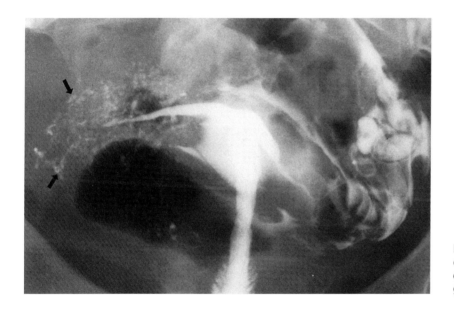

FIG. 10-20. Uterine cavity is distorted by adenomyosis *(arrows)*, diagnosable because contrast agent fills the numerous abnormal glandular structures within the mass.

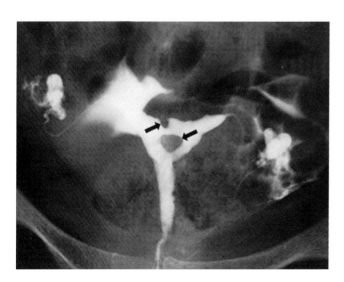

FIG. 10-21. Small irregular filling defects in the uterine cavity are synechiae *(arrows)*.

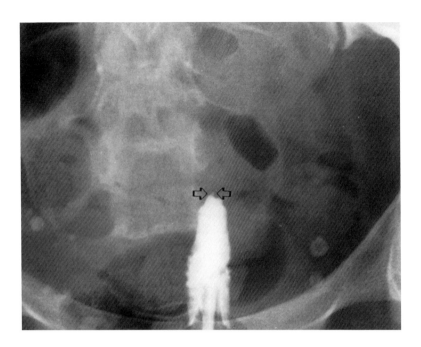

FIG. 10-22. A synechia at the cervical uterine junction *(open arrows)* results in filling of the cervical canal only, and is accompanied by absent menses and infertility (Asherman's Syndrome).

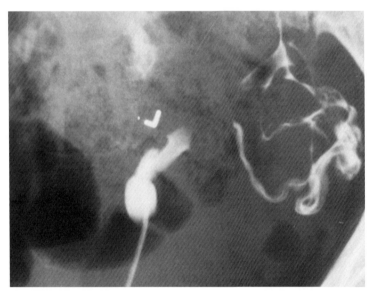

FIG. 10-23. Left unicornuate uterus. The differential diagnosis includes bicornuate uterus with a right non-communicating rudimentary horn (which would likely be visible by sonography), and uterus didelphys (in which case a separate right vagina and cervix should be present).

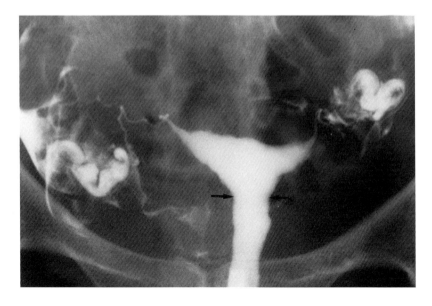

FIG. 10-24. The widened internal os region *(arrows)*, which gives a funnel shape to the uterine cavity and cervical canal would be difficult to appreciate with ultrasound, and is confirmatory of incompetent cervix in this woman with a history of four painless second-trimester fetal losses.

vagina. Bicornuate uterus is associated with a low incidence of fertility and pregnancy complications and therefore is usually not treated. Class V (septate uterus) consists of two uterine cavities and a single fundus. The septum can involve the cervix and vagina as well. Of the correctable lesions a uterine septum has the highest incidence of fertility and pregnancy problems and for this reason the septum is usually removed hysteroscopically. Class VI (arcurate uterus) is probably a normal variant and looks like a small septum.) Class VII (T-shaped uterus) is caused by diethylstilbesterol (DES) exposure in utero. In addition to a small, T-shaped uterus that is difficult to define sonographically, these women may have a mucosal ridge or hood superior to their external cervix and clear cell adenocarcinoma of the vagina. They do have fertility and pregnancy problems and no definite treatment is known.

In general, uterine shape abnormalities are better defined by conventional HSG than any other imaging test. An internal os wider than 1 cm or a funnel-shaped uterus and cervix (Figure 10-24) in a woman with painless second-trimester pregnancy losses is confirmatory of incompetent cervix.

REFERENCES

1. Winfield AC, Wentz AC. Diagnostic imaging in infertility. 2nd ed. Baltimore: Williams and Wilkins, 1992.
2. Margolin FR. A new cannula for hysterosalpingography. AJR 1988; 151:729.
3. Sholkoff SD. Balloon hysterosalpingography catheter. AJR 1987;149: 995.
4. Thurmond AS, Uchida BT, Rosch J. Device for hysterosalpingography and fallopian tube catheterization. Radiology 1990;174:571.
5. Soules MR, Spadoni LR. Oil versus aqueous media for hysterosalpingography: a continuing debate based on many opinions and few facts. Fertil Steril 1982;38:1.
6. Pittaay DE, Winfield AC, Maxson W, Daniell J, Herbert C, Wentz AC. Prevention of acute pelvic inflammatory disease after hysterosalpingography: efficacy of doxycycline prophylaxis. Am J Obstet Gynecol 1983;147:623.
7. Schuitemaker NWE, Helmerhorst FM, Tjon A, Tham RTO, van Saase JLC. Late anaphylactic shock after hysterosalpingography. Fertil Steril 1990;54:535.
8. Justesen P, Rasmussen F, Anderson PE Jr. Inadvertently performed hysterosalpingography during early pregnancy. Acta Radiol Diag 1986; 27:711.
9. Rasmussen F, Lindequist S, Larsen C, Justesen P. Therapeutic effect of hysterosalpingography: oil- versus water-soluble contrast media—a randomized prospective study. Radiology 1991;179:75.
10. Buttram VC. The American Fertility Society classification of adnexal adhesions, distal tubal occlusion, tubal occlusion secondary to tubal ligation, tubal pregnancies, müllerian anomalies and intrauterine adhesions. Fertil Steril 1988;49:944

Transabdominal and Transvaginal Sonographic-Guided Procedures

Arthur C. Fleischer, MD

Both transabdominal and transvaginal sonography afford accurate guidance for a variety of guided procedures. Most common among these are follicular aspiration and cyst aspiration. Both of these procedures require the use of a needle guide, which affords accurate and real-time determination of the location of the needle tip. The needle path is displayed on the monitor. The tip of the needle is usually scored to provide increased echogenicity, thereby enhancing its visualization.

Once the probe is covered with a sterile sheath or condom, the vaginal wall is cleaned and anesthetized (Fig. 10-25). The needle path as seen on the monitor is lined up with the structure of interest and the needle is introduced (Fig. 10-26). Deflation or aspiration of the contents can be observed on the monitor and then the needle is removed.

Some clinicians prefer the spring-loaded needle to the standard needle with an internal stylet because less pain is experienced with a quick and decisive needle excursion.[1]

Transabdominal approach may be preferable if the area of interest is superior to the pelvic area. Needle guides are also available for transabdominal transducers. Because of the standoff, the initial 1 to 1.5 cm may not be depicted, however.

The reader is referred to other articles for detailed descriptions of this technique.[2]

The most common indications for transvaginal sonographic- or transabdominal sonographic-guided aspiration include the following:

- Cyst aspiration in patients undergoing ovulation induction (Fig. 10-27)
- Cystic mass aspiration in nonsurgical patients in whom the exact histology is needed to manage the patient properly (Fig. 10-28)
- Drainage of pyosalpinx or ovarian abscesses in patients nonresponsive to medical treatment (Fig. 10-29)
- Aspiration of masses with potential to torse or cause recurrent pain, such as endometriosis (Fig. 10-30)

Of these indications, transvaginal sonographic-guided aspiration is probably most efficacious in the treatment of recurrent endometriomas. Excellent palliation after aspiration has been reported.[3] Similarly, peritoneal cysts or

(text continued on page 342)

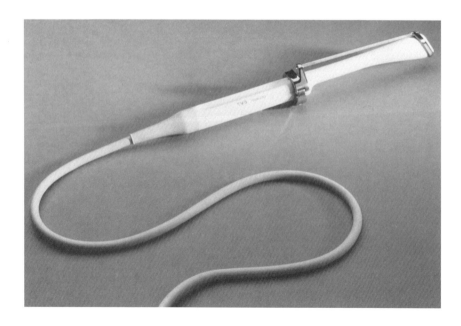

FIG. 10-25. Needle guide secured on shaft of transvaginal probe.

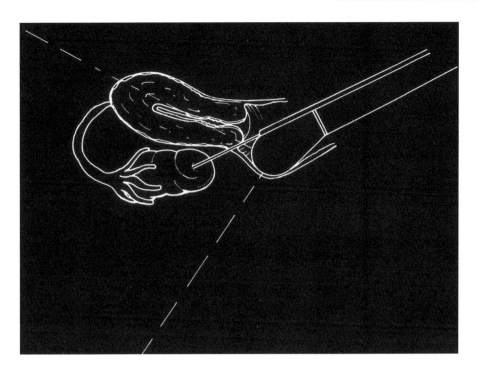

FIG. 10-26. Diagram of needle aspiration of mature follicle. It is important to avoid the major vessels, and this can be accomplished when transvaginal color Doppler sonography is used to delineate them before puncture.

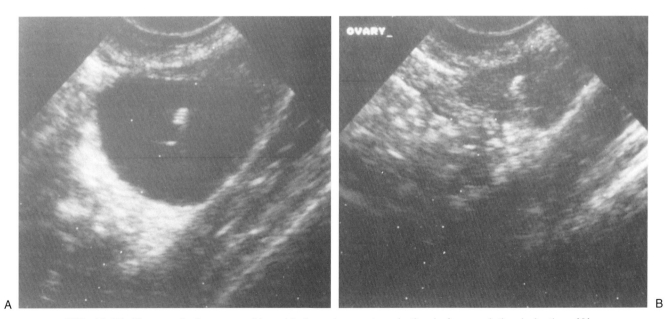

A   B

FIG. 10-27. Transvaginal sonographic-guided ovarian cyst aspiration before ovulation induction. **(A)** The needle tip is seen within the cyst. **(B)** Complete collapse of cyst after aspiration.

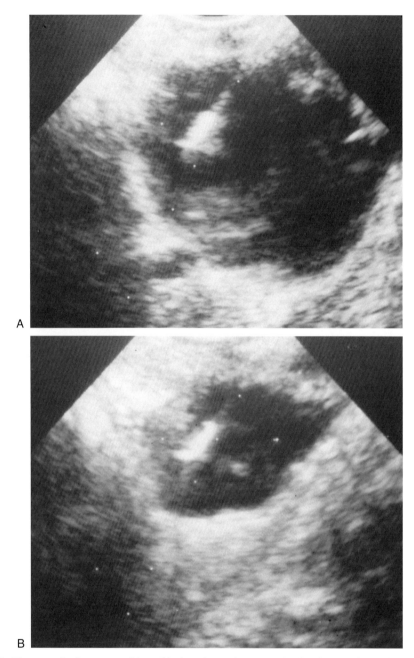

FIG. 10-28. Transvaginal sonographic-guided peritoneal cyst aspiration in a patient with postoperative pelvic pain. **(A)** The irregularly shaped cystic mass is entered. **(B)** Image taken after half of the fluid was aspirated.

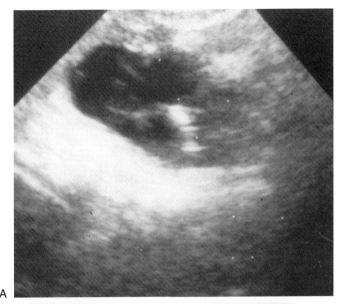

A

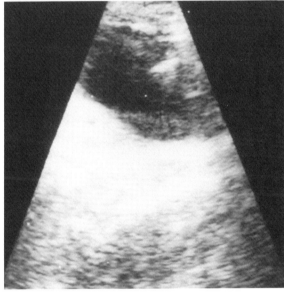

B

FIG. 10-29. Transvaginal sonographic-guided aspiration of intraovarian abscess in a patient who was refractive to antibiotic treatment. **(A)** Before aspiration, the abscess was localized. **(B)** Image taken during aspiration. This patient's fever disappeared 2 days after the drainage.

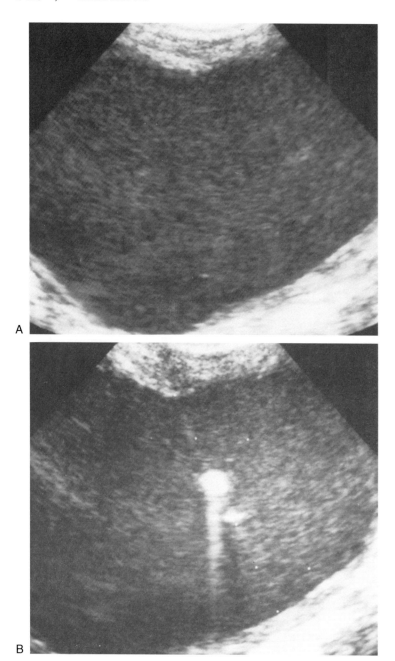

A

B

FIG. 10-30. Transvaginal sonographic-guided aspiration of an endometrioma. **(A)** Before aspiration, the volume of hemorrhage was calculated by the prolate ellipsoid approximations (length × width × height × 0.5) to be 150 mL. **(B)** Image taken during aspiration showing needle to be centrally located within the endometrioma.

postoperative lymphoceles may be aspirated with good chance for symptomatic relief (see Fig. 10-41). Cystic masses tend to reaccumulate their fluid in over a half of the patients studied in one series.[4] Another potential problem is the aspiration of suspected ovarian neoplasms. One large series of patients with ovarian tumors inadvertently aspirated showed no cases of peritoneal spread.[5] We recommended as a precaution that CA 125 titers be drawn before aspiration, even though no complications have been reported in 11 ovarian cancers whose solid areas were purposefully sampled.[6] Cytologic evaluation of the aspirate may not be accurate in the detection of ovarian malignancy.[7] Because of the frequency of adnexal cysts in postmenopausal women, aspiration of these cysts should be limited only to those that are

persistent and symptomatic or those with irregular or sonographically suspicious areas.[8,9] Percutaneous drainage of tuboovarian abscesses or pelvic fluid collections can be an important part of the definitive treatment of these conditions.[10,11] Cyst aspiration in women undergoing ovulation induction may decrease intrinsic pressure within the ovary, thereby allowing better flow.[10,12] One thousand women who underwent guided aspirations or biopsies showed no significant long- or short-term complications.[13]

REFERENCES

1. Quigley MJ. Use of automated needle biopsy gun for the first step in transvaginal catheter placement. AJR 1993;161:877.

2. Goldstein S, Timor-Tritsch IE. Ultrasound in gynecology. New York: Churchill Livingstone, 1995.

3. Aboulghar MA, Mansour RT, Serour GI, Rizk B. Ultrasonic transvaginal aspiration of endometriotic cysts: an optional line of treatment in selected cases of endometriosis. Hum Reprod 1991;6:1408.

4. Dordoni D, Zaglio S, Zucca S. Role of sonographically guided aspiration in the clinical management of ovarian cysts. J Ultrasound Med 1993;12:27.

5. Maiman M, Seltzer V, Boyce J. Laparoscopic excision of ovarian neoplasms subsequently found to be malignant. Obstet Gynecol 1991;77:563.

6. Bret PM, Guibaud L, Atri M, et al. Transvaginal US-guided aspiration of ovarian cysts and solid pelvic masses. Radiology 1992;185:377.

7. Granberg S, Norstrum A, Wikland M. Comparison of endovaginal and cystological evaluation of cystic masses. J Ultrasound Med 1991;10:9.

8. Wolf SI, Gosink BB, Feldesman MR, et al. Prevalence of simple adnexal cysts in postmenopausal women. Radiology 1991;80:65.

9. Levine D, Gosink BB, Wolf SI, et al. Simple adnexal cysts: the natural history in postmenopausal women. Radiology 1992;184:653.

10. Casola G, vanSonnenberg E, D'Agostino HB, et al. Percutaneous drainage of tubo-ovarian abscesses. Radiology 1992;182:399.

11. Abbitt PL, Goldwag S, Urbanski S. Endovaginal sonography for guidance in draining pelvic fluid collections. AJR 1990; 154:849–850.

12. Aboulghar MA, Mansour RT, Serour GI, et al. Transvaginal ultrasonic needle guided aspiration of pelvic inflammatory cystic masses before ovulation induction for in vitro fertilization. Fertil Steril 1990;53:311.

13. Zanetta G, Trio D, Lissoni A, et al. Early and short-term complications after US-guided puncture of gynecologic lesions: evaluation after 1,000 consecutive cases. Radiology 1993;189:161.

Transvaginal Sonographic-Guided Intervention

Miles Reid, MD and Mostafa Atri, MD

The advent of cross-sectional imaging of the pelvis has led to imaging-guided procedures such as biopsies and aspiration and drainage of fluid collections. For pathologic processes situated in the pelvis, a transabdominal approach is occasionally not feasible, owing to the interposition of structures such as the bowel, bladder, or uterus. Alternative techniques that have been developed include the transabdominal transcystic approach,[1] transrectal sonographic-guided approach,[2] a CT-guided approach through the greater sciatic foramen,[3] and the transvaginal approach.[4–6]

The transcystic approach involves transabdominal sonography and a transabdominal puncture where the needle passes through the urinary bladder. Disadvantages of the transcystic approach include a greater distance between the transducer and the target as well as the necessity of a double-wall puncture of a viscus. This technique is limited to biopsy, because one does not wish to risk introducing infection from an abscess into the bladder. As well, a catheter cannot be placed from this route. When used for biopsy, this technique has been shown to be safe.[1]

The transrectal approach is another alternative technique that is more limited in terms of access. This approach is mainly used for abscess drainage because there is a risk of introducing infection when this approach is used to perform a biopsy or for cyst or fluid aspiration. A drawback to this approach for draining abscesses is catheter expulsion.[2]

An approach from the greater sciatic foramen[3] requires CT guidance; therefore, it exposes the patient to ionizing radiation. Because there is much soft tissue to transgress (ie, the gluteal muscles), this technique is also relatively painful. Catheter kinking after insertion is another disadvantage. In addition, there is the risk of neurovascular complications involving the sciatic nerve or its roots and injury of branches of the internal iliac artery.

Transvaginal sonographic-guided interventional techniques offer many benefits. The bowel or bladder is far less commonly interposed between the transducer and the structure of interest, affording improved visualization as well as a shorter, direct path for needles or catheters. The proximity to the target allows a higher frequency probe to be used, resulting in improved resolution. Although limited to 50% of the population, transvaginal sonographic-guided intervention has proved useful for many indications, such as diagnostic aspiration, abscess drainage, cyst aspiration, cyst scle-

rosis, biopsy of masses, ectopic pregnancy termination, selective pregnancy reduction, oocyte retrieval for in vitro fertilization, and fetal interventional techniques. In this chapter, these indications are discussed individually, with the exception of the last two topics.

TECHNIQUE

The patient with an empty bladder is placed in the lithotomy position. A combination of intravenous diazepam and fentanyl is used for sedation and analgesia. Antibiotics are not routinely used. After sterile preparation of the vulva and the vagina with chlorhexidine, an endovaginal probe ranging in frequency from 5 to 7.5 MHz sterilized with glutaral (Cidex) and covered with a sterile condom is used for these procedures. The probe is equipped with a sterile guide. The software-derived dotted line, representing the needle path, is then aligned with the target (eg, cyst, mass) (Fig. 10-31). The needle or catheter is then advanced under sonographic guidance. Figure 10-32 shows the equipment used for transvaginal interventions.

DIAGNOSTIC ASPIRATION AND ABSCESS DRAINAGE

Diagnostic aspiration of pelvic fluid collections allows for characterization of the fluid. If pus is aspirated, a drainage catheter may be inserted at that time. Otherwise, the fluid should be sent for Gram stain, culture, and sensitivity. If the fluid is suspected to be of a particular origin (eg, from the kidney, pancreas, or lymphatics) then appropriate biochemical testing (eg, creatinine, amylase, triglyceride) may be done as well. If malignancy is suspected, fluid should be sent for cytologic study.

Earlier investigators[6] had reported transvaginal aspiration and drainages using sonographic guidance with a transabdominal probe, but transvaginal sonographic guidance is clearly better. Aspiration may be performed with needles ranging in caliber from 19 to 22 gauge. If pus is aspirated, a drainage catheter may be inserted.[5] This can be accomplished either by the trochar or Seldinger technique. Catheter types include locking and nonlocking pigtail catheters in

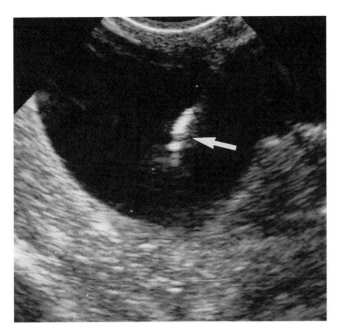

FIG. 10-31. Endovaginal sonogram of a needle *(arrow)* within a pelvic cyst, following the software-derived needle path *(small white dots)*. Shown is a 20-gauge amniocentesis needle, the tip of which is scored for increased echogenicity.

sizes from 7F to 12F. A scalpel nick in the vaginal wall is sometimes necessary. For cases in which placement of a catheter through the vaginal wall is very difficult, Eschelman and associates[7] suggest using a Colapinto needle as a dilator or as a stiffening cannula for the passage of a fascial dilator. We often use the trochar technique with the assistance of a guide that we have developed (Fig. 10-33). This guide replaces the manufacturer's guide and allows placement of a catheter up to 14F. The whole procedure is performed under sonographic guidance. Fluoroscopy is used to aid placement of the catheter in some cases using the Seldinger technique. We always suture the tube to the vaginal wall or inner aspect

of the thigh as is recommended by other authors for the nonlocking catheters.[5] Pelvic fluid collections and abscesses from many causes may be drained, including postoperative collections, appendicitis, Crohn's disease, diverticulitis, and pelvic inflammatory disease (Fig. 10-34).

Transvaginal abscess drainage for nongynecologic causes is usually an alternative to the transabdominal approach when there is no safe access or to the transgluteal approach with similar indications. However, the indication for the drainage of tuboovarian abscesses or pyosalpinges is not as straightforward. These conditions are generally treated by intravenous antibiotics; and if there is no response within 72 hours, surgical or radiologic drainage is contemplated.[8] Success rates of 86% (14 pelvic fluid collections of different causes) and 78% (27 pelvic abscesses of different causes) have been reported by van Sonnenberg and co-workers[9] and Feld and colleagues[10] for transvaginal drainage. Casola and associates[11] had an 81.2% success rate for drainage of tuboovarian abscesses in a group of 16 patients who had failed to respond to intravenously administered antibiotics using different approaches. They concluded that their preferred route of drainage for deep pelvic collections was transvaginal rather than transgluteal, based on the two cases of sciatic nerve injury that developed in their series of patients.

Aboulghar and associates[12] reported a series of 15 patients with acute pelvic inflammatory disease, all of whom had either a pyosalpinx or tuboovarian abscess on sonography. These patients were treated with needle aspiration and instillation of an antibiotic but no drainage catheter. They all received systemic antibiotics. All patients defervesced in 72 hours or less and were free of pain within 72 hours as well. Unfortunately, there was no control group and long-term fertility was not assessed.

Several studies have shown sonographic-guided transvaginal drainage to be both safe and effective. The only complication reported in a series published on transvaginal catheter drainage is a vaginal fistula in a group of 18 patients drained transvaginally.[10]

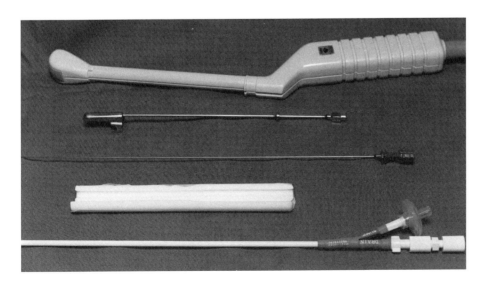

FIG. 10-32. Shown from top to bottom are the ultrasound transducer, needle guide, needle, catheter guide (in open position), and drainage catheter.

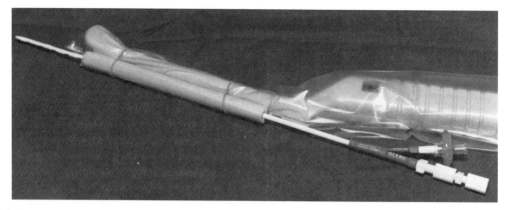

FIG. 10-33. The probe is shown with a sterile cover. The catheter guide is attached to it with sterile elastic bands, and the drainage catheter is inserted within. Once the catheter has been inserted, the guide is hinged open (see Fig. 10-32) to allow its removal from the catheter.

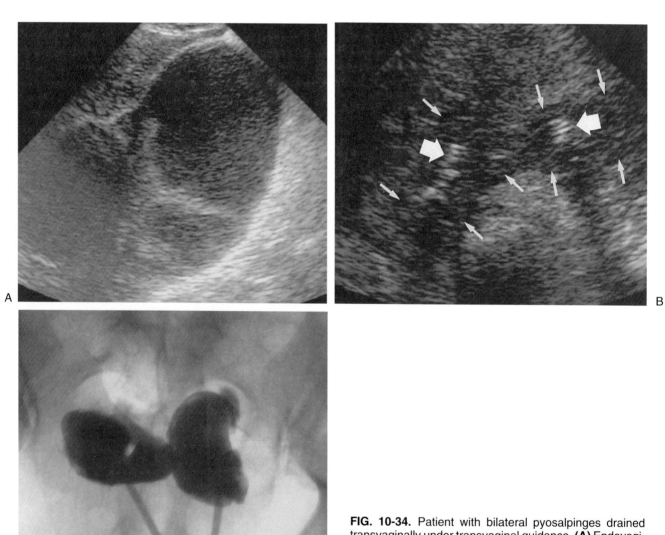

FIG. 10-34. Patient with bilateral pyosalpinges drained transvaginally under transvaginal guidance. **(A)** Endovaginal sonogram of one pyosalpinx. **(B)** Endovaginal sonogram after insertion of a 10F drainage tube into each pyosalpinx demonstrates collapsed fallopian tubes *(small arrows)*. Large arrows indicate the drainage catheters. **(C)** Abscessogram performed through each tube 2 days later shows drainage catheters coursing from the vagina into each contrast medium—filled fallopian tube.

ECTOPIC, HETEROTOPIC, AND MULTIFETAL PREGNANCIES

Ectopic pregnancy occurs in approximately 1 in 100 pregnancies. More than 99% of ectopic pregnancies are tubal. The major complication is hemorrhaging, with the result that ectopic pregnancy is the most common cause of maternal death during the first half of pregnancy.[13] Treatment of ruptured ectopic pregnancy and ectopic pregnancies in unstable patients is surgical, whereas alternative treatment options including medical and expectant management are offered in addition to surgery for early nonruptured ectopic pregnancies.

Different substances have been used for the medical treatment of ectopic pregnancy, including prostaglandin $F_{2\alpha}$, potassium chloride, hypertonic glucose, and methotrexate.[14–19] Among these substances, methotrexate is the most widely used. Methotrexate is administered both locally by the transvaginal, laparoscopic, and transcervical approaches[18–21] and systemically by intramuscular injection.[22] The initial regimens for systemic administration of methotrexate necessitated several injections, causing some side effects. This prompted direct injection of the ectopic pregnancy by some investigators, which prevented these systemic side effects.[15–19,21] The technique uses sonography to guide a needle (19 gauge) into the gestational sac or the localized hematosalpinx. The contents of the sac, if present, are partially aspirated and then methotrexate (1 mg/kg) is injected.[20] The use of color Doppler imaging during injection helps localize the needle tip (Fig. 10-35).

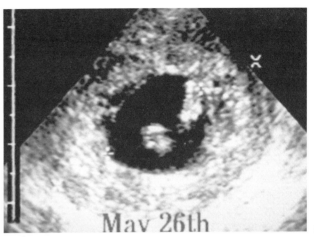

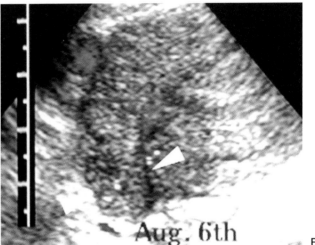

FIG. 10-36. (A) Advanced live ectopic pregnancy on the day of methotrexate injection. **(B)** Remnant of ectopic pregnancy *(between arrowheads)* 3 months after methotrexate injection. (From Atri, Bret PM, Tulandi T, et al. Ectopic pregnancy: evolution after treatment with transvaginal methotrexate. Radiology 1992:185:749.)

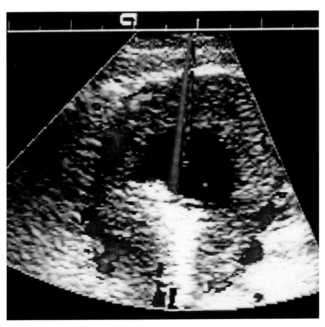

FIG. 10-35. Color Doppler image of methotrexate being injected into ectopic gestational sac. The exact course of needle is marked by color Doppler imaging as the drug is being injected.

We conducted a prospective study in a group of high-risk women with a transvaginal sonographic diagnosis of ectopic pregnancy. Patients who were symptomatic or had declining serum β-human chorionic gonadotropin (hCG) levels and ruptured or heterotopic ectopic pregnancies were excluded. We considered a 15% or more decline of the serum β-hCG level in the 24 to 48 hours after transvaginal injection as proof of a successful treatment. In our first 25 ectopic pregnancies treated with transvaginal injection of methotrexate, 19 (76%) were successfully treated (Fig. 10-36).[20] The other 6 were operated, 4 of these because of abdominal pain the day after injection and 2 because of abdominal pain and vaginal bleeding at a later date despite dropping serum β-hCG levels. Surgery performed on the failed group revealed only one ruptured ectopic pregnancy. In our series of ectopic pregnancies treated by the transvaginal approach, our success rate was not significantly altered by the initial β-hCG level nor by the ectopic pregnancy appearance, vascularity, or size.[20] Despite a positive response to treatment, our series demonstrated that 63% of the ectopic pregnancies treated with methotrexate increased in size and 68% became more vascular during the course of resolution.[20] The only complication was several days of abdominal cramps in one patient. Perhaps the main disadvantage of transvaginal methotrexate administration compared with surgery is the long follow-up, which involves serial β-hCG measurements until they are undetectable. The mean follow-up duration was 35 days in our series. If the patient develops new symptoms, follow-up transvaginal sonography is helpful in determining the cause.

The direct injection of an ectopic pregnancy with methotrexate or other substances has been replaced by a single-dose systemic administration of methotrexate by intramuscular injection. In a literature review of 306 ectopic pregnancies treated with systemic methotrexate and 295 with direct injection, the mean success rate was 94% versus 83%; the mean tubal patency after treatment was 81% versus 88%; and the mean pregnancy rate was 71% versus 82.5%, with 11% of those pregnancies being ectopic in the systemic injection group versus 6% in the direct injection group.[23]

Heterotopic pregnancy is the coexistence of an intrauterine pregnancy with an ectopic pregnancy and occurs with a reported incidence ranging from 1 in 2,600 to 1 in 30,000 pregnancies. The incidence increases in pregnancies achieved through assisted reproduction such as in vitro fertil-

ization. The problem of heterotopic pregnancy may be managed by transvaginal sonographic-guided intervention. The technique is similar to that described for treatment of ectopic pregnancy except that potassium chloride or hypertonic glucose (50% concentration) rather than methotrexate is used to spare the intrauterine pregnancy. Fernandez and co-workers[24] reported a series of six cases of heterotopic pregnancy. Three patients chose the option of expectant management, and three were treated with a potassium chloride injection into the ectopic sac. Four ectopic pregnancies were interstitial, including the three treated with potassium chloride. The technique involved insertion of an 18-gauge needle into the ectopic sac and aspiration, followed by injection of potassium chloride (2 mEq in a 2-ml volume). Asystole was then looked for on sonography. All cases but one were successfully treated. The one failure was in the expectant management group, and the patient underwent laparoscopic salpingectomy. The intrauterine pregnancies went on to term in three of five of the successfully treated patients; however, in two cases the intrauterine pregnancy aborted spontaneously. Because of the continuous secretion of β-hCG by the intrauterine pregnancy, follow-up must be sonographic.

A similar technique is used for the reduction of multifetal pregnancies, usually in the setting of assisted reproduction. Transvaginal sonography is used to guide a needle into the thorax of the embryo, and potassium chloride is injected.[25] Comparable results to those of the transabdominal approach have been reported with this technique.[26]

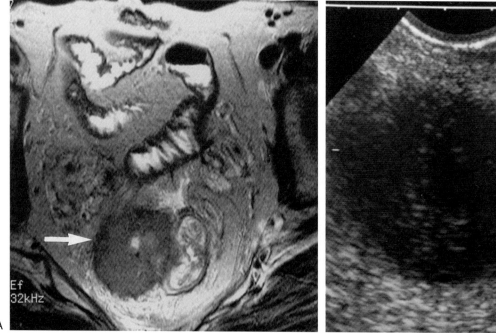
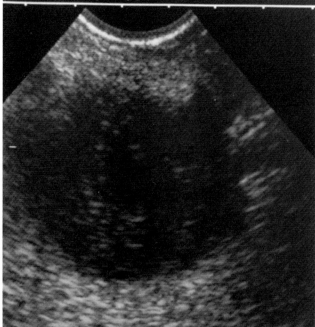

A   B

FIG. 10-37. Ovarian carcinoma recurrence. **(A)** MRI demonstrates mass *(arrow)* adjacent to rectosigmoid. Anteriorly located bowel loops limit transabdominal biopsy approach. **(B)** Endovaginal sonogram shows proximity of lesion to probe, allowing for easy biopsy with a 22-gauge needle.

PELVIC CYSTS, CYSTIC NEOPLASMS, AND SOLID NEOPLASMS

Management of suspected primary malignant ovarian neoplasms precludes biopsy in favor of total resection due to concern regarding the possibility of peritoneal seeding. Thus the role of biopsy is reserved for (1) cases for which disease recurrence[4] or metastases from ovarian cancer is suspected, (2) patients with a known primary and strong indication of metastatic disease in the pelvis, and (3) masses with a very low index of suspicion for malignancy on transvaginal sonography as a complementary test. The use of this procedure may spare patients in this group unnecessary operations.

A transvaginal route is chosen when it provides the best approach, which is common in the setting of ovarian pathology or recurrent disease from cervical or uterine malignancy. The basic technique is described earlier. For cytologic aspiration, needles from 19 to 22 gauge may be used, and aspiration is performed with a 20-ml syringe and aspiration gun. The needle is inserted and withdrawn several centimeters repetitively while aspirating. Core biopsies may be obtained with an 18-gauge biopsy needle and gun. Color Doppler imaging can be used to avoid puncturing a vascular structure.

Biopsy of pelvic lesions is safe with a low rate of complication that is comparable to that of the currently well-established abdominal biopsy.[27,28] Bret and associates[27] reported one minor complication in a group of 61 aspirations and biopsies, and Zanetta and colleagues[28] mentioned 3.9% minor complications and 0.7% major complications requiring surgery in a group of 893 patients. Zanetta and colleagues used both transabdominal and transvaginal approaches and found a higher complication rate with the transabdominal approach. In the early part of their study they had a higher complication rate with aspiration of dermoid cysts and endometriomas, presumably because of peritoneal irritation from spillage of the content of these cysts. Their complication rate dropped with the avoidance of aspiration of these two lesions. Aspiration of dermoid cysts can be avoided because most have characteristic appearances on transvaginal sonography.[29]

In a study by Bret and associates,[27] sonographic-guided aspiration of solid pelvic masses was performed in 13 patients, 11 of whom had a history of carcinoma. Eleven of 13 were proven to have a malignancy (Fig. 10-37). Nine (82%) of these showed true-positive results, and there were two false-negative results. There were no false-positive results and no complications.

A number of studies have identified those cysts with very low malignant potential.[30–32] There are now scoring systems available to separate cysts with low malignant potential from those with high malignant potential.[33] In general, unilocular cysts or cysts with a few thin septa are almost always benign.[34] Cysts considered for aspiration must have a benign sonographic appearance, resembling simple or hemorrhagic cysts. Cysts with thick walls, nodules, or multiple septations are excluded. Although the role of transvaginal sonographic-guided cyst aspiration has not been determined, some poten-

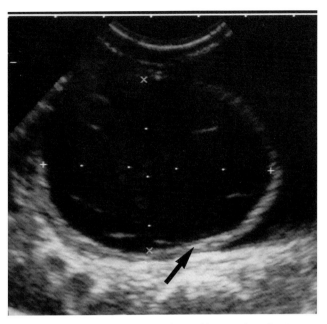

FIG. 10-38. Premenopausal patient with a previous hysterectomy for fibroids. A persistent right ovarian thin-walled cyst with few internal echoes is seen. It is surrounded partially by a rim of ovarian tissue *(arrow)* and some fluid in the pelvis (F). This cyst was aspirated completely and clear fluid was obtained. There was no recurrence on follow-up 2 months later.

tial indications exist, in particular, in the premenopausal age group. They include apparent functional cysts that are symptomatic or persist after two cycles (Fig. 10-38). Occasionally, hormonal therapy is given to patients to suppress development of functional cysts while allowing the older cysts to regress. The conventional treatment for cysts that fail to resolve is surgical.[35] Transvaginal needle aspiration of symptomatic benign-appearing cysts or persistent functional cysts can potentially reduce the number of surgical procedures or hormonal replacement in this age group.[27,36] Ovarian remnant syndrome is another indication of cyst aspiration in this age group. These are women who have had difficult oophorectomies because of underlying adhesions resulting in residual ovarian tissue.[37] These patients tend to present with pain because of the development of a functional cyst (Fig. 10-39). The reluctance of gynecologists to reoperate on these patients makes transvaginal cyst aspiration an ideal alternative treatment.

With the advent of transvaginal sonography, benign-appearing postmenopausal cysts are more frequently recognized. Transvaginal sonographic studies have shown that simple-appearing cysts are quite common in postmenopausal women (a reported prevalence as high as 17%).[38,39] This has changed the traditional surgical treatment of these cysts to a more conservative approach. The indications for cyst aspiration in this age group is less clear. In our experience, postmenopausal cyst intervention is requested in two groups of patients: (1) those with benign-appearing symptomatic cysts and (2) those with persistent postmenopausal cysts larger than 3 cm who are anxious or whose physicians choose inter-

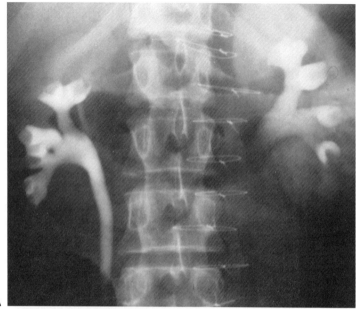

A

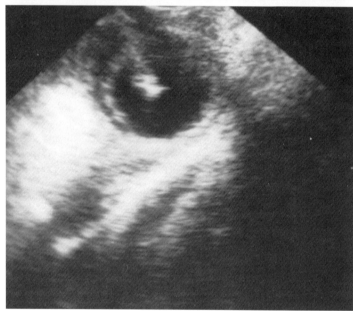

B

FIG. 10-39. Premenopausal patient with ovarian remnant syndrome after oophorectomy for endometriosis. **(A)** Intravenous pyelogram showing left hydronephrosis, a result of ureteral obstruction due to a cyst from an ovarian remnant. **(B)** Sonogram demonstrating tip of needle in this 2-cm cyst. Symptoms and hydronephrosis resolved after aspiration.

vention over long-term follow-up examination. Although a negative cytologic result confirms the sonographic diagnosis, cytology of the aspirate has a sensitivity of only 47% for detecting malignancy, with a negative predictive value that is 81% at best.[40]

Under transvaginal sonographic guidance and using needles ranging in caliber from 19G to 22G, the sonologist introduces the needle into the cyst, which is then evacuated as completely as possible. We often use a 20-gauge amniocentesis needle for aspirating cystic lesions because the tip is very echogenic and side holes facilitate aspiration. Specimens are sent for microbiologic and cytologic evaluation. A normal serum CA 125 level is documented before all ovarian cyst aspirations.

After ovarian cyst aspiration in premenopausal patients,

up to 48% may recur.[27] The cyst recurrence rate in the postmenopausal group appears to be even higher, at least 62%.[27] This poor result has prompted us to perform cyst sclerosis with ethanol to prevent recurrence (Fig. 10-40).[41] This would only be done in postmenopausal women owing to the risk of causing infertility from ethanol spillage in younger women. When aspiration of simple-appearing postmenopausal cysts is requested, we sclerose the cyst immediately after aspiration because of the high recurrence rate of aspiration alone. Sclerosis is done as an outpatient procedure. Approximately two thirds of the aspirated cysts content is replaced with 100% alcohol that is left in place for 20 minutes and then aspirated. Of the first seven postmenopausal cysts that were sclerosed because of initial recurrences after aspiration alone, four resolved and three recurred. There were no com-

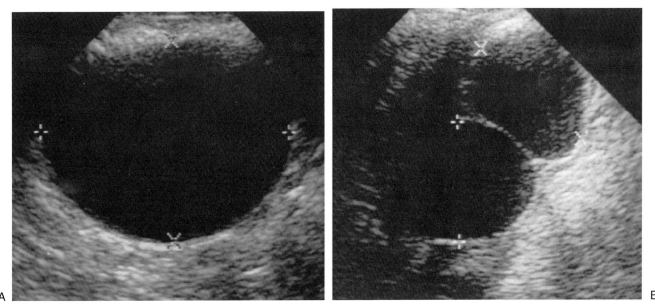

A

B

FIG. 10-40. This postmenopausal patient initially had **(A)** a 5-cm thin-walled, unilocular, right ovarian cyst that was aspirated and sclerosed. There was no recurrence on 2-year follow-up. **(B)** She later developed two cysts on the left ovary, one measuring 3.7 cm and the other 3 cm. These were aspirated and sclerosed. No recurrence was seen after 1-year of follow-up.

plications.[41] One of the drawbacks of cyst sclerosis is their complex appearance after alcohol instillation. This causes difficulty in follow-up of these cysts if they do not resolve (Fig. 10-41).

CONCLUSION

Transvaginal sonographic-guided intervention is a safe technique with a low complication rate. It has proven to be useful for many indications involving pelvic pathologic processes and has demonstrated advantages over alternatives such as transabdominal, transcystic, and transrectal sonographic-guided techniques and the CT-guided approach through the greater sciatic foramen. It frequently provides the best imaging of deep pelvic lesions as well as the most direct and closest route of access, free of intervening structures. The established indications include diagnostic aspiration of pelvic fluid, abscess drainage, biopsy of masses, ectopic pregnancy termination, and selective pregnancy reduction. The role that transvaginal sonographic-guided interventional techniques play in ovarian cyst management needs to be more clearly defined.

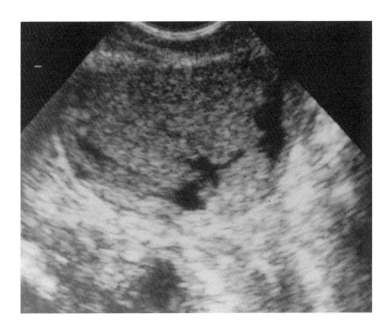

FIG. 10-41. Sonogram showing complex, mostly solid appearance of a benign cyst that had undergone sclerosis. (From Atri M, Nazarnia S, Bret PM, et al. Endovaginal sonographic appearance of benign ovarian masses. Radiographics 1994;14:747.)

REFERENCES

1. Steiner E, Mueller PR, Simeone JF, et al. Transcystic biopsy: a new approach to posterior pelvic lesions. AJR 1987;149:93.
2. Nosher JL, Needell GS, Amorosa JK, Krasna IH. Transrectal pelvic abscess drainage with sonographic guidance. AJR 1986;146:1047.
3. Butch RJ, Mueller PR, Ferrucci JT Jr, et al. Drainage of pelvic abscesses through the greater sciatic foramen. Radiology 1986;158:487.
4. Fornage BD, O'Keefe F. Ultrasound guided transvaginal biopsy of malignant cystic pelvic mass. J Ultrasound Med 1990;9:53.
5. Abbitt PL, Goldwag S, Urbanski S. Endovaginal sonography for guidance in draining pelvic fluid collections. AJR 1990;154:849.
6. Nosher JL, Winchman HK, Needell GS. Transvaginal pelvic abscess drainage with US guidance. Radiology 1987;165:872.
7. Eschelman DJ, Sullivan KL. Use of a Colapinto needle in US-guided transvaginal drainage of pelvic abscesses. Radiology 1993;186:893.
8. Soper DE. Upper genital tract infections. In: LJ Copeland, ed. Textbook of gynecology. Philadelphia, WB Saunders, 1993;517.
9. van Sonnenberg E, D'Agostino HB, Casola G, et al. US guided transvaginal drainage of pelvic abscesses and fluid collections. Radiology 1991;181:53.
10. Feld R, Eschelman DJ, Sagerman JE, et al. Treatment of pelvic abscesses and other fluid collections: efficacy of transvaginal sonographically guided aspiration and drainage. AJR 1994;163:1141.
11. Casola G, van Sonnenberg E, D'Agostino HB, et al. Percutaneous drainage of tubo-ovarian abscesses. Radiology 1992;182:399.
12. Aboulghar MA, Mansour RT, Serour GI. Ultrasonographically guided transvaginal aspiration of tuboovarian abscesses and pyosalpinges: an optional treatment for acute pelvic inflammatory disease. Am J Obstet Gynecol 1995;172:1501.
13. Hammond CB, Bachus KE. Ectopic pregnancy. In: Scott JR, DiSaia PJ, Hammond CB, Spellacy WN, eds. Danforth's Obstetrics and Gynecology, ed 7. Philadelphia, JB Lippincott, 1994:187.
14. Timor-Tritsch I, Baxi L, Peisner DB. Transvaginal salpingocentesis: a new technique for treating ectopic pregnancy. Am J Obstet Gynecol 1989;160:459.
15. Ory SJ, Villaneuva AL, Sand PK, et al. Conservative treatment of ectopic pregnancy with methotrexate. Am J Obstet Gynecol 1986;154:1299.
16. Tulandi T, Atri M, Bret PM, et al. Transvaginal intratubal methotrexate treatment of ectopic pregnancy. Fertil Steril 1992;58:98.
17. Vejtorp M, Vejerslev LO, Ruge S. Local prostaglandin treatment of ectopic pregnancy. Hum Reprod 1989;4:464.
18. Lang PF, Weiss PA, Mayer HO, et al. Conservative treatment of ectopic pregnancy with local injection of hyperosmolar glucose solution or prostaglandin-F2 alpha: a prospective randomized study. Lancet 1990;14:336:78.
19. Aboulghar MA, Mansour RT, Serour GI. Transvaginal injection of potassium chloride and methotrexate for the treatment of tubal pregnancy with a live fetus. Hum Reprod 1990;5:887.
20. Atri M, Bret PM, Tulandi T, et al. Ectopic pregnancy: evolution after treatment with transvaginal methotrexate. Radiology 1992;185:749.
21. Risquez F, Forman R, Maleika F, et al. Transcervical cannulation of the fallopian tube for the management of ectopic pregnancy: prospective multicenter study. Fertil Steril 1992;58:1131.
22. Stovall TG, Ling FW, Gray LA. Single dose methotrexate for treatment of ectopic pregnancy. Obstet Gynecol 1991;77:754.
23. Carson SA, Buster JE. Ectopic pregnancy. N Engl J Med 1993;329:1174.
24. Fernandez H, Lelaidier C, Doumerc S, et al. Nonsurgical treatment of heterotopic pregnancy: a report of six cases. Fertil Steril 1993;60:428.
25. Bollen N, Camus M, Tournaye H, et al. Embryo reduction in triplet pregnancies after assisted procreation: a comparative study. Fertil Steril 1993;60:504.
26. Timor-Tritsch IE, Peisner DB, Monteagudo A, et al. Multifetal pregnancy reduction by transvaginal puncture: evaluation of the technique used in 134 cases. Am J Obstet Gynecol 1993;168:799.
27. Bret PM, Guibaud L, Atri M, et al. Transvaginal US-guided aspiration of ovarian cysts and solid pelvic masses. Radiology 1992;185:377.
28. Zanetta G, Trio D, Lissoni A, et al. Early and short term complications after US guided puncture of gynecologic lesions: evaluation after 1,000 consecutive cases. Radiology 1993;189:161.
29. Atri M, Nazarnia S, Bret PM, et al. Endovaginal sonographic appearance of benign ovarian masses. Radiographics 1994;14:747.
30. Hermann UJ, Locher GW, Goldhirsch A. Sonographic patterns of ovarian tumor: prediction of malignancy. Obstet Gynecol 1987;69:777.
31. Meire HB, Ferrant P, Guha T. Distinction of benign from malignant ovarian cysts by ultrasound. Br J Obstet Gynecol 1978;85:893.
32. Andolf E, Jorgensen C. Simple adnexal cysts diagnosed by ultrasound in postmenopausal women. J Clin Ultrasound 1988;16:301.
33. Lerner JP, Timor-Tritsch IE, Federman A, Abramovich G. Transvaginal ultrasonographic characterization of ovarian masses with an improved weighted scoring system. Am J Obstet Gynecol 1994;170:81.
34. Granberg S, Wikland M, Jansson I, Macroscopic characterization of ovarian tumors and the relation to the histological diagnosis: criteria to be used for ultrasound evaluation. Gynecol Oncol 1989;35:139.
35. DiSaia PJ. Ovarian neoplasms. In: Scott JR, DiSaia PJ, Hammond CB, Spellacy WN, eds. Danforth's Obstetrics and Gynecology, ed 7. Philadelphia, JB Lippincott, 1994:969.
36. Yee H, Greenebaum E, Lerner J, et al. Transvaginal sonographic characterization combined with cytologic evaluation in the diagnosis of ovarian and adnexal cysts. Diagn Cytopathol 1994;10:107.
37. Pettit PD. Lee RA. Ovarian remnant syndrome: diagnostic dilemma and surgical challenge. Obstet Gynecol 1988;71:580.
38. Wolf SI, Gosink BB, Feldesman MR, et al. Prevalence of simple adnexal cysts in postmenopausal women. Radiology 1991;180:65.
39. Levine D, Gosink BB, Wolf SI, et al. Simple adnexal cysts in postmenopausal women. Radiology 1992;184:653.
40. Granberg S, Norstrom A, Wikland M. Comparison of endovaginal ultrasound and cytological evaluation of cystic ovarian tumors. J Ultrasound Med 1991;10:9.
41. Bret PM, Atri M, Guibaud L, et al. Ovarian cysts in postmenopausal women: preliminary results with transvaginal alcohol sclerosis: work in progress. Radiology 1992;184:661.

Intraoperative and Postoperative Guidance with Transrectal and Transperineal Sonography

Arthur C. Fleischer, MD

Transrectal sonography can provide guidance for difficult dilatation and curettage, intracavitary tandem placement, and cerclage placement. The biplane transrectal probe is recommended because one can image in the sagittal plane as well as axially, thereby confirming the position of a dilator or tandem in two planes (Fig. 10-42). Transrectal sonography is particularly helpful in patients whose external cervical os cannot be adequately visualized owing to extensive cervical cancer or vaginal stenosis, for example.

The biplane transrectal probe is covered with a condom, and fluid is introduced within the condom. The covered probe is introduced into the rectum after K-Y jelly is spread over the tip and anterior surface of the condom. This provides optimal contact with the rectal wall. The cervix is usually imaged initially in the longitudinal plane followed by selected images in the axial orientation.

If one is interested in localization of the external os, the endocervical canal can be identified on longitudinal views (Fig. 10-43). Once the dilator is introduced into the cervix, its central location can be confirmed with the axial scan. If perforation is suspected, it can be documented with transrectal sonography (Fig. 10-44).

My colleagues and I have had experience with over 25 cases in which transrectal sonography was useful in guiding dilatation and curettage, intrauterine tandem placement, or cerclage suture placement (Fig. 10-45).[1] Transrectal sonography can also be used for guiding biopsy or aspiration (see Figs. 10-46, 10-47, 10-50, 10-51, and 10-53).[2,3]

If transrectal sonography is used intraoperatively, the transducer is held by the operator and a sterile towel is placed over the operator's hand. The retractors are placed to the side walls of the vagina, allowing ultrasound to be transmitted through the rectum in a long-axis plane. The study should be videotaped for documentation purposes.

I observed a few cases of uterine perforation (Fig. 10-46). The dilator or tandem could be identified as being extrauterine in both cases. For cerclage placement, the relative position of the sutures within the cervix can be identified (Fig. 10-48).

In some cases, a transperineal approach is needed. This is particularly true in patients who have undergone pelvic exenteration. In some cases the transvaginal probe with a needle guide was used for guided aspiration (Fig. 10-50).

Transabdominal and transvaginal sonography can be used to detect and evaluate postoperative hematoma. Initially these may appear hypoechoic, but after they organize are isoechoic to hyperechoic (Figure 10-52).

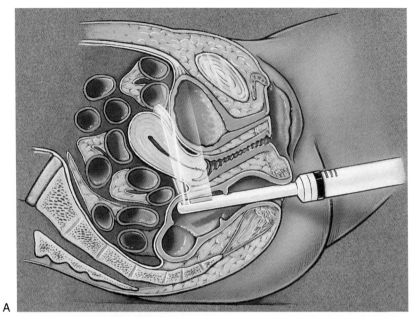

A

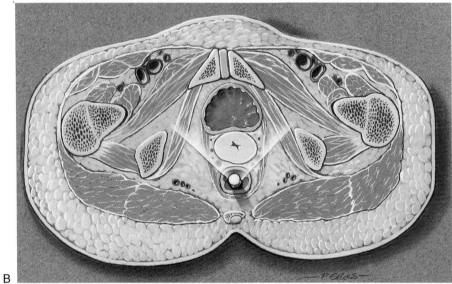

B

FIG. 10-42. Transrectal sonography of the uterus and cervix. **(A)** Diagram showing imaging planes of transrectal sonographic probe. **(B)** Diagram of axial field of view seen with axially oriented transducer elements localized at tip of the probe.

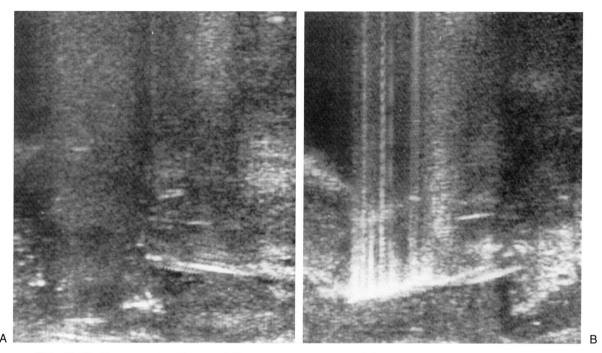

FIG. 10-43. Transrectal guidance of dilatation and curettage. **(A)** Initially the dilator was directed too anteriorly. **(B)** After redirection posteriorly, the dilator entered the endometrial lumen through the cervix.

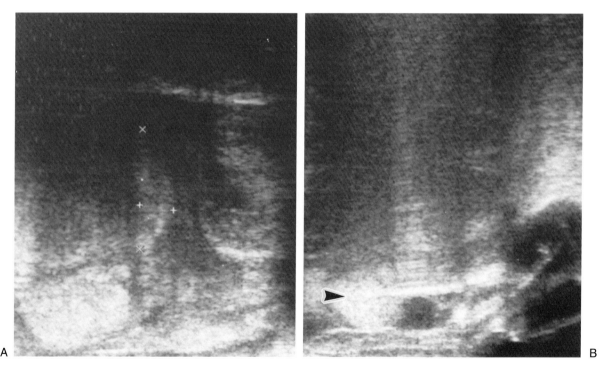

FIG. 10-44. Uterine perforation documented by transrectal sonography. **(A)** The uterus was severely anteflexed. The cursors outline the endometrium. **(B)** On introduction of the dilator it extended into a bowel loop within the cul-de-sac *(arrowhead)*.

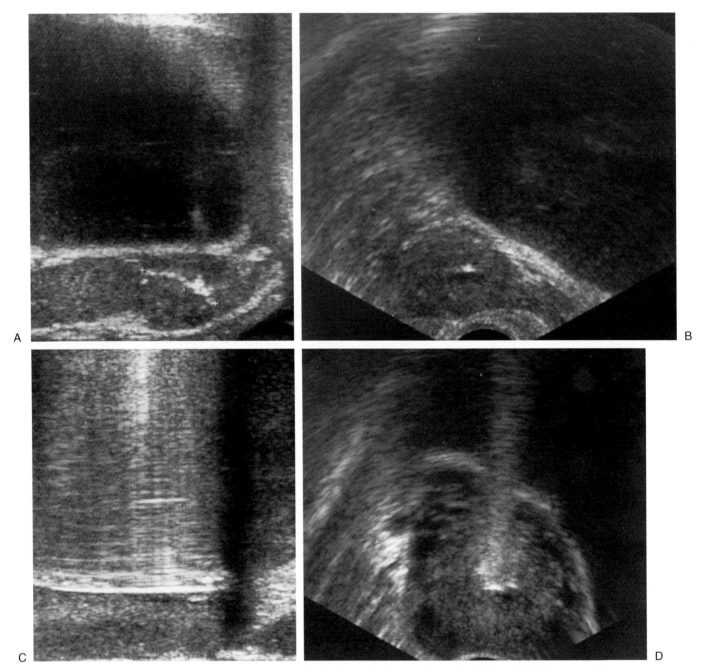

FIG. 10-45. Optimal placement of intrauterine tandem for intracavitary irradiation. Initial transrectal sonography in long- **(A)** and short- **(B)** axis of the cervix. The cervix could not be identified by visual inspection. **(C)** Long-axis view showing tandem centrally located within the uterus. **(D)** Axial scan demonstrating tandem to be centrally located within the uterine lumen.

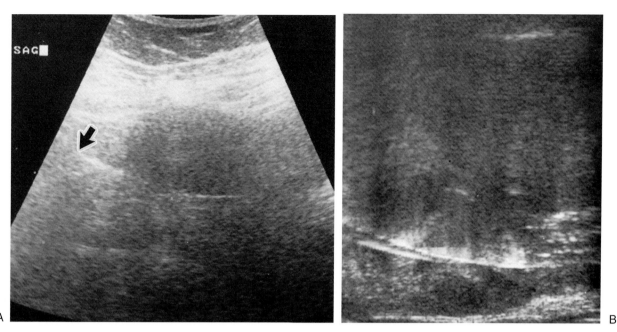

FIG. 10-46. Guidance after uterine perforation of tandem. **(A)** Transabdominal scan showing tandem to extend outside the uterus *(arrow).* **(B)** Transrectal sonography showing tandem to be centrally located after its repositioning.

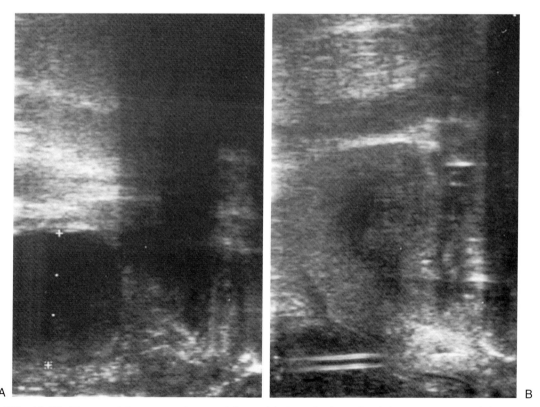

FIG. 10-47. Transrectal sonography used for guided aspiration of cul-de-sac abscess. **(A)** Initial transrectal sonogram showing 3-cm abscess collection in the cul-de-sac. **(B)** Drainage catheter within aspirated abscess.

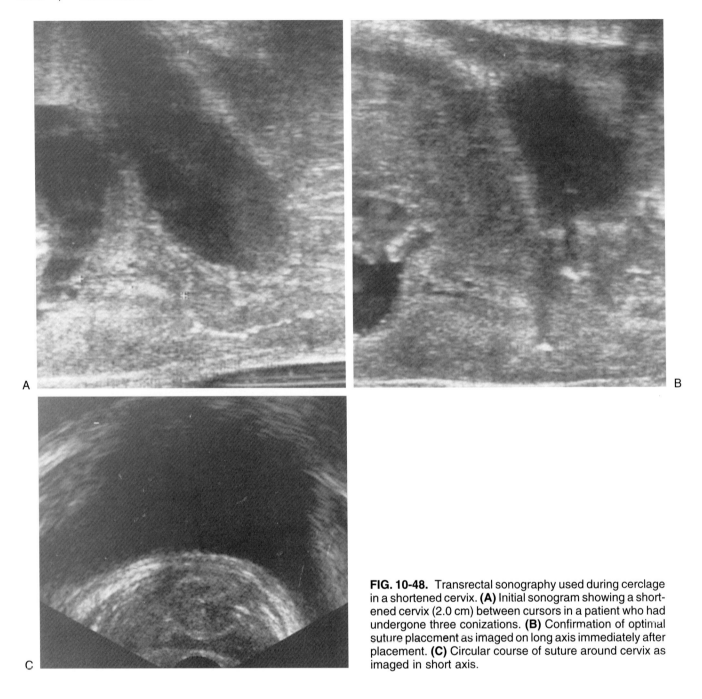

FIG. 10-48. Transrectal sonography used during cerclage in a shortened cervix. **(A)** Initial sonogram showing a shortened cervix (2.0 cm) between cursors in a patient who had undergone three conizations. **(B)** Confirmation of optimal suture placement as imaged on long axis immediately after placement. **(C)** Circular course of suture around cervix as imaged in short axis.

FIG. 10-50. Transperineal aspiration of perirectal abscess in a patient status post pelvic exenteration. **(A)** Pelvic CT scan showing multiloculated perirectal abscess. **(B)** Transperineal transvaginal sonogram showing multiloculated abscess. **(C)** Same abscess after aspiration. Needle tip is seen within deflated abscess cavity.

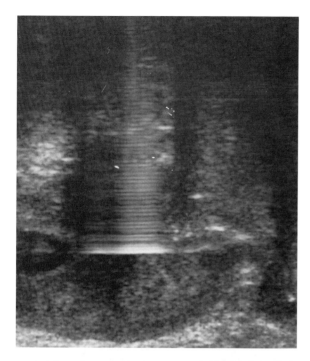

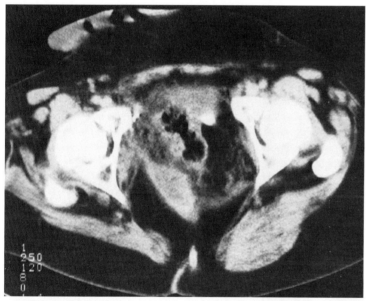

FIG. 10-49. Transrectal sonography used for guidance of needle aspiration of fistula within blind pouch of bicornuate uterus.

A

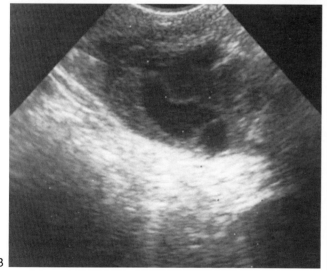

B

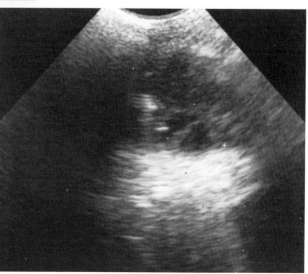

C

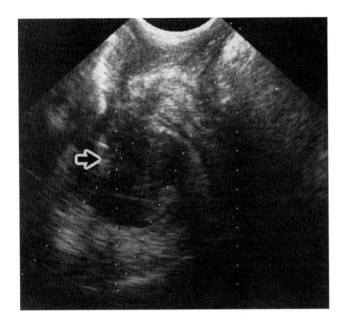

FIG. 10-51. Transperineal guided biopsy of recurrent gestational trophoblastic disease. The biopsy needle *(arrow)* is seen within the mass.

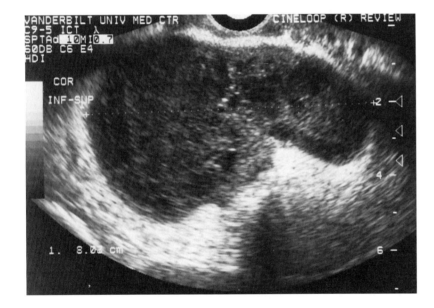

FIG. 10-52. Transvaginal sonogram of pelvic hematoma immediately after a vaginal hysterectomy.

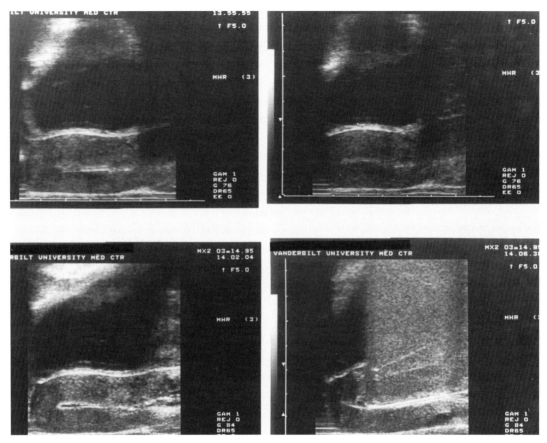

FIG. 10-53. Composite of transrectal sonographic-guided dilatation and curettage in a patient with possible myometrial abnormality. *(Top left)* Initial placement of dilator. *(Top right)* Removal of dilator. *(Bottom left)* Before curettage. *(Bottom right)* During curettage.

REFERENCES

1. Fleischer A, Burnett L, Jones H, Cullinan J. Transrectal and transperineal sonography for guided intrauterine procedures. J Ultrasound Med 1995; 14:135.
2. Savader B, Hamper U, Sheth S, et al. Pelvic masses: aspiration biopsy with transrectal sonography. Radiology 1990;176:351.
3. Alexander A, Eschelman D, Nazarian L. Transrectal sonographically guided drainage of deep pelvic abscesses. AJR 1994;112:1227.

Postoperative Complications: Computed Tomography

R. Brooke Jeffrey Jr., MD

Computed tomography is often a pivotal examination in the evaluation of patients with postoperative complications after pelvic surgery. CT is quite accurate for diagnosing postoperative fluid collections, such as abscesses or lymphoceles. In addition, CT-guided percutaneous drainage is often the treatment of choice for these conditions. CT may also prove invaluable for diagnosing other postoperative complications, such as bowel and ureteral obstruction and venous thrombosis.

ABSCESS

Computed tomography is often the primary imaging method for the diagnosis of postoperative pelvic abscesses. Postoperative sonography is often limited by poor transducer contact owing to open wounds and surgical drains. In addition, overlying bowel gas due to paralytic ileus may compromise sonographic evaluation. The imaging hallmark of an abscess on CT is a complex fluid that demonstrates mass effect (Fig. 10-54).[1,2-6] Noninfected fluid collections typically lack mass effect and rarely displace adjacent bowel loops or solid viscera. Compared with sonography, one clear advantage of CT is the ability to image the entire intraperitoneal and extraperitoneal pelvic compartments. CT is also exquisitely sensitive for small gas bubbles. Gas bubbles, however, are an infrequent finding in most abdominal abscesses and are demonstrated in probably only one third of patients.[2] Therefore, the CT appearance of an abscess is often nonspecific and may be mimicked by other complex fluid collections, such as a hematoma, lymphocele, seroma, or pancreatic pseudocyst. In selected patients, diagnostic needle aspiration must be performed for precise diagnosis.

Contrast medium enhancement often facilitates identifying pelvic abscesses and distinguishing solid inflammatory masses (ie, phlegmon) from liquefied pus.[6] If a pelvic hematoma is suspected on the basis of clinical findings and a falling hematocrit, preliminary noncontrast CT scans are helpful to identify areas of high attenuation (30–60 Hounsfield units [HU]). With contrast medium enhancement most pelvic abscesses are low attenuating lesions, generally on the order of 15 to 25 HU. Areas of phlegmon typically enhance with contrast medium administration and may approx-

imate the attenuation of adjacent muscle (25–50 HU). Contrast medium enhancement may also prove valuable in identifying enhancing membranes around the periphery of an abscess due to its fibrocapillary network. Noninfected fluid collections typically do not demonstrate enhancing peripheral membranes.

On CT, the presence of an air-fluid level within an abscess indicates either a gas-forming organism or an underlying enteric fistula.[7] Fistulas to the small bowel may occur after inadvertent enterotomy (Fig. 10-55). Because of the low bacterial content of small bowel fluid, patients with small bowel perforation may have an indolent course and present 5 to 10 days postoperatively with low-grade fevers.

One of the main values of CT is guidance for percutaneous drainage of pelvic abscesses.[8-10] CT can often clearly define a safe abscess route for catheter insertion by identifying adjacent bowel loops and major vascular structures (Fig. 10-56). The majority of pelvic abscesses can be drained by either CT or sonographic guidance, thus avoiding surgery.

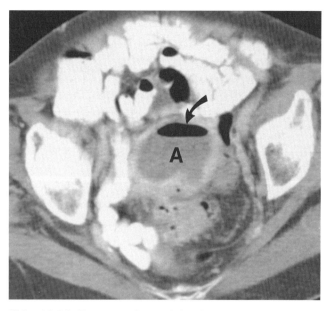

FIG. 10-54. Postoperative pelvic abscess demonstrating mass effect and air—fluid level. Note well-defined abscess (A) with air—fluid level *(curved arrow)*. Note displacement of opacified bowel loops by the abscess.

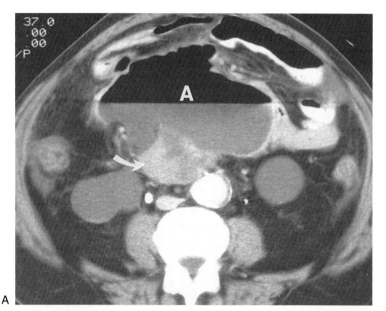

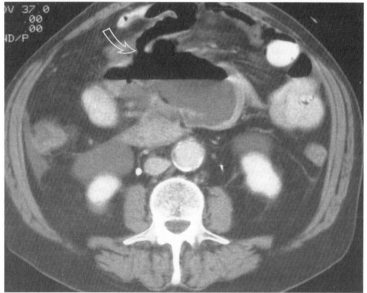

FIG. 10-55. Enteric abscess due to perforation of the small bowel at surgery. **(A)** Note large abscess cavity with air—fluid level (A). Note residual tumor mass in the mesentery *(arrow)*. **(B)** Direct communication to the small bowel is visualized *(arrow)*.

CT may also prove valuable for diagnosing other conditions that present as fever and leukocytosis that may clinically mimic a pelvic abscess. These include superficial wound infections (Fig. 10-57), pseudomembranous colitis, pyonephrosis, and septic pelvic thrombophlebitis (Fig. 10-58). Colonic wall thickening in a postoperative patient receiving antibiotics may be the only evidence for *Clostridium difficile* infection because some patients do not present with diarrhea.[11] On CT, colonic wall thickening is present in 60% of patients with pseudomembranous colitis.[11] Marked dilation of the collecting system in a febrile patient should suggest ureteral obstruction and possible pyonephrosis (Fig. 10-59). In a febrile patient low attenuating thrombus within pelvic veins suggests the diagnosis of septic thrombophlebitis (Fig. 10-60).

LYMPHOCELE

Postoperative collections of lymphatic fluid are common 2 to 4 weeks after radical lymphadenectomy.[12,13] The majority of lymphoceles are asymptomatic and are ultimately resorbed without sequela. In a small percentage of patients, lymphoceles may encapsulate and cause pelvic pain, venous thrombosis, or signs and symptoms of infection. On CT, lymphoceles appear as low attenuation lesions that may mimic the appearance of an abscess. Attenuation values of lymphoceles, in fact, may be less than water (typically − 5 to − 15 HU), owing to the lipid content of lymphatic fluid, which has negative attenuation values. Lymphoceles have a characteristic location along the anatomic pathway of major lymphatic chains.

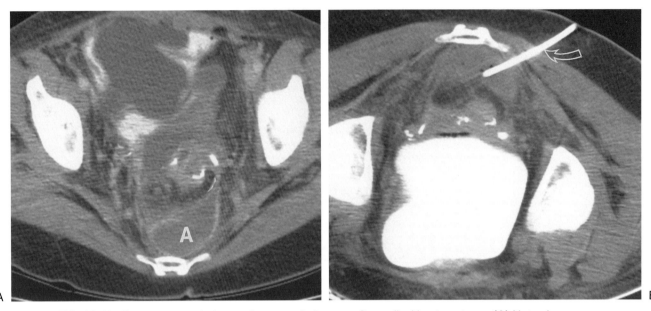

FIG. 10-56. Percutaneous drainage of presacral abscess after radical hysterectomy. **(A)** Note abscess cavity with enhancing membranes (A). **(B)** A catheter *(curved arrow)* was inserted into the presacral abscess in the prone position. The abscess completely resolved with percutaneous drainage.

Symptomatic pelvic lymphoceles may be treated with needle aspiration or catheter drainage and sclerotherapy using an antibiotic solution or absolute alcohol. Fotiou and associates[12] reported a 5.5% incidence of lymphoceles after modified radical hysterectomy in 88 patients.[12] Of the five cases, four developed within 2 months after surgery and presented as pelvic pain, fever, or symptoms of pressure. Radiologic-guided needle aspiration was successful in treating four of the five cases. Akhan and colleagues[13] successfully treated seven of eight lymphoceles using percutaneous sclerotherapy with absolute alcohol (Fig. 10-61).

SMALL BOWEL OBSTRUCTION

Postoperative adhesions commonly develop after gynecologic surgery and are a major cause of small bowel obstruction. Monk and coworkers[14] reported a 2% to 3% incidence of small bowel obstruction related to adhesions in patients undergoing hysterectomy. This incidence increased to 5% in patients undergoing radical hysterectomy.[14] Postoperative adhesions appear to be the result of impaired fibrinolysis. Fibrin and cellular exudate routinely accompany intraperitoneal surgery. They may evolve into fibrous adhesions if there

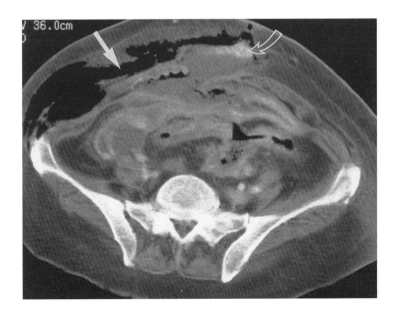

FIG. 10-57. Superficial wound infection diagnosed by CT. Note extensive gas-forming infection of the abdominal wall after laparotomy for ovarian carcinoma *(arrow)*. Extravasation of oral contrast *(curved arrow)* indicates associated bowel perforation from inadvertent enterotomy.

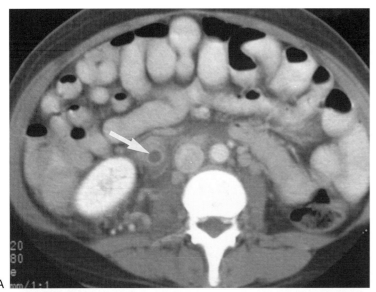

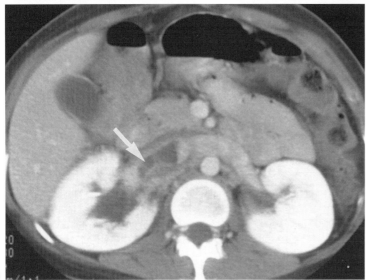

FIG. 10-58. Septic thrombosis of the gonadal vein after pelvic surgery. Note low-attenuation thrombus in the gonadal vein in **(A)** *(arrow)*. Thrombus extends into the inferior vena cava in **(B)** *(arrow)*.

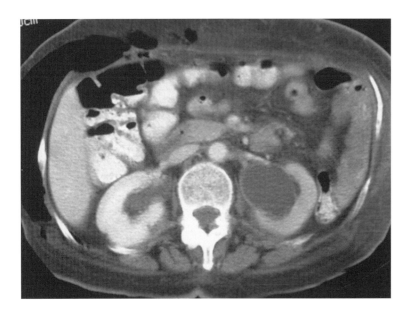

FIG. 10-59. Postoperative ureteral obstruction and pyonephrosis. Same patient as Figure 10-70. Note marked left hydronephrosis due to an obstructed left ureter. There is an extensive gas forming infection in the soft tissues of the abdominal wall. Percutaneous nephrostomy revealed pus in left collecting system.

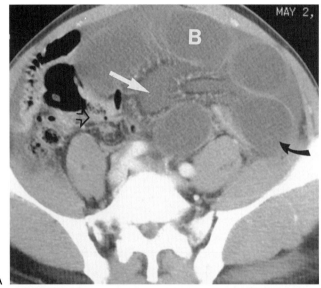

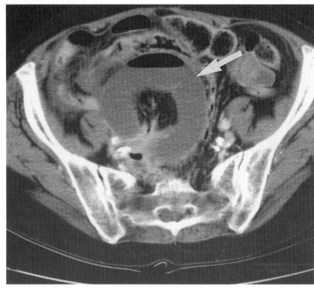

FIG. 10-60. Strangulated closed-loop obstruction in two patients. In **(A)** note marked dilatation of the small bowel (B). There is a high-density hematoma in the mesentery *(straight arrow)* and poor contrast enhancement of the bowel wall in focal areas *(curved arrow)* due to ischemia. Note collapsed distal bowel in the right lower quadrant *(open arrow).* At surgery strangulated obstruction was noted with bowel necrosis. In another patient **(B),** note characteristic U-shaped configuration of dilated segment of bowel closed-loop obstruction *(arrow).*

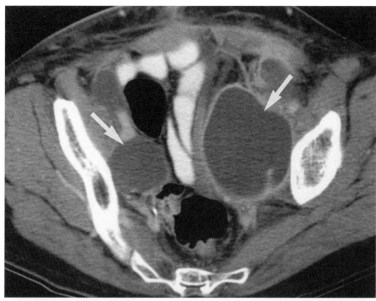

A

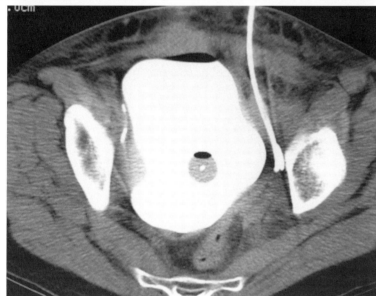

B

FIG. 10-61. Bilateral pelvic lymphoceles successfully treated with percutaneous sclerotherapy. **(A)** Note bilateral lymphoceles after radical lymphadenectomy *(arrows).* **(B)** Note catheter inserted into large left pelvic lymphocele. After sclerotherapy with absolute alcohol, the lymphoceles resolved.

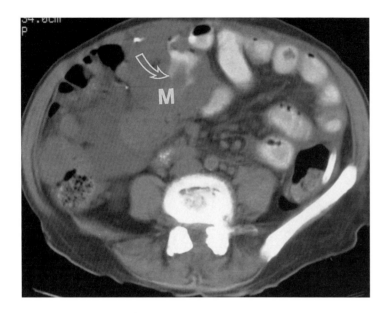

FIG. 10-62. Partial small bowel obstruction due to recurrent tumor from metastatic carcinoma of the cervix. Note large tumor mass (M) with erosion into the small bowel and a leakage of contrast medium into the tumor mass *(curved arrow)*. Note that no oral contrast medium is seen distal to the tumor mass. At surgery, partial small bowel obstruction due to recurrent tumor was found.

is impaired fibrinolysis. Fibrinolysis may be impeded by inadequate blood supply, thermal injury, radiation-induced arteritis, or the presence of foreign bodies.

CT may be of clinical value in the assessment of patients with signs and symptoms suggesting small bowel obstruction (Fig. 10-62).[15–18] CT may accurately distinguish paralytic ileus from obstruction by demonstrating an abrupt transition between dilated and nondilated segments of bowel. Compared with barium studies, such as enteroclysis, CT is better tolerated and can be performed more rapidly. In addition, CT may identify specific types of small bowel obstructions, such as closed-loop and strangulated obstruction, internal hernias, or obstruction due to recurrent tumor.[19] In patients with adhesions there is no evidence of a mass at the point of transition. The hallmark of closed-loop obstruction CT is identification of a U-shaped dilated segment of bowel that has a characteristic beak sign due to torsion and volvulus of the dilated segment.[19]

REFERENCES

1. Wolverson MK, Jagannadharao B, Sundaram M, et al. CT as a primary diagnostic method in evaluating intraabdominal abscess. AJR 1979; 133:1089.
2. Callen PW. Computed tomographic evaluation of abdominal and pelvic abscesses. Radiology 1979;131:171.
3. Haaga JR, Alfidi RJ, Havrilla TR, et al. CT detection and aspiration of abdominal abscesses. AJR 1977;128:465.
4. Chiu LC, Schapiro RL, Yiu VS. Abdominal abscess: computed tomographic appearance, differential diagnosis and pitfalls in diagnosis. J Comput Assist Tomogr 1978;2:195.
5. Jeffrey RB Jr, Grendell JH, Federle MP, et al. Improved survival with early CT diagnosis of pancreatic abscess. Gastrointest Radiol 1987;12: 26.
6. Jeffrey RB Jr, Tolentino CS, Federle MP, Laing FC. Percutaneous drainage of periappendiceal abscesses: review of 20 patients. AJR 1987; 149:59.
7. Kerlan RJ, Jeffrey RB Jr, Pogany AC, Ring EJ. Abdominal abscess with low-output fistula: successful percutaneous drainage. Radiology 1985;155:73.
8. vanSonnenberg E, Ferrucci JJ, Mueller PR, et al. Percutaneous drainage of abscesses and fluid collections: technique, results, and applications. Radiology 1982;142:1.
9. vanSonnenberg E, Mueller PR, Ferrucci JJ. Percutaneous drainage of 250 abdominal abscesses and fluid collections: I. Results, failures, and complications. Radiology 1984;151:337.
10. Mueller PR, vanSonnenberg E, Ferrucci JJ. Percutaneous drainage of 250 abdominal abscesses and fluid collections. II. Current procedural concepts. Radiology 1984;151:343.
11. Boland GW, Lee MJ, Cats AM, et al. Antibiotic-induced diarrhea: specificity of abdominal CT for the diagnosis of *Clostridium difficile* disease. Radiology 1994;191:103.
12. Fotiou SK, Tserkezoglou AJ, Steinhauer G, et al. Pelvic lymphocysts after radical hysterectomy and lymphadenectomy. Eur J Gynaecol Oncol 1994;15:449.
13. Akhan O, Cekirge S, Ozmen M, Besim A. Percutaneous transcatheter ethanol sclerotherapy of postoperative pelvic lymphoceles. Cardiovasc Intervent Radiol 1992;15:224.
14. Monk BJ, Berman ML, Montz FJ. Adhesions after extensive gynecologic surgery: clinical significance, etiology, and prevention. Am J Obstet Gynecol 1994;170:1396.
15. Megibow AJ, Balthazar EJ, Cho KC, et al. Bowel obstruction: evaluation with CT [see comments]. Radiology 1991;180:313.
16. Fukuya T, Hawes DR, Lu CC, et al. CT diagnosis of small-bowel obstruction: efficacy in 60 patients. AJR 1992;158:765; discussion 771.
17. Maglinte DD, Gage SN, Harmon BH, et al. Obstruction of the small intestine: accuracy and role of CT in diagnosis. Radiology 1993;188: 61.
18. Balthazar EJ. George W. Holmes Lecture. CT of small-bowel obstruction. AJR 1994;162:255.
19. Balthazar EJ, Bauman JS, Megibow AJ. CT diagnosis of closed loop obstruction. J Comput Assist Tomogr 1985;9:953.

Clinical Gynecologic Imaging, edited
by Arthur C. Fleischer, Marcia C. Javitt,
R. Brooke Jeffrey, Jr., and Howard W. Jones III,
Lippincott-Raven Publishers, Philadelphia © 1997.

CHAPTER 11

Imaging of the Lower Urinary Tract

Martin Quinn, MD, MRCOG and Mike Bourne, FRCR

**Magnetic Resonance Imaging Anatomy of the
    Lower Urinary Tract**
Sonographic Anatomy of the Lower Urinary Tract
**Magnetic Resonance Imaging of Urinary Stress
    Incontinence**

**Sonographic Imaging of Urinary Stress
    Incontinence**
Summary

The precise anatomy of the lower urinary tract has been a controversial subject for over 40 years, although recent studies of serial histologic sections have substantially clarified many issues.[1–5] Absence of suitable imaging techniques has ensured that much of the detailed anatomy remained obscure. The development of sophisticated MRI techniques has eliminated many of the problems associated with sonographic techniques[6–9] and enabled soft tissue imaging in vivo in nulliparous subjects.[10] MRI techniques provide a detailed account of nulliparous anatomy in contrast to preceding descriptions that have depended on cadaveric dissection of (parous) cadavers.[1–5]

The original description of the pathoanatomy of stress incontinence used indirect imaging techniques (bead-chain cystourethrography) to describe the anatomic features associated with an increase in intraabdominal pressure (ie, posterior and inferior rotation of the urethrovesical junction).[11–14] The loss of anatomic support of the urethrovesical junction was originally termed *anatomic stress incontinence,* although the anatomic lesion or lesions could not be imaged directly.[11,12] The pathoanatomy of genital prolapse has been similarly elusive.[15–18]

What structures prevent downward displacement of the vesical neck in continent nulliparous subjects? A stable suburethral "hammock" comprising the anterior vaginal wall and pubocervical fascia with intact lateral attachments provides important primary support.[5] The pubovesical components of the anterior suspensory mechanism may limit downward displacement with an increase in intraabdominal pressure by virtue of their attachment to the inferior border of the pubis. Finally, the cervix provides important support for the upper vagina because it is suspended from the sacrum

and pelvic sidewall by the uterosacral and cardinal ligaments, respectively, and may contribute indirectly to the support of the vesical neck.

Traditional views of female continence have depended on the "pressure transmission theory of female continence"[19] in which the urethra is divided into intraabdominal and extraabdominal portions by the pelvic floor (Fig. 11-1). Any increase in intraabdominal pressure is transmitted to the proximal urethra contemporaneously, and continence is preserved. There is no anatomic feature related to the urethra that serves this function (see serial MRI sections, Figs. 11-9 and 11-10), and there are many patients with prolapse of the anterior vaginal wall who remain continent despite displacement of the urethrovesical junction. DeLancey[5] has proposed the "hammock hypothesis" of female continence, in which the urethra is compressed against a stable layer of the anterior vaginal wall and pubocervical fascia by an increase in intraabdominal pressure. Stability of the supporting layer that "prevents downward displacement of the urethrovesical junction" is preserved by its attachments: (1) laterally to the pelvic sidewall by virtue of insertions into the arcus tendineus fasciae pelvis and the pubococcygeus; (2) anteriorly to the pubis by means of the anterior suspensory mechanism of the vesical neck and the arcus tendineus fasciae pelvis; and (3) posteriorly to the uterine cervix and the uterosacral-cardinal ligament complex of endopelvic fasciae, through the pericervical connective tissue.

Variations in the nomenclature of these features have contributed to some of the confusion that has arisen in previous discussions of this topic. DeLancey's nomenclature is used where appropriate throughout this discussion of the anatomy of the lower urinary tract.[1]

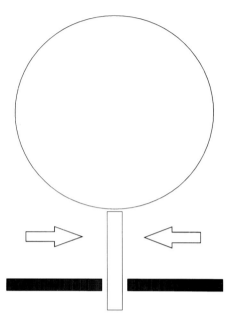

FIG. 11-1. The pressure transmission hypothesis of female continence depends on the transmission of any increase in intraabdominal pressure to the intraabdominal proxima urethra to maintain continence. There is no anatomic feature that separates the intraabdominal urethra from the extraabdominal urethra (see Fig. 9-10); in particular, the pubococcygeus has only an indirect relationship with the urethra itself.

Unfamiliar anatomy of the retropubic space in a nulliparous cadaver illustrates the complex of supporting structures that comprise the anterior suspensory mechanism of the vesical neck (Fig. 11-2).[20,21] This complex of structures includes a ''pubourethral'' component (sometimes termed *the pubourethral ligaments*), a ''pubovesical'' component (sometimes termed *the pubovesical ligaments*), and its continuation as the arcus tendineus fasciae pelvis (''white line'' over

the obturator fascia). The precise function of the anterior suspensory mechanism remains unclear, although it is a substantial feature in nulliparas and is appropriately placed to prevent downward displacement of the urethrovesical junction during an increase in intraabdominal pressure.

The *external striated sphincter* is the term applied to the striated muscle associated with the urethra and includes the external, circular layer of striated muscle of the urethra, the compressor urethrae, and the urethrovaginal sphincter. The compressor urethrae and urethrovaginal sphincter are minor striated components associated with the distal urethra proximal to the perineal membrane whose function is unclear though may be concerned with voluntary interruption of flow, emptying the distal urethra, or some circumstances in which continence is threatened.

MAGNETIC RESONANCE IMAGING ANATOMY OF THE LOWER URINARY TRACT

Normal anatomy of the lower urinary tract has been defined in vivo using MRI techniques in a series of asymptomatic nulliparous women (Figs. 11-4 through 11-11). Previous studies[22–26] have described some features of the pathoanatomy of urinary stress incontinence, although controlled studies of the anatomic effects of vaginal delivery are awaited. Serial axial and sagittal images of 4-mm thickness demonstrate the urethra and its adjacent, soft tissue supporting structures in nulliparous subjects (imaging with a pelvic surface coil and a parent unit; General Electric Signa, 1.5T, Milwaukee, WI, using fast spin-echo techniques with T2 weighting of the imaging sequences). Three important axial sections have been defined (see Figs. 11-4 through 11-7): (1) the ischial spines, (2) the proximal urethra, and (3) the perineal membrane.

The ischial spines define an important axial plane that

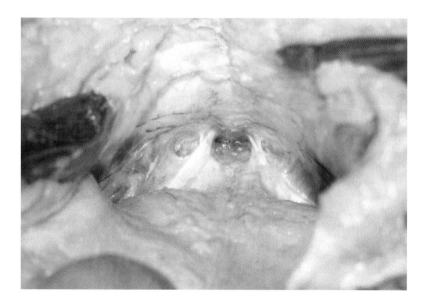

FIG. 11-2. The retropubic space of a nulliparous cadaver. The anterior suspensory mechanism of the vesical neck is clearly demonstrated and connects the posterior surface of the pubis, the anterior surface of the vesical neck, the urethra, and the pubococcygeus. The pubovesical component extends posteriorly to the ischial spines as the arcus tendineus fasciae pelvis, otherwise known as the "white line" over the obturator internus. The anterior suspensory mechanism primarily contains smooth muscle fibers, although its precise function remains controversial.

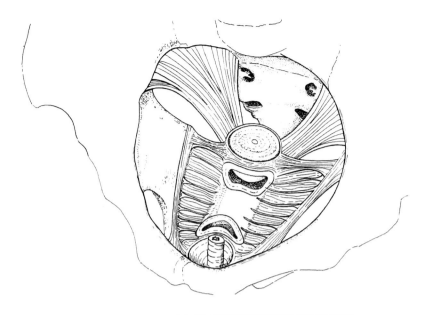

FIG. 11-3. Transvaginal shelf. The vagina is successively suspended, attached, and fused by the uterosacral ligaments, pubocervical fascia and perineal structures, respectively.

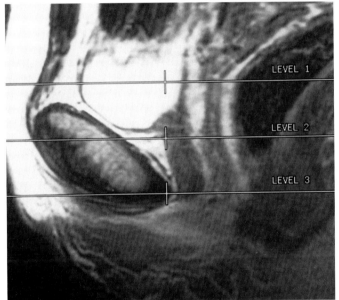

FIG. 11-4. The important axial landmarks of the lower genital tract are the ischial spines (see Fig. 11-5), the proximal urethra (see Fig. 11-6), and the perineal membrane (see Fig. 11-7).

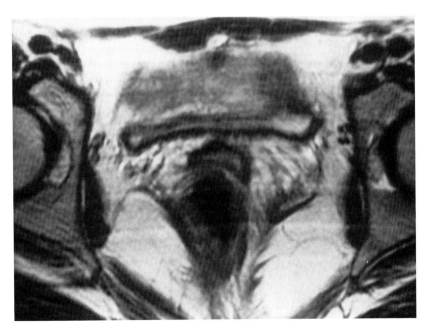

FIG. 11-5. An axial section of the lower genital tract at the level of the ischial spines demonstrating the uterine cervix and the vagina. The ischiococcygeus connects the ischial spines and the tip of the coccyx. The upper vagina is a horizontal feature that is supported by the lateral cervical and uterosacral ligaments.

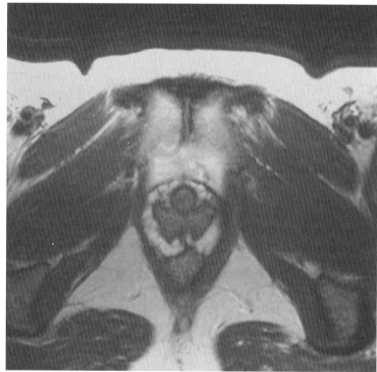

A

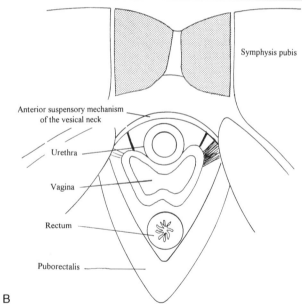

Symphysis pubis

Anterior suspensory mechanism
of the vesical neck

Urethra

Vagina

Rectum

Puborectalis

B

FIG. 11-6. Axial MRI of the anterior pelvis at the level of the proximal urethra **(A)** with diagram **(B).** The urethra, vagina, and the rectum are enclosed within the sling of pubococcygeus. The anterior suspensory mechanism occupies the retropubic space and inserts between the pubococcygei anterior to the urethra. The prominent feature is the butterfly shape of the nulliparous vagina that is formed by the insertion of the anterior horns into the pubococcygei (see Fig. 11-8, *plates 2* through *4*) and the posterior horns into the rectum (see Fig. 11-8, *plates 4* and *5*).

includes the uterine cervix and the lateral cervical ligaments (see Fig. 11-5). The second axial plane associated with the proximal urethra is identified by the increased ratio of longitudinal smooth muscle to circular striated muscle (see Fig. 11-6). The prominent soft tissue landmark associated with the distal urethra is the perineal membrane, which provides a platform for the external genitalia and serves as the distal anchor for the midline viscera (see Fig. 11-7).

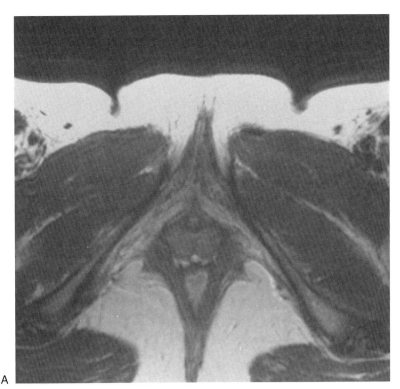

A

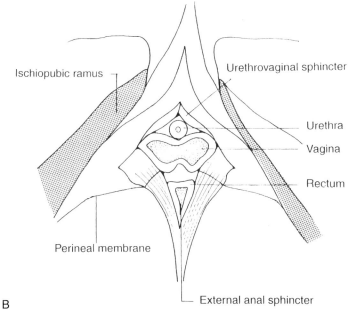

B

Ischiopubic ramus

Urethrovaginal sphincter

Urethra

Vagina

Rectum

Perineal membrane

External anal sphincter

FIG. 11-7. An axial section of the anterior pelvis at the level of the perineal membrane **(A)** and diagram **(B).** The urethra, vagina, and rectum penetrate the triangular shape of the perineal membrane whose posterior free edge is observed on each side of the rectum. The bulbo-cavernosi occupy the lateral edge of the perineal membrane adjacent to the ischiopubic rami. The perineal body is not a prominent feature, and striated muscle fibers arising from the external anal sphincter insert into the posterior edge of the perineal membrane.

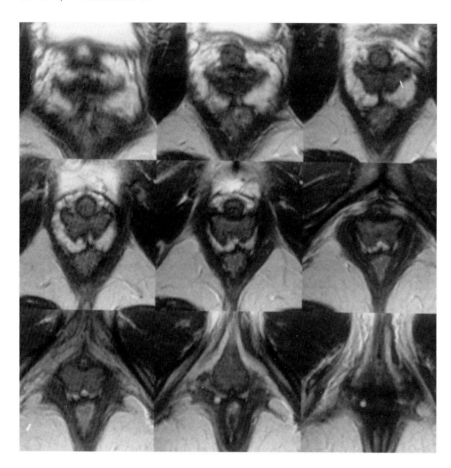

FIG. 11-8. Serial sections of the anterior pelvis at 4-mm intervals from the vesical neck *(plate 1)* to the perineal membrane *(plate 5)* in a nulliparous subject. The "hammock" of the anterior vaginal wall provides inferior support for the proximal urethra by virtue of its lateral attachments to the arcus tendineus fasciae pelvis *(plate 2)* and the pubococcygeus *(plates 3 and 4)*. Components of the anterior suspensory mechanism are demonstrated in plates 1 through 4.

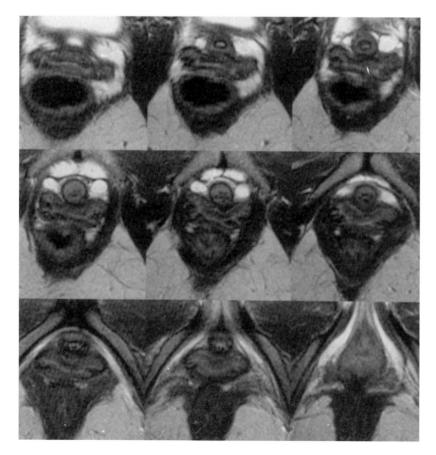

FIG. 11-9. Serial sections of the anterior pelvis at 4-mm intervals from the vesical neck *(plate 2)* to the perineal membrane *(plate 6)* in a nulliparous subject. The proximal urethra is identified by the ratio of smooth to striated urethral muscle *(plate 3)*, the compressor urethrae passes anterior to the urethra between the ischiopubic rami *(plate 5)*, and the urethrovaginal sphincter is a minor feature *(plate 6)*.

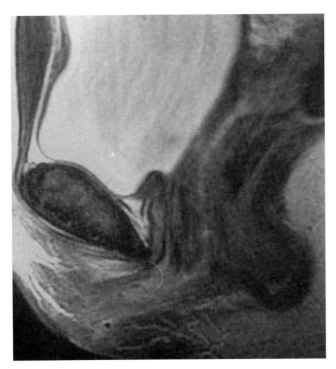

FIG. 11-10. Midline sagittal section of the anterior female pelvis. The symphysis pubis is a secondary cartilaginous joint with an intervening pad of cartilage between the two bony surfaces. The urethral mucosa and the circular and longitudinal layers of urethral muscle are apparent. Components of the anterior suspensory mechanism are visible in the retropubic space.

The prominent anatomic feature of the lower female pelvis is the characteristic H-shape of the nulliparous vagina that is formed by the anterior attachments to the medial border of pubococcygeus and the posterior attachments to the rectum through the rectovaginal "pillars" (see Fig. 11-6). The important supports of the vagina are the cardinal ligaments at the level of the cervix at its upper extent and the perineal membrane at its lower extent. Between these attachments it is connected to the arcus tendinei by the suburethral endopelvic fasciae and medial part of the pubococcygeus (see Fig. 11-3). These lateral attachments, together with the vaginolevator attachment, stabilize the anterior vaginal wall and pubocervical fascia, against which the urethra may be compressed by an increase in intraabdominal pressure.

MRI techniques provide reliable and consistent imaging of the components of the levator ani at different levels of the pelvis with the sling of pubococcygeus prominent in all sections of the lower pelvis. Relaxation of the pubococcygeus before voiding causes opening of the vesical neck and proximal urethra because of the direct connection between the anterior vaginal wall and the proximal urethra. Contraction of the detrusor muscle and the longitudinal smooth muscle of the urethra causes bladder emptying through an open urethra. Pudendal neuropathy resulting from vaginal delivery may have an impact on the function of the levator ani and presents as disturbances of urinary or bowel function.

Previously, invasive techniques have been required to demonstrate these effects, and the literature remains controversial on the precise impact of such lesions.

The perineal membrane separates the pelvic viscera, contained posteriorly by pubococcygeus, from the external genitalia, and extends between the medial borders of the ischiopubic rami to occupy a horizontal plane with the patient in an erect position. Direct support is provided for the distal vagina and urethra, and the posterior fibers insert into the perineal body. Both the compressor urethrae and the urethrovaginal sphincter are paraurethral structures that are composed of striated muscle and occupy a position immediately proximal to the perineal membrane. They may act as secondary components in the female continence mechanism in some circumstances. Important anatomic features in the posterior compartment of the pelvis include the external anal sphincter and the insertion of some of its fibers into the perineal membrane.[27] MRI of the perineum confirms their origin from the external anal sphincter and perineal body to insert into the perineal membrane (see Figs. 11-8 and 11-9), although the "perineal body" is not a substantive feature of perineal anatomy and has a limited role in the prevention of genital prolapse.

The anatomy of the anterior suspensory mechanism of the vesical neck has been a controversial subject for many years.[20,21] There have been few opportunities to study the

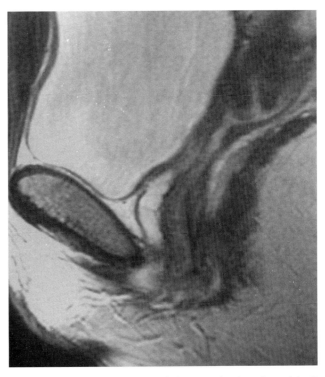

FIG. 11-11. Sagittal section of the anterior female pelvis 8 mm to the left of the midline. The pubic ramus is demonstrated in detail with an outer layer of cortical bone and the pubovesical and pubourethral components of the anterior suspensory mechanism in the retropubic space. Some aspects of the external genitalia are demonstrated.

retropubic space in continent nulliparous subjects, and it is rare to see significant remnants of this structure at retropubic urethropexy because they have been disrupted or attenuated at vaginal delivery. Identified anatomic features of the anterior suspensory mechanism of the vesical neck have been awarded a variety of terms, including *the pubourethral ligaments, pubovesical ligaments, pubovesical muscle,* and *urethropelvic ligaments.* Some variations in anatomy may account for the apparent discordance, although MRI in continent, nulliparous subjects provides insights into the precise anatomic arrangements (see Figs. 11-8 and 11-9). Parasagittal sections confirm the presence of bilateral structures arising from the anterior surface of the bladder and inserting into the posterior surface of the pubis (see Fig. 11-5). Axial sections demonstrate their close association with the proximal urethra (see Figs. 11-10 and 11-11) and the component that inserts into the medial border of the pubococcygeus (see Fig. 11-8). The function of the anterior suspensory mechanism of the vesical neck is controversial because it contains predominantly smooth muscle fibers and the origin is above the insertion with the patient in the erect position, suggesting that it is unlikely that the bladder neck is "suspended" from the inferior border of the pubis.[3] It seems placed to prevent downward displacement of the vesical neck with an increase in intraabdominal pressure, although the anterior vaginal wall and pubococcygeus also contribute to that function. Disruption of the anterior suspensory mechanism after traumatic vaginal delivery is associated with excessive mobility of the entire urethra and early onset of urinary stress incontinence in the puerperium, although both lateral and suburethral supports may also be disrupted in such circumstances. Occupying symmetric positions in the pelvis in similar fashion to the anterior suspensory mechanism are two additional pairs of ligaments that insert into the uterine cervix: the lateral cervical (cardinal) ligaments and the uterosacral ligaments. Removal of the uterine cervix at hysterectomy has been associated with the subsequent onset of urinary stress incontinence and genital prolapse, although this association has not been tested in controlled studies.

SONOGRAPHIC ANATOMY OF THE LOWER URINARY TRACT

Abdominal, vaginal, perineal, and rectal sonography have been used to image the lower urinary tract.[6,7,28–32] At present, vaginal and perineal techniques provide adequate resolution of the anatomic features in a noninvasive, patient-acceptable fashion. Perineal sonography may be limited by the acoustic impedance of the symphysis pubis, the lack of a consistent relationship of the transducer to the anatomic features, and the inability of the technique to be used for dynamic studies with the patient in the sitting position, although it is a simple technique for observing the effects of

retrograde filling cystometry on the bladder neck and proximal urethra.

Vaginal sonography may be used with the patient in either supine or sitting positions to image the consequences of provocative maneuvers and suprapubic surgery on the continence mechanism. A potential disadvantage of the vaginal route is the opportunity for displacement of the anterior vaginal wall in patients with significant genital prolapse (type B),[11] although enhanced resolution and patient acceptance are significant advantages of the technique. Vaginal sonography is the optimal technique for the evaluation of patients after suprapubic surgery in which anatomic objectives are achieved by successful operations and abnormal anatomy is often a feature of unsuccessful procedures.[7,9]

Sonographic appearances of the lower urinary tract depend on the different acoustic impedances of the adjacent tissues, including cartilage (symphysis pubis), bone (pubic rami), urine, and soft tissues (Figs. 11-12 through 11-14). Additional information may be obtained by urethral catheterization or combining the sonographic technique with concurrent measurement of intravesical and intraurethral pressures (video-cystosonography). Imaging in both clinical applications (ie, preoperative evaluation of the incontinent patient and evaluation of the postoperative anatomic result) has been consistently achieved with a high-frequency (7 MHz), mechanical sector scanner (Bruel & Kjaer 8537) that has reduced external dimensions (diameter 18 mm) and a wide field angle (112 degrees) that enables imaging in both supine

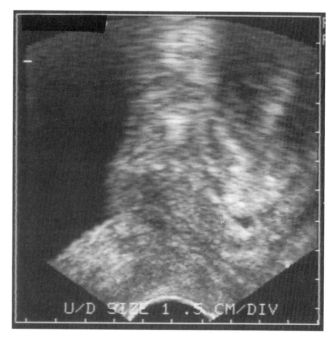

FIG. 11-12. The midline sagittal plane of the pelvis demonstrated with vaginal ultrasound. The symphysis pubis is a hyperechoic feature that appears in the same midline plane as the urethrovesical junction and the urethra. The bladder neck and the urethra are clearly demonstrated.

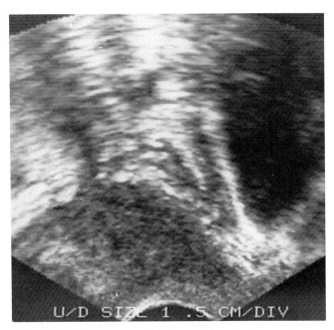

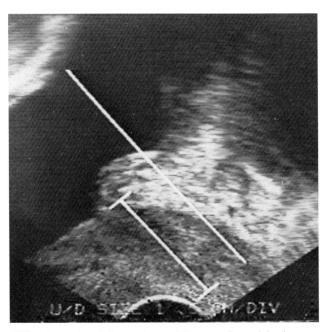

FIG. 11-13. The parasagittal plane of the anterior pelvis demonstrating the same anatomic features as Figure 11-12 except for the hypoechoic appearance of the pubic ramus in a plane adjacent to the midline sagittal plane. The urethra and bladder are demonstrated in similar fashion to Figure 11-12.

FIG. 11-14. An oblique plane of the anterior pelvis demonstrating the hyperechoic appearances of the anterior suspensory mechanism of the vesical neck. The craniocaudal axis of the patient is indicated because the transducer of the probe is offset at 45 degrees to the horizontal.

and sitting positions, at rest, and during provocative maneuvers (see Fig. 11-4).

The midline sagittal plane of the pelvis is defined by the symphysis pubis, the urethra, and the urethrovesical junction. The symphysis pubis is a secondary cartilaginous joint with sonographic appearances that are determined by the pad of cartilage connecting the pubic bones (see Fig. 11-1). Cartilage appears as a homogeneous, hyperechoic pattern that is differentiated from adjacent connective tissue by the shape of its inferior border and its immobility during provocative maneuvers. The inferior border of the symphysis pubis is a fixed reference point from which reproducible, anatomic observations may be made. The midline sagittal plane is clearly defined and is distinguished from the pubic bones by its characteristic appearance. The pubic bones are composed of trabecular bone that has a hypoechoic appearance with a dense inferior edge that has a contrasting hyperechoic appearance (see Fig. 11-13). In the oblique plane the pubovesical component of the anterior suspensory mechanism of the vesical neck may be defined between the anterior surface of the bladder and the inferior border of the pubic ramus (see Fig. 11-14). The bladder is clearly defined by the characteristic hypoechoic appearances of the stored urine. The urethrovesical junction is identified by its characteristic shape, and the course of the urethra is indicated by the appearances of the apposed epithelial surfaces. Additional information may be obtained with biplanar endoprobes that enable imaging in sagittal and coronal planes.

MAGNETIC RESONANCE IMAGING ANATOMY OF URINARY STRESS INCONTINENCE

Previous descriptions of the MRI anatomy of urinary stress incontinence have described alterations of the pubococcygeus[25] and disruption of the vaginolevator attachments.[23] In a series of consecutive patients with "genuine" stress incontinence similar anatomic abnormalities have been noted (Figs. 11-15 through 11-18).

Disruption of the anterior suspensory mechanism and vaginolevator attachments at all levels of the lower pelvis are demonstrated in a patient with "genuine" stress incontinence (see Figs. 11-15 and 11-16). The vagina has taken on an "∩" shape as compared with the nulliparous "H" shape, and the stabilizing layer of the anterior vaginal wall and pubocervical fascia has been disrupted. The sling of pubococcygeus remains intact. In a second patient with "genuine" stress incontinence and fecal urgency after the spontaneous delivery of a newborn weighing 5080 g, anatomic features were associated with denervation of the lower pelvis (see Figs. 11-17 and 11-18). The abnormal anatomic features include disruption of the anterior suspensory mechanism of the vesical neck, absence of a normal vaginal configuration ("H" shape) with attenuation of the vagina at all levels of the pelvis (see Fig. 11-16), and attenuation of pubococcygeus in both shape and dimensions with a maximum thickness of 2 mm.

Further studies in sagittal, axial, and coronal planes are

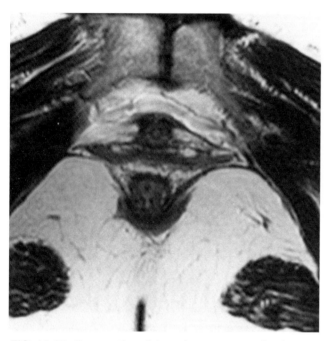

FIG. 11-15. Denervation of the pubococcygeus after forceps delivery in a patient with fecal urgency and urinary stress incontinence. The vagina is reduced in both shape and dimension (compare with Fig. 11-6), and the pubococcygeus has lost its usual sling conformation and is markedly atrophied. These observations were noted at all levels of the urethra.

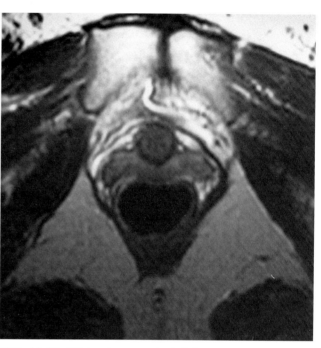

FIG. 11-17. Bilateral paravaginal defects. Disruption of the lateral attachments of the vagina in a patient with genuine stress incontinence. There is disorganization of the retropubic space, scarring of the anterior vaginal wall, and an altered vaginal configuration caused by loss of the insertions into the arcus tendineus fasciae pelvis and the pubococcygeus.

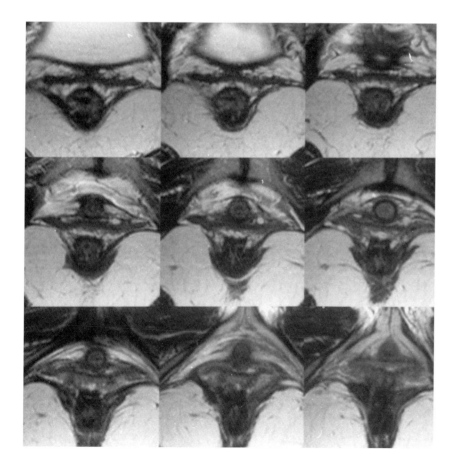

FIG. 11-16. Denervation of the pubococcygeus after forceps delivery in a patient with fecal urgency and urinary stress incontinence. The vagina is reduced in both shape and dimension (compared with Fig. 11-6), and the pubococcygeus has lost its usual sling conformation and is markedly atrophied. These observations were noted at all levels of the urethra.

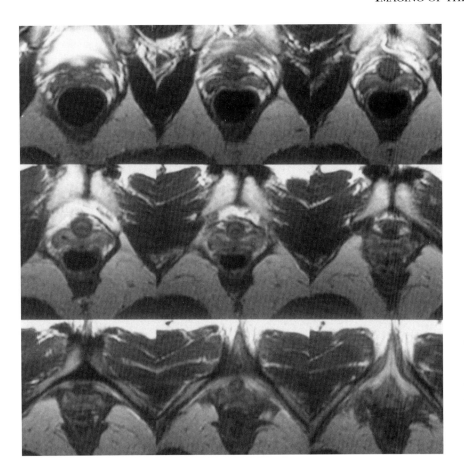

FIG. 11-18. Bilateral paravaginal defects. Disruption of the lateral attachments of the vagina in a patient with genuine stress incontinence. There is disorganization of the retropubic space, scarring of the anterior vaginal wall, and an altered vaginal configuration caused by loss of the insertions into the arcus tendineus fasciae pelvis and the pubococcygeus.

required to delineate the anatomic damage associated with vaginal delivery, hysterectomy, and subsequent onset of urinary stress incontinence and genital prolapse.

SONOGRAPHIC IMAGING OF URINARY STRESS INCONTINENCE

Comprehensive evaluation of the lower urinary tract requires sonographic equipment that is capable of dynamic imaging in real time (> 15 frames per second) with the patient in supine and sitting positions, at rest, and during provocative maneuvers (eg, a cough or Valsalva maneuver), so as to image urinary leakage concurrent with a cough (ie, "genuine" stress incontinence).[6] Many endoprobes have technical specifications that do not fulfil these requirements, although most systems may be used for the evaluation of the anatomic effects of suprapubic operations (eg, colposuspension and bladder neck), needle suspension operations, in which the evaluation depends on imaging the anatomic features at rest, and after a Valsalva maneuver. In patients without urinary symptoms sonography demonstrates minor downward and posterior rotation of the urethrovesical junction; there is no demonstrable urinary leakage in either supine or sitting positions.[6,9]

After clinical history and physical examination, including the demonstration of urinary incontinence concurrent with a cough, additional noninvasive investigations including urine culture, frequency-volume chart, urinary flow rate, and perineal pad-weighing tests may contribute to an overall evaluation of the lower urinary tract. Urodynamic studies including filling cystometry may be considered or may be combined with sonography of the lower urinary tract (video-cystosonography). The study may be completed by voiding to completion to establish the bladder volume and urine flow rate and final sonographic evaluation to demonstrate the absence of significant residual urine.

In patients with genuine stress incontinence, sonography demonstrates passive opening of the bladder neck and proximal urethra concurrent with a cough (Fig. 11-19). Few patients demonstrate these findings in the supine position, although they may be conveniently demonstrated with the patient in the sitting position. Almost invariably there is significant posteroinferior rotation of the urethrovesical junction that is characteristic of "anatomic" stress incontinence and has been demonstrated using indirect radiologic techniques including bead-chain cystourethrography.[11–14] Patients with a "fixed" urethra are rare and have invariably had multiple unsuccessful surgical procedures. Patients with neurologic symptoms require formal evaluation with cystometry and concurrent measurement of intravesical and intraabdominal pressures. Additional sonographic configura-

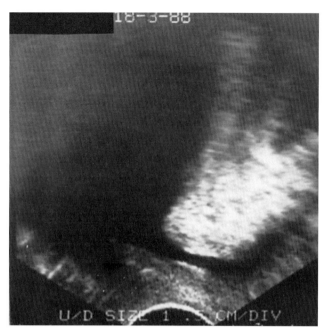

FIG. 11-19. Genuine stress incontinence. Concurrent opening of the bladder neck and proximal urethra with urinary leakage concurrent with a cough. Urinary incontinence is almost invariably associated with posteroinferior rotation of the urethrovesical junction.

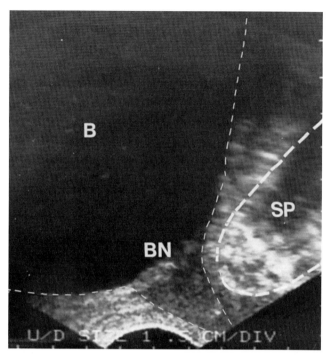

FIG. 11-20. Disruption of the anterior suspensory mechanism of the bladder neck (BN) after traumatic vaginal delivery. There is no evidence of the anterior suspensory mechanism in the retropubic space, and the anterior surface of the bladder (B) rests against the posterior surface of the symphysis pubis (SP). Suburethral supports have also been disrupted so that an increase in intraabdominal pressure is associated with marked downward displacement of the vesical neck and concurrent urinary stress incontinence.

tions associated with urinary stress incontinence include disruption of the anterior suspensory mechanism of the vesical neck (Fig. 11-20) and post-hysterectomy incontinence (Fig. 11-21). Disruption of the anterior suspensory mechanism (and suburethral supports) occurs after traumatic vaginal delivery and is associated with forceps delivery, epidural analgesia, and malpositions of the vertex. Post-hysterectomy configurations have not been validated in systematic studies, although division of the lateral cervical and uterosacral ligaments at the time of hysterectomy may result in an unsupported bladder base. Increases in intra-abdominal pressure displace the bladder base and ''strip open'' the posterior leaf of the proximal urethra.

Urinary incontinence associated with detrusor instability may be differentiated from genuine stress incontinence by the nature and timing of urinary leakage relative to the cough (Fig. 11-22). Urinary leakage is delayed relative to the cough and is associated with active contraction of the detrusor muscle that accounts for the phasic increase in intravesical pressure. In a prospective comparison of traditional urodynamic techniques and vaginal sonography the sonographic technique was both sensitive and specific for the diagnosis of genuine stress incontinence without the necessity for urethral and rectal catheterization.[8,9] Imaging studies to detect the effects of detrusor instability on the continence mechanism have not been performed because additional provocative maneuvers including retrograde bladder filling may be required to provoke detrusor activity whose clinical significance remains uncertain.

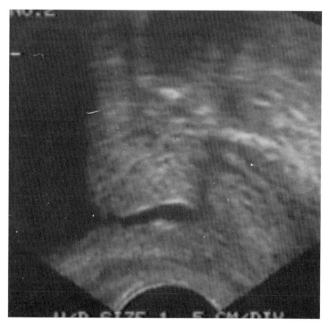

FIG. 11-21. Post-hysterectomy stress incontinence. Division of the uterosacral and lateral cervical ligaments is associated with loss of support of the upper vagina and bladder base. An increase in intraabdominal pressure is associated with opening of the posterior wall of the proximal urethra and subsequent urinary stress incontinence.

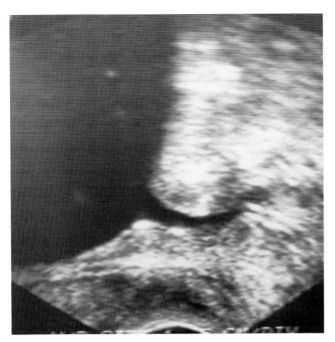

FIG. 11-22. Detrusor incontinence. The nature and timing of urinary incontinence associated with detrusor instability is different from that associated with genuine stress incontinence. Urinary incontinence is delayed relative to the cough.

Surgical treatment of genuine stress incontinence has included many different surgical procedures, although they divide into three approaches: (1) colposuspension,[33,34] (2) needle suspension operations, [35,36] and (3) sling procedures.[37]

Laparoscopic techniques for colposuspension are becoming increasingly popular because they combine surgical accuracy with reduced morbidity.[38] The central principle of suprapubic surgery for genuine stress incontinence—elevation of the bladder neck—has been based on theories of pressure transmission so that a displaced urethrovesical junction is restored to an "intraabdominal pressure zone." This approach has been associated with successful treatment of primary stress incontinence, although this has been accompanied by significant rates of postoperative detrusor instability and voiding difficulties.[39–42] Clinical and experimental observations have indicated potential problems with this hypothesis; there is no anatomic feature that differentiates the intraabdominal urethra from the extraabdominal urethra; there are many continent patients with significant degrees of genital prolapse, and successful surgical treatment is frequently associated with pressure transmission ratios in excess of 100% of the preoperative value. The "hammock" hypothesis proposes that the condition commonly results from loss of support of the urethrovesical junction and that successful surgery, particularly for primary stress incontinence, restores the support of the urethrovesical junction.[5]

The "prevention of downward displacement" of the urethrovesical junction (with secondary "elevation" of the vesical neck) by the interposition of a vaginal shelf, needle

suspension, or sling is a subtle, but important, shift in surgical approach that may be associated with comparable success rates without the additional morbidity associated with voiding difficulties and postoperative detrusor instability. In practical terms this approach entails avoidance of overtightening the supporting sutures between the vaginal fornices and the iliopectineal ligament at colposuspension or overtightening an interposed sling. Alternative approaches may be required in patients with recurrent stress incontinence, and prolonged observations of the surgical outcomes will be necessary.

Vaginal sonography of the postoperative results of suprapubic surgery is a simple, noninvasive, clinical technique that confirms that the anatomic objectives of the operation have been achieved.[7,9] In addition, it demonstrates to the patient early in the postoperative period that she has an accurate surgical result that has converted a mobile, incontinent mechanism into a stable, continent configuration. Reproducible anatomic observations in the midline sagittal plane are independent of bladder volume because the vaginal fornices have been secured in a fixed, permanent configuration that prevents downward displacement of the urethrovesical junction. Accurate postoperative configurations after colposuspension demonstrate absence of downward displacement of the urethrovesical junction with an increase in intraabdominal pressure and absence of fixed indentations of the trigone or bladder base (Fig. 11-23).

Abnormal postoperative configurations after colposuspension may be identified by mobility of the urethrovesical junction or by fixed indentations of the trigone and bladder base.

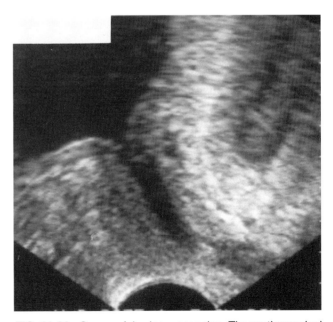

FIG. 11-23. Successful colposuspension. The urethrovesical junction is supported by the fixation of the vaginal fornices to the iliopectinal ligaments by nonabsorbable sutures. An increase in intraabdominal pressure is associated with no displacement of the urethrovesical junction.

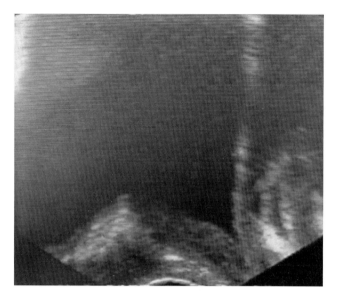

FIG. 11-24. Persistent stress incontinence after colposuspension. The supporting sutures have been placed too high on the endopelvic fascia so that when tied to the iliopectineal ligament the vaginal fornices indent the bladder base. There has been no effect on the urethrovesical junction, and an increase in intraabdominal pressure produces urinary incontinence concurrent with a cough.

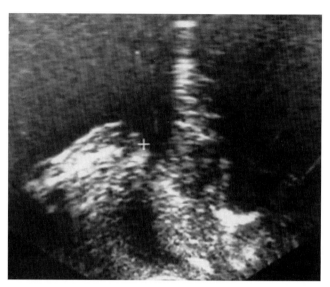

FIG. 11-25. Frequency-urgency syndrome after colposuspension. The supporting sutures have been placed too high on the endopelvic fascia, producing a vaginal shelf that underpins the trigone. The bladder neck has been supported so that continence is preserved although the patient had a debilitating urge syndrome associated with de novo postoperative detrusor instability.

Abnormal mobility of the urethrovesical junction may be observed in association with recurrent stress incontinence, whereas fixed indentations are associated with frequency-urgency syndrome (Fig. 11-24), postoperative detrusor instability, or persistent stress incontinence (Fig. 11-25). Recurrent stress incontinence may occur in the "immediate" postoperative period or be "delayed" until the climacteric. In both circumstances excessive mobility of the urethrovesical junction (>10 mm with a Valsalva maneuver) occurs with an increase in intraabdominal pressure. Fixed indentations of the bladder base are associated with inaccurate placement of the supporting sutures (and possibly excessive elevation of the vaginal fornices toward the iliopectineal ligaments). If the sutures are placed at the level of the vaginal vault, then no support is afforded to the urethrovesical junction and the patient has persistent stress incontinence; suture placement beneath the trigone is associated with persistent urge syndrome and postoperative detrusor instability.

CONCLUSION

Traditional concepts of continence based on theories of "pressure transmission to an intraabdominal urethra" have been overemphasized, and anatomic concepts are being reexamined. MRI techniques have provided new insights into the precise anatomy of the paraurethral soft tissues. "Structure" and "function" are distinct and separate entities, although a thorough understanding of the precise anatomic features will form the basis for new hypotheses regarding the function

of the female continence mechanism that can be tested in appropriate clinical settings. One of the primary benefits of improved imaging techniques includes the adoption of consistent anatomic terms that enable radiologic, gynecologic, urologic, and colorectal clinicians to discuss overlapping (Fig. 11-26) problems using the same vocabulary.

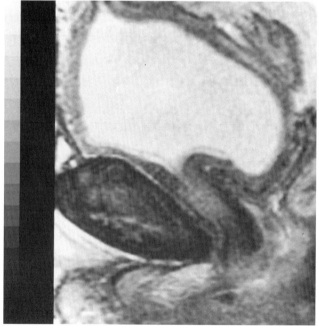

FIG. 11-26. MR image of a successful colposuspcusion. The vaginal shelf supports the bladder neck the vagina and is "forked" by the surgical procedure.

MRI has provided an important description of the soft tissue anatomy of the lower urinary tract in nulliparous subjects, and some gross anatomic abnormalities have been described in patients with urinary stress incontinence. Further sophistication may be introduced with three-dimensional imaging protocols. Many of these observations may be replicated with contemporary multiplanar sonographic techniques. Vaginal sonography enables dynamic studies of the effects of provocative maneuvers on the continence mechanism and high-resolution views of the postoperative anatomy after suprapubic surgery. The technique is simple, noninvasive, and acceptable to patients. Further studies using biplanar and three-dimensional sonographic techniques to examine the etiology and pathoanatomy of urinary stress incontinence and genital prolapse are anticipated in the near future.

REFERENCES

1. Delancey JOL. Correlative study of paraurethral anatomy. Obstet Gynecol 1986;68:91.
2. Delancey JOL. Structural aspects of the extrinsic continence mechanism. Obstet Gynecol 1988;72:296.
3. Delancey JOL. Pubovesical ligament: a separate structure from the urethral supports (pubourethral ligaments). Neurourol Urodynam 1989;8:53.
4. Delancey JOL. Anatomy of the urethral sphincters and supports. In: Drife JO, Hilton P, Stanton SL, eds. Micturition. New York, Springer-Verlag, 1990:3.
5. Delancey JOL. The hammock hypothesis. Am J Obstet Gynecol 1994;170:1713.
6. Quinn MJ, Beynon J, Mortensen NM, Smith PJB. Transvaginal endosonography in the assessment of urinary stress incontinence. Br J Urol 1988;62:414.
7. Quinn MJ, Beynon J, Mortensen NM, Smith PJB. Vaginal endosonography in the postoperative assessment of colposuspension. Br J Urol 19889;63:295.
8. Quinn MJ, Farnsworth BA, Pollard WJ, et al. Vaginal ultrasound in the diagnosis of stress incontinence: a prospective comparison to urodynamic investigations. Neurourol Urodynam 1989;8:291.
9. Quinn MJ. Vaginal ultrasound of the lower urinary tract, MD Thesis, University of Bristol, 1994.
10. Quinn MJ, Harrison S, Bourne M. Magnetic resonance imaging of the lower urinary tract in nulliparous subjects. Am J Obstet Gynaecol, in press.
11. Green TH. Development of a plan for the diagnosis and treatment of urinary stress incontinence. Am J Obstet Gynecol 1962;83:632.
12. Green TH. Urinary stress incontinence: differential diagnosis, pathophysiology and management. Am J Obstet Gynecol 1975;122:368.
13. Hodgkinson CP. Relationships of the female urethra in urinary incontinence. Am J Obstet Gynecol 1953;65:560.
14. Hodgkinson CP. Urethrocystogram: metallic bead-chain technique. Clin Obstet Gynecol 1958;1:668.
15. Richardson AC, Lyon JB, Williams NL. A new look at pelvic relaxation. Am J Obstet Gynecol 1976;126:568.
16. Richardson AC, Edmonds PB, Williams NL. Treatment of stress urinary incontinence due to paravaginal fascial defect. Obstet Gynecol 1981;57:357.
17. Shull R, Benn SJ, Kuehl TJ. Surgical management of prolapse of the anterior vaginal segment: an analysis of support defects, operative morbidity and anatomic outcome. Am J Obstet Gynecol 1994;171:1429.
18. Shull R, Capen CV, Riggs MW, Kuehl TJ. Preoperative and postoperative analysis of site-specific pelvic support defects in 81 women treated with sacrospinous ligament suspension and pelvic reconstruction. Am J Obstet Gynecol
19. Enhorning G. Simultaneous recording of intravesical and intraurethral pressure. Acta Chir Scand (Suppl) 1961;276:1.
20. Zacharin RF. The suspensory mechanism of the female urethra. J Anat 1963;97:423.
21. Zacharin RF. The anatomic supports of the female urethra. Obstet Gynecol 1968;32:754.
22. Klutke C, Golomb J, Barbaric Z, Raz S. The anatomy of stress incontinence: magnetic resonance imaging of the female bladder neck and urethra. J Urol 1990;143:563.
23. Huddlestone HT, Dunnihoo DR, Huddleston PM, Meyers PC. Magnetic resonance imaging of defects in DeLancey's vaginal support levels I, II and III. Am J Obstet Gynecol 1995;172:1778.
24. Hricak H, Secaf E, Buckley DW, et al. Female urethra: MR Imaging. Radiology 1991;178:527
25. Kirschner-Hermanns R, Wein B, Niehaus S, et al. The contribution of magnetic resonance imaging of the pelvic floor to the understanding of urinary incontinence. Br J Urol 1993;72:715.
26. Plattner V, Leborgne J, Heloury Y, et al. MRI evaluation of the levator ani muscle: anatomic correlations and practical applications. Surg Radiol Anat 1991;13:129.
27. Snell RL. Clinical anatomy. Boston, Little, Brown & Co, 1981.
28. Clark AL, Creighton SM, Pearce JM, Stanton SL. Localisation of the bladder neck by perineal ultrasound; methodology and applications. Neurourol Urodynam 1990;9:394.
29. Creighton SM, Pearce JM, Stanton SL. Perineal video-ultrasonography in the assessment of vaginal prolapse: early observations. Br J Obstet Gynaecol 1992;99:310.
30. Koelbl H, Bernaschek G. A new method for sonographic urethrocystography and simultaneous pressure-flow studies. Obstet Gynecol 1989;74:417.
31. Koelbl H, Bernaschek G, Deutinger J. Assessment of female urinary incontinence by introital sonography. J Clin Ultrasound 1990;18:370.
32. Kohorn EI, Scioscia AL, Jeanty P, Hobbins JC. Ultrasound cystourethrography by perineal scanning for the assessment of female stress urinary incontinence. Obstet Gynecol 1986;68:269.
33. Burch JC. Urethrovaginal fixation to Cooper's ligament for correction of stress incontinence, cystocoele and prolapse. Am J Obstet Gynecol 1961;117:805.
34. Stanton SL. The colposuspension operation for urinary incontinence. Br J Obstet Gynaecol 1976;83:890.
35. Raz S. Modified bladder neck suspension for female stress incontinence J Urol 1981;18:82.
36. Stamey T. Endoscopic suspension of the vesical neck for urinary stress incontinence. Surg Gynecol Obstet 1973;136:547.
37. Richmond DH, Sutherst JR. Burch colposuspension or sling for stress incontinence? A prospective study using transrectal ultrasound. Br J Urol 1989;64:600.
38. Lyons TL. Laparoscopic colposuspension. In: Reich H, ed. Laparoscopic hysterectomy. 1993
39. Stanton SL, Cardozo LD. Results of the colposuspension operation for incontinence and prolapse. Br J Obstet Gynaecol 1978;86:693.
40. Cardozo LD, Stanton SL, Williams JE. Detrusor instability following surgery for genuine stress incontinence. Br J Urol 1979;51:204.
41. Galloway NTM, Davies N, Stephenson TP. The complications of colposuspension. Br J Urol 1987;60:122.
42. Steel SA, Cox C, Stanton SL. Long term follow up of detrusor instability following colposuspension. Br J Urol 1985;58:138.

Clinical Gynecologic Imaging, edited
by Arthur C. Fleischer, Marcia C. Javitt,
R. Brooke Jeffrey, Jr., and Howard W. Jones III,
Lippincott-Raven Publishers, Philadelphia © 1997.

CHAPTER 12

Pediatric Gynecologic Imaging

Marta Hernanz-Schulman, MD

The use of pediatric pelvic sonography has largely paralleled that in adult women, eliminating more invasive radiologic procedures and decreasing gonadal radiation dose. However, there are differences in the application of this modality to the female infant and prepubertal child. These differences are both technical and interpretative, based on differences in anatomy and in the physiologic and pathologic processes that affect the reproductive tract of the young girl. In this chapter the techniques involved in pediatric pelvic imaging, pediatric genital anatomy and its evolution through puberty, and the sonographic evaluation of pathologic states distinct to the pediatric population are discussed. Conditions that are characteristically present in adolescent and adult women, such as pelvic inflammatory disease, are discussed elsewhere in this text.

TECHNIQUE

Routine pediatric pelvic imaging is performed through the transabdominal approach, which requires a filled urinary bladder. In continent children, this is accomplished in a manner similar to that in adults, by requesting that the patient drink a noncarbonated beverage approximately 30 minutes before the scheduled examination. Infants, on the other hand, void frequently and may not retain maximum bladder distention. However, examination in these patients is facilitated by maintaining a generous state of hydration, because adequate bladder filling will occur relatively quickly. Transvaginal imaging is not part of the routine pelvic examination in the girl before the initiation of sexual activity.

Transperineal scanning can supplement the transabdominal examination when necessary, especially in young infants. This technique is usually carried out with a 5- to 10-MHz linear transducer placed in the midline of the perineum. As in transvaginal scanning, the transducer is placed within a sterile glove for scanning, and it is cleansed in a sterilizing solution before and after completion of the examination (Fig. 12-1).

NORMAL ANATOMY

The normal female pelvic anatomy varies with age, reflecting the changes in hormonal influence on both ovarian and uterine morphology. In the neonate, maternal hormonal stimulation induces ovarian enlargement and folliculogenesis; over time, involution occurs and genital anatomy remains static until activation of the pituitary-gonadal axis preceding puberty.

Neonatal Anatomy

(Fig. 12-2)

Uterus

The uterus in the term neonate measures approximately 2 cm in length. Uterine size in the newborn is only slightly smaller than that in the older, prepubertal child; thus, the ratio of uterine size to body size is much greater. The cervix and the fundus are approximately equal in size, and they can be distinguished with difficulty or not at all. Endometrial hypertrophy occurs in response to maternal hormones, a fact that is reflected in an echogenic or bilayered uterine lumen on sonographic images (see Fig. 12-2A).[1]

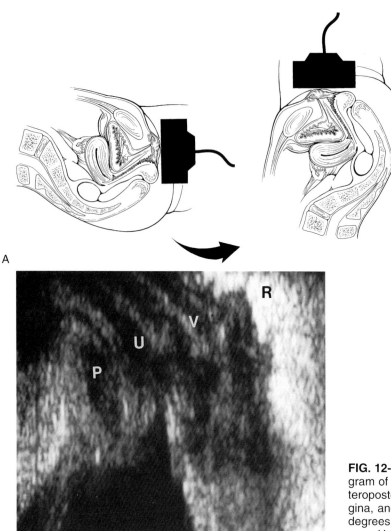

A

B

FIG. 12-1. Transperineal technique and anatomy. **(A)** Diagram of transperineal scan. The transducer is oriented anteroposteriorly along the perineum, outlining the urethra, vagina, and rectum. The sonographic depiction is rotated 90 degrees counterclockwise. **(B)** Neonatal transperineal anatomy. Urethra (U), vagina (V) and rectum (R) are well outlined. P, cartilaginous portion of symphysis pubis.

Ovaries

The neonatal ovaries exhibit considerable variability in size and morphology. They are relatively hypoechoic when compared with the older, prepubertal girl, and typically can be identified by the presence of cysts of variable size (see Fig. 12-2D).

Prepubertal Anatomy

(Fig. 12-3)

Uterus

After the neonatal period, the uterus is characterized by the preponderance of the cervix over the fundus, which becomes very thin and gives the organ a tonguelike appearance.[2] It is best found by identifying the vagina in the midline

and following this structure cephalad into the uterus itself. The fundocervical length is 2 to 3 cm. Endometrial echoes are never present (Fig. 12-3A).

The vagina is represented by two closely apposed linear mucosal echoes. The normal vagina is always collapsed, although immediately after micturition urine routinely enters the vagina; this is a normal finding.

Ovaries

The prepubertal ovary is relatively hyperechoic, with an echogenicity similar to that of the uterus. Ovarian volume is approximated by measuring the ovary in three planes and using a simplified formula for calculating the volume of a prolate ellipsoid: (length × width × depth) ÷ 2. The normal prepubertal ovarian volume is 1 to 2 mL. Cysts are usually minute (1 to 2 mm) or not visible. These characteristics may render the normal prepubertal ovary difficult to recognize. One method is to identify the broad ligaments of the uterus in

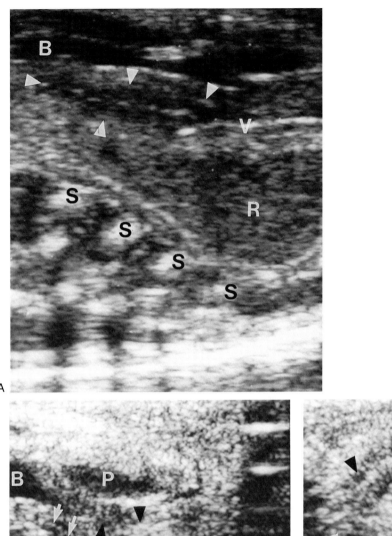

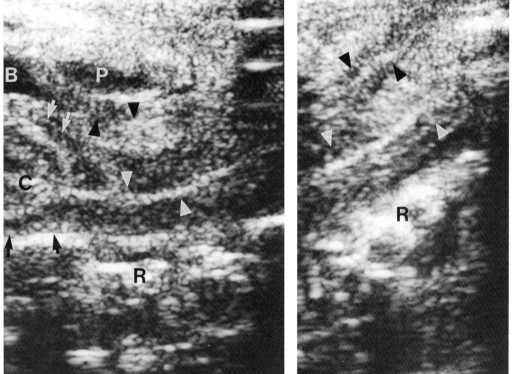

FIG. 12-2. Neonatal anatomy. **(A)** Sagittal scan of newborn pelvis. Bladder (B) is nearly empty. Arrowheads outline the uterus; note the more prominent cervix caudad and the presence of an endometrial stripe. V, vagina; R, rectum, coursing caudad anterior to sacrum (S). **(B)** Enlarged view of the cervical region *(left)* and the perineum *(right)* obtained with a different transducer demonstrates the anatomic detail that may be obtained in these infants. On the left, note the vaginal vault *(arrows)* surrounding the uterine cervix (C). A central white stripe *(white arrowheads)* outlines the apposed vaginal mucosal surfaces. P, cartilaginous symphysis pubis; B, bladder, ending in urethra *(black arrowheads)*. R, rectum. On the right, the scan is continued transperineally, outlining the urethra *(black arrowheads)*, the vagina *(white arrowheads)*, and the rectum (R).

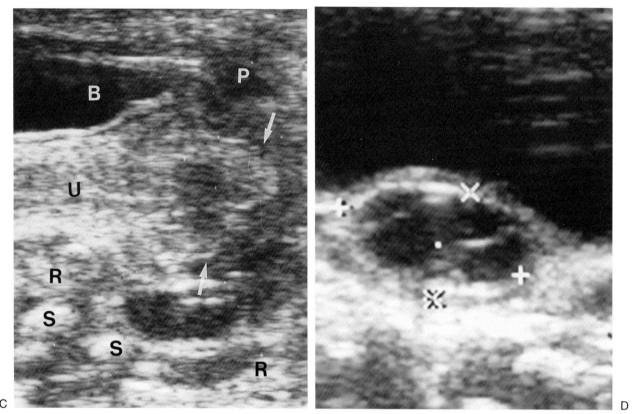

C

D

FIG. 12-2. *Continued.* **(C)** Sagittal scan of 1500-g infant. Note the prominent cervical lips *(arrows)* protruding into the vaginal vault caudad to the uterus (U). B, bladder; S, sacrum; R, rectum; P, cartilaginous portion of symphysis pubis. **(D)** Sonogram illustrating a typical appearance of neonatal ovary, outlined by calipers. Note the multiple cysts.

the transverse plane and to follow these structures laterally until a normal ovary is encountered (see Fig. 12-3B).

Although cysts are not typically found in the normal prepubertal ovaries, the presence of cysts is not indicative of pathology. Single cysts as large as 9 mm can be present normally in the prepubertal ovary (see Fig. 12-3C and D). However, the presence and persistence of multiple large cysts, especially when coupled with increased ovarian volume, is abnormal in this age group.[2]

As the child matures and enters the immediate premenarchal stage, pelvic anatomy assumes an intermediate conformation between prepubertal and adult norms. In these children, ovarian cysts are normal and commonplace and ovarian volume is intermediate between prepubertal and adult values.

Pubertal Anatomy

(Fig. 12-4)

Uterus

After puberty fundal growth invests the uterus with the typical pear shape seen in adult women. Before childbearing, the uterus generally measures 6 to 7 cm in length (see Fig. 12-4A) After parity, the uterus is usually somewhat larger and the fundus more dominant (see Fig. 12-4B).

Ovaries

The average size of the postpubertal ovary is approximately 10 cm^3.[3] Several cysts are characteristic (see Fig. 12-4C).[4] This is covered at length elsewhere in this text.

Transperineal Anatomy

In transperineal imaging, a sagittal scan is produced with the external perineum adjacent to the transducer face in the near-field, and progressively deeper or more cephalad structures are depicted within the image. Conventionally, the anterior aspect of the patient is depicted on the left side of the image, coinciding with the conventional illustration of the right side in transaxial scanning. Thus, the urethra, vagina, and rectum are sequentially illustrated from the viewer's left-to-right on the final image (see Fig. 12-1 and 12-2B).

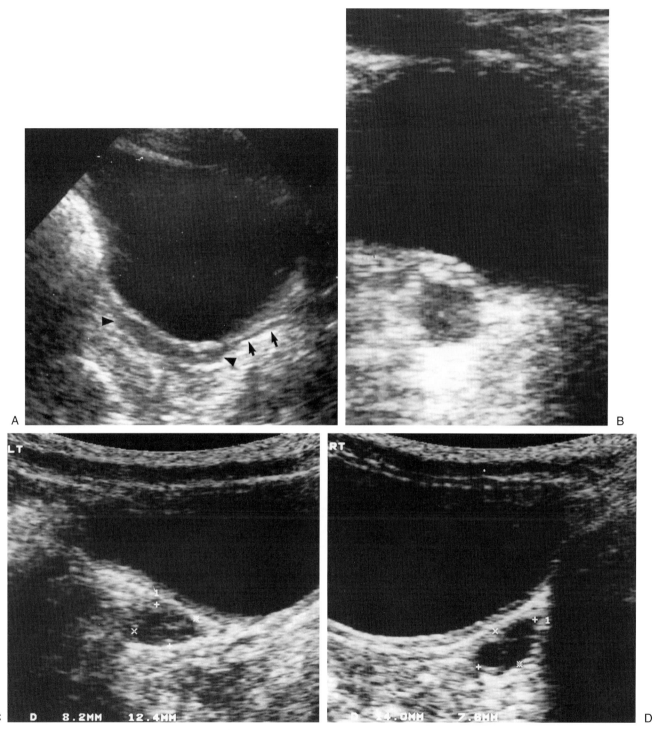

FIG. 12-3. Prepubertal anatomy. **(A)** Longitudinal sonogram of prepubertal uterus. Note the inconspicuous appearance of the uterus in this 4-year-old girl. The fundocervical length *(arrowheads)* is 3.2 cm. Arrows point to the vaginal stripe. **(B** through **D)** These figures illustrate a spectrum of the normal prepubertal ovary. The appearance is commonly afollicular and relatively hyperechoic **(B)** but can range to include multiple cysts of varying size **(C** and **D)**.

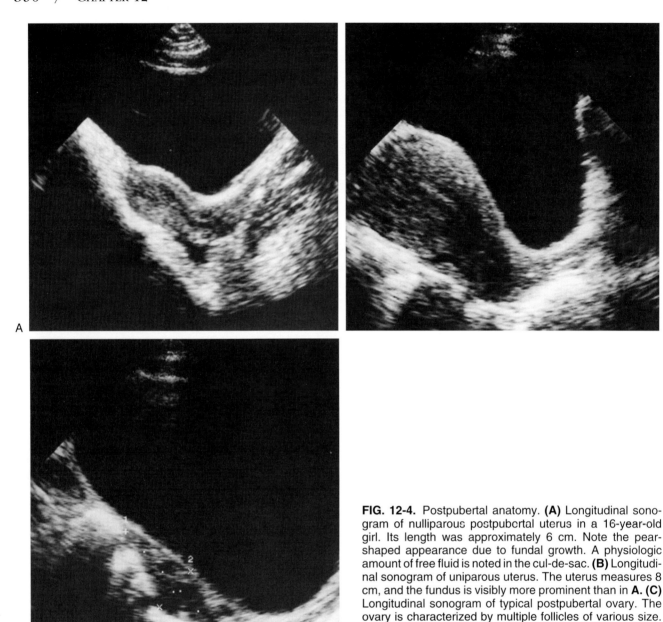

A

B

C 48.5MM 17.9MM

FIG. 12-4. Postpubertal anatomy. **(A)** Longitudinal sonogram of nulliparous postpubertal uterus in a 16-year-old girl. Its length was approximately 6 cm. Note the pear-shaped appearance due to fundal growth. A physiologic amount of free fluid is noted in the cul-de-sac. **(B)** Longitudinal sonogram of uniparous uterus. The uterus measures 8 cm, and the fundus is visibly more prominent than in **A.** **(C)** Longitudinal sonogram of typical postpubertal ovary. The ovary is characterized by multiple follicles of various size. The most distinct difference when compared with the child is its larger size.

CONGENITAL ABNORMALITIES

Ambiguous Genitalia

In humans, testicular development originates in the sex-determining region of the Y chromosome.[5] The pre-Sertoli cells of the primordial testis elaborate antimüllerian hormone, which in turn induces regression of the paramesonephric or müllerian ducts, the precursors of the internal female genitalia. The testis secretes testosterone, which governs the development of the genital primordia into the external male phenotype. Thus, in the absence of a Y chromosome, or of the sex-determining region of the Y chromosome, there will be no regression of the müllerian system, and a normal internal female genital apparatus will develop; similarly, in the absence of testosterone elaborated by a fetal testis, the external genital primordia will evolve into a normal female phenotype.

Patients with ambiguous external genitalia are referred to the radiologist for evaluation of the internal genital apparatus. An accurate assessment is based on an understanding of these conditions and of the difference between true and pseudo hermaphroditism.

True hermaphrodites are rare individuals, often 45X/46XY, 46XX/47XXY, or 46XX/46XY mosaics, who have both ovarian and testicular tissue, at times in the form of an ovotestis, and who may have partial formation of a uterine horn or a vas deferens.

A pseudohermaphrodite is defined as an individual whose external genitalia are in varying discordance with the internal genital apparatus and the chromosomal sex. The adjectives "male" and "female" refer to the chromosomal sex.

In a male pseudohermaphrodite, defective hormone production by the fetal testis, or end-organ insensitivity to the effects of testosterone, results in variable feminization of the external genitalia. Because male pseudohermaphrodites possess testes that elaborate antimüllerian hormone, these individuals are characterized by absence of paramesonephric or müllerian derivatives and lack a uterus. The most common and least severe form of male pseudohermaphroditism is hypospadias.

A rare but well-developed form of this condition is termed *testicular feminization syndrome,* in which there is complete end-organ insensitivity to the effects of testosterone. The end result is a woman who is genetically male, with normal male internal apparatus but complete feminization of the external sexual characteristics. Because the external feminization is complete, these patients do not present with ambiguous genitalia; they may present with inguinal hernias, and a normal testis may be found incidentally within the hernial sac, leading to the unsuspected diagnosis and ensuing psychosocial implications.

Female pseudohermaphrodites, on the other hand, are the result of overabundance of virilizing androgens. These can be produced by the adrenal glands in cases of congenital adrenal hyperplasia or adrenal carcinoma[6] or occasionally by maternal administration of virilizing progestin compounds (Fig. 12-5A and B). Because testes are absent, antimüllerian hormone is not produced, and the internal genitalia are normally differentiated into female phenotype. Examination of the adrenal glands is thus essential in infants with ambiguous genitalia in whom a uterus is identified. The hypertrophied neonatal adrenal loses its "λ" configuration; instead, it resembles multiple coils of rope, as the enlarged adrenal copes to fit within its suprarenal space (see Fig. 12-5C). This appearance has been termed the *cerebriform pattern.*[7] Some investigators have cautioned that a normal appearance of the adrenal does not exclude this diagnosis.[8]

In summary, in a child with ambiguous or masculinized genitalia, the presence of a uterus would imply absence of fetal elaboration of antimüllerian hormone and, by implication, absence of testes. Absence of a uterus, on the other hand, would infer fetal elaboration of antimüllerian hormone, presence of testes, and a defect in testicular testosterone production or end-organ testosterone insensitivity, leading to feminization of the external genital primordia. Although unequivocal characterization of a gonad is dependent on histology, the gonad of a true hermaphrodite may have mixed sonographic characteristics[9] with the development of cysts at puberty and is prone to develop neoplasms, such as gonadoblastoma. Thus, the major use of sonography in patients with ambiguous genitalia lies in the demonstration of the uterus. Uterine assessment is easiest in the neonatal period, when maternal hormonal stimulation renders it most visible. Midsagittal images at the level of the symphysis pubis allow identification of the upper vagina, which is continuous with the uterine cervix (see Fig. 12-2A and B).

Hydrometrocolpos and Uterine Duplication Anomalies

Hydrometrocolpos refers to the distention of the uterus and vagina by mucus and blood. Hydrometrocolpos may be simple; secondary to imperforate hymen, vaginal atresia, or uterine cervical dysplasia and stenosis; or encountered in association with uterine duplication anomalies.

Simple Hydrometrocolpos

Because uterine and vaginal distention is produced by hormonal stimulation, there are two windows during which the condition of simple hydrometrocolpos is discovered: at menarche or in the immediate neonatal period. The older patient typically presents with cyclical episodes of abdominal pain and failure to menstruate despite having reached an appropriate Tanner stage.

Sonography is an ideal modality to evaluate this condition noninvasively, relatively inexpensively, yet nonetheless accurately. Midline sagittal images, again at the level of the pubic symphysis, will demonstrate the distended vagina, capped by the uterus. The uterine lumen is distended with fluid, an appearance that is never seen in the normal nonpregnant patient. Vaginal and uterine distention are variable and largely dependent on the duration of symptoms; however, vaginal dilatation is usually much greater than that of the uterus (Fig. 12-6).[10]

The condition is caused by an imperforate hymen in the majority of cases. In the remainder, vaginal stenosis or vaginal atresia may be present. If the vaginal atresia is complete, the resulting dilatation involves solely the uterine cavity and is then termed *hematometra.* In patients with hematometra, only the uterus is dilated with mucus and blood products. This rarer anomaly is due to primary dysgenesis and stenosis of the uterine cervix.

Hydrometrocolpos may be found in association with caudal regression syndrome (ie, anal atresia and urogenital sinus anomalies) (Figs. 12-7 and 12-8). Caudal regression syndrome refers to the variable aplasia or agenesis of the fetal "tail end." Thus, this syndrome encompasses a wide spectrum, including patients with isolated anorectal atresia and patients with lumbosacral agenesis. In these children, the internal genitalia should be examined during the initial sonographic investigation of the kidneys and spinal cord.

In cases of simple imperforate hymen, the sonographic diagnosis is complemented by the physical examination, which reveals a bulging hymen. If the latter is not present on physical examination, and hematometrocolpos is present, the diagnosis is therefore distal vaginal atresia. The atretic segment can be identified and measured with transperineal sonography in these cases (see Fig. 12-7B).[11]

Text continues on p. 396

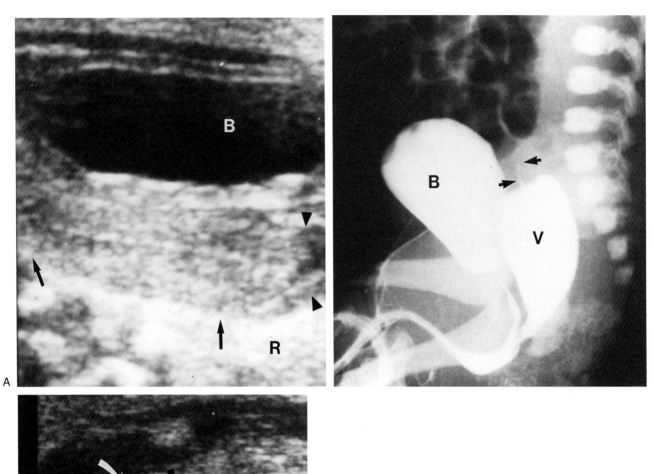

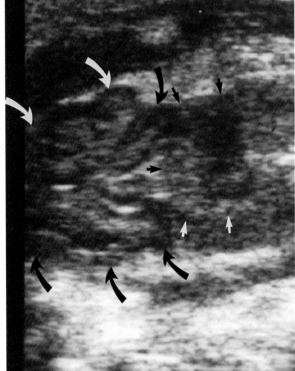

FIG. 12-5. Congenital adrenal hyperplasia. **(A)** Midsagittal scan of a "baby boy" with ambiguous genitalia demonstrates a normal uterus *(arrows)* with central endometrial strip. B, bladder; R, air in rectum. There is a small amount of fluid in the vaginal vault *(arrowheads)*. **(B)** Voiding cystourethrogram on same infant. Note the elongated, masculinized urethra. The proximal portion of the urethra receives the vaginal perineal termination, through which contrast medium enters and outlines the vagina (V) and endocervical canal *(arrows)*. B, bladder. **(C)** Adrenal gland of same infant. Arrows outline renal upper pole; curved arrows point to hypertrophied adrenal gland. The appearance was similar bilaterally.

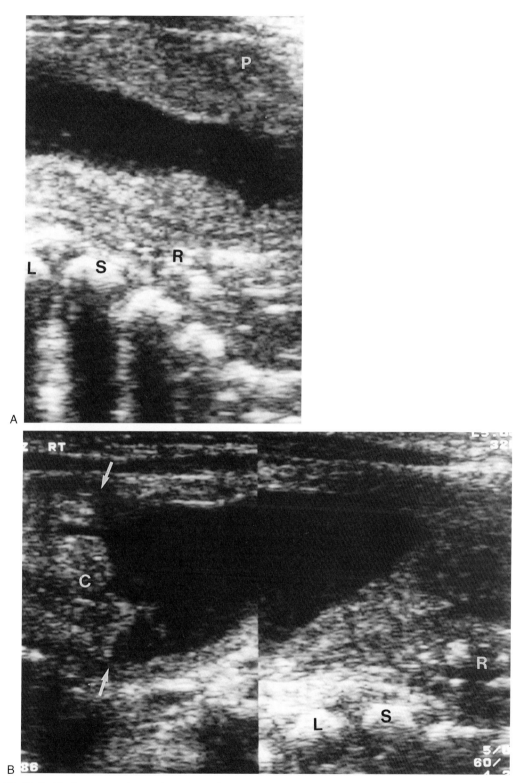

FIG. 12-6. Hydrometrocolpos. A newborn failed to pass urine; renal examination revealed small, dysplastic kidneys. **(A)** Sagittal pelvic scan fails to identify a bladder anteriorly. Instead, a fluid-filled structure lies anterior to the rectum (R). Note that the structure extends outside the pelvis, above the lumbosacral lordosis (L, L5; S, S1). P, cartilaginous symphysis pubis. **(B)** Composite, dual-screen image of the fluid-filled structure illustrated in **A** demonstrating its appearance more cephalad. Note the diagnostic, characteristic cup-shaped vaginal vault *(arrows)* outlining the cervical lips (C).

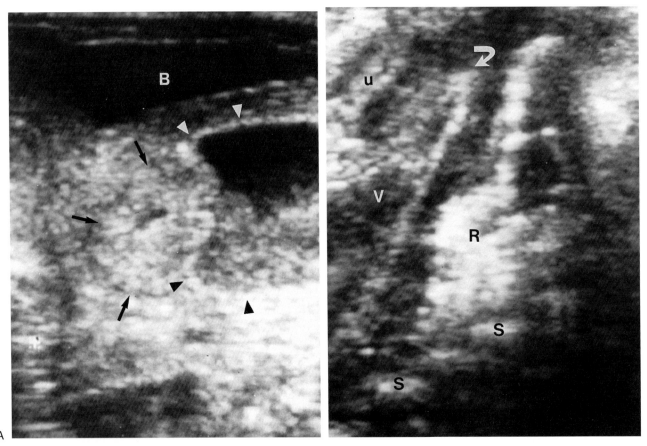

FIG. 12-7. Urogenital sinus anomaly with distal vaginal atresia. **(A)** Sagittal scan through the infraumbilical area in neonate with distal vaginal atresia. The vaginal vault *(arrowheads)* outlines the cervical lips of the uterus *(arrows)*. A small amount of fluid is seen within the endometrial canal of the uterus. The distended vagina, which contains dependent debris compresses and elevates base of bladder (B). **(B)** Transperineal scan of same infant as depicted in **A.** Note the anterior urethra (u), distended vagina (V) with blind termination *(curved arrow),* the posterior rectum (R) filled with hyperechoic material, and the sacral vertebrae (S).

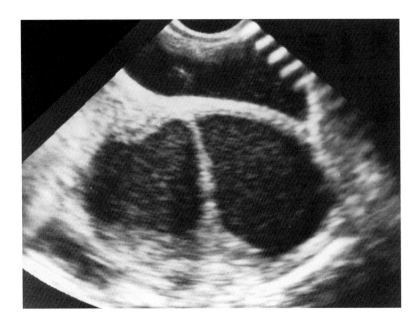

FIG. 12-8. Obstructed uterovaginal duplication; anal atresia. Transverse sonogram through the lower abdomen in neonate with anal atresia and abdominal distention. The sonogram illustrates markedly dilated, duplicated vaginas. The marked dilatation was secondary to a distal rectovaginal fistula.

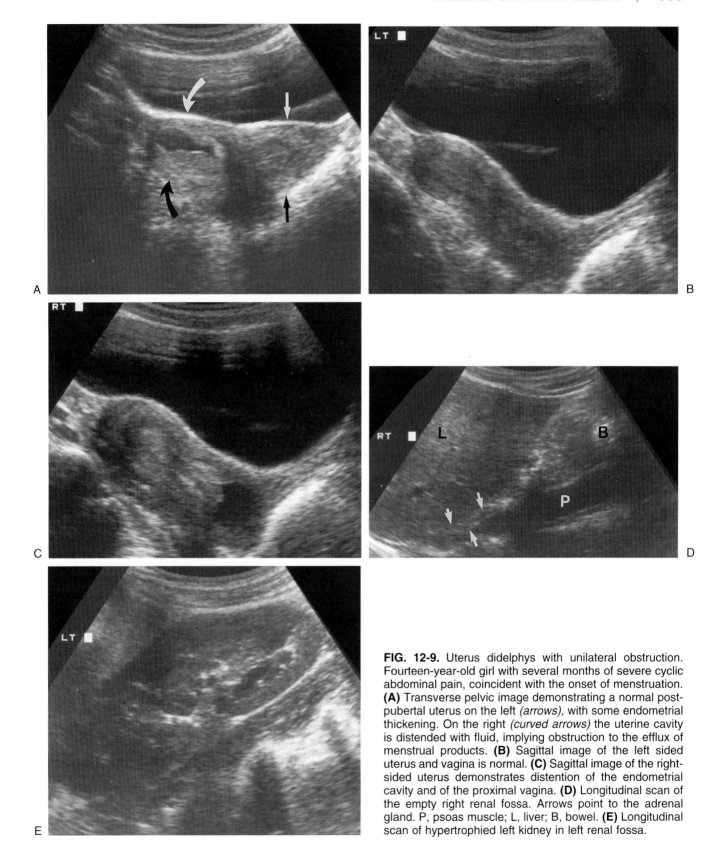

FIG. 12-9. Uterus didelphys with unilateral obstruction. Fourteen-year-old girl with several months of severe cyclic abdominal pain, coincident with the onset of menstruation. **(A)** Transverse pelvic image demonstrating a normal post-pubertal uterus on the left *(arrows),* with some endometrial thickening. On the right *(curved arrows)* the uterine cavity is distended with fluid, implying obstruction to the efflux of menstrual products. **(B)** Sagittal image of the left sided uterus and vagina is normal. **(C)** Sagittal image of the right-sided uterus demonstrates distention of the endometrial cavity and of the proximal vagina. **(D)** Longitudinal scan of the empty right renal fossa. Arrows point to the adrenal gland. P, psoas muscle; L, liver; B, bowel. **(E)** Longitudinal scan of hypertrophied left kidney in left renal fossa.

Hydrometrocolpos with Uterine Duplication Anomalies

The normal single uterus and vagina are the result of fusion of the paramesonephric or müllerian ducts. Failure of fusion of a variable portion results in variable duplication of the uterus. Uterus didelphys refers to complete duplication of the uterus, cervix, and upper vagina. Duplication of the uterus alone is termed *uterus duplex bicollis*; duplication of the fundus sparing the cervix is termed *uterus duplex unicollis*, or *bicornuate*. The septate uterus refers to a septum within the uterine lumen. Simple duplication without distal obstruction may affect fertility and the ability to carry a pregnancy to term. Uterine duplication complicated by distal obstruction of one moiety is invariably associated with ipsilateral renal agenesis or dysgenesis, likely resulting from the complex interaction of the affected paramesonephric (müllerian) duct with the ipsilateral metanephric (wolffian) duct, the precursor of the kidney (Fig. 12-9).

ACQUIRED ABNORMALITIES

Precocious Puberty

Precocious puberty refers to the abnormally early onset of maturation of the external sexual characteristics in response to premature activation of the pituitary gonadal axis. A majority of these cases are idiopathic, although the syndrome can be secondary to central nervous system lesions originating in the pituitary or hypothalamus. Pseudoprecocious puberty, on the other hand, refers to the onset of external sexual maturation without activation of the pituitary gonadal axis and does not lead to ovulation. These patients are affected by autonomous neoplastic adrenal or gonadal lesions, which may be benign or malignant. These include adrenal adenomas and carcinomas and ovarian lesions such as cysts, granulosa-theca cell tumors, embryonal carcinoma, and choriocarcinomas (Fig. 12-10).

Sonography plays an important role in the evaluation of children with premature sexual development. In patients with true precocious puberty, the maturation of the internal genitalia is assessed and response to therapy can be monitored.[2] In those girls with pseudoprecocious puberty, the offending lesion can be identified and characterized so that therapy can be directed appropriately.

Ovarian Lesions

Adnexal Torsion

As discussed in previous sections, adnexal torsion often occurs in association with an ovarian mass lesion, such as a cyst. It can occur in utero or in the prepubertal child. If undiscovered, the necrotic ovary may undergo calcification and present as a migratory, partly calcified abdominal mass.

In the neonate, ovarian torsion is likely to present as an extrapelvic mass lesion with cystic and solid elements and internal hemorrhage (Figs. 12-11 and 12-12). In the older child presenting during the acute event, the sonographic findings are relatively nonspecific. The ovary is enlarged and may demonstrate multiple peripheral follicles.[12,13] On Doppler interrogation, intraovarian flow may be absent; however, presence of both venous and arterial flow in no

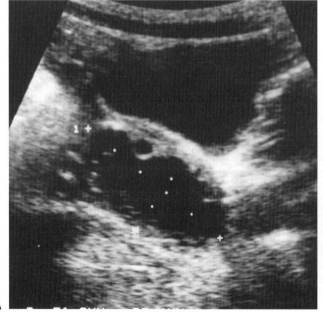

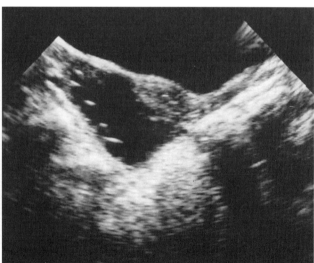

FIG. 12-10. Pseudoprecocious puberty. (**A** and **B**) Parasagittal scans of left ovary of a 6-year-old girl presenting with the rapid onset of somatic sexual maturation and vaginal bleeding. The ovary *(cursors in A)* is markedly enlarged with a dominant cyst. Multiple small follicles, best seen in **B,** were distributed along the periphery of the dominant cyst. Pathologically, this lesion proved to be a benign follicular cyst with stimulated follicles along its periphery.

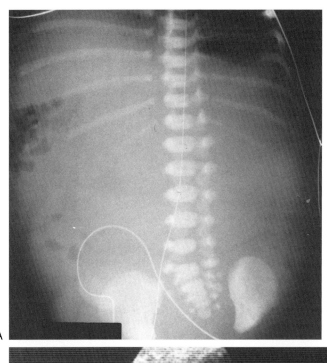

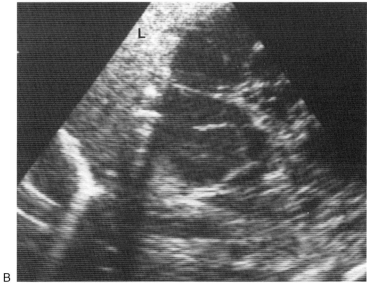

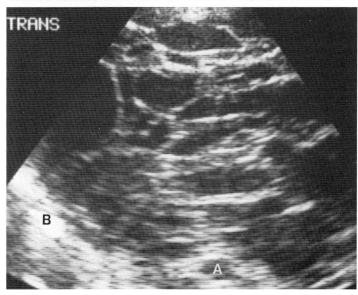

FIG. 12-11. Neonatal torsed ovarian cyst. (A) Abdominal radiograph of newborn with distended abdomen. The film demonstrates a water-density mass displacing normal loops of bowel to the right. Upper sagittal (B) and mid-abdominal transverse image (C) of the infant's abdomen reveals that the mass extends superiorly to the liver's edge (L) and fills the abdomen, displacing gas-filled bowel (B) to the right. A, aorta.

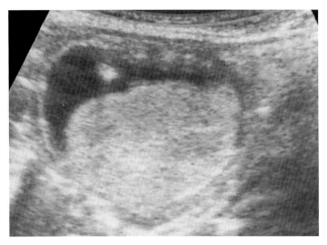

FIG. 12-12. Neonatal torsed ovary. Sonogram of the lower abdomen in a newborn, in whom a mass had been discovered incidentally in utero. The mass is cystic and contained freely mobile internal material. A torsed ovary was removed at surgery.

way excludes this diagnosis.[14,15] Central or peripheral flow signal may be present in as many as 80% of patients, depending on age.[16]

Benign Ovarian Masses

Cysts

Follicular and corpus luteum cysts are an integral part of the normal ovarian cycle of folliculogenesis and atrophy. Abnormally large ovarian cysts result from failure of involution of the normally occurring follicular and corpus luteum cysts.

As previously outlined in this chapter, ovarian cysts in neonates are the result of stimulation of the infant's ovaries by maternal hormones. These cysts can reach a very large size, may be found anywhere in the pelvis or abdomen, and can undergo torsion or hemorrhage (see Figs. 12-11 and 12-12). Ovarian cysts should be part of the differential diagnosis of any large cystic or complex mass encountered in a female infant. These cysts can lead to torsion of the ovary. Most smaller cysts found incidentally will resolve spontaneously over a course of several months.[17,18] Pathologic enlargement of follicular and corpus luteum cysts occurring in young girls after puberty is discussed in detail in Chapter 2.

Neoplasms

Approximately two thirds of childhood ovarian neoplasms are benign, and approximately one third are malignant. Ovarian malignancies are uncommon, comprising less than 1% of malignant lesions in children.[19]

Nearly one half of childhood ovarian tumors are dermoids or teratomas, and 90% to 95% of these are mature or benign (Figs. 12-13 and 12-14). Because of the multiplicity of tissues that may be present in these tumors, their sonographic appearance is variable but may be characteristic. Fat is usually echogenic, and hair often produces considerable shadowing. The tumor may be entirely cystic or entirely solid; calcification may be present.[20] The demonstration of fat and calcium by CT or abdominal radiograph may confirm the preoperative diagnosis if necessary.

Cystadenomas present as ovarian cysts that range from relatively small (4 to 5 cm) to very large. Malignant transformation into cystadenocarcinoma may occur (Fig. 12-15).

Malignant Ovarian Masses

These lesions can be categorized as epithelial tumors, sex cord–stromal tumors, germ cell tumors, and lesions occurring in the ambiguous gonad. Sonographically, they are usually of mixed echogenicity, with solid and cystic elements with thickened internal septa. Peritoneal fluid and implants may be present.

Epithelial tumors derive from the epithelial investment of the ovary. As discussed earlier, these may be benign (cystadenoma) or malignant (cystadenocarcinoma) (see Fig. 12-15).

Sex cord–stromal tumors are derived from the embryonic mesenchyma that will develop into the supporting tissue of the ovary (granulosa-theca cells) or of the testis (Sertoli-Leydig cells). Most of these tumors are hormonally active and clinically present with pseudoprecocious puberty or virilization. Although these tumors are generally slow growing, remote postoperative recurrences can occur.[21]

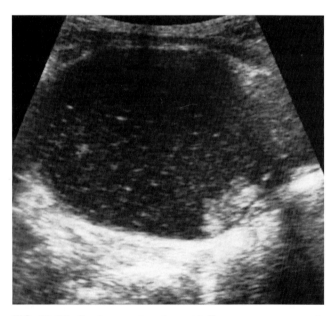

FIG. 12-13. Benign ovarian dermoid. Transverse supravesical scan of a 6-year-old girl presenting with pelvic pain. A cystic mass contains speckled material that was actively swirling on real-time examination. There is a dependent conglomerate of material on the left.

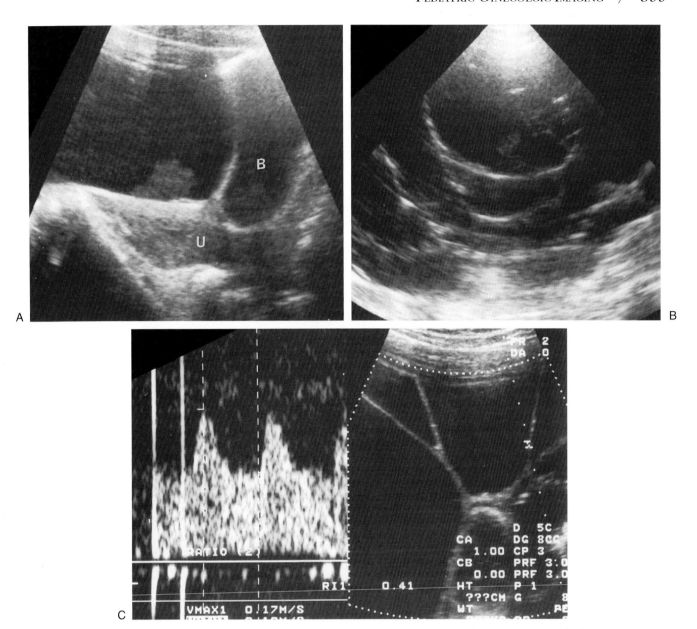

FIG. 12-14. Benign ovarian dermoid. **(A)** Mid-sagittal examination in teenaged girl complaining of urinary frequency demonstrates a large cystic mass with posterior nodule, compressing the bladder (B) caudad. U, uterus. **(B)** Supraumbilical scan reveals that the mass extends cephalad to occupy a large portion of the abdomen; in this area, it is multiseptated. **(C)** Doppler interrogation of the septa demonstrates flow, indicating that they consist of vascularized tissue, rather than septations within internal hemorrhage. Pathologically, this was shown to be a very large, but mature, teratoma.

Germ cell tumors comprise a variety of ovarian neoplasms with a wide range of malignancy; these are the more common of the ovarian malignant tumors.

Dysgerminoma is the most common type of ovarian malignancy and usually presents in the second or third decade of life.[21] Endodermal sinus tumors are aggressive, malignant lesions that produce α-fetoprotein. Embryonal carcinoma is also an aggressive tumor that can be hormonally active, elaborating both α-fetoprotein and human chorionic gonadotro-

pin. Human chorionic gonadotropin may also be secreted by choriocarcinoma; hormonal production by both embryonal carcinoma and choriocarcinoma may lead to the clinical presentation of pseudoprecocious puberty. The malignant potential of teratomas is directly related to the percentage of immature or embryonal tissue contained within the tumor and is inversely proportional to age at presentation.[21]

Gonadoblastomas, as discussed earlier in this chapter, are prone to occur in dysgenetic gonads, such as streak gonads,

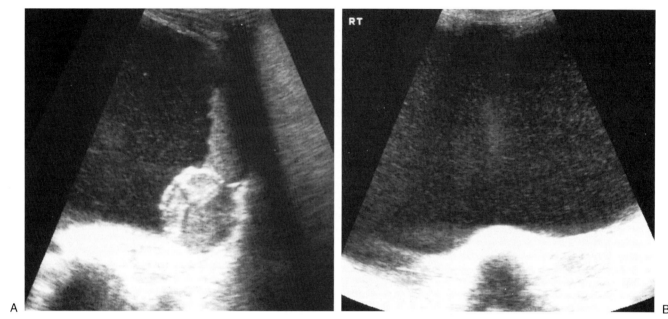

FIG. 12-15. Cystadenoma/cystadenocarcinoma. **(A)** Examination of the pelvis in this adolescent girl demonstrates a cystic mass with solid peripheral component. Multiple speckled internal echoes are present within the mass. **(B)** Transverse infraumbilical image demonstrates the large size of the mass and its relatively homogeneous internal contents. Pathologic diagnosis was epithelioid tumor of borderline malignancy.

and in male pseudohermaphrodites. The malignant potential of these tumors is variable.

Uterine and Vaginal Neoplasms

Neoplasms of the uterus and vagina are rare in children. The most common uterine or vaginal neoplasm in this age group is rhabdomyosarcoma. The tumor presents as a solid mass within the vaginal cavity or enlarging and distorting the uterus. Adenocarcinoma is a rarer tumor, which may be seen in young adolescents with a history of maternal exposure to diethylstilbestrol.[6] Germ cell tumors also occur in this region; these tumors comprise approximately 3% of malignant diseases in children and adolescents, and approximately 1% of these will be located in this anatomic region. The clinical presentation is usually blood-tinged vaginal discharge in a girl younger than 3 years old.[22]

Transperineal scanning facilitates identification of the

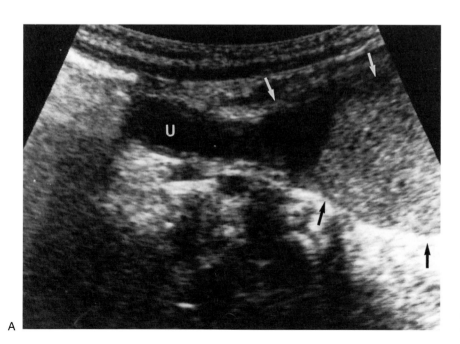

FIG. 12-16. Solid vaginal neoplasm. **(A)** Sagittal sonogram of a 14-month-old girl presenting with vaginal bleeding demonstrates distention of the vagina *(arrows)* with echogenic material lacking a fluid—fluid interface. The cavity of the prepubertal uterus (U) is distended.

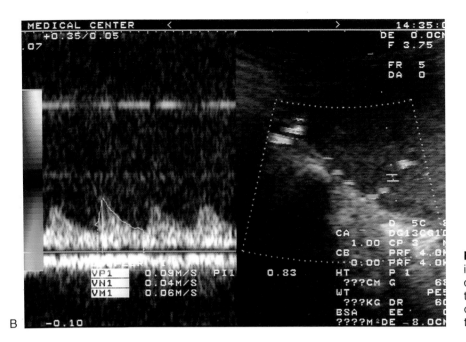

FIG. 12-16. *Continued.* **(B)** Doppler interrogation of the vaginal material demonstrates arterial flow, confirming that it is a solid mass. Final pathologic diagnosis was endodermal sinus tumor.

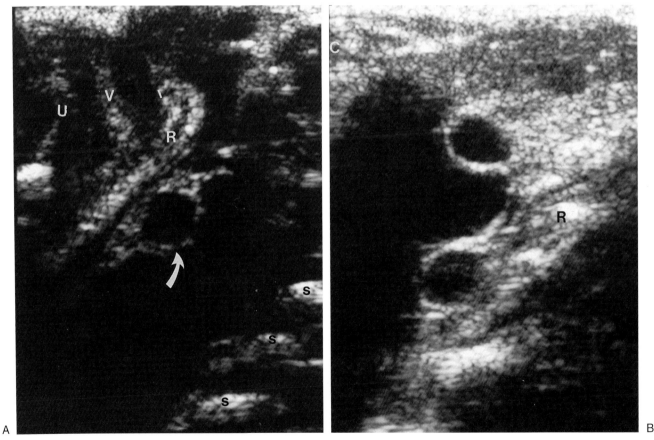

FIG. 12-17. Cystic sacrococcygeal teratoma. **(A)** Transperineal scan of newborn with large cystic pelvic mass discovered in utero. The postnatal examination demonstrates that the mass is retrorectal and extends to the transducer face at the perineum. The mass is anechoic, with smaller cysts abutting the rectum anteriorly *(arrow)*. U, urethra; V, vagina; R, rectum; s, sacral vertebrae. **(B)** Longitudinal midline scan along the lower back on same patient as illustrated in **A.** The precoccygeal (C), retrorectal (R) location of the cyst is demonstrated again. Note again the smaller retrorectal cysts. Final pathologic diagnosis was mature teratoma.

anatomic origin of the tumor mass. Doppler interrogation confirms the solid nature of the vaginal lesion (Fig. 12-16).[23]

OTHER PELVIC MASSES

The evaluation of pediatric pelvic masses is greatly simplified by determining their position relative to the rectum. This approach streamlines the differential diagnosis and guides subsequent imaging and therapy. Masses that are located anterior to the rectum are those that relate to the genitourinary tract, such as ovarian neoplasms. Sacrococcygeal teratoma, neuroblastoma, anterior meningocele, and rectal duplication are all found posterior to the rectum.

The relationship of a mass to the rectum can be delineated with transperineal sonography (Fig. 12-17), which also outlines its relationship to the vagina, uterus, and urethra. If necessary, confirmation of the location of the rectum with respect to the mass can be obtained by placing a small amount of contrast medium in the rectum under radiographic fluoroscopic control.

CONCLUSION

Sonography is a powerful tool in the evaluation of the little girl's pelvis. Through the morphologic illustration of the pelvic organs, important information is obtained in patients with ambiguous genitalia, congenital urogenital anomalies, and pelvic neoplastic disease.

REFERENCES

1. Nussbaum AR, Sanders RC, Jones MD. Neonatal uterine morphology as seen on real-time US. Radiology 1986;160:641.
2. Ambrosino M, Sklar C, Davis R, et al. Sonographic evaluation of the efficacy of medical treatment for precocious puberty: a comparative clinical and imaging study. J Ultrasound Med 1994;13:501.
3. Cohen HL, Tice HM, Mandel FS. Ovarian volumes measured by US: bigger than we think. Radiology 1990;177:189.
4. Pache TD, Wladimiroff JW, Hop WC, Fauser BC. How to discriminate between normal and polycystic ovaries: transvaginal US study. Radiology 1992;183:421.
5. McLaren A. What makes a man a man? Nature (London) 1990;346:216.
6. Pratt CB, Douglass ED. Management of the less common cancers of childhood. In: Pizzo PA, Poplack DG, eds. Principles and practice of pediatric oncology. Philadelphia, JB Lippincott, 1989.
7. Avni EF, Rypens F, Smet MH, Galetty E. Sonographic demonstration of congenital adrenal hyperplasia in the neonate: the cerebriform pattern. Pediatr Radiol 1993;23:88.
8. Bryan PJ, Caldamone AA, Morrison SC, et al. Ultrasound findings in the adreno-genital syndrome (congenital adrenal hyperplasia). J Ultrasound Med 1988;7:675.
9. Eberenz W, Rosenberg HK, Moshang T, et al. True hermaphroditism: sonographic demonstration of ovotestes. Radiology 1991;179:429.
10. Blask AR, Sanders RC, Rock JA. Obstructed uterovaginal anomalies: demonstration with sonography: II. Teenagers. Radiology 1991;179:84.
11. Scanlan KA, Pozniak MA, Fagerholm M, Shapiro S. Value of transperineal sonography in the assessment of vaginal atresia. AJR 1990;154:545.
12. Graif M, Itzchak Y. Sonographic evaluation of ovarian torsion in childhood and adolescence. AJR 1988;150:647.
13. Graif M, Shalev J, Strauss S, et al. Torsion of the ovary: sonographic features. AJR 1984;143:1331.
14. Quillin SP, Siegel MJ. Transabdominal color Doppler ultrasonography of the painful adolescent ovary. J Ultrasound Med 1994;13:549.
15. Rosado W Jr, Trambert MA, Gosink BB, and Pretorius DH. Adnexal torsion: diagnosis by using Doppler sonography. AJR 1992;159:1251.
16. Stark JE, Siegel MJ. Ovarian torsion in prepubertal and pubertal girls: sonographic findings. AJR 1994;163:1479.
17. Nussbaum A, Sanders RC, Hartman DS, et al. Neonatal ovarian cysts: sonographic-pathologic correlation. Radiology 1988;168):817.
18. Nussbaum AR, Sanders RC, Benator RM, et al. Spontaneous resolution of neonatal ovarian cysts. AJR 1987;148:175.
19. Breem JL, Bonam JF, Maxson WS. Genital tract tumors in children. Pediatr Clin North Am 1981;28:355.
20. Sisler CL, Siegel MJ. Ovarian teratoma: a comparison of the sonographic appearance in prepubertal and postpubertal girls. AJR 1990;154:139.
21. King DR. Ovarian cysts and tumors. In: Welch KW, Randolph JG, Ravitch JA Jr, et al, eds. Pediatric surgery, ed 4, vol 2. Chicago, Year Book Medical Publishers, 1986:1341.
22. Ablin A, Isaacs H Jr. Germ cell tumors. In: Pizzo PA, Poplack DG, eds. Principles and practice of pediatric oncology. Philadelphia, JB Lippincott, 1989.
23. Hernanz-Schulman M. State of the art: applications of Doppler sonography to extracranial pediatric diagnosis. Radiology 1993;189:1.

Clinical Gynecologic Imaging, edited
by Arthur C. Fleischer, Marcia C. Javitt,
R. Brooke Jeffrey, Jr., and Howard W. Jones III,
Lippincott-Raven Publishers, Philadelphia © 1997.

CHAPTER 13

Future Developments in Gynecologic Imaging

Future Developments in Gynecologic Sonography
Arthur C. Fleischer, MD
   Amplitude Color Doppler Sonography
   Contrast Agents
   Three-Dimensional Sonography
   Other Uses
   Conclusion
Future Developments in Magnetic Resonance
   Imaging of the Female Pelvis

Marcia C. Javitt, MD
New Developments in Computed Tomography
R. Brooke Jeffrey, Jr., MD
   Spiral Computed Tomography
   Three-Dimensional Computed Tomographic
     Angiography
   Virtual Reality Applications of Three-Dimensional
     Spiral Computed Tomography

Future Developments in Gynecologic Sonography

Arthur C. Fleischer, MD

The versatile nature of diagnostic sonography affords many new innovations, including the depiction of blood flow. Blood flow estimations can, in turn, be considered an approximation of function and possibly reflect response to certain treatment regimens. The most recent technologic advance in sonography involves improved depiction of blood flow by amplitude or power color Doppler sonography. This, coupled with refinement of sonographic contrast agents, may result in more physiologic depiction of flow than is currently available with standard color Doppler sonography.

AMPLITUDE COLOR DOPPLER SONOGRAPHY

Amplitude or power color Doppler sonography detects the presence or absence of a Doppler shift from blood flow and displays this information in shades of orange. The advantage of amplitude color Doppler sonography over frequency shift color Doppler sonography is the detection of minute amounts

of very slowly flowing blood due to a three to four times enhancement in sensitivity.[1] This enhancement is related to improved signal-to-noise ratio for amplitude-based Doppler shifts over frequency-based color Doppler imaging (Fig. 13-1). As opposed to frequency color Doppler sonography in which detection of frequency shift is angle dependent, power Doppler is angle independent and not as susceptible to confusing signals created by aliasing (Table 13-1). However, disadvantages of amplitude color Doppler sonography include increased persistence, which sometimes blurs the image and does not allow for accurate temporal resolution when used in conjunction with contrast medium injection.

What amplitude color Doppler imaging reveals is the relative vascularity of organs such as the placenta, uterus, and ovaries. Arterial and venous vessels down to a fraction of a millimeter (40 μm) can be detected with the use of contrast medium injection with the receiver tuned to the second harmonic coupled with power color Doppler imaging. This approach may allow depiction of vascular flow patterns within

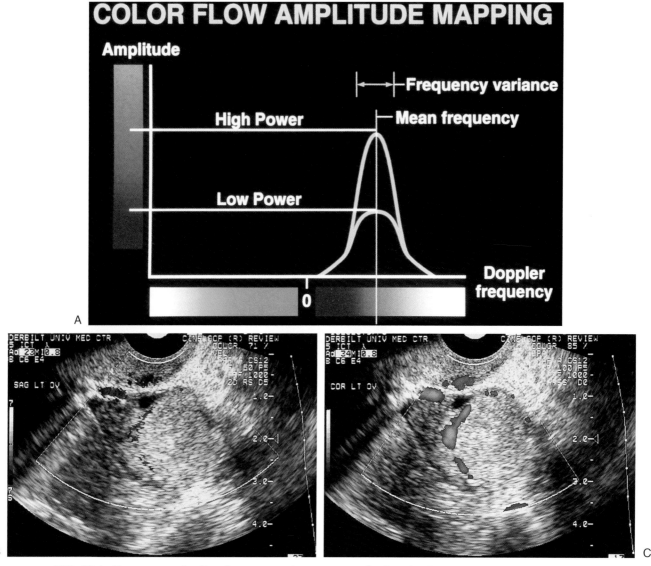

FIG. 13-1. Frequency color Doppler sonography versus amplitude color Doppler sonography. **(A)** Diagram depicting the differences of frequency versus amplitude and color Doppler sonography. A greater difference in the signal can be obtained with amplitude or power of signal versus frequency. **(B)** Frequency color Doppler sonogram of solid intraovarian mass. **(C)** Color Doppler sonogram of same mass in **B** showing peripheral blood flow pattern.

masses. The data so obtained may be displayed in time-activity curves similar to those used in dynamic nuclear medicine studies that plot "perfusion" over time. This technique may have implications in distinguishing benign versus malignant lesions because the vascularity of benign lesions is derived from a normal vascular bed with predictable branching patterns whereas tumors inside a chaotic network of vessels have several intratumoral shunts.[2] The relative perfusion in different areas of a region of interest might also be depicted by amplitude color Doppler sonography. This, in turn, may be helpful in determining the relative probability of tumor versus infarction.

TABLE 13-1. *Relative advantages and disadvantages of amplitude color Doppler sonography over frequency shift color Doppler sonography*

Advantages	Disadvantages
Improved sensitivity	Prone to blooming with increased persistence
Angle independent, less prone to aliasing	Does not provide velocity, direction information
Not as susceptible to flash artifacts	Prone to flash artifacts

CONTRAST AGENTS

The potential use of contrast agents coupled with amplitude color Doppler sonography affords the assessment of blood flow within tissue, which in turn might be related to function and malignant potential. It is well known, for example, that malignant tumors have more vessels per area than most benign counterparts. This parameter is potentially quantifiable with technical refinements in color Doppler sonography. It is indeed propitious that the development of sonographic contrast agents has occurred concomitantly with improved color Doppler sonographic capabilities with the use of amplitude color Doppler processing. There are several types of contrast agents that have and are in the process of being available for use in sonography. These include ones consisting of microbubbles suspended between albumen (Albunex), galactose microparticles (Levovist and Echovist), perfluorocarbon, and other substances that become gas as they enter the bloodstream.[3,4] One symposium that was devoted entirely to sonographic contrast agents attested to the widespread interest in this topic and its potential applications. In a few years, use of contrast agents in sonographic examinations may become as routine as it is now in certain radiographic studies, such as excretory urography or computed tomography.

Cosgrove and coworkers[5] and Duda and associates[6] have documented the enhancement patterns of breast and prostate tumors, and the uptake is longer and the dwell time is greater in malignancy (Fig. 13-2; Table 13-2). In addition to a higher number of microscopic vessels in tumors, there are several areas of intratumoral shunts.[7] This topic is being investigated along with changes in blood flow that occur during treatment with an antitoxin.

Burns[8] described improved resolution with detection of the second harmonic frequency after a contrast medium is introduced. He reports visualization of vessels as small as 40 μm. Improved signal fidelity with the use of the second harmonic has improved signal-to-noise ratio over the primary frequency or fundamental. Scanners may require software modification to adequately image those parameters.

The future for depiction of flow with contrast medium–enhanced color Doppler imaging seems promising. In gynecology, possible clinical applications include improved tumor detection and more accurate recognition of hyperfused areas

TABLE 13-2. *Color Doppler sonographic features of malignant neovascularization*

Feature	Benign	Malignant
Number of vessels	Scanty	Many
Position	Radial	Circumferential
Tortuosity	+/−	+ + + +
Shunts	0	+
Time to peak	>1 min	<1 min
Washout time	~3 min	~6 min

From Cosgrove D. Levovist in breast and prostate cancer. In: Syllabus from symposium with ultrasound agents. Thomas Jefferson University Symposium, Atlantic City, NJ, May 1995, pp 47–49.

or tumor that are known to be vascular, such as gestational trophoblastic and ectopic pregnancy. Future improvements in depiction of tumor vascularity will involve quantification of the amplitude color Doppler sonography.[9] This technique uses a software program that quantifies and weighs pixel density arising from areas of vascularity. This parameter correlates to the microvessel count, which has been shown to be of predictive value for malignant potential. The use of contrast media with quantified CDS may further improve assessment of vascularity, which may also correlate to tumor response to therapy. This technique may also reveal differences in vessel branching patterns in benign versus malignant tumors.

THREE-DIMENSIONAL SONOGRAPHY

In gynecology, three-dimensional sonography may afford improved depiction of complicated anatomy such as the pedicle of a polyp or the relationship of a tumor to surrounding tissue.[10,11] Three-dimensional sonography requires stepped imaging in one plane and another orthogonal to the original plane. It has been reported to improve the observer's appreciation of complex uterine malformations and certain endometrial disorders.[12] For those worried about the additional cost of a 3-D system, a "poor man's" third dimension can be achieved with the use of a single plastic lens.[13] Three-dimensional scanning may become available in technologically sophisticated scanners. The color Doppler sonographic data obtained with amplitude color Doppler imaging can be superimposed in three dimensions to graphically depict the configuration of blood flow.

OTHER USES

Endoscopic probes can be fitted with transducers to depict anatomic details from within a structure. This technology can be used for laparoscopic sonography or endoluminal gastrointestinal applications (Fig. 13-3). Laparoscopic and endoluminal sonography allows the examiner to visualize structures close to the surface of the organ. For example, laparoscopic sonography provides information concerning the extent of involvement of bowel tumors.[14]

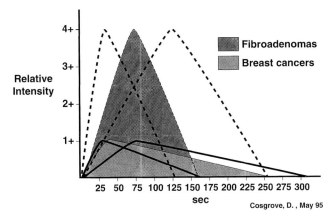

FIG. 13-2. Approximate time activity curves for tumor versus benign breast mass. Tumors seem to have longer uptake and longer dwell time when compared with fibroadenoma. (Adapted from David Cosgrove, MD.)

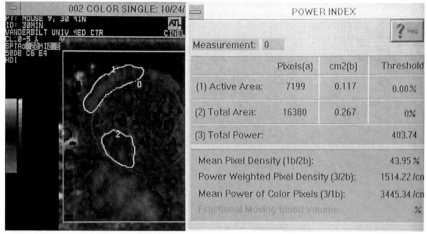

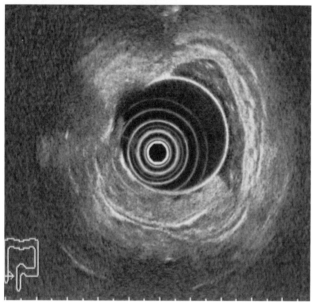

FIG. 13-3. (A) Quantified color Doppler sonography of tumor showing areas of vascularity and their power-weighted pixel density. **(B)** Endoluminal ultrasound showing noninvasive tumor in cecum. **((B)** Courtesy of Howard Merz, MD, and Wui Chong, MD.)

CONCLUSION

The future use of gynecologic sonography is currently and will continue to be enhanced by these and other technologic developments. It is hoped that improved technology can be reflected in improved care of gynecologic patients.

REFERENCES

1. Rubin JM, Bude RO, Carson PL, et al. Power Doppler US: a potentially useful alternative to mean frequency-based color Doppler US. Radiology 1994;190:853.
2. Less JR, Skalak TC, Sevick EM, Jain RK. Microvascular architecture in a mammary carcinoma: branching patterns and vessel dimensions. Cancer Res 1991;51:265.
3. Goldberg BB, Liu JB, Burns PN, et al. Galactose-based intravenous sonographic contrast agent: experimental studies. J Ultrasound Med 1993;12:463.
4. Schwarz KQ, Becher H, Schimpfky C, et al. Doppler enhancement with SH U 508A in multiple vascular regions. Radiology 1994;193: 195.
5. Cosgrove D. Levovist in breast and prostate cancer. In: Syllabus from symposium with ultrasound contrast agents. Thomas Jefferson University Symposium, Atlantic City, NJ, May 1995, pp 47–49.
6. Duda VF, Rode G, Schlief R. Echocontrast agent enhanced color flow imaging of the breast. Ultrasound Obstet Gynecol 1993;3:191.
7. Schoenfeld A, Levavi H, Tepper R, et al. Assessment of tumor-induced angiogenesis by three-dimensional display: confusing Doppler signals in ovarian cancer screening? Letters to the Editor. Ultrasound Obstet Gynecol 1994;4:515.
8. Burns PN. Harmonic imaging adds to ultrasound capabilities. Diagn Imaging Suppl 1995;May:AU7.
9. Meyerowitz C, Fleischer A, Browsky A, et al. Correlation of color Doppler sonography to tumor vascularity (submitted, 1996).
10. Fenster A, Downey D, Rankin R. 3-D allows interactive slicing of sonograms. Diagn Imaging Suppl 1995;May:AU11.
11. Pretorius DH, Nelson TR. Three-dimensional ultrasound. Ultrasound Obstet Gynecol 1995;5:219.
12. Jurkovic D, Geipel A, Gruboeck K, et al. Three-dimensional ultrasound for the assessment of uterine anatomy and detection of congenital anomalies: a comparison with hysterosalpingography and two-dimensional sonography. Ultrasound Obstet Gynecol 1995;5:233.
13. Kossoff G. Three-dimensional ultrasound: technology push or market pull? Editorial. Ultrasound Obstet Gynecol 1995;5:217.
14. Wojtowycz A, Spirt B, Kaplan D, Roy A. Endoscopic US of the gastrointestinal tract with endoscopic radiographic and pathologic correlation. Radiographics 1995;15:735.

Future Developments in Magnetic Resonance Imaging of the Female Pelvis

Marcia C. Javitt, MD

Despite many important recent technologic advances in MRI, the clinical utilization of pelvic MRI has lagged behind expectations based on careful reading of the radiology literature. Improved pelvic coil technology, including pelvic phased-array multicoils, provide better signal-to-noise ratios than ever before. The use of gadolinium for enhanced scans with fat suppression or chemical shift imaging has yielded more accurate evaluation in extent of disease workups for malignancies and better tissue characterization. Fast scanning methods permit greater patient throughput than ever before, especially with the advent of fast spin-echo techniques for T2-weighted scans. With these developmens, pelvic MRI is the study of choice for staging of gynecologic malignancies.

In the future, new and improved pulse sequences will be tested for improved efficiency that must be weighed against accuracy in diagnosis. With an eye toward controlling costs in the new era of managed care, cost-effectiveness of new techniques, software, and hardware will necessarily be tested before changes can be implemented.

Future developments on the horizon will probably include three-dimensional rendering of tissues, perhaps even with holographic techniques. Even faster scanning methods will likely result in "real time" MRI, thereby permitting new and improved functional and dynamic scanning. Faster magnetic resonance angiography and blood flow sensitive techniques will undoubtedly play a role in pelvic imaging but will have an even greater impact on cerebrovascular and cardiac disease evaluation. Endoluminal MRI may be performed within vessels, in the ureters, as well as in hollow organs of all descriptions.

Subtraction and image registration techniques may well result in improved multimodality approaches, improved identification of vascular structures, and surgical and radiation treatment planning.

Spectroscopy, which has not yet been widely available for clinical applications, may come into its own. As refinements in technology provide improved signal-to-noise ratios, perhaps even higher field strength magnets may potentiate the clinical use of spectroscopy.

New safe and nontoxic contrast materials will undoubtedly be developed that can provide more prolonged enhancement of tissues with better soft tissue contrast to differentiate normal from abnormal tissues.

Scanning will become filmless and completely digital, with reading rendered entirely from monitors. Biopsies and even selected forms of treatment or ablation may become automated and machine driven from prescriptions rendered by the radiologist or radiation therapist.

With these improvements, the speed and accuracy of pelvic MRI will improve. The standard of care will likely be adjusted, and utilization will increase in response. Ultimately this will result in cost savings: patient workups are better tailored to make diagnoses. Problem-solving after other imaging techniques such as sonography or CT is better achieved. Treatment planning and surveillance for tumors can best be accomplished.

New Developments in Computed Tomography

R. Brooke Jeffrey Jr., MD

SPIRAL COMPUTED TOMOGRAPHY

The single most important new advancement in CT has been the development of spiral (helical) CT. The unique feature of spiral CT is its slip-ring technology, which combines continuous scan acquisition with continuous table translation.[1–3] Conventional dynamic scanners require a fixed interscan delay as a single scan is first acquired and then the patient is moved to a new position. By virtue of a continuous table feed, spiral CT completely eliminates any interscan delay. Thus acquisition of a spiral CT data set is four to nine times faster than conventional CT.[1] The most important clinical implication for spiral CT is the ability to perform breath-held imaging.[4,5] An entire anatomic region can, therefore, be imaged without motion or respiratory artifacts. Spiral CT data can be viewed as a "volumetric data set" that can be edited to provide exquisite three-dimensional images of the skeletal system, soft tissues, and vascular structures.

THREE-DIMENSIONAL COMPUTED TOMOGRAPHIC ANGIOGRAPHY

After intravenous injection of contrast medium, a spiral CT data set can be acquired to coincide with peak arterial enhancement. Specific editing techniques such as shaded surface display or maximum intensity projection can then be used to create three-dimensional images of the vascular system that have exquisite anatomic resolution (Figs. 13-4 through 13-7).[6–10] These images are in essence "subtraction angiograms" because extraneous tissues are edited out of the data set. Unlike MRI angiography, three-dimensional CT angiography (CTA) is not encumbered by flow or phase artifacts that are caused by turbulence or vessel tortuosity. In addition, CTA, unlike MRI, can demonstrate calcifications that are important in the assessment of atherosclerosis. Finally, CTA can clearly depict metallic intravascular stents and stent grafts by use of curved planar re-formations (Fig. 13-7). Susceptibility artifacts preclude imaging of metallic stents with MRI angiography.

Potential clinical applications for three-dimensional CT of the pelvis include evaluation of atherosclerotic disease, arteriovenous malformations, metallic stents and stent-grafts, and congenital anomalies. By simply delaying the timing of scan acquisition to the venous phase, it may be possible to evaluate venous structures with three-dimensional CT venography as well. This may be of value in the future to diagnose entities such as pelvic thrombophlebitis and anomalies of the iliac veins or inferior vena cava.

VIRTUAL REALITY APPLICATIONS OF THREE-DIMENSIONAL SPIRAL COMPUTED TOMOGRAPHY

Developments in software have made possible a variety of "virtual reality" applications of three-dimensional spiral CT. These include virtual endoscopy and virtual angioscopy. Although a number of editing techniques have been developed for virtual reality applications, the most promising is perspective volume rendering.[11–14] By using this editing technique each voxel within the data set is assigned opacity and color. Images are rendered to display perspective so that close objects appear larger than identical objects farther from a fixed point of view. In addition, specialized software allows an observer to "fly through" the CT data set to perform "virtual endoscopy." To date this has been performed in the tracheobronchial tree (virtual bronchoscopy), the vascular system (virtual angioscopy), and the colon (virtual colonoscopy) (Fig. 13-8).[14–16] Specific color maps are generated for anatomic regions such as the colonic mucosa to simulate the actual visual experience of clinical endoscopy. The software is interactive and thus the flight plan can be generated to fly in or out of the specific area that the observer chooses. High soft tissue contrast medium enhancement is required to fly through a hollow viscus. For example, to perform virtual colonoscopy, air must be insufflated into the section to distend the colon before the "fly through." Similarly, virtual angioscopy requires high intravascular contrast enhancement with an intravenous bolus injection.

The ability to perform virtual endoscopic manipulation of three-dimensional data sets creates a new era for three-dimensional imaging. It may be possible within a single examination to perform CT angiography, virtual colonoscopy, as well as review of the two-dimensional axial images. It is anticipated with the increasing speed and capacity of newer

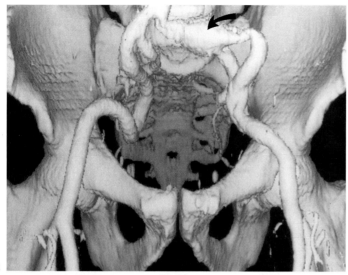

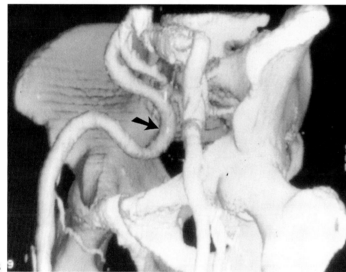

FIG. 13-4. Three-dimensional CT angiogram. A shaded surface display of the pelvis **(A)** demonstrates an aneurysm of the left common iliac *(arrow)*. **(B)** Note the tortuosity of the right iliac vessels seen on the oblique view *(arrow)*.

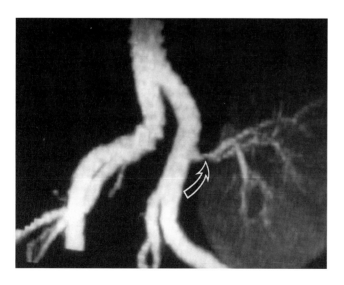

FIG. 13-5. Three-dimensional CT angiogram of renal transplant artery stenosis. Maximal intensity projection demonstrates stenosis of proximal renal transplant artery *(arrow)*.

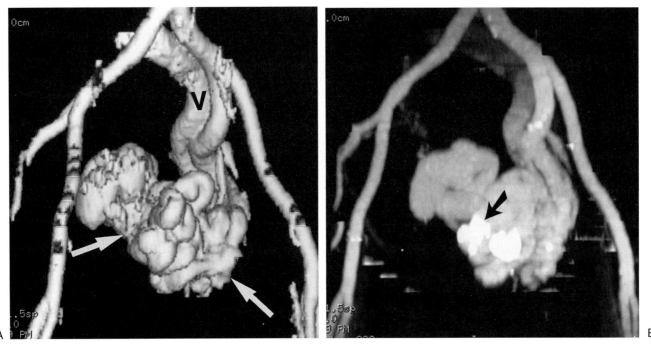

FIG. 13-6. Three-dimensional CT angiogram of pelvic arteriovenous malformation. **(A)** Shaded surface display demonstrates large lesion *(arrows)* with prominent early-draining left common iliac vein (V). **(B)** Maximal intensity projection demonstrates areas of calcification within the arteriovenous malformation *(arrow).*

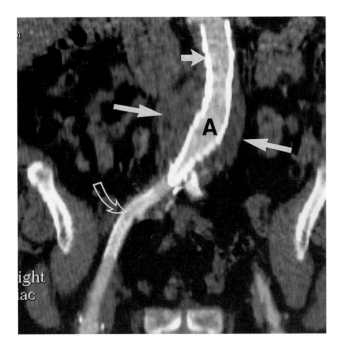

FIG. 13-7. Curved planar re-formation of aortic and iliac artery stent grafts. A curved planar re-formation through the aorta and right common iliac artery demonstrates patency of the aortic lumen (A). Note the high-density metallic portion of the stent graft *(small arrow).* Note thrombus within aortic aneurysm *(large arrows).* A patent left common iliac stent is noted *(curved open arrow).*

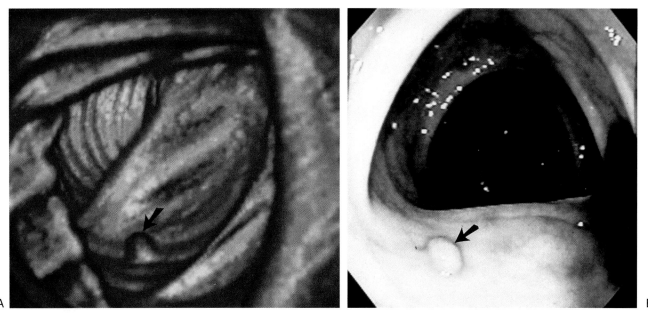

FIG. 13-8. Comparison of virtual colonoscopy and clinical colonoscopy. **(A)** Virtual colonoscopy demonstrates a small polyp in the ascending colon *(arrow)*. **(B)** This is confirmed with endoscopy *(arrow)*.

computer systems that virtual reality applications will become increasingly important for many types of pelvic imaging.

REFERENCES

1. Napel SA. Basic principles of spiral CT. In: Fishman EK, Jeffrey RBJ, eds. Spiral CT: principles, techniques and clinical applications. New York, Raven Press, 1995:1.
2. Kalender WA, Polacin A. Physical performance characteristics of spiral CT scanning. Med Phys 1991;18:910.
3. Kalender WA, Seissler W, Klotz E, Vock P. Spiral volumetric CT with single-breath-hold technique, continuous transport, and continuous scanner rotation. Radiology 1990;176:181.
4. Remy JM, Remy J, Giraud F, Marquette CH. Pulmonary nodules: detection with thick-section spiral CT versus conventional CT. Radiology 1993;187:513.
5. Costello P, Dupuy DE, Ecker CP, Tello R. Spiral CT of the thorax with reduced volume of contrast material: a comparative study. Radiology 1992;183:663.
6. Napel S, Marks MP, Rubin GD, et al. CT angiography with spiral CT and maximum intensity projection. Radiology 1992;185:607.
7. Aoki S, Sasaki Y, Machida T, et al. Cerebral aneurysms: detection and delineation using 3D-CT angiography. AJNR 1992;13:1115.
8. Marks MP, Napel S, Jordan JE, Enzmann DR. Diagnosis of carotid artery disease: preliminary experience with maximum-intensity-projection spiral CT angiography. AJR 1993;160:1267.
9. Rubin GD, Walker PJ, Dake MD, et al. Three-dimensional spiral computed tomographic angiography: an alternative imaging modality for the abdominal aorta and its branches. J Vasc Surg 1993;18:656; discussion 665.
10. Rubin GD, Dake MD, Napel SA, et al. Three-dimensional spiral CT angiography of the abdomen: initial clinical experience. Radiology 1993;186:147.
11. Fishman EK, Drebin B, Magid D, et al. Volumetric rendering techniques: applications for three-dimensional imaging of the hip. Radiology 1987;163:737.
12. Drebin RA, Carpenter L, Hanrahan P. Volume rendering. Comput Graphics 1988;22:65.
13. Rusinek H, Mourino MR, Firooznia H, et al. Volumetric rendering of MR images. Radiology 1989;171:269.
14. Beaulieu CF, Baker ME, Chotas HG, et al. Volume rendering for 3D helical CT of abdominal aorta. Radiology 1993;189:173.
15. Vining DJ, Shifrin RY, Haponik EF, et al. Virtual bronchoscopy. Radiology 1994;193:261.
16. Vining DJ, Shifrin RY, Grishaw EK, et al. Virtual colonoscopy. Radiology 1994;193:446.

Index

An *f* after a page number denotes a figure or diagram; a *t* denotes a table.
Abbreviations used: CT = computed tomography; MRI = magnetic resonance imaging.

413